SURGICAL ANATOMY

JOHN E. HEALEY, Jr., M.D. (DECEASED)

Former Professor of Anatomy, The University of Texas Graduate School of Biomedical Sciences and Chief of Experimental Surgery, The University of Texas M.D. Anderson Hospital and Tumor Institute at Houston.

In collaboration with

JOSEPH HODGE, M.D.

Adjunct Clinical Professor of Surgery, Jefferson Medical College of The Thomas Jefferson University, Philadelphia, Pennsylvania; Department of Surgery, Spartanburg Regional Medical Center and Doctors Memorial Hospital; Adjunct Professor of Surgery and Anatomy, Mary Black Memorial Hospital School of Nursing, University of South Carolina, Spartanburg, South Carolina

Illustrated by
DONALD JOHNSON, WILLIAM A. OSBURN,
AND JEANET DRESKIN

SECOND EDITION

1990 • B.C. Decker Inc., Publisher
Toronto • Philadelphia

Publisher

B.C. Decker Inc
3228 South Service Road
Burlington, Ontario   L7N 3H8

B.C. Decker Inc
320 Walnut Street
Suite 400
Philadelphia, Pennsylvania   19106

Sales and Distribution

United States and Puerto Rico
The C.V. Mosby Company
11830 Westline Industrial Drive
Saint Louis, Missouri   63146

Canada
McAinsh & Co. Ltd.
2760 Old Leslie Street
Willowdale, Ontario   M2K 2X5

Australia
McGraw-Hill Book Company
Australia Pty. Ltd.
4 Barcoo Street
Roseville East 2069
New South Wales, Australia

Brazil
Editora McGraw-Hill do Brasil, Ltda.
rua Tabapua, 1.105, Itaim-Bibi
Sao Paulo, S.P. Brasil

Colombia
Interamericana/McGraw-Hill
de Colombia, S.A.
Apartado Aereo 81078
Bogota, D.E. Colombia

Europe
McGraw-Hill Book Company GmbH
Lademannbogen 136
D-2000 Hamburg 63
West Germany

France
MEDSI/McGraw-Hill
6, avenue Daniel Lesueur
75007 Paris, France

Hong Kong and China
McGraw-Hill Book Company
Suite 618, Ocean Centre
5 Canton Road
Tsimshatsui, Kowloon
Hong Kong

India
Tata McGraw-Hill Publishing
Company, Ltd.
12/4 Asaf Ali Road, 3rd Floor
New Delhi 110002, India

Indonesia
P.O. Box 122/JAT
Jakarta, 1300 Indonesia

Italy
McGraw-Hill Libri Italia, s.r.l.
Piazza Emilia, 5
1-20129 Milano MI
Italy

Japan
Igaku-Shoin Ltd.
Tokyo International P.O. Box 5063
1-28-36 Hongo, Bunkyo-ku,
Tokyo 113, Japan

Korea
C.P.O. Box 10583
Seoul, Korea

Malaysia
No. 8 Jalan SS 7/6B
Kelana Jaya
47301 Petaling Jaya
Selangor, Malaysia

Mexico
Interamericana/McGraw-Hill de
Mexico, S.A. de C.V.
Cedro 512, Colonia Atlampa
(Apartado Postal 26370)
06450 Mexico, D.F., Mexico

New Zealand
McGraw-Hill Book Co.
New Zealand Ltd.
5 Joval Place, Wiri
Manukau City, New Zealand

Panama
Editorial McGraw-Hill
Latinoamericana, S.A.
Apartado Postal 2036
Zona Libre de Colon
Colon, Republica de Panama

Portugal
Editoria McGraw-Hill de Portugal, Ltda.
Rua Rosa Damasceno 11A–B
1900 Lisboa, Portugal

South Africa
Libriger Book Distributors
Warehouse Number 8
"Die Ou Looiery"
Tannery Road
Hamilton, Bloemfontein 9300

Southeast Asia
McGraw-Hill Book Co.
348 Jalan Boon Lay
Jurong, Singapore 2261

Spain
McGraw-Hill/Interamericana
de Espana, S.A.
Manuel Ferrero, 13
28020 Madrid, Spain

Taiwan
P.O. Box 87-601
Taipei, Taiwan

Thailand
632/5 Phaholyothin Road
Sapan Kwai
Bangkok 10400
Thailand

United Kingdom, Middle East and Africa
McGraw-Hill Book Company (U.K.) Ltd.
Shoppenhangers Road
Maidenhead, Berkshire
SL6 2QL England

Venezuela
McGraw-Hill/Interamericana, C.A.
2da. calle Bello Monte
(entre avenida Casanova y Sabana Grande)
Apartado Aereo 50785
Caracas 1050, Venezuela

NOTICE

The authors and publisher have made every effort to ensure that the patient care recommended herein, including choice of drugs and drug dosages, is in accord with the accepted standards and practice at the time of publication. However, since research and regulation constantly change clinical standards, the reader is urged to check the product information sheet included in the package of each drug, which includes recommended doses, warnings, and contraindications. This is particularly important with new or infrequently used drugs.

Surgical Anatomy—2

ISBN 1-55664–127-3

Printed in Hong Kong

Library of Congress catalog card number: 89–50083

10 9 8 7 6 5 4 3 2 1

Dedicated to

Our Mentors and Friends

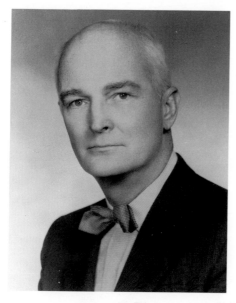

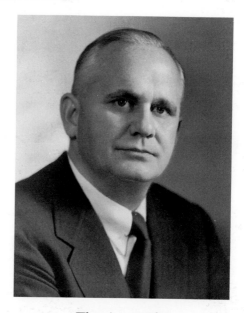

The Surgeon
John H. Gibbon, Jr. (1903–1973)

Graduate of Princeton University (1923) and Jefferson Medical College (1927). Became Professor of Surgery and Director of Surgical Research in 1946 and in 1954 was named Samuel D. Gross Professor and Chairman of the Department of Surgery at Jefferson.

The Anatomist
George A. Bennett (1904–1958)

Graduate of Wabash College (1923). Doctor of Medicine, University of Munich (1937). Became Professor and Chairman of the Department of Anatomy and Director of the Daniel Baugh Institute of Anatomy, Jefferson Medical College, in 1948, and in 1950 was appointed Dean of the College.

Preface

For many years, physicians have argued that a large amount of the anatomical material presented to the medical student in the preclinical years was of little practical value in ensuing clinical training and practice of medicine. This argument is not completely valid. The practical material *was* included, but because of the tremendous amount of information presented, particularly in the area of gross anatomy, the student was usually lost in a maze of detail. Anatomy faculties today are sorely lacking in gross anatomists who have the clinical experience which would enable them to enlighten the students to differentiate impractical details from the essential practical facts of gross anatomy.

With the tremendous information explosion which has occurred in the medical sciences in recent years, it became imperative that a change be made in the traditional medical curriculum. The curriculum is changing, but primarily at the expense of courses in gross anatomy. There are many individuals in the field of medical education who advocate the complete subjugation of anatomy to the college premedical level. Anatomy, particularly gross anatomy, should be streamlined to meet the required adjustments in the medical curriculum but certainly not eliminated!

Over the past years in teaching graduate medical students, I have observed a very interesting phenomenon. Whereas, in earlier years, the applicants for graduate courses in regional anatomy were invariably surgeons preparing for their surgical board examinations, during recent years, applications have been received from physicians of practically all specialties—all, that is, except specialists in psychiatry and dermatology. This, I feel, is an expression of the physicians' awareness of their lack of and need for anatomical training in the practice of medicine.

From my experience in teaching graduate medical students, it became obvious that there was a need for a concise anatomic descriptive text with an accompanying atlas. It was also apparent that they wanted not only a regional descriptive anatomy but also some practical applications of the anatomical knowledge. With these needs as our goal, the task of assembling this book was initiated.

I well realize that this book has its shortcomings. It was designed as a concise anatomy of areas in which the *general* surgeon plays an important therapeutic role. It is for this reason that many areas are included, particularly those related to the special senses, i.e. eye, ear, nose, and throat. The areas covered in this book, however, are anatomical regions with which all physicians should be thoroughly familiar.

I have oversimplified the descriptive anatomy in several areas, but only to enable the reader to understand an almost incomprehensible concept. I have avoided full discussions of variational patterns but instead have tried to present a method by which the reader may establish a norm which will aid in the recognition of a variant pattern. The anatomical terminology can also be criticized by the purist. I have not followed a strict nomenclature but have used anatomical terms most commonly used by the clinician.

One of the most difficult chores in writing this book was the selection of surgical considerations to be discussed. What is presented is only a small particle of what could be presented. The material was limited in order to retain a concise text and should not imply that anything omitted is not of anatomical significance. In the discussions of surgical considerations involving operative procedures, we have tried to circumvent detailed surgical technique and have emphasized the surgical anatomical principles involved. What I regret most is the lack of individual reference to information contained in this book. If such references were made, the bibliography would require more pages than the entire text-atlas.

Acknowledgments

I wish to express my appreciation to my collaborator, Dr. Joseph Hodge. Dr. Hodge was named prosector in anatomy under Dr. George Bennett at the Daniel Baugh Institute of Anatomy at the same time that I joined the faculty of the Institute. He then entered Jefferson Medical College and after graduation took his surgical training under Dr. John H. Gibbon, Jr. He has contributed a great deal in the sections of surgical considerations of the neck, thorax, abdomen, and peripheral vascular procedures.

My thanks are also offered to Dr. William D. Seybold, former Clinical Associate Professor of Surgery, Baylor University College of Medicine, and Senior Surgeon, Kelsey-Seybold Clinic, Houston. He is truly a surgeon and an anatomist—a lost breed today. His assistance was most significant, particularly in the section on the thorax. Despite his heavy clinical chores, he always found time to assist me in questions regarding the clinical considerations of the various anatomical areas. I personally gained much in the knowledge of applied surgical anatomy from our association.

Dr. John McKeown, former Clinical Professor of Surgery of the Jefferson Medical College has aided me in the surgical considerations of the parotid region.

To the surgical staff of the University of Texas, M.D. Anderson Hospital and Tumor Institute at Houston, I must also give thanks. Unknown to them, their brains were picked on many occasions in order to obtain information incorporated in this book.

To the artists, Mr. Don Johnson, Mr. Bill Osburn, and Mrs. Jeanet Dreskin, I wish to express my gratitude for a job well done.

Also, my special appreciation goes to Mr. Robert Rowan, Executive Editor, B. C. Decker Inc., Publisher, for his assistance and encouragement in the preparation of this book.

No book, regardless of its size, can be accomplished without secretarial assistance. My appreciation is extended to Mrs. Maria Maloney, Mrs. Janie Breed, Miss Dixie Knight, Mrs. Betty Herndon, and Mrs. Mary Kunak.

JOHN E. HEALEY, JR., M.D.

Publisher's Note
Sadly, Jack Healey slipped away quietly just when this new edition was about to be published. A dedicated family man, he was also a man of multiple and broad talents, holding the many posts listed on the title page.

Foreword

Jack Healey and I first met in 1947 in Dr. John H. Gibbon, Jr.'s Surgical Research Laboratory at Jefferson where, as a medical student, he first demonstrated the interest in research that characterized his long and productive career. He and George Bennett, to whom this second edition of this book is dedicated, were among the finest teachers of anatomy that I have known. It is fitting that their names be linked in this improved and augmented version.

In the competitive world of medical school curriculum committees, when more and more material must be squeezed into the limited time available, it is natural that the opportunity for students to learn gross anatomy has been limited, perhaps too severely. Human anatomy has changed little over the millennia and its study holds few challenges for the brilliant investigator. Yet an understanding of it is essential to every physician, nurse, and other deliverers of health care, and when a new technique is developed, additional vital details come to light. At the same time the needs of the clinician differ greatly from those of the pure anatomist. It is this gulf that Dr. Healey has bridged so well, offering an eminently readable description of the human body correlated with practical application. This book will be read with pleasure and benefit by all who look forward to or participate in patient care.

JOHN Y. TEMPLETON, III, M.D.
Emeritus Professor of Surgery
Jefferson Medical College

Contents

SURGICAL
ANATOMY

The Parotid Space

The parotid space, or retromandibular space, is of clinical importance because of the presence of the parotid gland. The frequency of operative procedures upon this gland plus the fact that this area is one of the main passageways between the head and neck makes it necessary that the surgeon possess a knowledge of its anatomic relations.

BOUNDARIES (Figs. 1 and 2):

Anterior — masseter muscle; ramus of the mandible; internal pterygoid muscle.

Posterior — mastoid process; sternocleidomastoid muscle.

Superior — external auditory meatus; temporomandibular joint.

Inferior — sternocleidomastoid muscle; posterior belly of the digastric muscle.

Lateral — skin; superficial fascia; superficial layer of parotid fascia.

Medial — deep layer of parotid fascia; styloid process and related muscles; internal jugular vein; internal carotid artery; pharyngeal wall.

FASCIAL RELATIONSHIP (Fig. 2):

The superficial (investing) layer of deep cervical fascia ascends and splits around the inferior border of the parotid gland into a superficial and a deep layer of *parotid fascia*.

The *superficial layer of parotid fascia* is a dense fibrous tissue layer which attaches to the zygomatic process above, and is continuous with the fascia covering the sternocleidomastoid muscle behind, and the masseter muscle in front.

The *deep layer of parotid fascia* extends along the medial surface of the gland and attaches to the base of the skull. It is not as dense as the superficial layer except for that portion extending between the styloid process and the angle of the mandible which thickens to form the *stylomandibular* ligament. The deep layer is especially thin along its medial surface where it is related directly to the pharyngeal wall.

PAROTID GLAND PROPER (Fig. 2, and Fig. 1, page 5):

The parotid gland, the largest of the salivary glands, occupies the entire parotid space; its boundaries, therefore, are in general identical with the boundaries of that space. Portions of the gland, however, may extend in various directions beyond these boundaries.

A prolongation of the gland may be related to the medial surface of the internal pterygoid muscle, the *pterygoid lobe* (Fig. 2). A medial extension between the internal carotid artery and styloid process, sometimes quite isolated, is referred to as the *carotid lobe* (Fig. 2). A prolongation into the posterior portion of the glenoid fossa immediately in front of the external auditory meatus is termed the *glenoid lobe* (Fig. 1, page 5). The largest and most common extension, however, is the *socia parotidis*, or *accessory parotid gland*, which is located anterior in position between the parotid duct and the zygomatic arch (Fig. 1, page 5). This lobe may be entirely detached from the main portion of the gland.

PAROTID DUCT (Fig. 1, page 5):

The duct of the parotid gland, *Stensen's duct*, extends from the anterior margin of the gland and proceeds forward over the masseter muscle about a finger's breadth below the zygomatic arch. It makes an abrupt turn at the anterior border of the masseter muscle and pierces the buccal fat pad, the buccinator muscle, and the mucous membrane of the mouth. The termination of the duct is on the summit of a papilla located opposite the crown of the second upper molar tooth (Fig. 2, page 9).

BILOBE CONCEPT (Fig. 2, page 5):

As early as 1912, the concept was put forth that the parotid gland is fundamentally divisible into two lobes, a *superficial* and a *deep*. The main branches of the facial nerve pass between these lobes in a fascial plane. The two lobes are joined by an isthmus of varying size, behind which the main trunk of the facial nerve divides; the zygomaticofacial division passes above the isthmus, and the cervicofacial division below.

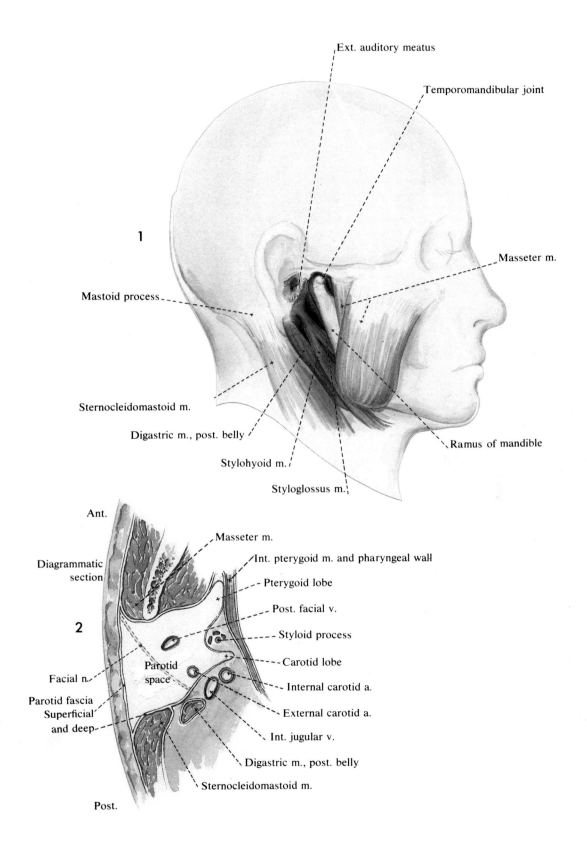

1

Ext. auditory meatus

Temporomandibular joint

Masseter m.

Mastoid process

Sternocleidomastoid m.

Digastric m., post. belly

Stylohyoid m.

Styloglossus m.

Ramus of mandible

Ant.

Diagrammatic section

2

Facial n.

Parotid fascia
Superficial
and deep

Parotid space

Post.

Masseter m.

Int. pterygoid m. and pharyngeal wall

Pterygoid lobe

Post. facial v.

Styloid process

Carotid lobe

Internal carotid a.

External carotid a.

Int. jugular v.

Digastric m., post. belly

Sternocleidomastoid m.

RELATED STRUCTURES (Figs. 1 and 2):

One can define a superior, anterior, inferior, and posterior border of the parotid gland, and to each border are related certain important anatomic structures. The main structure is the *facial nerve*. This nerve enters the parotid space via the stylomastoid foramen. After giving off the posterior auricular nerve and the nerve to the stylohyoid and posterior belly of the digastric, it extends forward to the posterior surface of the isthmus. Here it divides into *zygomaticofacial* and *cervicofacial* divisions. The zygomaticofacial division further divides into temporal and zygomatic branches; the cervicofacial gives off the buccal, mandibular, and cervical branches. The terminal branches of the facial nerve freely communicate with each other and with branches of the trigeminal nerve.

In addition to the facial nerve, certain other structures are intimately related to the gland—namely, the external carotid artery and its branches, the external jugular vein and its tributaries, the auriculotemporal nerve, and the great auricular nerve.

**Structures Related to the
Superior Border:**

Posterior to Anterior:

1. **Auriculotemporal Nerve**—is a branch of the mandibular division of the trigeminal, carrying secretory fibers to the gland from the otic ganglion, and sensory fibers from the skin of the ear, external auditory meatus, mandibular joint, and temporal region of the scalp.
2. **Superficial Temporal Artery**—arises at the neck of the mandible as a terminal branch of the external carotid.
3. **Superficial Temporal Vein**—joins the internal maxillary in the parotid space to form the posterior facial vein.
4. **Temporal Branch of the Facial Nerve**—usually multiple, innervates the frontalis and orbicularis oculi muscles.

**Structures Related to the
Anterior Border:**

Superior to Inferior:

1. **Zygomatic Branch of the Facial Nerve**—extends forward to innervate the orbicularis oculi and the zygomaticus muscles.
2. **Transverse Facial Vein**—drains into the posterior facial vein.
3. **Transverse Facial Artery**—is the largest collateral branch of the superficial temporal artery.
4. **Parotid Duct**—runs transversally across the masseter muscle about a finger's breadth below the zygomatic arch.
5. **Buccal Branch of the Facial Nerve**—parallels the duct but lies just below it. It may at times arise from the zygomaticofacial division rather than the cervicofacial.

It innervates the muscles of the nose and angle of the mouth, as well as the buccinator.

6. **Mandibular Branch of the Facial Nerve**—supplies the quadratus labii inferioris and the mentalis muscles.

**Structures Related to the
Inferior Border:**

Anterior to Posterior:

1. **Cervical Branch of the Facial Nerve**—may be readily identified at the angle of the mandible. Although its main supply is to the platysma muscle, this nerve should be preserved, for it frequently gives rise to a marginal-mandibular branch which turns upward along the anterior border of the masseter to innervate the muscles at the angle of the mouth.
2. **External Jugular Vein**—is formed at the lower border of the gland by the union of the posterior auricular and the posterior division of the posterior facial veins. It serves as a good guide to the facial plane between the superficial and deep parotid lobes.
3. **Great Auricular Nerve**—arises from C_2 and C_3, via the superficial cervical plexus. It ascends parallel to and slightly behind the external jugular vein and carries sensory fibers from the skin over the mastoid, back of the ear, and the skin and fascia covering the parotid gland.

**Structures Related to the
Posterior Border:**

Inferior to Superior:

1. **Posterior Auricular Vein**—joins the posterior division of the posterior facial to form the external jugular.
2. **Posterior Auricular Artery**—is given off at the upper border of the posterior belly of the digastric muscle and is one of the posterior branches of the external carotid.
3. **Posterior Auricular Nerve**—is the first branch of the facial nerve after its exit from the stylomastoid foramen. It supplies the posterior auricular and occipitalis muscles.

REMOVAL OF THE SUPERFICIAL LOBE
(Fig. 3):

After removal of the superficial lobe of the parotid, the isthmus of the gland can be visualized with its relationship to the facial nerve and its terminal branches. Lying just deep to the facial nerve branches may be seen the posterior facial vein and its important tributaries as well as the formation of the external jugular vein. The latter is formed by the posterior auricular and the posterior division of the posterior facial. The anterior division of the posterior facial joins the anterior facial to form the common facial.

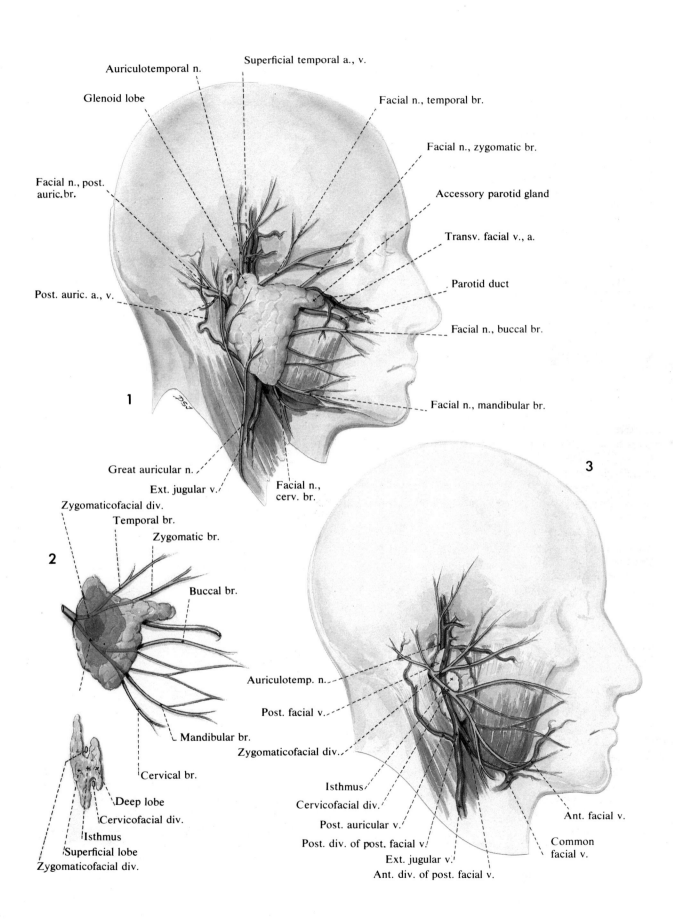

Auriculotemporal n.

Superficial temporal a., v.

Glenoid lobe

Facial n., temporal br.

Facial n., zygomatic br.

Facial n., post.
auric. br.

Accessory parotid gland

Transv. facial v., a.

Parotid duct

Post. auric. a., v.

Facial n., buccal br.

Facial n., mandibular br.

1

Great auricular n.

3

Ext. jugular v.

Facial n.,
cerv. br.

2

Zygomaticofacial div.

Temporal br.

Zygomatic br.

Buccal br.

Auriculotemp. n.

Post. facial v.

Zygomaticofacial div.

Mandibular br.

Cervical br.

Isthmus

Cervicofacial div.

Deep lobe

Post. auricular v.

Cervicofacial div.

Post. div. of post. facial v.

Ant. facial v.

Isthmus

Ext. jugular v.

Common
facial v.

Superficial lobe

Ant. div. of post. facial v.

Zygomaticofacial div.

REMOVAL OF THE DEEP LOBE:

The Parotid Bed (Fig. 1):

With the removal of the deep lobe of the parotid gland, the structures which constitute the parotid bed may be observed.

1. **External Carotid Artery** — this artery is the most superficial of the structures in the parotid bed, frequently being imbedded in the deep lobe of the gland. After removal of this lobe, the terminal branches, the *superficial temporal* and *internal maxillary,* may be seen arising from the main trunk at the neck of the mandible.

2. **Styloid Process and Its Related Muscles** (Fig. 2) — these include the following muscles from above downward: the *styloglossus, stylopharyngeus,* and the *stylohyoid.* The latter passes superficial to the external carotid; the other two muscles lie deep to this vessel.

3. **Internal Jugular Vein** — lies posterior in position in the parotid bed, just medial to the styloid process. It receives no important tributaries in this immediate area.

4. **Internal Carotid Artery** — is located just anterior to the internal jugular vein and gives off no branches in the parotid area.

5. **Glossopharyngeal (IX) Nerve** (Fig. 2) — may be identified as it courses around the inferior border of the stylopharyngeus muscle, which lies deep to and between the styloglossus above and the stylohyoid below.

6. **Vagus (X) Nerve** — occupies a position between the internal jugular vein and internal carotid artery and deep to these structures. It descends directly through the space and gives rise to the deep-lying superior laryngeal branch at this level.

7. **Spinal Accessory (XI) Nerve** — is superficial to the carotid sheath and as it descends is directed posteriorly deep to the posterior belly of the digastric and the sternocleidomastoid, innervating the latter, as well as the trapezius.

8. **Hypoglossal (XII) Nerve** — lies in about the same position as the spinal accessory, but as it descends it is directed anteriorly to the tongue.

Lymphatics of the Parotid Area (Fig. 3):

Lymph nodes related to the parotid gland may be divided into two groups, superficial and deep.

1. **Superficial Group** — these nodes are often referred to as the preauricular nodes and lie in the superficial fascia of this area. They are variable in number and receive lymph channels from areas adjacent to the parotid space, i.e., the upper part of the face, the temporal area of the scalp, and the anterior portion of the auricle. These nodes all drain into the chain of nodes lying along the external jugular vein.

2. **Deep Group** — these nodes are located in the substance of the parotid gland. In addition to receiving channels from the gland, they receive drainage from parts of the nasopharynx and from the nose, palate, eustachian tube, middle ear, and external auditory meatus. The lymph channels from these nodes extend caudalward to the *subparotid node,* from which channels pass to the chain along the internal jugular vein and the nodes associated with the spinal accessory nerve.

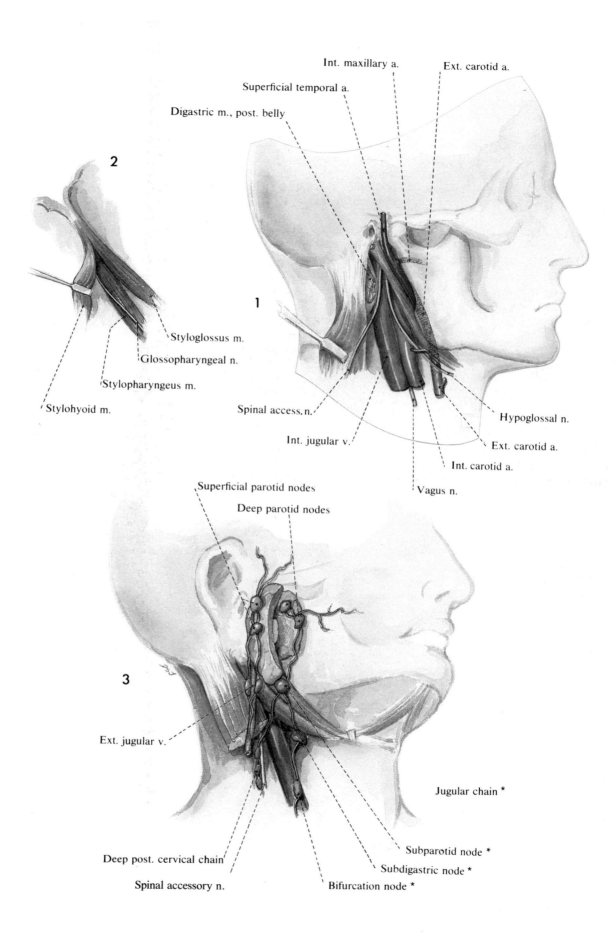

1

2

3

Int. maxillary a.

Ext. carotid a.

Superficial temporal a.

Digastric m., post. belly

Styloglossus m.

Glossopharyngeal n.

Stylopharyngeus m.

Stylohyoid m.

Spinal access. n.

Int. jugular v.

Hypoglossal n.

Ext. carotid a.

Int. carotid a.

Vagus n.

Superficial parotid nodes

Deep parotid nodes

Ext. jugular v.

Jugular chain *

Deep post. cervical chain

Spinal accessory n.

Bifurcation node *

Subdigastric node *

Subparotid node *

CLINICAL CONSIDERATIONS:

The most common inflammatory lesion of the parotid gland is *parotitis* due to mumps. The incidence of postoperative or surgical parotitis has steadily decreased since the introduction of the sulfonamide drugs and antibiotics. However, with the emergence of antibiotic-resistant strains of staphylococci, parotitis may proceed to actual suppuration and abscess formation. Suppuration of the gland may extend superiorly with perforation into the external auditory meatus and involvement of the temporomandibular joint (Fig. 1, page 3). Deep-seated abscesses may project and drain into the pharynx (Fig. 2, page 3).

As in any abscess, drainage is indicated over the site of fluctuation, or where pus has been localized. External drainage can be accomplished through a short transverse or oblique incision parallel to the radiating fibers of the facial nerve and the parotid duct (Fig. 1a). If the suppurative process extends posteriorly or superiorly, a vertical preauricular incision may be made just anterior to the ear from above the tragus to the angle of the mandible (Fig. 1b). Internal drainage may be accomplished from within the oral pharynx (Fig. 2).

Calculus Formation:

Calculi (sialoliths) can form in the major ducts of the three major salivary glands, but occur most commonly in the duct of the submaxillary gland. Obstruction of the parotid (Stensen's) duct by a calculus may be associated with recurrent or chronic parotitis and is best treated by excision of part or all of the parotid gland. Injection of radiopaque solutions into the duct orifice is utilized to confirm the presence of calculi by radiographic methods (sialography).

Salivary Fistulas:

Salivary fistulas may result from surgical procedures in the vicinity of or upon the parotid gland and duct. Various techniques have been advocated for conversion of external salivary fistulas to internal ones with a high percentage of failures due to occlusion. The majority of salivary fistulas will close spontaneously. Ligation of the parotid duct from within the mouth has been advocated to control salivary incontinence after radical surgery for malignant tumors of the floor of the mouth. Ligation of the parotid duct proximal to a fistula has been performed without adverse effects.

Neoplasms:

Mixed tumors form the most common group of neoplasms of salivary glands, and the parotid, the largest salivary gland, is the site of 85 to 90 per cent of mixed tumors which affect the salivary system. A mixed tumor of the parotid may involve the superficial lobe alone, rarely the deep lobe alone, or both lobes. Treatment of a mixed tumor of the parotid consists of excision of the tumor with a considerable margin of normal gland. For this reason, tumors involving the deep lobe frequently require total parotidectomy. Mixed tumors are notorious for high recurrence rates, mainly owing to inadequate excision with residual tumor in the remaining gland. A less significant number of recurrences may be due to implantation of tumor tissue into the wound and possibly to multiple foci of origin. The microscopic pattern of a benign mixed tumor is not a significant factor in determining whether or not a mixed tumor is likely to recur. From 5 to 12 per cent of mixed tumors show evidence of malignancy, whereas 30 per cent of all parotid tumors are malignant.

Parotidectomy:

In performing a partial or total parotidectomy adequate exposure is essential. This may be accomplished by making a vertical preauricular incision (Fig. 1b) and extending this posteriorly toward the mastoid and anteriorly in the submandibular area (Figs. 1c and d).

The most important step in doing a parotidectomy is the identification, dissection, isolation, and preservation of the facial nerve. The incidence of injury to the facial nerve can be minimized by careful dissection and by exposing and isolating it before removing the tumor. Some surgeons find the use of a stimulating electrode of great value in identifying branches of the facial nerve. Others commence by exposing the cervical branch at the angle of the jaw and following it back to the main trunk. One may also utilize the posterior facial vein as a guide to the fascial plane between the superficial and deep lobe. The safest procedure is exposure of the main trunk of the facial after its exit from the stylomastoid foramen. Three anatomic structures should be identified: the mastoid process, the angle of the mandible, and the cartilaginous ear canal. The main trunk may be identified about midway between the latter two structures (Fig. 3). After isolation of the facial nerve, removal of the deep lobe is carried out (Fig. 4), keeping in mind the relationship of the structures in the parotid bed (Fig. 1, page 7).

In the presence of a malignant tumor of the parotid gland, it may be necessary to sacrifice the facial nerve or its branches. Nerve grafts have been utilized successfully to repair such defects. The presence of tumor in lymph nodes below the parotid tumor or elsewhere in the neck is an indication for extension of the operative procedure to include a radical neck dissection.

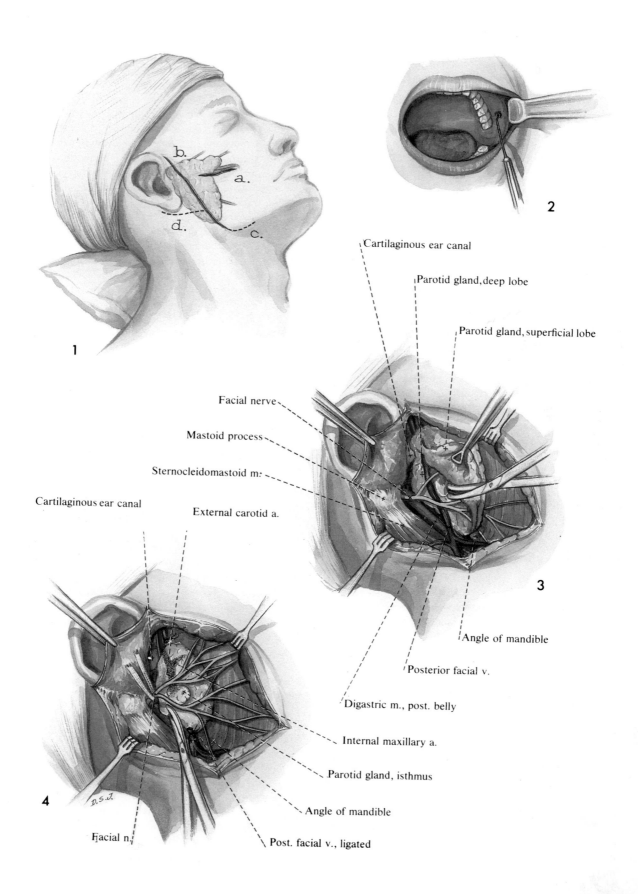

Cartilaginous ear canal

Parotid gland, deep lobe

Parotid gland, superficial lobe

Facial nerve

Mastoid process

Sternocleidomastoid m.

Cartilaginous ear canal

External carotid a.

Angle of mandible

Posterior facial v.

Digastric m., post. belly

Internal maxillary a.

Parotid gland, isthmus

Angle of mandible

Facial n.

Post. facial v., ligated

D.S.J.

The Neck

GENERAL CONSIDERATIONS:

Before discussing the regional anatomy of the neck, it is important to know its topographic divisions and surface markings in order to simplify the areas of surgical importance.

Topography (Fig. 1):

The main topographic landmark in the neck is the sternocleidomastoid muscle. This muscle and the midline of the neck along with the anterior border of the trapezius divide the neck into an anterior and a posterior triangle.

The Anterior Triangle — is bounded anteriorly by the midline of the neck and posteriorly by the sternocleidomastoid muscle. Its superior boundary is formed by the lower border of the mandible and a line drawn from the angle of the mandible to the tip of the mastoid process. This triangle may be subdivided as follows:

1. Submandibular triangle
2. Submental triangle
3. Carotid triangle
4. Muscular triangle

The Posterior Triangle — is limited anteriorly by the sternocleidomastoid, posteriorly by the trapezius, and below by the middle third of the clavicle. This is further divided by the posterior belly of the omohyoid into:

5. Occipital triangle
6. Subclavian triangle

Surface Markings (Fig. 1):

In addition to the aforementioned sternocleidomastoid muscle and its bony attachments, other conspicuous and palpable structures in the neck include:

1. **Thyroid Cartilage** — is especially prominent where the right and left laminae of this cartilage fuse in the upper midline of the neck and is referred to as the laryngeal prominence or Adam's apple.
2. **Hyoid Bone** — is located in the midline about 1 inch above the laryngeal prominence and in line with the lower border of the third cervical vertebra. If followed laterally, the greater cornu may be palpated. Its tip lies about midway between the laryngeal prominence and the mastoid process and is an important surgical landmark for the ligation of the lingual artery.
3. **Cricoid Cartilage** — lies just below the thyroid cartilage and at the level of the sixth cervical vertebra.

Skin of the Neck:

The skin of the neck is of particular importance to the surgeon in regard to the cosmetic effect following incisions in this area. The fibers of the corium course predominantly in the planes of the body surface and display prevailing directions that differ strikingly in different regions of the body. These are the *Langer's lines*. In the neck, they run in a transverse direction, and incisions should be made accordingly; for example, the collar incision for thyroidectomy.

Superficial Fascia (Fig. 2):

This subcutaneous layer of the neck, like that elsewhere in the body, is made up of loose areolar connective tissue and contains superficial blood vessels and nerves. In the neck, in addition to these structures, one finds a voluntary muscle, the *platysma*; this muscle is one of facial expression, therefore innervated by the facial nerve. In incisions in the neck, it is always imperative that the severed ends of this muscle be reapproximated in order to overcome unsightly postoperative defects. The superficial cervical veins and nerves are located deep to the platysma muscle.

1. **External Jugular Vein** — its origin has already been discussed (page 4). The vein descends superficial to the sternocleidomastoid muscle and pierces the deep cervical fascia in the posterior triangle to empty into the subclavian vein. The deep fascia is firmly attached to the vein wall as this vein pierces the fascia. This prevents collapse of the vein if it is accidentally cut.

2. **Anterior Jugular Vein** — begins in the suprahyoid region and descends near the midline parallel with its partner of the opposite side. Just above the clavicle it pierces the deep fascia, passes beneath the sternocleidomastoid, and empties into the external jugular. It is often connected with the vein of the opposite side above the sternal notch, forming the *jugular venous arch*.

3. **Vein of Kocher** — frequently arises from the branches of the common facial vein, descends along the anterior border of the sternocleidomastoid, and drains into the jugular venous arch or the internal jugular. If the anterior jugular is absent, this vein is usually of large size.

4. **Superficial Cervical Plexus** — arises from the anterior primary divisions of cervical segments C_2 to C_4.

a. LESSER OCCIPITAL (C_2) — hooks around the spinal accessory, ascends along the posterior border of the sternocleidomastoid muscle, and terminates in auricular, mastoid, and occipital branches.

b. GREAT AURICULAR (C_2 to C_3) — takes exit from under the middle of the posterior border of the sternocleidomastoid, and extends upward posterior to and parallel with the external jugular vein. Its distribution has already been discussed (page 4).

c. TRANSVERSE CERVICAL (C_2 to C_3) — exits just below the great auricular and extends across the sternocleidomastoid to the anterior triangle where it fans out to supply the skin between mentum and sternum.

d. SUPRACLAVICULAR (C_3 to C_4) — exits from the middle of the posterior border of the sternocleidomastoid and divides into three terminal branches:

(1) *Anterior* — extends downward, innervating the skin as far as the second intercostal space and the sternoclavicular joint.

(2) *Middle* — descends over the middle third of the clavicle, at times piercing this bone, thereby causing persistent neuralgia if involved in the callus following fractures of the clavicle.

(3) *Posterior* — is distributed to the skin over the upper two-thirds of the deltoid and the acromioclavicular joint.

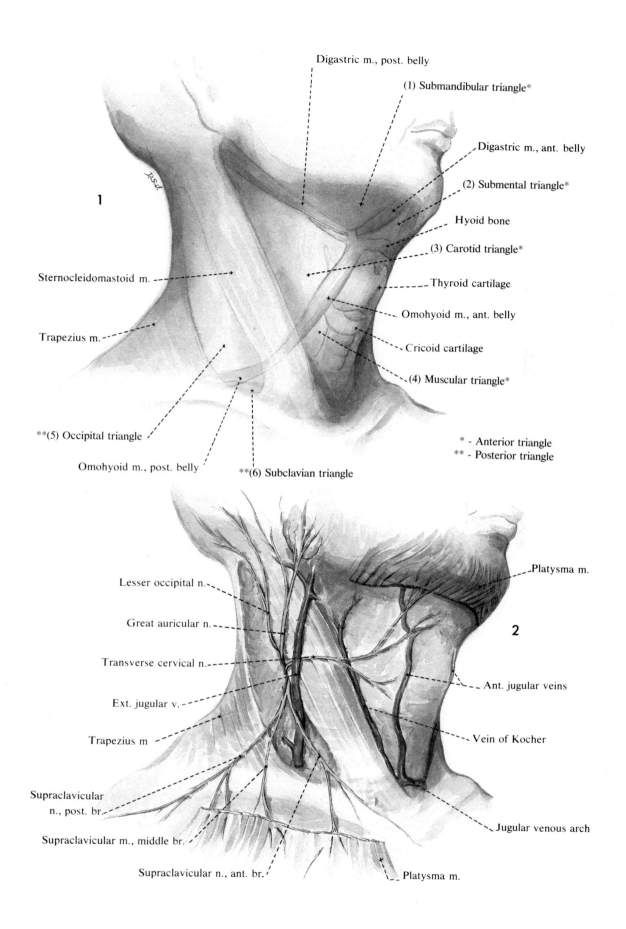

1

Digastric m., post. belly

(1) Submandibular triangle*

Digastric m., ant. belly

(2) Submental triangle*

Hyoid bone

(3) Carotid triangle*

Thyroid cartilage

Omohyoid m., ant. belly

Cricoid cartilage

(4) Muscular triangle*

Sternocleidomastoid m.

Trapezius m.

**(5) Occipital triangle

Omohyoid m., post. belly

**(6) Subclavian triangle

* - Anterior triangle
** - Posterior triangle

2

Platysma m.

Lesser occipital n.

Great auricular n.

Transverse cervical n.

Ext. jugular v.

Trapezius m

Supraclavicular
n., post. br.

Supraclavicular m., middle br.

Supraclavicular n., ant. br.

Ant. jugular veins

Vein of Kocher

Jugular venous arch

Platysma m.

THE SUBMANDIBULAR TRIANGLE:

The submandibular triangle is also referred to as the submaxillary or digastric triangle. The main structure within the triangle is the submaxillary gland. Also of surgical significance is the presence of the submandibular lymph nodes which may be involved in malignant disease of the areas which they drain.

Boundaries and Muscular Contents (Fig. 1):

The boundaries of the triangle are formed by the anterior and posterior bellies of the digastric and the inferior border of the mandible. In the floor are found three muscles, each lying at a slightly deeper level than the other, and because of the very distinct direction of their fibers, these muscles may be utilized as important surgical landmarks. From superficial to deep, they are as follows:

1. **Mylohyoid**—arises from the mylohyoid ridge of the mandible and inserts on the hyoid bone and into a median raphe extending from the hyoid to the mandible. It is innervated by the mylohyoid nerve, a branch of the mandibular division of the trigeminal.

2. **Hyoglossus**—takes origin from the greater cornu and part of the body of the hyoid and inserts into fibrous framework of the tongue. This muscle is innervated by the hypoglossal.

3. **Superior Constrictor of the Pharynx**—the lowermost fibers of this muscle may be seen in the submandibular triangle. They arise from the root of the tongue, posterior portion of the mylohyoid ridge of the mandible, and pterygomandibular raphe and insert in a median raphe in the posterior midline of the pharynx. The muscle receives its innervation from branches of the glossopharyngeal and vagus nerves.

Within the space are found the afore-described styloid muscles (Fig. 2, page 7).

Superficial Contents (Fig. 2):

In the superficial fascia of this region are found the following structures:

1. **Cervical Branch of the Facial Nerve**—descends into the submandibular triangle at the angle of the mandible and innervates the platysma muscle. It sends a branch *(pars mandibularis)* which sweeps upward at the anterior border of the masseter muscle to supply some of the muscles at the angle of the mouth.

2. **Anterior Facial Vein**—after receiving tributaries from the region of the face, this vein descends at the anterior border of the masseter and extends posteriorly through the submandibular triangle to join the anterior division of the posterior facial vein. This union forms the *common facial vein.*

Submaxillary Fascia (Fig. 3):

The deep fascia roofing the triangle is formed by the superficial or investing layer of deep cervical fascia. It splits around the gland to form a superficial and deep layer of submaxillary fascia.

The *superficial layer* of submaxillary fascia attaches to the inferior border of the mandible, and is rather taut. In order to palpate the gland or nodes in this area, it is necessary to depress the mandible somewhat in order to relax the fascial covering.

The *deep layer* of the submaxillary fascia extends upward on the medial surface of the mandible and attaches to the mylohyoid ridge.

The submaxillary fascia is not as intimately related to the submaxillary gland as is the parotid fascia to the parotid gland. Its surgical enucleation may therefore be carried out more readily than that of the parotid.

Submaxillary Gland (Figs. 2 and 3 and Fig. 1, page 15):

The submaxillary gland is a racemose gland and occupies the major portion of the submandibular triangle. A part of the gland extends beyond the space, between the mylohyoid and the hyoglossus muscles. It passes forward for a varying distance toward the floor of the mouth, closely associated with the submaxillary duct. This extension is referred to as the deep process (Fig. 1, page 15). The remainder of the gland is described as the *superficial part* (Fig. 2).

Related Structures (Fig. 2):

As already mentioned, only two structures lie in the superficial fascia of the submandibular area, the *cervical branch* of the *facial nerve* and the *anterior facial vein.*

The superficial veins are the only structures crossing superficial to the posterior belly of the digastric in this region. Incisions may be made directly upon this muscle without the sacrifice of any structures of surgical significance.

Deep to the submaxillary fascia are found the following structures closely related to the gland:

1. **External Maxillary (Facial) Artery**—is most intimately related to the submaxillary gland. This artery arises in the carotid triangle and is the uppermost of the three anterior branches of the external carotid artery. It passes upward deep to the posterior belly of the digastric and stylohyoid, then loops forward following a tortuous course to the face at the anterior border of the masseter. In the submandibular space it gives rise to branches supplying the soft palate, the faucial tonsils, the submaxillary gland, and the submental triangle.

2. **Mylohyoid Nerve**—is seen in this area extending from the anterior border of the gland and traveling in association with the submental vessels to innervate the mylohyoid and the anterior belly of the digastric. It is a branch of the inferior alveolar branch of the mandibular division of the trigeminal.

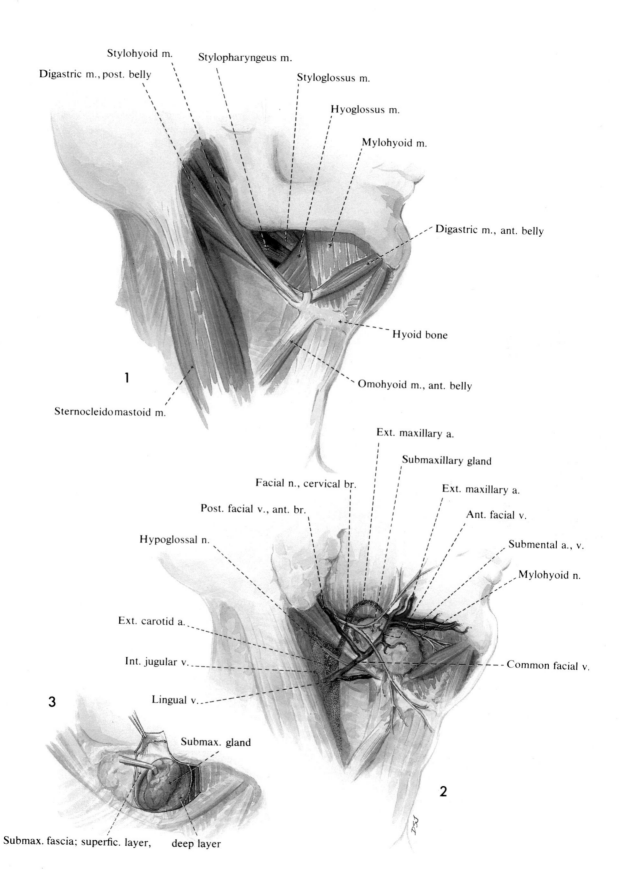

Stylohyoid m.

Digastric m., post. belly

Stylopharyngeus m.

Styloglossus m.

Hyoglossus m.

Mylohyoid m.

Digastric m., ant. belly

Hyoid bone

Omohyoid m., ant. belly

1

Sternocleidomastoid m.

Ext. maxillary a.

Submaxillary gland

Facial n., cervical br.

Ext. maxillary a.

Post. facial v., ant. br.

Ant. facial v.

Hypoglossal n.

Submental a., v.

Mylohyoid n.

Ext. carotid a.

Int. jugular v.

Common facial v.

Lingual v.

3

Submax. gland

2

Submax. fascia; superfic. layer, deep layer

Removal of the Submaxillary Gland
(Fig. 1):

After removal of the superficial portion of the gland, the structures related to the floor of the space may be visualized. The related muscles have already been shown (Fig. 1, page 13). In addition, the submaxillary duct, certain important nerves, and blood vessels are present.

1. **Submaxillary (Wharton's) Duct** — arises from the medial aspect of the gland and passes between the mylohyoid and hyoglossus. Here it lies in a very important relationship with two nerves of the tongue, the lingual above and the hypoglossal below. The duct terminates in the floor of the mouth on a small papilla at the side of the frenulum of the tongue.

2. **Lingual Nerve** — is a branch of the mandibular division of the trigeminal. This nerve is usually not seen in the operative field, unless pulled downward by excessive traction on the gland. It crosses the superior constrictor and the hyoglossus, then deep to the mylohyoid, at which point it lies just above Wharton's duct. It carries general sensory fibers from the mucous membrane of the floor of the mouth and anterior two-thirds of the tongue. Running incorporated in it are the fibers of the *chorda tympani*, a branch of the facial. The latter carries taste fibers from the anterior two-thirds of the tongue and efferent parasympathetic fibers to the *submaxillary ganglion*, from which autonomic secretory fibers are distributed to the submaxillary and sublingual glands and mucous membrane of the floor of the mouth.

3. **Glossopharyngeal Nerve** — is a mixed nerve carrying motor fibers to the stylopharyngeus and constrictor muscles, and sensory fibers from the middle ear, pharynx, and posterior one-third of the tongue as well as the carotid body. Its relationship with the stylopharyngeus has already been described (page 6). It enters the pharyngeal wall in the interval between the superior and middle constrictors along with the stylopharyngeus muscle.

4. **Vagus Nerve** — remains between the internal carotid artery and internal jugular vein as described in the parotid bed.

5. **Spinal Accessory Nerve** — extends posteriorly superficial to the internal jugular and deep to the posterior belly of the digastric and sternocleidomastoid muscles.

6. **Hypoglossal Nerve** — extends through the parotid space into the submandibular triangle superficial to the carotid sheath. It descends into the carotid triangle and swings forward to return to the submandibular triangle deep to the posterior belly of the digastric where it disappears between the mylohyoid and hyoglossus. It supplies the styloglossus and hyoglossus in this area, then proceeds forward to innervate all remaining extrinsic and intrinsic muscles of the tongue.

7. **Superior Cervical Sympathetic Ganglion** — lies medial (deep) to the carotid sheath at the angle of the mandible. This large, spindle-shaped ganglion gives rise to postganglionic sympathetic fibers destined to blood vessels, glands, and pilomotor muscles of the head and upper neck.

8. **Lingual Artery** — the second of the three anterior branches of the external carotid, is given off just below the origin of the external maxillary in the carotid triangle, frequently as a common trunk with the latter. It extends forward near the tip of the greater cornu of the hyoid bone, a fairly constant relationship. It then passes deep to the hyoglossus to give off its terminal branches, the *dorsal lingual*, *sublingual*, and *deep lingual* arteries.

9. **Posterior Auricular Artery** — is one of three posterior branches of the external carotid and is given off just above the posterior belly of the digastric and runs along its superior border.

10. **Internal Carotid Artery** — remains deep to the styloid muscles in the carotid sheath and gives off no branches in this area.

11. **Lingual Vein** — exits beneath the hyoglossus with the lingual artery and descends into the carotid triangle to empty into the internal jugular vein or common facial vein.

12. **Internal Jugular Vein** — remains unchanged in position from that seen in the parotid area (Fig. 1, page 7).

Submental Triangle (Figs. 1 and 2):

The submental triangle is bounded by the midline of the neck, the hyoid bone, and the anterior belly of the digastric. The floor is formed by the mylohyoid muscle. The only contents of the triangle are the submental lymph nodes, which drain the skin of the chin, the lower lip, the floor of the mouth, and the tip of the tongue. Efferent channels pass to submandibular nodes or to the carotid and omohyoid nodes of the jugular chain.

Lymphatics of the Submandibular Area (Fig. 2):

Lymph nodes of the submandibular area may be divided into three groups designated as: (1) *preglandular*, (2) *prevascular*, and (3) *retrovascular*. The submandibular nodes receive afferent channels from the submental nodes, oral cavity, and anterior face. Efferent channels from the submandibular nodes drain primarily into the jugulodigastric (subdigastric), jugulocarotid (bifurcation), and jugulo-omohyoid nodes of the chain along the internal jugular vein. A few channels pass via the subparotid node into the chain along the spinal accessory nerve (deep posterior cervical nodes).

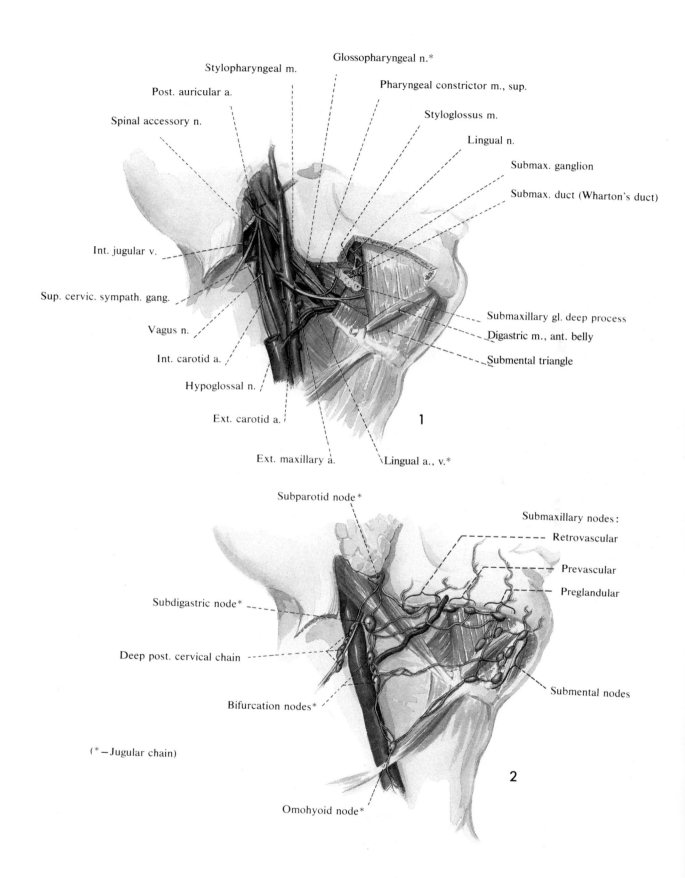

Stylopharyngeal m.

Glossopharyngeal n.*

Post. auricular a.

Pharyngeal constrictor m., sup.

Spinal accessory n.

Styloglossus m.

Lingual n.

Submax. ganglion

Submax. duct (Wharton's duct)

Int. jugular v.

Sup. cervic. sympath. gang.

Submaxillary gl. deep process

Vagus n.

Digastric m., ant. belly

Int. carotid a.

Submental triangle

Hypoglossal n.

Ext. carotid a.

Ext. maxillary a.

Lingual a., v.*

1

Subparotid node*

Submaxillary nodes:

Retrovascular

Prevascular

Subdigastric node*

Preglandular

Deep post. cervical chain

Submental nodes

Bifurcation nodes*

(*—Jugular chain)

2

Omohyoid node*

THE CAROTID TRIANGLE:

This triangle is so named and is of surgical significance because it contains all parts of the carotid arterial system.

Boundaries and Muscular Contents (Fig. 1):

The area is bounded by the posterior belly of the digastric above, the anterior belly of the omohyoid below, and the sternocleidomastoid behind.

In the floor of the triangle are found the following muscles:

1. **Hyoglossus**—which has already been seen in the submandibular area, may be visualized near the apex of this triangle arising from the upper border of the greater cornu of the hyoid bone.

2. **Thyrohyoid**—lies on the same plane as the hyoglossus and arises from the oblique line of thyroid cartilage. It is one of the strap muscles of the neck, and therefore innervated by branches of the deep cervical plexus (page 18).

3. **Middle Constrictor of the Pharynx**—lies more lateral in position and deep to the two muscles just described. It arises from the hyoid bone and inserts in a median raphe in the posterior midline of the pharynx.

4. **Inferior Constrictor of the Pharynx**—is located on the same plane as the middle constrictor, its superior fibers, however, overlapping the lowermost fibers of the middle constrictor. This fan-shaped muscle arises from the thyroid and cricoid cartilages and inserts in the median raphe of the pharynx. The pharyngeal muscles are innervated by the pharyngeal branches of the glossopharyngeal and vagus nerves.

5. **Longus Capitus**—is the deepest muscle in the carotid triangle, one of the prevertebral group, lying anterior to the vertebral column.

Superficial Fascia (Fig. 2, page 11):

As already described in the general discussion of the superficial fascia of the neck, one finds in this area the platysma muscle, deep to which lie the transverse cervical nerve, the vein of Kocher, and the anterior jugular vein.

Deep Fascia (Fig. 2):

The deep fascia of the neck may be conveniently divided into three distinct layers: a superficial, a middle, and a deep layer. There is still a great deal of controversy in regard to these fascial planes, particularly to the extension of the middle layer of fascia. In addition to these layers, one must consider the fascia related directly to the pharynx.

1. **Superficial (Investing) Layer**—completely encircles the neck and in so doing invests the sternocleidomastoid and trapezius muscles. It is this same layer that invested the two glands previously described, the parotid and the submaxillary.

2. **Middle (Pretracheal) Layer**—a rather complex layer that may be differentiated into two laminae: an *anterior lamina*, which invests the strap muscles of the neck and extends laterally to the omohyoid muscles and superiorly to the hyoid bone, and a *posterior lamina*, which splits around the thyroid gland, forming the false or surgical capsule of the thyroid gland.

3. **Deep (Prevertebral) Layer**—this fascial layer covers the prevertebral muscles of the anterior triangle, the longus capitus and cervicus, as well as the muscle in the floor of the posterior triangle.

4. **Buccopharyngeal Fascia**—a thin fibrous sheath which extends from the base of the skull covering the constrictor muscles over the lateral and posterior surfaces of the pharynx. It is continuous with the fascia covering the buccinator muscle.

5. **Carotid Sheath**—a tubular fascial structure extending from the base of the skull to the root of the neck and formed by fascial extensions from the superficial, middle, and deep layers of cervical fascia. It encases three important structures: the internal jugular vein laterally, the common carotid artery medially, and the vagus nerve posteriorly and between the other two structures.

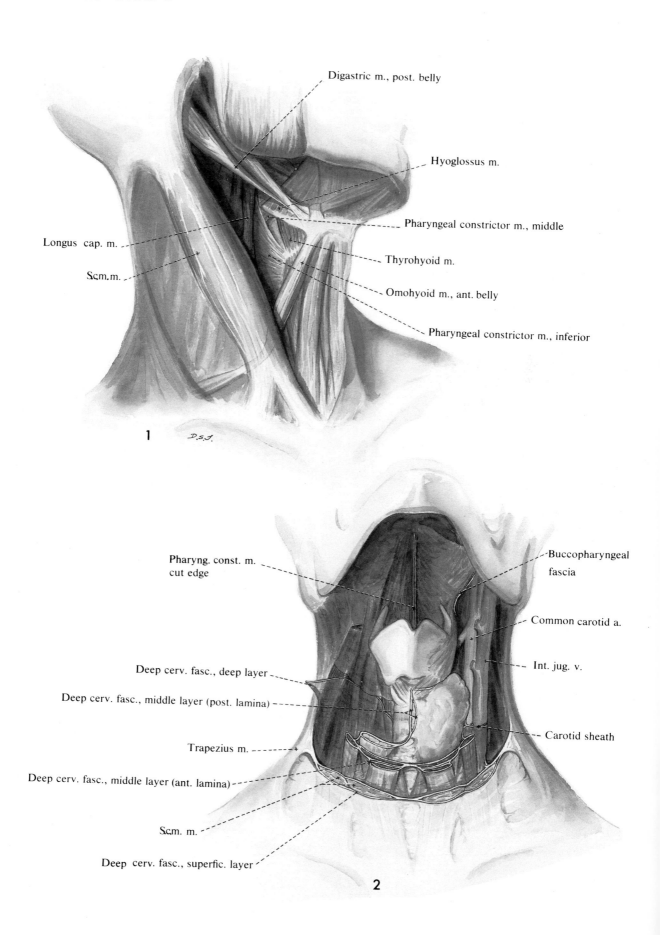

Digastric m., post. belly

Hyoglossus m.

Pharyngeal constrictor m., middle

Longus cap. m.

Thyrohyoid m.

Scm.m.

Omohyoid m., ant. belly

Pharyngeal constrictor m., inferior

D.S.J.

1

Pharyng. const. m. cut edge

Buccopharyngeal fascia

Common carotid a.

Int. jug. v.

Deep cerv. fasc., deep layer

Deep cerv. fasc., middle layer (post. lamina)

Carotid sheath

Trapezius m.

Deep cerv. fasc., middle layer (ant. lamina)

Scm. m.

Deep cerv. fasc., superfic. layer

2

Carotid Arterial System (Fig. 1):

1. **Common Carotid** — the right common carotid arises as a terminal branch of the innominate artery, whereas the left common carotid arises directly from the arch of the aorta. In the carotid triangle it is superficial in position and therefore readily palpable at the anterior border of the sternocleidomastoid, which partly overlaps it in the lower portion of the triangle. Only a few tributaries of the internal jugular vein, branches of the cervical plexus, and the omohyoid cross superficial to the artery. Digital compression to halt the flow of blood is placed at the anterior border of the sternocleidomastoid at the level of the cricoid, with pressure exerted posteriorly against the carotid tubercle on the transverse process of the sixth cervical vertebra *(tubercle of Chassaignac)*. The artery gives off no branches in the neck and ascends to a point 1/2 inch below and behind the greater cornu of the hyoid, or approximately at the upper border of the thyroid cartilage, where it terminates by dividing into the internal and external carotid arteries.

2. **Internal Carotid** — continues upward in the carotid sheath through the submandibular and parotid spaces to enter the cranial cavity via the carotid canal. It gives off no branches in the neck.

3. **External Carotid** — ascends through the submandibular and parotid spaces to terminate at the neck of the mandible. During its course, it gives rise to nine branches, some of which have already been described. These branches may be divided into anterior, posterior, and ascending branches:

    A. Anterior:
        1. External maxillary
        2. Lingual
        3. Superior thyroid
    B. Posterior:
        1. Posterior auricular
        2. Occipital
        3. Sternocleidomastoid
    C. Ascending:
        1. Superficial temporal
        2. Internal maxillary
        3. Ascending pharyngeal (not illustrated)

Related Structures (Fig. 1):

1. **Internal Jugular Vein** — in the upper part of the carotid triangle, this vein receives the common facial, lingual, and superior thyroid veins. In the lower portion of the triangle, the middle thyroid vein empties into it. The venous pattern in this area is extremely variable.

2. **Vagus Nerve** — gives off an important branch in the submandibular triangle: the *superior laryngeal*, the branches of which may be seen here. The *internal branch* may be identified piercing the thyrohyoid membrane at the lateral border of the thyrohyoid muscle. It carries sensory fibers from the larynx above the vocal cords. The *external branch* descends in association with the superior thyroid artery and innervates the cricothyroid and some fibers of the inferior constrictor.

3. **Spinal Accessory Nerve** — extends posteriorly deep to the sternocleidomastoid. Running with the nerve is the sternocleidomastoid artery, which may arise either from the external carotid or from the occipital artery.

4. **Hypoglossal Nerve** — winds forward under the occipital artery in the upper part of the triangle and proceeds into the submandibular triangle. It appears to give off a branch to the thyrohyoid, but this is actually a branch of the deep cervical plexus which will be discussed below (Fig. 2).

5. **Cervical Sympathetic Trunk** — lies in the same position as in the submandibular triangle, posterior to the carotid sheath. This is not shown in the accompanying illustration.

Cervical Plexus (Figs. 1 and 2):

The cervical plexus arises from the anterior primary divisions of C_1 to C_4. The *superficial* portion of the plexus has already been described (Fig. 2, page 11) and is purely sensory. The *deep cervical plexus* gives rise to some important motor nerves — mainly those to the strap muscles of the neck and the diaphragm, the latter via the phrenic nerve. Figure 2 illustrates diagrammatically the main branches of this plexus.

1. **Ansa Hypoglossi** — a branch from C_1 joins the hypoglossal nerve and after a short course divides into a branch supplying the thyrohyoid and geniohyoid and a descending branch, the *descendens hypoglossi*. Descending branches from C_2 to C_3 form the *descendens cervicalis*. These two branches join to form the *ansa hypoglossi*, which usually lies anterior to the carotid sheath. It is from these cervical branches that the strap muscles receive their innervation.

2. **Phrenic Nerve** — arises primarily from the anterior primary division of C_4, but may receive slips from C_3 or C_5. This is discussed more fully on page 26.

Lymphatics of Carotid Triangle (Fig. 2, page 15):

The main lymph nodes of the carotid triangle are those located along the course of the internal jugular vein, some of which are placed within the carotid sheath. They receive afferents either directly or indirectly from the submandibular and submental nodes, deep parotid nodes, and anterior and posterior deep cervical nodes. Efferents pass to the supraclavicular nodes. The nodes of the carotid triangle include the *jugulodigastric (subdigastric) nodes, jugulocarotid (bifurcation) nodes,* and *jugulo-omohyoid nodes.*

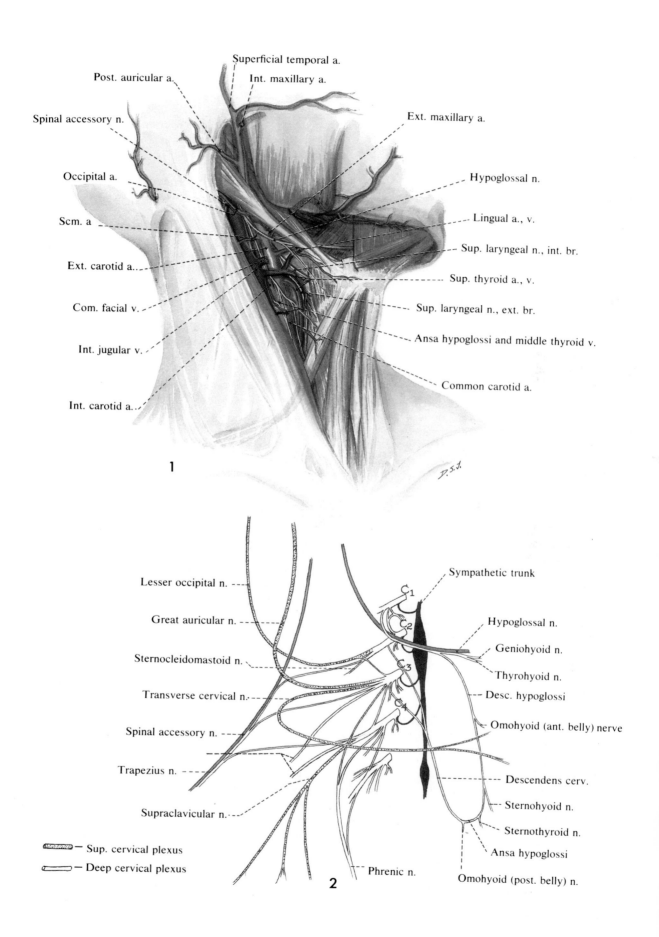

1

Post. auricular a.
Superficial temporal a.
Int. maxillary a.
Spinal accessory n.
Ext. maxillary a.
Occipital a.
Hypoglossal n.
Scm. a
Lingual a., v.
Ext. carotid a.
Sup. laryngeal n., int. br.
Com. facial v.
Sup. thyroid a., v.
Int. jugular v.
Sup. laryngeal n., ext. br.
Ansa hypoglossi and middle thyroid v.
Int. carotid a.
Common carotid a.

2

Lesser occipital n.
Sympathetic trunk
Great auricular n.
Hypoglossal n.
Geniohyoid n.
Sternocleidomastoid n.
Thyrohyoid n.
Transverse cervical n.
Desc. hypoglossi
Spinal accessory n.
Omohyoid (ant. belly) nerve
Trapezius n.
Descendens cerv.
Sternohyoid n.
Supraclavicular n.
Sternothyroid n.
Ansa hypoglossi
Phrenic n.
Omohyoid (post. belly) n.

— Sup. cervical plexus
— Deep cervical plexus

THE MUSCULAR TRIANGLE:

The presence of the thyroid gland renders this triangle extremely important to the surgeon. Its name is derived from the fact that it is covered superficially by the strap muscles of the neck.

Boundaries and Muscular Contents (Fig. 1):

The triangle is bounded by the midline of the neck, the sternocleidomastoid, and the *anterior belly of the omohyoid*. Within the triangle is found a superficial muscle, the *sternohyoid*, and two deep muscles, the *sternothyroid* the *thyrohyoid*. The latter four muscles are known as the strap or ribbon muscles and are innervated by the deep cervical plexus (Fig. 2, page 19). Another muscle, the *cricothyroid*, is not a strap muscle, but a tensor of the vocal cords and is innervated by the external branch of the superior laryngeal nerve. The origin and insertion of these muscles are obvious from their nomenclature.

Superficial Fascia (Fig. 2, page 11):

Deep Fascia (Fig. 2, page 17):

In the muscular triangle may be found all three layers of the deep cervical fascia, as well as the buccopharyngeal fascia and the carotid sheath (page 16).

Thyroid Gland (Fig. 2):

The gland consists of two lateral lobes, an isthmus, and, in some, a pyramidal lobe. Topographically, the *lateral lobes* may extend upward to the midpoint of the thyroid cartilage and inferiorly to the level of the sixth tracheal ring. The *isthmus* usually overlies the second to the fourth tracheal ring. The *pyramidal lobe* extends upward from the left side of the isthmus for a variable distance. The thyroid gland is overlapped by the strap muscles, which frequently must be cut to expose the gland adequately. If this procedure is necessary, the muscles should be severed high, to preserve their innervation. Medially, the gland is related to the cervical viscera, i.e., the pharynx, esophagus, larynx, and trachea. Posterolaterally, it is in contact with the structures of the carotid sheath.

The gland is completely enclosed in a delicate connective tissue sheath which adheres firmly to the gland, the *true capsule*. Also surrounding the gland is an extension from the middle layer of deep cervical fascia which forms the *false (surgical) capsule*. Between the two capsules are found the arterial, venous, and lymphatic plexuses, and sometimes the parathyroids (Fig. 1, page 37).

Related Structures (Fig. 2):

1. **Superior Thyroid Artery** — is the most inferior of the three anterior branches of the external carotid. It gives off the *superior laryngeal* branch, which pierces the thyrohyoid membrane with the internal branch of the superior laryngeal nerve (Fig. 1, page 19). It then descends to the superior pole of the thyroid gland, where it divides into three branches: one extends over the anterolateral surface, one to the posteromedial surface, and a third to the isthmus. It is closely associated with the external branch of the superior laryngeal nerve on its medial side; however, the nerve loses this relationship as it approaches the gland. It is for this reason that ligation of the artery at the superior pole of the gland is usually not associated with damage to that nerve.

2. **Inferior Thyroid Artery** — arises from the thyrocervical trunk of the first portion of the subclavian artery. It passes behind the carotid sheath to the posteromedial surface of the gland (not to the inferior pole) and sends off anastomotic branches to the superior thyroid, as well as tracheal and esophageal branches. It has a very important relationship with the recurrent laryngeal nerve, as discussed below.

3. **Thyroidea Ima Artery** — an inconstant branch to the gland which may arise from the innominate, arch of the aorta, or right common carotid.

4. **Internal Jugular Vein** — lies in the carotid sheath. Its superior thyroid tributary drains either directly or indirectly into the jugular in the upper portion of the triangle. The *middle thyroid* extends from the midportion of the gland, directly into the jugular; the *inferior thyroid* arises from the lower pole and drains into the innominate vein, or sometimes, as shown in Figure 2, into the jugular.

5. **External Branch of the Superior Laryngeal Nerve** — runs in relation to the superior thyroid artery but leaves it before reaching the upper pole. It innervates a portion of the inferior constrictor and the cricothyroid. Since the cricothyroid is a tensor of the cords, temporary hoarseness may result from injury to this nerve during thyroid surgery.

6. **Recurrent Laryngeal Nerve** — is a branch of the vagus which, on the left side, recurs around the arch of the aorta and on the right, around the subclavian artery. The direction of the nerves differ as they approach the gland; the left is located in the tracheo-esophageal groove, whereas the right approaches it in a more oblique direction. It is the main motor nerve of the larynx. It may pass in front of, behind, or between the branches of the inferior thyroid artery.

7. **Parathyroid Glands** — are extremely variable in position, size, and number. Usually four such glands are present, two superior and two inferior. The superior ones are found more medial in position and at about the level of the cricoid cartilage. In most instances they lie between the true and false capsules of the thyroid glands. The inferior glands lie close to the inferior pole of the thyroid in close approximation to the inferior thyroid artery. Their fascial relationships are more variable than those of the superior glands in that they may be between the two capsules of the thyroid, outside the surgical capsule, or imbedded within the thyroid tissue. They receive their blood supply from both the superior and inferior thyroid arteries (Fig. 2, page 39).

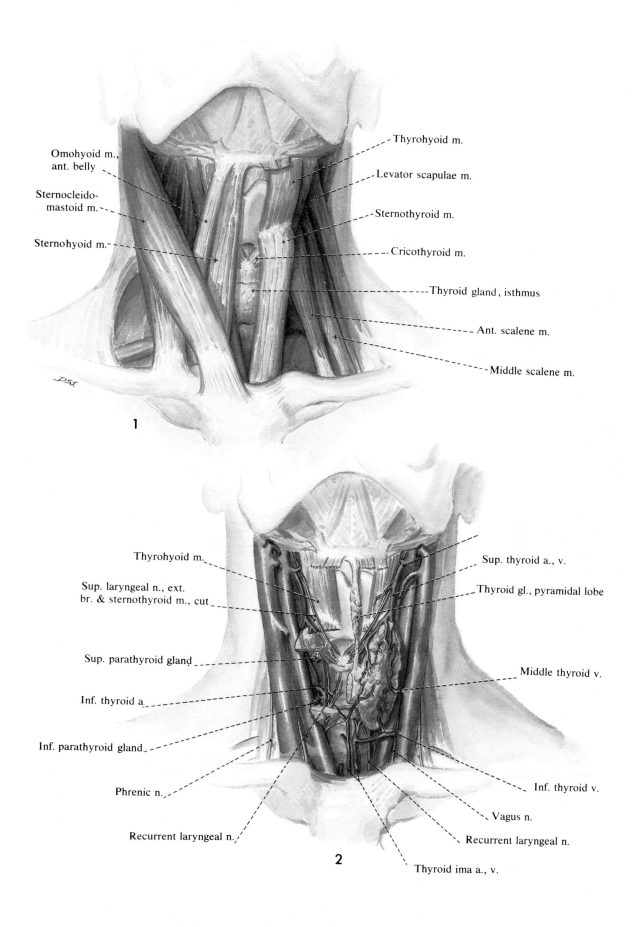

Omohyoid m., ant. belly

Sternocleido-mastoid m.

Sternohyoid m.

Thyrohyoid m.

Levator scapulae m.

Sternothyroid m.

Cricothyroid m.

Thyroid gland, isthmus

Ant. scalene m.

Middle scalene m.

1

Thyrohyoid m.

Sup. laryngeal n., ext. br. & sternothyroid m., cut

Sup. parathyroid gland

Inf. thyroid a.

Inf. parathyroid gland

Phrenic n.

Recurrent laryngeal n.

Sup. thyroid a., v.

Thyroid gl., pyramidal lobe

Middle thyroid v.

Inf. thyroid v.

Vagus n.

Recurrent laryngeal n.

Thyroid ima a., v.

2

Retrothyroid Area (Fig. 1):

After removal of the thyroid gland, the medially related cervical viscera may be visualized. The larynx and pharynx are located above the level of the cricoid cartilage. Neither of these structures will be discussed here. Below the cricoid level one finds the cervical trachea and esophagus.

1. **Cervical Trachea**—descends superficially in the midline of the neck, but is directed slightly posteriorly, so that, at the suprasternal notch, it lies about 1½ inches deep to the skin surface. Immediately in front of the trachea lies the thyroid isthmus (second to fourth ring) and the inferior thyroid veins. The thyroid ima vessels may also lie in this position (Fig. 2, page 21).

2. **Cervical Esophagus**—commences at the sixth cervical level (lower border of the cricoid cartilage) in continuity with the hypopharynx. It deviates toward the left side and for this reason the cervical esophagus is approached surgically from the left side. Owing to the deficiency of the longitudinal fibers in the posterior midline of the esophagus (*Laimer's area*), a potentially weak space exists. It was thought that this was the site of cervical diverticula. It has been shown, however, that they usually occur in *Zenker's triangle*, an interval between the transverse and oblique fibers of the lower portion of the inferior constrictor of the pharynx, the *cricopharyngeus* (Fig. 2).

3. **Recurrent Laryngeal Nerve**—can be seen after removal of the thyroid gland. It may be intimately related to the fascial attachment of the lateral thyroid lobe to the upper rings of the trachea (ligament of Berry), as shown in Figure 2, and may be pulled into the operative field during forward retraction of the gland.

4. **Sympathetic Trunk** (Fig. 1)—lies behind the carotid sheath, and in this area the remaining two cervical ganglia may be seen. The *middle ganglion* is usually small and related to the inferior thyroid artery at the level of C_6. The *inferior ganglion* lies at the neck of the first rib, just medial to the vertebral artery. It is frequently fused with the first thoracic ganglia, in which case they are collectively termed the *stellate ganglion*.

Lymphatics of the Muscular Triangle (Fig. 3):

The lymphatics of the muscular triangle are essentially those draining the thyroid gland. The thyroid drainage may be divided into a superior and an inferior group, each of which may be further divided into medial and lateral. The superior-medial drains into the *prelaryngeal (Delphian) node* located over the cricothyroid membrane. The superior lateral group drains into both the *bifurcation* and *omohyoid* group of nodes of the jugular chain. The inferior-medial drains into the *pretracheal* and *paratracheal nodes*; the inferior-lateral empties directly into the *supraclavicular* nodes.

The Root of the Neck (Fig. 1):

The structures of the root of the neck may be visualized only after retraction or removal of the sternocleidomastoid. The structures here consist of the first portion of the subclavian artery, the subclavian vein, the thoracic duct, and the dome of the pleura.

1. **Subclavian Vein**—begins at the lateral border of the first rib as a continuation of the axillary vein and terminates behind the sternoclavicular joint by joining the internal jugular to form the innominate vein. At the lateral border of the sternocleidomastoid it receives the external jugular. The subclavian vein lies superficial to its corresponding artery and slightly below it in this region.

2. **Subclavian Artery**—on the left side arises directly from the arch of the aorta and on the right, from the innominate. Only the first portion of the artery, lying medial to the anterior scalene muscle, is seen in this area. It gives off the following branches:

a. VERTEBRAL—is the largest branch of the subclavian and may be seen between the anterior scalene and the longus colli. It ascends vertically to the transverse foramen of C_6. No branches arise from this portion of the vertebral.

b. THYROCERVICAL TRUNK—arises near the medial border of the anterior scalene from the upper surface of the subclavian artery and gives off the following branches:

(1) *Inferior Thyroid*—loops upward, then medially behind the carotid sheath; its main distribution has already been discussed on page 20.

(2) *Transverse Cervical*—extends laterally in the root of the neck and passes in front of the anterior scalene.

(3) *Transverse Scapular*—takes a course similar to the transverse cervical, but slightly below it.

c. INTERNAL MAMMARY—arises from the lower surface of the subclavian, usually opposite the thyrocervical trunk, and in its cervical portion lies upon the pleura as it descends into the thoracic cage (not illustrated).

3. **Thoracic Duct**—may be seen on the left side as it ascends along the medial side of the left subclavian artery, arches anterior to the vertebral artery, and then descends to empty into the left subclavian vein near the union of the latter with the internal jugular. It may end here as a single trunk, but more frequently it breaks up into two or more smaller branches before its termination.

4. **Dome of the Pleura**—which covers the apex of the lung, extends upward into the root of the neck about 1½ inches above the border of the first rib anteriorly. It is supported and protected by a thickening of the deep cervical fascia, the *vertebropleural ligament (Sibson's fascia)* (not shown).

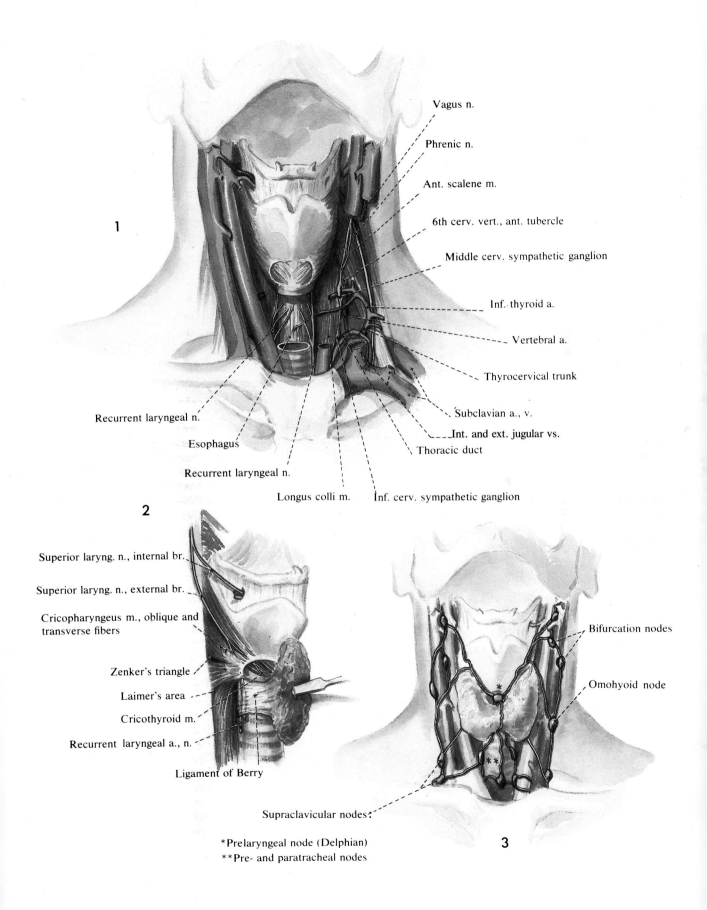

1

Vagus n.

Phrenic n.

Ant. scalene m.

6th cerv. vert., ant. tubercle

Middle cerv. sympathetic ganglion

Inf. thyroid a.

Vertebral a.

Thyrocervical trunk

Subclavian a., v.

Int. and ext. jugular vs.

Thoracic duct

Recurrent laryngeal n.

Esophagus

Recurrent laryngeal n.

Longus colli m.

Inf. cerv. sympathetic ganglion

2

Superior laryng. n., internal br.

Superior laryng. n., external br.

Cricopharyngeus m., oblique and transverse fibers

Zenker's triangle

Laimer's area

Cricothyroid m.

Recurrent laryngeal a., n.

Ligament of Berry

Bifurcation nodes

Omohyoid node

Supraclavicular nodes

*Prelaryngeal node (Delphian)
**Pre- and paratracheal nodes

3

THE POSTERIOR TRIANGLE:

The anterior scalene is the major landmark in this area, and the presence of the brachial plexus, phrenic nerve, and lymph nodes are of surgical importance.

Boundaries and Muscular Contents (Fig. 1):

The boundaries include the sternocleidomastoid, the trapezius, and the middle third of the clavicle. The posterior belly of the omohyoid divides the triangle into two smaller triangles, each of which is named according to the artery present, the *occipital* above and the *subclavian* below. Within the triangle the muscles listed below may be seen, from anterior to posterior:

1. **Anterior Scalene**—arises from the anterior tubercles of C_3 to C_6 and inserts on the scalene tubercle *(Lisfranc's)* on the upper surface of the first rib.

2. **Middle Scalene**—arises by slips from the transverse processes of C_1 to C_6 and is the largest of the scalenes. It also inserts on the first rib on a tubercle behind the groove for the subclavian artery.

3. **Posterior Scalene**—may be regarded as fibers of the middle scalene which gain attachment to the lateral surface of the second rib. Like the other scalenes these fibers are innervated by branches of the anterior rami of the cervical nerves.

4. **Levator Scapulae**—arises from the transverse processes of the first four cervical vertebrae and inserts on the vertebral border of the scapula. It is innervated by both the deep cervical plexus and the dorsal scapular branch of the brachial plexus.

In addition to the above muscles, the *splenius capitis* and the *semispinalis capitis* are present in the apex of the occipital triangle. Both belong to the spinal group of muscles and are innervated by the posterior primary divisions of the cervical nerves.

Superficial Fascia (Fig. 2, page 11):

Deep Fascia (Fig. 1):

All three layers of the deep cervical fascia are present in the posterior triangle. The *superficial layer* roofs the triangle and surrounds the two bounding muscles, the trapezius and sternocleidomastoid. The *middle layer,* its anterior lamella, extends laterally to the posterior belly of the omohyoid and is found, therefore, only in the subclavian triangle. It is a very distinct layer, anterior to which lies a pad of brownish fat, forming an important landmark in the approach to the anterior scalene. The *deep layer* covers the muscles in the floor of the triangle and is extremely important in radical neck dissections for, as will be seen, almost all important motor nerves lie deep to this fascial plane.

Brachial Plexus (Fig. 2):

The brachial plexus lies deep to the deep layer of fascia, as do all its branches. It may be divided into the following parts:

1. **Anterior Primary Divisions**—arise from C_5 through T_1 and are located behind the anterior scalene. Two main branches are given off from these parts, the *dorsal scapular* from C_5, which innervates the rhomboids and the levator scapulae, and the *long thoracic* from C_5, C_6, and C_7, which supplies the serratus anterior.

2. **Trunks**—form at the lateral border of the anterior scalene. The anterior primary divisions of C_5 and C_6 join to form the *upper trunk,* C_7 continues as the *middle trunk,* and C_8 and T_1 unite to form the *lower trunk.* The upper trunk is the only one that gives rise to any branches; these are the *suprascapular,* which extends into the scapular region to supply the supraspinatus and infraspinatus, and the *subclavius,* which innervates the subclavius muscle.

3. **Secondary Divisions**—arise just behind the clavicle, each trunk dividing into an *anterior* and a *posterior* secondary division.

4. **Cords**—are located in the axilla. All posterior secondary divisions join to form a *posterior cord.* The anterior secondary divisions of upper and middle trunks form the *anterolateral cord,* and the anterior secondary division of the lower trunk continues as the *anteromedial cord.* The cords and their terminal divisions are discussed on page 46.

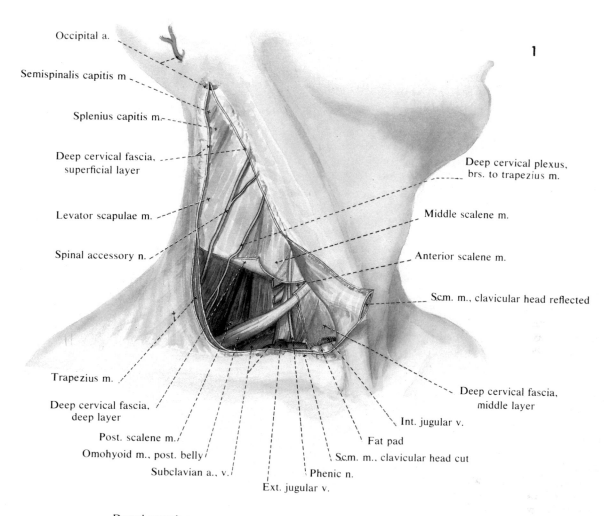

1

Occipital a.

Semispinalis capitis m

Splenius capitis m.

Deep cervical fascia, superficial layer

Levator scapulae m.

Spinal accessory n.

Deep cervical plexus, brs. to trapezius m.

Middle scalene m.

Anterior scalene m.

S.c.m. m., clavicular head reflected

Deep cervical fascia, middle layer

Trapezius m.

Deep cervical fascia, deep layer

Post. scalene m.

Omohyoid m., post. belly

Subclavian a., v.

Int. jugular v.

Fat pad

S.c.m. m., clavicular head cut

Phenic n.

Ext. jugular v.

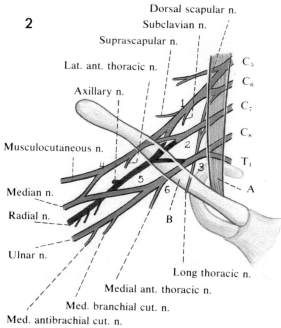

2

Dorsal scapular n.

Subclavian n.

Suprascapular n.

Lat. ant. thoracic n.

Axillary n.

Musculocutaneous n.

Median n.

Radial n.

Ulnar n.

C_5
C_6
C_7
C_8
T_1

A

B

Long thoracic n.

Medial ant. thoracic n.

Med. branchial cut. n.

Med. antibrachial cut. n.

* Subscapular nn.

KEY FOR FIG. 2

A. Anterior scalene muscle
   (Anterior 1° division behind)
   1. Upper trunk
   2. Middle trunk
   3. Lower trunk

B. Clavicle
   (Anterior and posterior 2° divisions behind)
   4. Anterolateral cord
   5. Posterior cord
   6. Anteromedial cord

Anterior Scalene Muscle (Fig. 1):

This muscle has gained great clinical significance because of its relationship with such structures as the subclavian artery, brachial plexus, and phrenic nerve. Spasm or contracture of the muscle leads to circulatory and neurological symptoms in the upper extremity which frequently necessitate surgical intervention. It is covered by the clavicular head of the sternocleidomastoid, and immediately in front of the muscle are found the subclavian vein, the transverse cervical and transverse scapular vessels, and the phrenic nerve. Behind are located the subclavian artery and the brachial plexus.

Related Structures (Fig. 1):

1. **Subclavian Vein** — lies superficial in position in front of the anterior scalene but usually does not rise above the clavicle. It receives the external jugular in the posterior triangle, and on the left side the thoracic duct may enter more lateral than usual, thereby passing anterior to the anterior scalene.

2. **Subclavian Artery** — lies behind the anterior scalene, the muscle dividing the artery into three parts, the first lying medial to the muscle, the second behind, and the third lateral to the muscle.

   a. FIRST PORTION — gives rise to three branches: the *vertebral, internal mammary,* and *thyrocervical trunk.* The first two vessels are discussed on page 22. The inferior thyroid branch of the thyrocervical trunk has already been considered on page 20. The remaining two branches from the trunk cross in front of the anterior scalene superficial to the deep layer of cervical fascia. The *transverse cervical* is superior in position and extends across the posterior triangle to the anterior border of the levator scapulae muscle, where it divides into an ascending and a descending *(posterior scapular)* branch. The *transverse scapular* also passes in front of the muscle and extends laterally behind the clavicle to the supraspinatus and infraspinatus fossae.

   b. SECOND PORTION — gives rise to only one branch, the *costocervical trunk,* which, because of its position behind the anterior scalene, is rarely of concern to the surgeon. This trunk gives rise to the deep cervical and superior intercostal arteries (not illustrated).

   c. THIRD PORTION — usually has no branches. However, one may find a transverse cervical (German) arising here, which, if present along with the transverse cervical of the first portion (British), becomes the posterior scapular or descending branch.

3. **Brachial Plexus** — anterior primary divisions of the plexus are located directly behind the anterior scalene and the trunks of the plexus at the lateral border of the muscle (page 24).

4. **Phrenic Nerve** — is of prime importance because it supplies the muscle fibers of the diaphragm. The diaphragm develops in the cervical region and migrates downward, thus explaining its cervical innervation. The nerve arises from the anterior primary division of C_4. However, it frequently receives fibers from C_3 and C_5. It takes a very characteristic course over the anterior scalene passing downward from lateral to medial and *deep* to the deep layer of fascia. In many cases an *accessory phrenic* is present. The three most frequent sites are: (1) a branch from C_5 passing downward lateral to the phrenic and joining it either in the root of the neck or in the subclavian triangle and thence into the thorax, (2) a branch from C_5 incorporated with the nerve to the subclavius and passing into the thorax anterior to the subclavian vein (Fig. 1), or (3) a branch from C_3 incorporated in the ansa hypoglossi and joining the phrenic in the thorax.

5. **Spinal Accessory Nerve** — is not directly related to the anterior scalene but is the uppermost structure of importance in the posterior triangle. It takes exit from under the sternocleidomastoid at the junction of its upper and middle third and descends parallel with the fibers of the levator scapulae. It then disappears beneath the trapezius, which it innervates. During its course, the nerve is joined by a communicating branch from the deep cervical plexus; running below and parallel to it are muscular branches from the deep cervical plexus to the trapezius muscle (Fig. 1, page 25). The latter nerves may be mistaken for the spinal accessory. The above mentioned nerves lie in a plane between the superficial and deep layers of cervical fascia. They are the only motor nerves that lie superficial to the deep layer of deep cervical fascia.

Lymphatics of the Posterior Triangle (Fig. 1):

The lymphatics in this area are part of the vertical and inferior horizontal group (page 28). The posterior cervical nodes of the vertical group are subdivided into a *superficial group* along the external jugular vein and a *deep group* accompanying the spinal accessory nerve. These nodes receive afferents from the subparotid node of the jugular chain, from the occipital and mastoid nodes, and from muscular and cutaneous channels in the neck. Efferents pass to the supraclavicular nodes. The deep nodes are intimately associated with the spinal accessory nerve, and in cases of malignant invasion of the nodes, the nerve must be sacrificed. The *inferior horizontal (supraclavicular) nodes* receive ascending channels from the upper extremity, axilla, and thorax, as well as descending channels from the posterior cervical, jugular, and visceral nodes. Their efferent vessels unite to form the subclavian trunk, which empties either directly or indirectly into the junction of the subclavian and internal jugular.

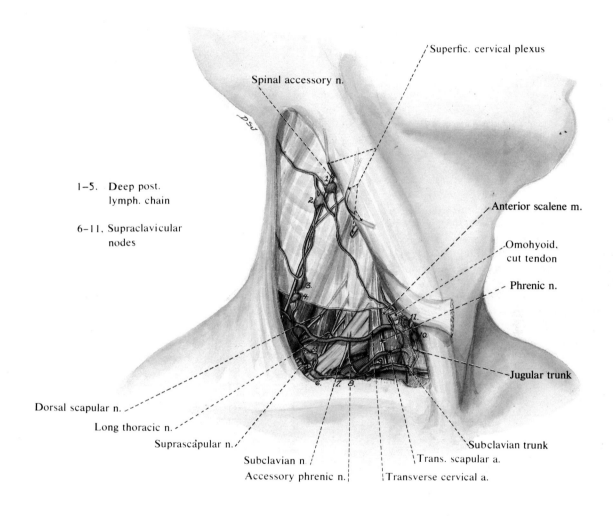

Superfic. cervical plexus

Spinal accessory n.

1–5. Deep post.
    lymph. chain

6–11. Supraclavicular
    nodes

Anterior scalene m.

Omohyoid,
cut tendon

Phrenic n.

Jugular trunk

Dorsal scapular n.

Long thoracic n.

Suprascapular n.

Subclavian n.

Accessory phrenic n.

Subclavian trunk

Trans. scapular a.

Transverse cervical a.

LYMPHATICS OF THE NECK:

The lymph nodes in this area of the body are given a more varied nomenclature than those in any other area. From the standpoint of diagnosis of the source of a disease process producing either inflammatory or malignant changes affecting a particular node or group of nodes, the knowledge of the drainage is of utmost importance. In a neck node dissection, however, it is imperative that one possess a knowledge of the anatomic location of all of these nodes so that total removal of these cervical nodes may be achieved. This nomenclature is an attempt to present to the surgeon an organized grouping of the cervical nodes in order to permit a surgical-anatomic approach to their removal. One can distinguish two horizontal chains and a vertical chain. The *horizontal chains* are divided into a *superior group* of nodes (Fig. 1*a*) and an *inferior group* (Fig. 1*c*). The vertical chain consists of the *posterior cervical nodes* (Fig. 1 *b*1), the *intermediate (jugular) nodes* (Fig. 1 *b*2), and the *anterior (visceral) nodes* (Fig. 1 *b*3).

Superior Horizontal Chain (Figs. 1*a* and 2)—consists of five groups of nodes encircling the base of the head. These groups are as follows:

1. Submental (Fig. 2 *a*1)
2. Submandibular (Fig. 2 *a*2)
3. Preauricular (parotid) (Fig. 2 *a*3)
4. Postauricular (mastoid) (Fig. 2 *a*4)
5. Occipital (Fig. 2 *a*5)

Vertical Chain (Figs. 1 and 2)—consists of three longitudinal groups of nodes extending through the cervical area.

1. POSTERIOR CERVICAL NODES (Fig. 1 *b*1)—are located in relation to two important landmarks of the posterior cervical triangle, the external jugular vein and the spinal accessory nerve. They are accordingly subdivided into a superficial and a deep group:

a. *Superficial*—extend along the course of the external jugular vein. They consist usually of one or two nodes along the external jugular vein as it crosses the sternocleidomastoid.

b. *Deep*—are in association with the spinal accessory nerve, particularly as the nerve enters the posterior triangle at the posterior border of the sternocleidomastoid deep to the investing layers of deep cervical fascia.

2. INTERMEDIATE (JUGULAR) NODES (Fig. 1 *b*2)—are the most important group extending along the course of the internal jugular vein and consist of:

a. *Juguloparotid (Subparotid)*—node located at the angle of the mandible.

b. *Jugulodigastric (Subdigastric)*—probably the most important node in the neck. This node is located at the junction of the common facial with the internal jugular.

c. *Jugulocarotid (Bifurcation)*—located at the bifurcation of the common carotid artery.

d. *Jugulo-omohyoid*—positioned at the crossing of the omohyoid over the internal jugular.

3. ANTERIOR (VISCERAL) NODES (Fig. 1 *b*3)—are related to the pharynx, esophagus, larynx, and trachea and drain the adjacent viscera.

a. *Parapharyngeal*—consists of nodes located along the lateral wall and in the retropharyngeal space which drain important structures in the deep face and upper digestive tract. Their efferent vessels connect with other anterior nodes or the intermediate (jugular) nodes.

b. *Paralaryngeal*—receives important afferents from the larynx and the thyroid gland.

c. *Paratracheal*—also receives afferents from the thyroid gland, as well as the trachea and esophagus.

d. *Prelaryngeal* (Delphian Node)—a solitary, fairly constant node located on the cricothyroid ligament. This node is important in lymphatic drainage of the thyroid and larynx.

e. *Pretracheal*—this nodal group is continuous with the mediastinal group of nodes, as is the paratracheal group.

Inferior Horizontal Chain (Figs. 1*c* and 2)—those nodes (supraclavicular nodes) lie in the subclavian triangle. They receive afferents from the upper extremity, the axilla, the thoracic wall, and the nodal groups of the vertical chain. Their efferents may enter either the jugular or subclavian trunks. Nodes of this group lying anterior to the anterior scalene muscle have become of clinical significance in the diagnosis of thoracic diseases since the bronchomediastinal trunk may drain into these nodes before entering the thoracic or right lymphatic duct. These nodes are clinically designated as the *scalene nodes*.

Right Lymphatic Duct—three terminal lymphatic trunks empty into the junction of the right subclavian and right internal jugular vein, either directly or indirectly. The trunks consist of the subclavian trunk from the supraclavicular nodes, the jugular trunk from the intermediate (jugular) nodes, and the bronchomediastinal trunk. It is rather rare that the three trunks coalesce to form a true right lymphatic duct. One or another may enter separately. Lymphatics from the right upper extremity, right side of head and neck, and right side of the thorax drain into the right lymphatic duct (Fig. 3).

Thoracic Duct—this is the chief collecting channel of the lymphatic system draining all lymphatics from below the diaphragm, from the left half of the thorax, from the left side of head and neck, and from the left upper extremity. It may receive the jugular, subclavian, and bronchomediastinal trunks on the left side. In some cases one or more of these trunks may enter separately (Fig. 3).

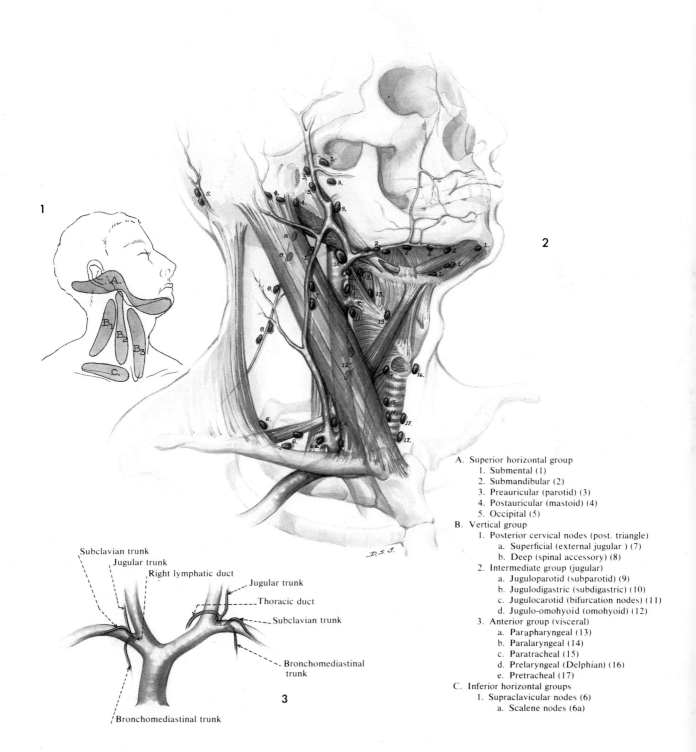

1

2

A. Superior horizontal group
  1. Submental (1)
  2. Submandibular (2)
  3. Preauricular (parotid) (3)
  4. Postauricular (mastoid) (4)
  5. Occipital (5)
B. Vertical group
  1. Posterior cervical nodes (post. triangle)
    a. Superficial (external jugular) (7)
    b. Deep (spinal accessory) (8)
  2. Intermediate group (jugular)
    a. Juguloparotid (subparotid) (9)
    b. Jugulodigastric (subdigastric) (10)
    c. Jugulocarotid (bifurcation nodes) (11)
    d. Jugulo-omohyoid (omohyoid) (12)
  3. Anterior group (visceral)
    a. Parapharyngeal (13)
    b. Paralaryngeal (14)
    c. Paratracheal (15)
    d. Prelaryngeal (Delphian) (16)
    e. Pretracheal (17)
C. Inferior horizontal groups
  1. Supraclavicular nodes (6)
    a. Scalene nodes (6a)

Subclavian trunk
Jugular trunk
Right lymphatic duct
Jugular trunk
Thoracic duct
Subclavian trunk
Bronchomediastinal trunk
Bronchomediastinal trunk

3

CLINICAL CONSIDERATIONS:

Topography:

The topography of the neck is shown on page 11. Of particular interest clinically are the topographic relationships of the common carotid artery and cricoid cartilage.

1. **Common Carotid Artery** — may be represented by a line drawn from the sternoclavicular joint to the point of its bifurcation which lies 1 cm. inferior and posterior to the tip of the greater cornu of the hyoid bone, or approximately at the level of the upper border of the thyroid cartilage.

2. **Cricoid Cartilage** — is palpable immediately below the thyroid cartilage at the level of C_6. It serves as a surgical guide to the approximate level of the following structures: (a) tendon of the omohyoid, (b) the passage of the inferior thyroid artery behind the common carotid artery, (c) the entrance of the vertebral artery into the transverse foramen of C_6, (d) the entrance of the recurrent laryngeal nerve into the larynx, (e) the middle cervical sympathetic ganglion, (f) the junction of the larynx and trachea, (g) the junction of the pharynx and esophagus, and (h) the opening of a pharyngo-esophageal (Zenker's) diverticulum.

Cervical Incisions:

Incisions should be carefully planned in order to gain adequate exposure yet yield the best cosmetic effect possible, since this is an exposed portion of the body. Incisions are therefore usually made parallel to the skin cleavage (Langer's) lines (see page 10). The cutaneous veins of the neck lie deep to the platysma in the subcutaneous tissue. Incisions in the neck bleed freely because the retraction of the platysma prevents collapse of the veins. When the incision is extended through the deep cervical fascia, however, the tension on the vein walls is relieved and the oozing reduced. In planning incisions in the suprahyoid area, care must be taken to preserve the *pars mandibularis of the cervical branch of the facial nerve* (page 12).

Cervical Nerve Blocks (Fig. 1):

Nerve blocks for local and regional anesthesia are frequently used for surgical procedures to infiltrate either superficial cervical plexus or brachial plexus.

1. **Superficial Cervical Plexus** — may be effectively blocked by infiltrating the anesthetic solution at multiple points along the posterior border of the sternocleidomastoid muscle. The main point of injection is at the junction of the upper and middle third of the posterior border.

2. **Brachial Plexus Block** — is carried out by inserting the needle above the mid-portion of the clavicle, directing it medially and downward toward the first rib. When paresthesias in the arm are felt, the area is infiltrated. The needle is then reinserted, directed from above and below. The index finger is usually placed at the upper border of the clavicle to depress the subclavian artery.

3. **Stellate Ganglion Block** — is utilized to treat various vasomotor dysfunctions of the upper extremity and neck. This ganglion is also termed the cervicothoracic ganglion since it is formed by the fusion of the inferior cervical sympathetic ganglion with the first thoracic ganglion. It lies on the neck of the first rib medial to the vertebral artery. With the head slightly extended, the sternocleidomastoid muscle and carotid sheath structures are displaced laterally by the index and middle fingers. The needle is inserted downward to make contact with the transverse process of the seventh cervical vertebra. When contact is made, the needle is withdrawn and deviated approximately 30 degrees medially and the anesthetic agent injected (not illustrated).

Carotid Arteriography (Fig. 2):

This is used for roentgen localization of extracranial arterial obstructions and intracranial lesions, both vascular and nonvascular. The dye may be injected through a needle introduced into the common carotid artery anywhere along its course in the neck (see Topography, above). The artery may best be approached in the carotid triangle where it is covered by skin and superficial and deep fascia. It is overlapped somewhat laterally by the anterior border of the sternocleidomastoid muscle. The common carotid may be fixed in this area between the thumb and index finger, the thumb acting to retract the sternocleidomastoid laterally.

Deep Cervical Fascial Spaces:

These are of significance in their role in the location and extension of deep infections in the neck. These potential spaces are located between layers of deep cervical fascia which are produced by stresses placed on primitive connective tissue embedding the developing organs in the fetus, resulting in these fibrous lamellae.

1. **Retrovisceral Space** (Fig. 3) — is the major pathway for spread of infection from the neck to the thorax. It extends from the base of the skull to the mediastinum and is bounded behind by the prevertebral layer of deep cervical fascia, and in front by the buccopharyngeal fascia covering the pharynx and esophagus. Because of its relationship to the latter structures this same space may also be referred to as *retropharyngeal* or *retroesophageal space*. An abscess in this space may be approached by an incision made parallel to the flexion creases at the level of the cricoid. The sternocleidomastoid and carotid sheath are retracted laterally, and the lateral lobe of the thyroid anteriorly and medially. This is the same approach used for excision of a pharyngo-esophageal diverticulum.

2. **Pretracheal Space** (Fig. 4) — is a potential area located between the middle layer of deep cervical fascia (posterior lamina) in front and the trachea behind. It is limited above at the attachment of the middle layer of fascia to the thyroid cartilage and continues into the mediastinum to the level of the pericardium. Surgical infections are rarely limited to this space, but if present may be approached through a midline incision in the neck.

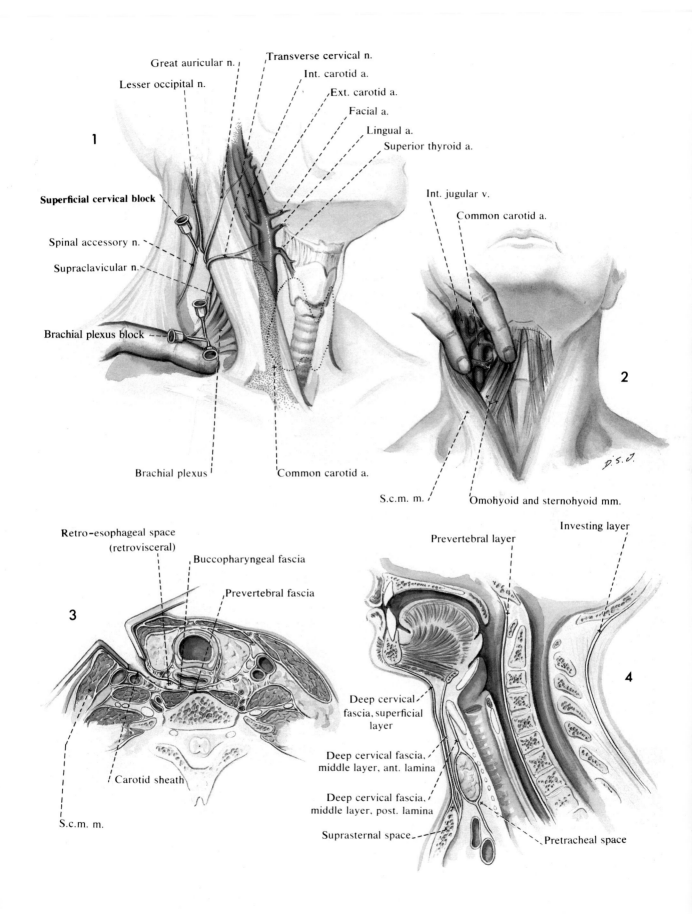

1

Great auricular n.

Transverse cervical n.

Lesser occipital n.

Int. carotid a.

Ext. carotid a.

Facial a.

Lingual a.

Superior thyroid a.

Superficial cervical block

Int. jugular v.

Common carotid a.

Spinal accessory n.

Supraclavicular n.

Brachial plexus block

Brachial plexus

Common carotid a.

2

S.c.m. m.

Omohyoid and sternohyoid mm.

Retro-esophageal space
(retrovisceral)

Buccopharyngeal fascia

Prevertebral fascia

3

Carotid sheath

S.c.m. m.

Prevertebral layer

Investing layer

Deep cervical
fascia, superficial
layer

Deep cervical fascia,
middle layer, ant. lamina

Deep cervical fascia,
middle layer, post. lamina

Suprasternal space

Pretracheal space

4

THE CAROTID ARTERIAL SYSTEM:

The common carotid artery and its internal and external branches are clinically important in occlusive disease because of atherosclerosis, thrombosis, emboli, trauma, and ligation for intracranial aneurysms. The popularity of carotid endarterectomy has waned appreciably in recent years.

To expose these vessels in the neck (Fig. 1), an incision is made along the anterior border of the sternocleidomastoid muscle from the angle of the jaw to the level of the lower border of the thyroid cartilage. The platysma muscle and superficial layer of the deep cervical fascia are incised, exposing the internal jugular vein. The common facial and superior thyroid tributaries are ligated and divided. The descending branch of the hypoglossal nerve and the superior laryngeal nerve must be identified and preserved at the upper end of the incision. The carotid vessels are dissected and an incision made in the anterolateral surface of the common carotid extending upward beyond the point of occlusion. (N.B.: The common carotid bifurcates at the upper border of the thyroid cartilage.)

Major Venous Channels:

1. **Subclavian Vein**—begins at the lateral border of the first rib as a continuation of the axillary vein and terminates behind the sternoclavicular joint by joining the internal jugular to form the innominate vein. At the root of the neck, the vein lies deep to the insertion of the sternocleidomastoid. It is superficial to the subclavian artery with the insertion of the anterior scalene intervening between the two structures.

The subclavian vein has gained great clinical significance since *intravenous hyperalimentation* has come to play such an important role in medicine. It is also utilized for the purposes of monitoring central venous pressure, obtaining central venous access for chemotherapy, and introducing intravenous pacemakers.

The vessels are entered by percutaneous needle injection under local anesthesia using a careful sterile technique. The approach may be either an infraclavicular or a supraclavicular puncture.

The infraclavicular approach (Fig. 2A) is usually preferred, with the patient lying in bed in a moderate (15 degrees) Trendelenburg position in order to obtain maximum filling of the vein. The head should be turned to the opposite side and the ipsilateral shoulder hyperextended. With a special needle and syringe, puncture is made through the skin at the midpoint of the lower border of the clavicle. It is directed medially in a horizontal plane toward the posterior aspect of the sternal notch. When the venipuncture is complete, the syringe is removed and an intravenous catheter introduced through the needle into the superior vena cava, a distance of 5 to 6 inches.

In the supraclavicular approach (Fig. 2B), the operator stands at the head of the patient and presses the index finger toward the feet behind the clavicular head of the sternocleidomastoid muscle. The needle is inserted in the horizontal plane parallel to the anterior scalene muscle into the vein which is medial to the subclavian artery and scalene tubercle.

2. **The Internal Jugular and Cephalic Veins**—are other major channels of clinical importance (Fig. 3). They are used as alternatives for the purposes described above for the subclavian vein.

An internal jugular venous puncture is made at the lateral border of the sternocleidomastoid muscle two fingerbreadths above the clavicle and directed toward the suprasternal notch. A second approach that may be used is to make the puncture in the interval between the sternal and clavicular heads of the sternocleidomastoid muscle.

The cephalic vein (page 45, Fig. 3) lies in the deltopectoral triangle and pierces the costocoracoid membrane to empty into the axillary vein above the pectoralis minor. It may be approached by an incision below the clavicle extending inferiorly in the deltopectoral triangle.

CHEMODECTOMAS:

Chemodectomas are tumors associated with the chemoreceptors in sympathetic nerves in the adventitia of blood vessels. They are also referred to as carotid body tumors, non-chromaffin paragangliomas, and chemoreceptomas. They are sensitive to temperature and chemical changes in the circulatory blood and may occur in various parts of the body. Such tumors in the region of the neck are rare, frequently multiple (10 per cent), have a familial tendency, and may become malignant. They are surgically significant in that, although slow growing, they are invasive and distort the associated blood vessels, involve various cranial nerves, and may present as a mass in the neck.

The most common sites in the neck are in the region of the jugular bulb in the jugular fossa at the base of the skull (glomus jugulare), at the bifurcation of the common carotid artery (carotid body), and along the vagus nerve either at the level of the nodose ganglion or along the cervical portion of the vagus nerve (glomus intravagale).

The lesions may bulge into the pharynx causing dysphagia, may produce paresis or paralysis of the regional cranial nerves, or may present as a mass in the neck. Carotid arteriography, venography, computed tomography, and ultrasonography are important in establishing a diagnosis. Surgery is the treatment of choice, although radiation therapy, either primary or adjuvant, has produced good results in some centers. Follow-up of these patients is extremely important because of possible recurrence or the development of a second chemodectoma. (Figure 5 illustrates the approach and anatomical structures related to a carotid body tumor.)

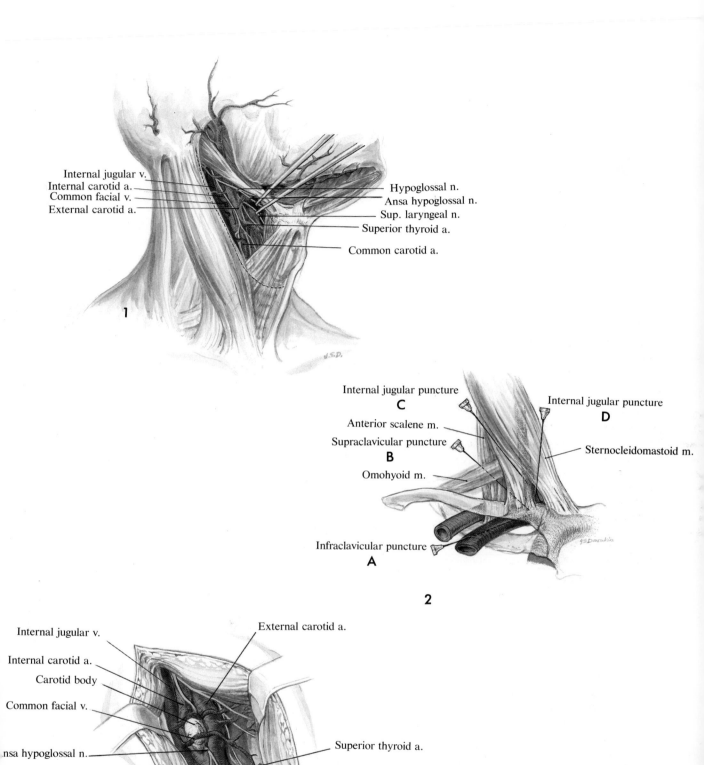

Internal jugular v.
Internal carotid a.
Common facial v.
External carotid a.

Hypoglossal n.
Ansa hypoglossal n.
Sup. laryngeal n.
Superior thyroid a.
Common carotid a.

1

Internal jugular puncture
C
Anterior scalene m.
Supraclavicular puncture
B
Omohyoid m.

Internal jugular puncture
D
Sternocleidomastoid m.

Infraclavicular puncture
A

2

Internal jugular v.
Internal carotid a.
Carotid body
Common facial v.
Ansa hypoglossal n.
Common carotid a.

External carotid a.

Superior thyroid a.
Superior thyroid v.

3

CONGENITAL ANOMALIES OF CLINICAL INTEREST:

Branchial Cyst and Fistula (Figs. 1 and 2):

These are embryologic defects usually associated with the second branchial arch. Five such arches are present in the embryo, each containing a plate of cartilage, a muscle mass, a nerve, and an artery. Between each arch is an internal depression, a *visceral pouch,* and an external depression, a *visceral cleft.* These structures are lined internally with columnar epithelium and externally with squamous epithelium.

1. **Branchial Cyst**—results from the rapid growth of the second arch, which comes to overlap the lower arches, forming a sinus between the down-growing arch and these lower arches *(cervical sinus).* The second arch ultimately fuses with the fifth arch, resulting in a squamous epithelium-lined space. This space eventually disappears as development proceeds, but if it remains it forms a *branchial cyst* (see Fig. 1, page 39). These cysts are located along the anterior border of the sterno-cleidomastoid muscle in the upper one-third of the neck.

2. **Branchial Fistula**—will result when the second arch fails to fuse with the fifth arch (Fig. 1, page 39). The internal opening of the fistula, when present, is located in the region of the palatine tonsil and the external opening along the anterior margin of the sternocleidomastoid muscle in the lower one-third of the neck (80 per cent). Since such a fistula lies below the second arch, whose artery is the external carotid, and above the third arch, whose artery is the internal carotid, the tract will obviously pass between these two arterial channels. The upper part of the tract is deep to the posterior belly of the digastric and stylohyoid muscles.

Branchial Fistula and Cyst Compared

Fistula	Cyst
1. Present at birth.	1. Appears in early adult life.
2. Situated in lower one-third of neck.	2. Situated in upper one-third of neck.
3. Lined with columnar epithelium, usually ciliated.	3. Lined with stratified squamous epithelium.
4. Exudes sticky mucous.	4. Filled with opaque fluid rich in cholesterol.

Thyroglossal Cyst (Figs. 1 and 3):

The thyroid gland appears in the early embryo as a median diverticulum in the floor of the pharynx between the first and second visceral pouch *(foramen caecum).* The diverticulum migrates caudad and takes the form of a small bilobed flask which is attached to the pharyngeal cavity by a narrow stalk, the *thyroglossal duct,* which lies anterior to the second arch mesoderm. In normal development the duct is completely reabsorbed, but it may persist in whole or in part. From this developmental history it is obvious that the tract should be anterior to the hyoid bone which develops in the second arch mesoderm. But its relation to this bone is complicated by growth changes which may bring part of the duct in contact with the deep surface of the hyoid (Fig. 3). Cystic remnants of the thyroglossal duct may occur anywhere along the course of migration from foramen caecum to the adult thyroid gland. The resultant *thyroglossal cyst* appears during childhood as a mass in the midline below the hyoid bone. Less frequently, however, it is located above the hyoid.

To insure complete removal, the central portion of the body of the hyoid must be removed, together with the cyst and entire stalk from the hyoid to the foramen caecum. The stalk passes upward and posteriorly from the hyoid at an angle of 45 degrees and may or may not be a well defined, easily recognizable structure.

Accessory and Ectopic Thyroids:

Accessory thyroid tissue may develop at any point along the original path of the thyroglossal duct. An ectopic thyroid is one in which all the thyroid tissue is located in an aberrant position. A frequent site for such ectopic thyroid tissue is at the base of the tongue *(lingual thyroid).*

Cervical Rib (Fig. 4):

The incidence of cervical ribs is reported as being 1 to 2 per cent, most of these being bilateral. The anterior extremity of a cervical rib extending from C_7 may terminate in one of several ways: (1) articulate with the sternum, (2) articulate or fuse with the first rib, (3) attach to the first rib by a fibrous band, or (4) present a free end. When it is well developed, both the subclavian artery and the lower trunk of the brachial plexus groove the anterior and upper surface of the cervical rib, and symptoms of vascular or nerve compression may be produced. Poststenotic aneurysm of the third part of the subclavian artery may also result. These changes develop because of impingement of the plexus and subclavian artery between the anterior scalene muscles and the cervical rib and its fibrous band or by angulation of the plexus and vessel over the cervical rib in their exit through the superior thoracic aperture. Treatment ranges from conservative muscular re-education to scalenotomy with or without resection of the rib.

Scalene Anticus Syndrome (Fig. 4):

Although this is not a true congenital defect, it may be best mentioned here, since it gives rise to symptoms identical to those of a cervical rib, but is due to spasm or hypertrophy of the scalene anticus muscle. Transection of the scalene at its insertion may be performed to alleviate this condition. During the procedure, the anterior relation of the subclavian vein and phrenic nerve should be recalled (page 26).

Thoracic Outlet Syndrome:

The cervical rib syndrome and the scalene anticus syndrome are two of many syndromes preferably called the thoracic outlet syndrome. The other syndromes included are the hyperabduction syndrome, the first thoracic rib syndrome, the pectoralis minor syndrome, and the costoclavicular syndrome. The symptoms produced by all these conditions are due to compression of

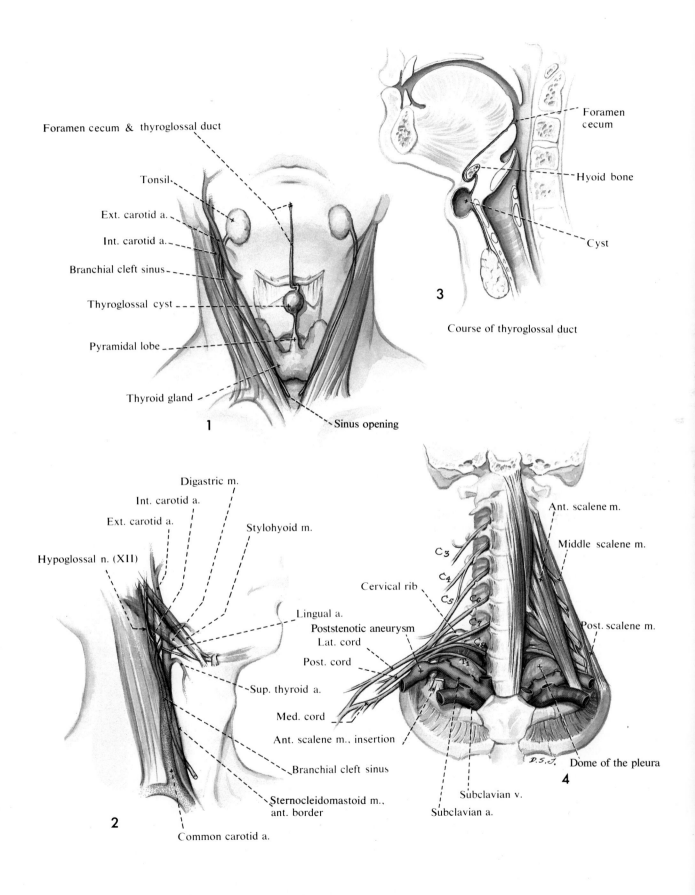

1

Foramen cecum & thyroglossal duct

Tonsil

Ext. carotid a.

Int. carotid a.

Branchial cleft sinus

Thyroglossal cyst

Pyramidal lobe

Thyroid gland

Sinus opening

3

Foramen cecum

Hyoid bone

Cyst

Course of thyroglossal duct

2

Digastric m.

Int. carotid a.

Ext. carotid a.

Hypoglossal n. (XII)

Stylohyoid m.

Lingual a.

Poststenotic aneurysm

Lat. cord

Post. cord

Sup. thyroid a.

Med. cord

Ant. scalene m., insertion

Branchial cleft sinus

Sternocleidomastoid m., ant. border

Common carotid a.

4

Ant. scalene m.

Middle scalene m.

C₃

C₄

Cervical rib

C₅

C₆

C₇

Post. scalene m.

C₈

T₁

Dome of the pleura

Subclavian v.

Subclavian a.

the neurovascular structures extending anywhere from the thoracic outlet to the insertion of the pectoralis minor muscle. They are characterized by neurological deficits and/or vascular (arterial or venous) changes in the upper extremity.

Most patients are relieved by nonoperative methods, including weight reduction and muscle exercise programs. In cases of vascular occlusion or aneurysmal formation in the subclavian artery, operative intervention is imperative. Operative procedures may include transaxillary resection of the first thoracic rib, division of the pectoralis minor tendon, or resection of the clavicle.

CLINICAL ANATOMY OF THE THYROID GLAND

Surgical Capsule (Fig. 1):

This is a thin layer of connective tissue investing the thyroid gland. It is also referred to by the following synonyms: *pretracheal fascia, middle layer of deep cervical fascia (posterior lamella), false thyroid capsule,* and *perithyroid sheath.* It is not the well defined layer shown semidiagrammatically in Figure 1, but a condensation of connective tissue about the thyroid, not to be confused with the *true capsule* of the gland. The latter is adherent to the gland surface, sending septa between the lobules. There is, however, a plane of easy dissection between the *true* and *surgical* capsules.

The relations of the parathyroid glands and recurrent laryngeal nerves to the surgical capsule are of importance. Both structures are frequently imbedded in the surgical capsule, but this relationship is not constant. In the so-called "adherent zone" at the posteromedial aspect of the gland (Fig. 4), the recurrent nerves enter for a short distance the substance of the gland in some (10 per cent) people. In Figure 1, the nerves are shown outside the surgical capsule, and the inferior parathyroid gland deep to the true capsule.

In the same illustration, the *lateral* relationship of the *middle thyroid vein* and the posterior relation of the *inferior thyroid artery* are apparent.

Surgical Approach (Fig. 2):

The approach to the thyroid is by a transverse (collar) incision placed midway between the upper end of the sternum and the upper border of the thyroid cartilage with the neck in a hyperextended position. The upper poles of the gland extend to mid-level of the thyroid cartilage and the lower pole to the sixth tracheal ring. The isthmus covers the second, third, and fourth tracheal rings (Fig. 2, page 21).

1. **Skin Flaps** (Fig. 3)—are constructed above and below, the upper flap extending to the thyroid notch and the lower, to the sternal notch. These flaps consist of skin, subcutaneous tissue, and platysma muscle.

2. **Fascial Incision** (Figs. 1 and 3)—is made in a vertical direction in the midline through the superficial layer of deep fascia (between the sternocleidomastoids), the middle layer, anterior lamella (between the sternohyoid muscles), and the middle layer, posterior lamella (between the sternothyroid muscles). The incision through the latter fascial layer opens the surgical capsule and brings into view the thyroid isthmus with the thyroid cartilage above and cricoid below. The three distinct fascial planes are usually not evident to the surgeon, and their division may be carried out by a single incision. The sternohyoid and sternothyroid muscles may be severed or retracted laterally to expose the anterior surface of the lateral lobes.

3. **Mobilization** (Fig. 4)—is facilitated by ligation and division of the middle thyroid vein. The anterior and medial displacement of the lateral lobe brings into view the following important structures: superior thyroid and inferior thyroid arteries, trachea, carotid sheath, inferior parathyroid glands, and recurrent laryngeal nerve. The structures have already been discussed on page 20, but the recurrent nerve warrants further consideration.

RECURRENT LARYNGEAL NERVE—may be injured during a thyroidectomy by clamping, cutting, ligating, or stretching. Accurate knowledge of its relationships to the trachea, the inferior thyroid artery, and thyroid gland is the surgeon's best insurance against accidental injury. The closeness of the relationship between the recurrent nerve and the inferior thyroid artery makes ligation of the artery near the gland dangerous to the nerve, but on the other hand, this close relation is useful to the surgeon in locating the nerve so that it may be seen and avoided. The relationship between the recurrent nerve and inferior thyroid artery is extremely variable, the nerve passing in front of, behind, or between branches of the artery. Usually the recurrent nerve lies outside of the surgical capsule, but this is an inconstant relationship, particularly at the level of the upper two or three tracheal rings. Here the gland is attached to the cricoid and trachea by a band of dense connective tissue (*adherent zone, ligament of Berry*). At this point, the nerve may lie against the posterior surface of the gland (Fig. 4), or in rare instances (10 per cent), it may pass through the thyroid tissue. It is in particular jeopardy in this area during complete thyroid lobectomy.

It must be kept in mind also that the recurrent nerve may not be a single trunk in the thyroid region, for frequently the nerve will have an extralaryngeal branching 0.5 cm. or more below its entrance into the larynx.

The recurrent course of the nerve depends upon its developmental relationship to the primitive aortic arches. On the right it recurs around the subclavian artery, and on the left, the ligamentum arteriosum (page 110). In the presence of an anomalous right subclavian artery arising from the aortic arch, the right recurrent nerve arises from the cervical portion of the vagus at the level of the larynx or thyroid and pursues a horizontal course to its point of entrance into the larynx, an *anomalous recurrent nerve.*

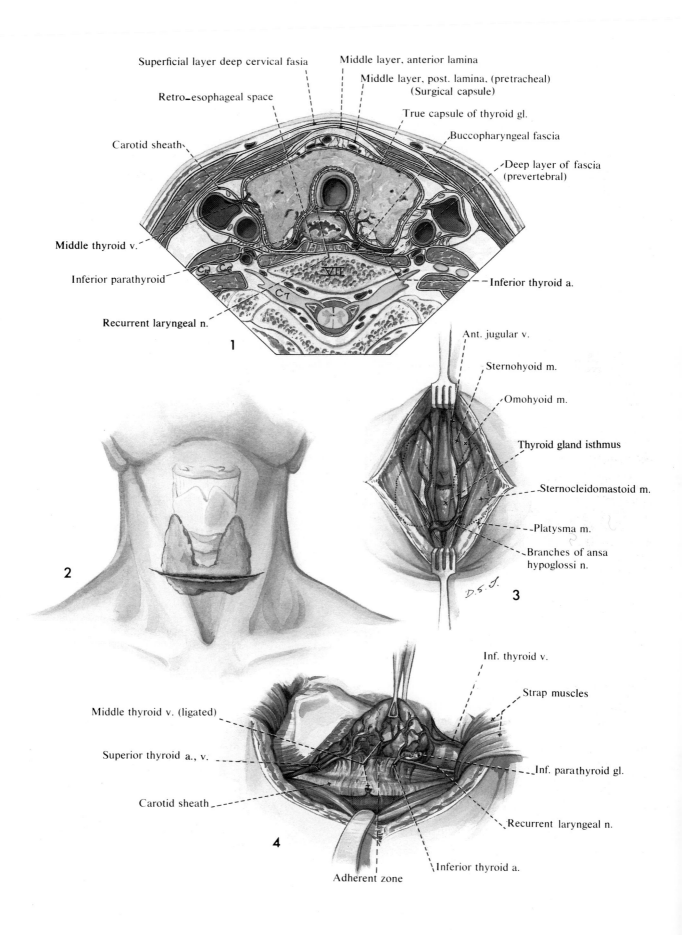

Superficial layer deep cervical fasia

Retro–esophageal space

Middle layer, anterior lamina

Middle layer, post. lamina, (pretracheal) (Surgical capsule)

True capsule of thyroid gl.

Buccopharyngeal fascia

Deep layer of fascia (prevertebral)

Carotid sheath

Middle thyroid v.

Inferior parathyroid

Recurrent laryngeal n.

Inferior thyroid a.

1

2

Ant. jugular v.

Sternohyoid m.

Omohyoid m.

Thyroid gland isthmus

Sternocleidomastoid m.

Platysma m.

Branches of ansa hypoglossi n.

D.S.I.

3

Inf. thyroid v.

Strap muscles

Middle thyroid v. (ligated)

Superior thyroid a., v.

Inf. parathyroid gl.

Carotid sheath

Recurrent laryngeal n.

Inferior thyroid a.

Adherent zone

4

PARATHYROID GLANDS:

Embryology (Fig. 1):

The parathyroid glands develop from the third and fourth pharyngeal pouches, and are designated as parathyroid III and parathyroid IV, respectively. Parathyroid III originates from the third pouch in conjunction with the thymic primordium. These primordia migrate caudalward so that parathyroid III (inferior parathyroids) comes to lie in a lower position in the neck than that of parathyroid IV (superior parathyroids), which are derived from the fourth pouch.

The relationship of parathyroid III to the thymus is of importance in understanding the variable position of the inferior parathyroid glands. There may be an early separation of these two structures so that the inferior glands may fail to migrate and develop in the upper neck as high as the hyoid level. On the other hand, the separation may be much delayed or may fail entirely, and the parathyroid may descend into the anterior mediastinum (Fig. 3). When normal separation occurs, the inferior parathyroid becomes related to the thyroid gland (see below).

Appearance:

The normal parathyroid gland weighs 30 to 40 mg. and measures some 6 mm. in length, 3 mm. in width, and 2 mm. in thickness. It is ovoid in shape with a smooth surface. In the adult, fine fibrous septa extending from the capsule into the parenchyma of the gland produce a very fine granular appearance. The color of the parathyroid varies with the fat content. Before puberty it contains no fat and varies from pinkish to coffee brown in color, but later there is an admixture of fat which may occupy one pole or completely surround the glandular tissue, producing a yellowish tint to the gland or the appearance of a fat globule.

Number and Location (Figs. 2 and 3):

Four parathyroid glands are usually present, but reports of numbers have varied from one to 12. When fewer than four glands are found, it is more probable that some have been missed in the dissection than that they are absent. More than four glands may result from a splitting of the original anlage.

Both superior (IV) and inferior (III) parathyroids are usually located on the posterior aspect of the lateral thyroid lobes, the superior near the junction of the upper and middle third of the thyroid, and inferior parathyroid near the lower pole of the thyroid (Fig. 2, page 21, and Fig. 4, page 37). There is much variation in position, particularly in regard to the inferior glands. Parathyroid tissue may occur anywhere in the visceral compartment of the anterior neck from the level of the carotid bifurcation to the anterior mediastinum. The superior glands are situated posterior and may be more intimately related to the pharynx or esophagus rather than to the thyroid. The inferior parathyroid lies in a more anterior plane than the superior and is usually situated anterior to the recurrent laryngeal nerve and the inferior thyroid artery. Parathyroids, particularly the inferior, may also be located on the lateral or anterior surface of the thyroid gland or imbedded in the thyroid tissue.

Blood Supply (Fig. 2):

The main supply to both superior and inferior glands is via the inferior thyroid artery. The superior glands receive in addition a branch from the superior thyroid artery which arises from the anastomotic channel between the two main thyroid arteries. These parathyroid vessels enter the gland at a definite hilus. The venous and lymphatic drainage is into the thyroid systems.

A thorough knowledge of the appearance, location, and blood supply of the parathyroids is necessary for their preservation not only during operations on the thyroid, but also in the search for parathyroid adenoma.

Cervical Trachea (Tracheostomy, Tracheotomy)

A surgical incision through the anterior wall of the cervical trachea is frequently performed as either an emergency or an elective procedure to maintain an adequate airway.

Incision (Fig. 4) for the approach to the cervical trachea may be made through either a transverse or a midline direction. Topographically, this portion of the trachea extends from the cricoid cartilage to the suprasternal notch. It should be recalled that at the latter level, the trachea is 1½ inches deep to the skin.

A vertical midline incision is most frequently used. In making such an approach the position of the *jugular venous arch* (Fig. 2, page 11) should be kept in mind. A short horizontal incision between the anterior borders of the sternocleidomastoid muscles produces a less conspicuous scar.

The *approach* through the skin and subcutaneous tissue is followed by a midline incision through the deep cervical fascia, permitting lateral retraction of the sternohyoid muscles, which exposes the cervical trachea. The isthmus of the thyroid gland overlies the second to fourth tracheal rings. The isthmus may be transected, retracted either superiorly or inferiorly to obtain adequate exposure of the rings which are to be divided.

A *high tracheostomy* is one performed above the level of the thyroid isthmus. Section of the cricoid, which will result in laryngeal stenosis, must be avoided.

A *low tracheostomy* is carried out at the level of the third to sixth tracheal rings. In this approach the inferior thyroid veins and thyroid ima vessels may be encountered (Fig. 2, page 21).

The *tracheal incision* (Fig. 5) is a vertical one, usually through the third, fourth, and fifth tracheal rings.

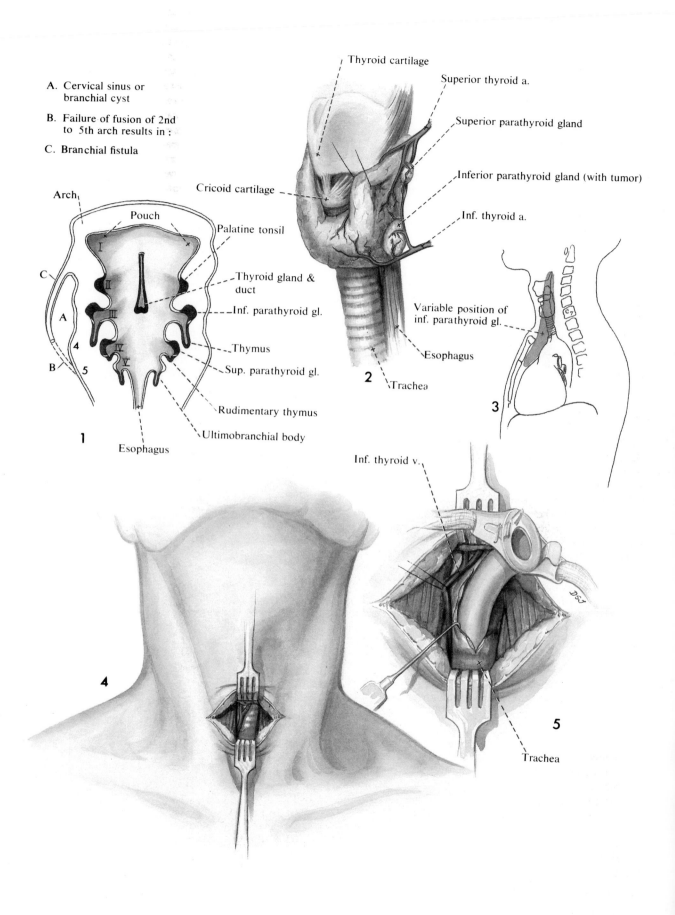

A. Cervical sinus or branchial cyst

B. Failure of fusion of 2nd to 5th arch results in :

C. Branchial fistula

Arch

Pouch

Palatine tonsil

C

I

Thyroid gland & duct

II

Inf. parathyroid gl.

A

III

4

Thymus

B

IV

5

V

Sup. parathyroid gl.

Rudimentary thymus

Ultimobranchial body

1

Esophagus

Thyroid cartilage

Superior thyroid a.

Superior parathyroid gland

Inferior parathyroid gland (with tumor)

Cricoid cartilage

Inf. thyroid a.

Variable position of inf. parathyroid gl.

Esophagus

2

Trachea

3

Inf. thyroid v.

4

5

Trachea

RADICAL NECK DISSECTION:

The purpose of a radical neck dissection is to remove the lymphatics in the drainage areas of primary cancers occurring in the region of the head and neck (Fig. 2, page 29). In applying the principle of regional lymphatic excision (radical dissection) in the surgery of cancer, the apparently normal tissue surrounding the lymph nodes and lymphatic vessels must be sacrificed to insure removal of tissues involved or likely to be involved by neoplasm. In addition to the lymphatics and areolar tissue, certain muscles, blood vessels, nerves, and glandular tissue must be sacrificed in order to gain proper access. In recent years a modified radical neck dissection has been advocated by some surgeons. In this procedure, the sternocleidomastoid muscle is preserved. It makes for a more tedious dissection and possible incomplete en-bloc removal of the nodal chains.

Incision (Fig. 1)—consists of a curved horizontal limb extending from the mastoid process to the mentum. The lower extension of the curve descends to about the hyoid level. A vertical limb extends from the center of the horizontal incision to the junction of the middle and inner third of the clavicle. This incision is carried through the platysma muscle.

This is the Crile approach, but many variations of this approach have been advocated. For better cosmetic result a MacFee incision may be used, consisting of upper and lower transverse incisions more in accord with Langer's lines (page 10).

Boundaries of Dissection (Figs. 2 and 3):

1. **Superior**—inferior margin of mandible, lower pole of the parotid gland, and mastoid process.
2. **Anterior**—midline of the neck.
3. **Inferior**—manubrium sterni, medial two-thirds of clavicle.
4. **Posterior**—anterior border of trapezius muscle.
5. **Superficial**—deep surface of platysma muscle.
6. **Deep**—deep layer (prevertebral) of deep cervical fascia.

N.B. All important motor nerves with the exception of the spinal accessory nerve and cervical branch of the facial lie *deep* to this fascial plane.

The *pars mandibularis of the cervical branch of the facial nerve* (Fig. 2, page 13) is readily injured in incisions near the angle of the mandible. Knowledge of its location will enable the surgeon to avoid this nerve. Its injury results in partial paralysis (depressor anguli oris and depressor labii inferioris muscles) of the lower lip.

The nerve lies deep to the platysma 1 cm. behind and below the angle of the mandible. It then extends forward parallel and inferior to the lower border of the mandible, and proceeding upward to the face, crosses the external maxillary (facial) artery and anterior facial vein at the anterior border of the masseter muscle. If these anatomic relations are kept in mind, injury to the nerve can be avoided during the development of the upper flap, which consists of skin, subcutaneous tissue, and platysma muscle.

Structures Removed (Figs. 2 and 3):

1. **Muscles**—sternocleidomastoid and omohyoid.

2. **Nerves**—superficial branches of the cervical plexus (great auricular, lesser occipital, transverse colli, and supraclavicular), ansa hypoglossi, and spinal accessory nerve.
3. **Vessels**—*Veins*—anterior, external, and internal jugular with its tributaries. *Arteries*—external maxillary (facial) artery.
4. **Glands**—submaxillary (deep process may be preserved) and lower pole of the parotid gland.
5. **Lymphatics and Areolar Tissue**—of the submental, submandibular, carotid, muscular, and posterior triangles.

Structures Preserved (Figs. 2 and 3):

1. **Muscles**—the platysma and all muscles in the floor of the anterior and posterior triangles, and the digastric and stylohyoid muscles (the latter two are sacrificed only in unusual circumstances).
2. **Nerves**—ramus mandibularis of cervical branch of the facial, hypoglossal (XII), lingual, phrenic, vagus, brachial plexus, and cervical sympathetic trunk.
3. **Vessels**—*Veins*—none. *Arteries*—All branches of the carotid systems except the external maxillary (facial) artery. (The superior thyroid and lingual arteries may be sacrificed if necessary.)
4. **Lymphatics**—thoracic duct (Fig. 1, page 23).

PARTIAL (UPPER) NECK DISSECTION:

This procedure is performed for much the same purpose as a radical neck dissection but is limited to the upper parts of the anterior triangle, namely, the submental, submandibular, and carotid triangles. *Supraomohyoid* or *suprahyoid* neck dissection are other terms used to identify this procedure.

Incision—the horizontal portion of the incision used for radical neck dissection is utilized in this partial neck dissection.

Boundaries of Dissection (Fig. 4):

1. **Superior**—lower margin of mandible, lower pole of the parotid gland.
2. **Anterior**—midline of the neck.
3. **Inferior and Posterior**—hyoid bone, anterior belly of omohyoid, and anterior border of the sternocleidomastoid.

Structures Removed:

1. **Muscles**—none.
2. **Nerves**—none.
3. **Vessels**—*Veins*—anterior facial vein and common facial vein. *Arteries*—external maxillary (facial) artery.
4. **Glands**—submaxillary and inferior pole of parotid gland.
5. **Lymphatics and Areolar Tissue**—of the submental, submandibular, and carotid triangles.

Structures Preserved:

1. **Muscles**—all muscles in the floor of the submental and submandibular triangles, as well as the platysma, digastric, and stylohyoid muscles.
2. **Nerves**—pars mandibularis of cervical branch of facial, hypoglossal (XII), and lingual nerves.
3. **Vessels**—*Veins*—internal jugular vein. *Arteries*—the carotid system.

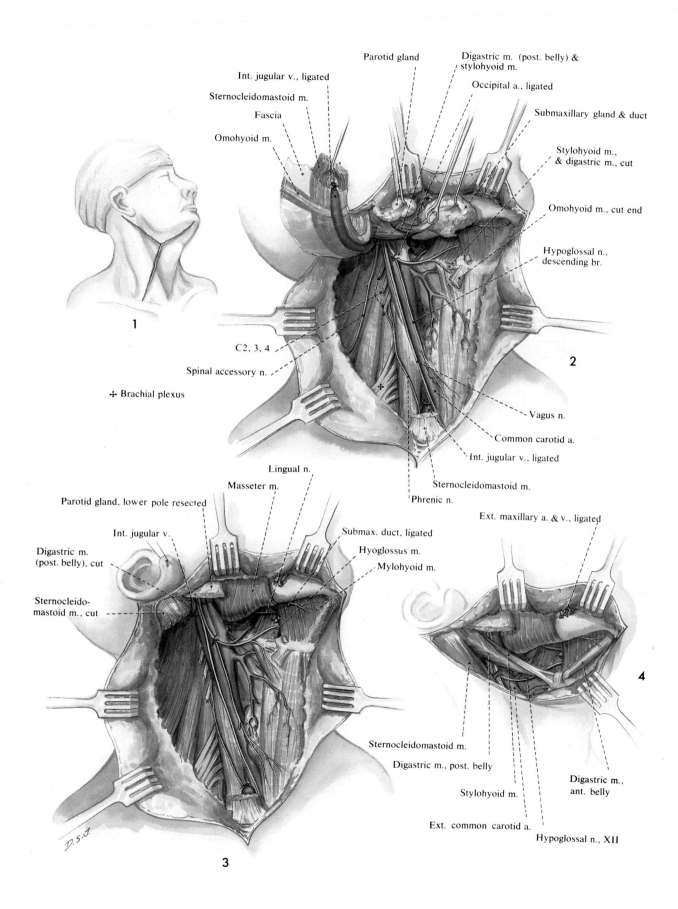

Parotid gland

Digastric m. (post. belly) &
stylohyoid m.

Occipital a., ligated

Int. jugular v., ligated

Sternocleidomastoid m.

Fascia

Omohyoid m.

Submaxillary gland & duct

Stylohyoid m.,
& digastric m., cut

Omohyoid m., cut end

Hypoglossal n.,
descending br.

C2, 3, 4

Spinal accessory n.

Brachial plexus

Vagus n.

Common carotid a.

Int. jugular v., ligated

Sternocleidomastoid m.

Phrenic n.

1

2

Lingual n.

Masseter m.

Parotid gland, lower pole resected

Int. jugular v.

Digastric m.
(post. belly), cut

Sternocleido-
mastoid m., cut

Submax. duct, ligated

Hyoglossus m.

Mylohyoid m.

Ext. maxillary a. & v., ligated

4

Sternocleidomastoid m.

Digastric m., post. belly

Stylohyoid m.

Ext. common carotid a.

Digastric m.,
ant. belly

Hypoglossal n., XII

3

The Breast and Axilla

THE BREAST:

The breasts, or *mammae,* are modified glands of cutaneous origin. They consist of three anatomical parts, a *cutaneous layer,* a *stroma* consisting of a subcutaneous fatty layer and a connective tissue supporting layer, and a *parenchyma,* or glandular tissue.

Topography:

The extensions of the breast are so variable in the adult female that precise topographic landmarks cannot be defined. Variations due to the gravid state, menstrual cycle, obesity, age, and other factors all alter the topographic contours. The parenchymal tissue usually extends beyond the protuberance of the breast. From a surgical point of view, the breast topography extends to the clavicle above, the midline medially, the seventh costal cartilage inferiorly, and the margin of the latissimus dorsi laterally. The breast parenchyma frequently extends into the axilla through an opening in the axillary fascia *(foramen of Langer)* as the *axillary tail of Spence* (Fig. 1). The parenchymal tissue usually extends beyond the protuberance of the breast.

Structure (Figs. 1 and 2):

1. **Cutaneous Layer** — is thinner than the skin of the axilla. It is covered by down-hairs associated with numerous sebaceous and sweat glands. Superficial veins may be prominent. It is more adherent to the underlying superficial fatty layer than in most areas, but is very flexible and elastic. Modifications of the skin are present over the center of the breast, namely, the areola and the nipple.

   a. AREOLA — consists of thin pigmented skin that varies with the natural coloring of the individual and pregnancy, being darker in brunettes and multipara. Elevations may be seen in the areola caused by underlying sebaceous glands and rudimentary milk glands *(areolar tubercles of Montgomery).* There is no fat in the corium of the areola.

   b. NIPPLE — varies in shape and position. It contains many sebaceous glands and numerous smooth muscle fibers. The skin is wrinkled and pigmented and contains 15 to 20 minute openings of the underlying lactiferous ducts.

2. **Stroma** — lies beneath the skin covering the whole gland except under the nipple and areola. It consists of superficial fascia which also extends deep to the parenchymal tissue and is therefore termed the *mammary adipose capsule.* It interposes itself between lobes and lobules and produces the smooth external appearance of the breast. Other connective tissue elements consist of strands which extend from the apices of the lobes to the corium of skin, the *retinacula mammae.* They are especially well developed in the upper quadrants of the breast and are termed the *suspensory ligaments of Cooper.*

3. **Parenchyma** — is a mass of glandular tissue, the *corpus mammae,* most prominent in the subareolar area. It is composed of 15 to 20 lobes of irregular pyramidal groups of glandular material. The apex of each lobe points toward the nipple. Each lobe possesses an *excretory (lactiferous) duct,* whose orifice is located in the nipple. Each duct is dilated in its subareolar position to form a *sinus lactiferus.*

Arterial Supply (Fig. 3):

The main supply to the breast comes from the internal mammary artery. The breast receives additional supply from branches of the axillary artery and aorta.

1. **Internal Mammary** — is a branch from the first portion of the subclavian artery. The second and fourth perforating branches are most important in the blood supply to the breast.

2. **Lateral Thoracic** — is a branch of the second portion of the axillary artery and supplies the lateral and caudal portions of the breast.

3. **Aortic Intercostals** — may send small branches to the breast by its lateral cutaneous rami.

Venous Drainage (Fig. 3, page 49):

Lymphatic Drainage:

The lymphatics of the breast may be divided into cutaneous and parenchymal drainage:

1. **Cutaneous Drainage** (Fig. 4) — radiates from a circumareolar plexus.

   a. LATERAL — to the anterior (pectoral) axillary nodes.

   b. SUPERIOR — to the medial axillary nodes and the apical (infraclavicular) nodes.

   c. MEDIAL — to the internal mammary nodes and to the cutaneous lymphatics of the opposite side.

   d. INFERIOR — to the cutaneous lymphatics of the upper abdominal wall and liver.

2. **Parenchymal Drainage** (Fig. 5) — receives channels from the breast proper as well as the skin of the nipple and areola. These afferent channels drain into the *subareolar plexus.* From this plexus two main efferent channels arise:

   a. SUPERIOR CHANNEL — receives tributaries from the outer portion of the gland and drains into the anterior axillary nodes.

   b. INFERIOR CHANNEL — receives tributaries from the inner portion of the gland and drains into the anterior axillary nodes.

   c. ACCESSORY CHANNELS — two major efferent channels extend from the subareolar plexus to the apical nodes of the axilla and to the lateral (brachial) nodes.

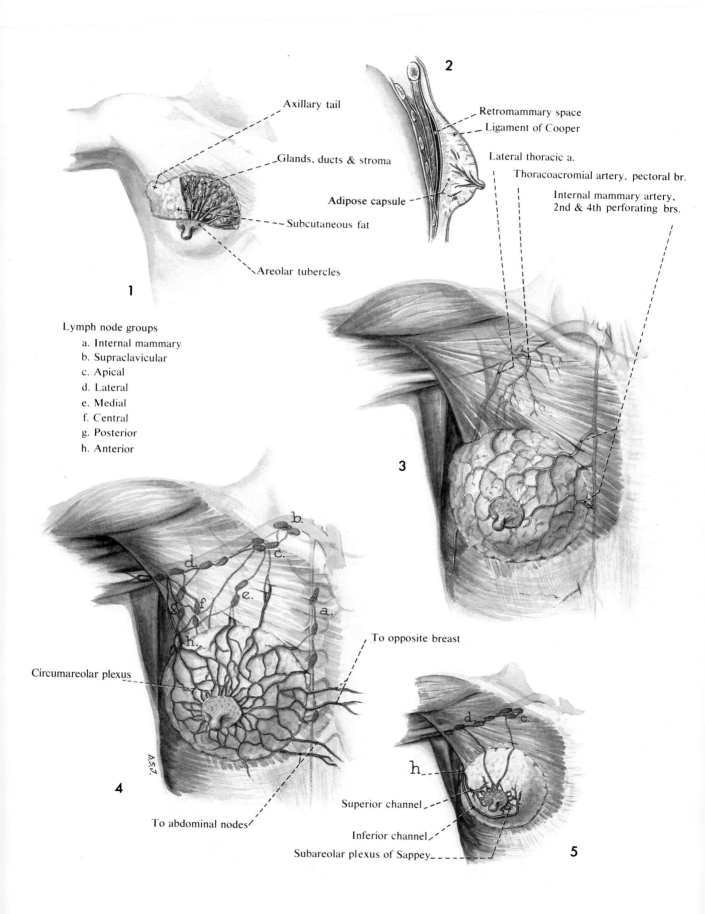

2

Axillary tail

Glands, ducts & stroma

Adipose capsule

Subcutaneous fat

Areolar tubercles

1

Retromammary space

Ligament of Cooper

Lateral thoracic a.

Thoracoacromial artery, pectoral br.

Internal mammary artery,
2nd & 4th perforating brs.

Lymph node groups
  a. Internal mammary
  b. Supraclavicular
  c. Apical
  d. Lateral
  e. Medial
  f. Central
  g. Posterior
  h. Anterior

3

Circumareolar plexus

To opposite breast

To abdominal nodes

4

Superior channel

Inferior channel

Subareolar plexus of Sappey

5

THE AXILLA:

The axilla, or armpit, is pyramidal in shape and, therefore, has an apex, base, and four muscular walls.

Boundaries (Fig. 1):

1. **Apex**—is formed by the clavicle, upper border of the first rib, and the superior border of the scapula.
2. **Base**—is made up of the skin of the axilla, the superficial fascia, and the axillary fascia, a continuation of the pectoral fascia.
3. **Anterior Wall**—consists of pectoralis major and minor and is innervated by the *anterior*-medial and *anterior*-lateral *cords* via medial and lateral anterior thoracic nerves.
    a. PECTORALIS MAJOR—arises by a clavicular, sternal, and abdominal head and inserts into the *lateral* lip of the bicipital groove.
    b. PECTORALIS MINOR—takes origin by slips from the second to fifth ribs and inserts on the coracoid process of the scapula.
4. **Posterior Wall**—is made up of three muscles which, from superior to inferior, are the subscapular, teres major, and latissimus dorsi, all of which are innervated by the *posterior cord* via the subscapular nerves.
    a. SUBSCAPULAR—arises in the subscapular fossa and inserts into the lesser tubercle of the humerus.
    b. TERES MAJOR—takes origin from the inferior angle of the scapula and extends to the *medial* lip of the bicipital groove.
    c. LATISSIMUS DORSI—has an extensive origin from the dorsum of the body and terminates *in* the bicipital groove.
5. **Lateral Wall**—consists of two muscles, the coracobrachialis and the short head of the biceps, both arising from the coracoid process and innervated by the anterior-*lateral cord* via the musculocutaneous nerve.
    a. CORACOBRACHIALIS—extends from the coracoid process to the middle third of the shaft of the humerus.
    b. SHORT HEAD OF THE BICEPS—arises in common with the coracobrachialis and inserts, after joining the long head, into the radius and the antibrachial fascia.
6. **Medial Wall**—is formed by the upper digitations of the serratus anterius. It is innervated by the *long thoracic nerve* from anterior primary divisions of the brachial plexus.
    SERRATUS ANTERIUS—arises from digitations from the upper nine ribs and inserts into the vertebral border of the scapula.

Deep Fascia (Fig. 2):

Since the anterior wall of the axilla is made up of two muscular strata, it necessitates two distinct deep fascial layers: one covers the pectoralis major, the *pectoral fascia*; the other covers the pectoralis minor, the *clavipectoral fascia*.

1. **Pectoral Fascia**—encloses the pectoralis major and extends from the lower border of the muscle to become *axillary* fascia extending posteriorly as the fascia of the latissimus dorsi. Laterally it is continuous with the investing fascia of the arm.
2. **Clavipectoral Fascia**—extends from the clavicle above to the axillary fascia below. It surrounds the subclavius and pectoralis minor muscles. Between the subclavius and pectoralis minor this fascia is thickened to form the *costocoracoid membrane* which is pierced by the cephalic vein, thoraco-acromial vessels, and the anterior thoracic nerves. After splitting around the pectoralis minor, the fascia fuses and joins the axillary fascia to form the *suspensory ligament* of the axilla.
3. **Axillary Sheath**—is a prolongation of the deep layer of the deep cervical fascia enclosing the axillary vessels and branches of the brachial plexus. It extends for a variable distance into the axilla.

Axillary Vein (Fig. 3):

With the upper extremity in the abducted position the main structure brought into view is the axillary vein and its tributaries. More superficial, however, are the lateral cutaneous branches of the upper intercostal nerves; that from T_2, passing to the medial side of the brachium, is termed the *intercostobrachial nerve*.

At the lower border of the teres major, the *basilic* vein joins the *brachial* veins to form the axillary vein which extends upward to the lower border of the first rib. Here the vein is termed the subclavian. Its tributaries follow the branches of the axillary artery except for the following:

1. **Cephalic Vein**—arises on the dorsum of the hand, passes upward in the superficial fascia of the upper extremity, and pierces the costocoracoid membrane at the deltopectoral triangle. It empties into the axillary vein above the pectoralis minor. This vessel serves as a collateral channel for venous return from the upper extremity following occlusion of the axillary vein. It also serves as a guide to the first portion of the axillary artery.
2. **Thoraco-epigastric Vein**—connects the superficial epigastric below with the lateral thoracic branch of the axillary above, thus serving as an important collateral pathway after obliteration of the inferior vena cava.

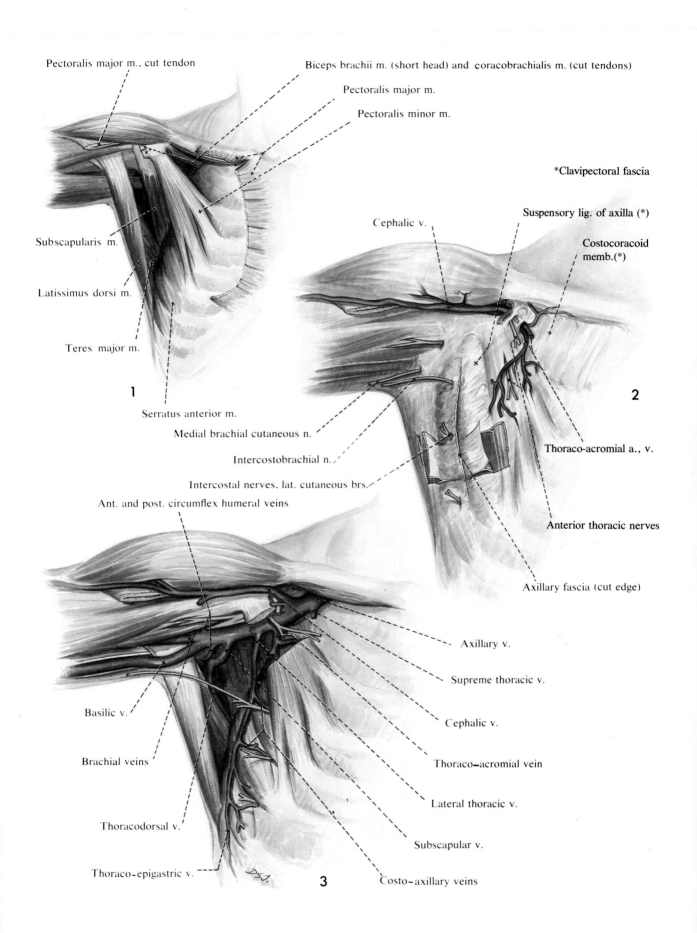

Pectoralis major m., cut tendon

Biceps brachii m. (short head) and coracobrachialis m. (cut tendons)

Pectoralis major m.

Pectoralis minor m.

*Clavipectoral fascia

Cephalic v.

Suspensory lig. of axilla (*)

Costocoracoid memb.(*)

Subscapularis m.

Latissimus dorsi m.

Teres major m.

1

Serratus anterior m.

Medial brachial cutaneous n.

Intercostobrachial n.

Intercostal nerves, lat. cutaneous brs.

Ant. and post. circumflex humeral veins

2

Thoraco-acromial a., v.

Anterior thoracic nerves

Axillary fascia (cut edge)

Axillary v.

Supreme thoracic v.

Basilic v.

Cephalic v.

Brachial veins

Thoraco–acromial vein

Lateral thoracic v.

Thoracodorsal v.

Subscapular v.

Thoraco-epigastric v.

3

Costo-axillary veins

Axillary Artery (Figs. 1 and 2):

After removal of the axillary vein, the artery is clearly visible along with the cords of the brachial plexus, which are named according to their relative position to the artery. The artery extends from the lower border of the first rib to the lower border of the teres major and is arbitrarily divided by the pectoralis minor into three parts:

1. **First Portion** — is located between the first rib and the upper border of the pectoralis minor and gives off one branch.

SUPREME THORACIC — passes behind the axillary vein and across the apex of the axilla to supply the structures in the first intercostal space.

2. **Second Portion** — is found behind the pectoralis minor and usually gives rise to two branches:

a. THORACO-ACROMIAL — pierces the costocoracoid membrane and divides into branches directed toward the clavicle, acromion process, and the deltoid and pectoral muscles.

b. LATERAL THORACIC — descends along the medial wall of the axilla, to about the fifth intercostal space. It sends branches to the muscles of the anterior and medial walls of the axilla and mammary gland.

3. **Third Portion** — extends from the lower border of the pectoralis minor to the lower border of teres major. There are three branches which arise from this third portion (Figs. 1 and 2):

a. SUBSCAPULAR — extends toward the posterior wall of the axilla and terminates as the *circumflex scapular* and *thoracodorsal*. The former pierces the posterior axillary wall through a muscular interval, bounded by the subscapular, teres major, and long head of the triceps *(triangular space)*, and reaches the infraspinatus fossa. The thoracodorsal continues through the axilla to the inferior scapular angle.

b. ANTERIOR CIRCUMFLEX HUMERAL — is a small branch which passes deep to the coracobrachial and biceps tendons and winds around the surgical neck of the humerus.

c. POSTERIOR CIRCUMFLEX HUMERAL — arises opposite the anterior circumflex branch and winds around the surgical neck of the humerus to anastomose with the anterior branch. It pierces the posterior wall of the axilla through a space bounded by the shaft of the humerus, teres minor, teres major, and long head of the triceps *(quadrilateral space)*. It is accompanied in this space by the axillary nerve. The artery gives off an important anastomotic branch to the profunda brachii.

Brachial Plexus (Figs. 1 and 2; Fig. 2, page 25):

1. **Anterolateral Cord:**

a. LATERAL-ANTERIOR THORACIC — pierces the costocoracoid membrane and supplies the pectoral muscles.

b. MUSCULOCUTANEOUS — is the most lateral of the terminal branches and innervates the muscles of the lateral wall of the axilla, the coracobrachialis, and the biceps. It pierces the coracobrachial as it descends to the arm.

c. LATERAL HEAD OF THE MEDIAN — forms the lateral component of the median nerve.

2. **Anteromedial Cord:**

a. MEDIAL-ANTERIOR THORACIC — joins the lateral anterior thoracic to innervate the pectoral muscles.

b. MEDIAN HEAD OF MEDIAN — passes obliquely over the third part of the axillary artery to join the lateral head from the anterolateral cord to form the median nerve. The latter lies along the lateral side of the artery.

c. ULNAR — is the largest of the medial cord branches and arises at the lower border of the pectoralis minor. It descends into the arm along the medial side of the axillary artery.

d. MEDIAL ANTIBRACHIAL CUTANEOUS — arises in close relation with the ulnar nerve.

e. MEDIAL BRACHIAL CUTANEOUS — lies medial to axillary vein in the lower axilla; pierces the deep fascia and is distributed to the skin of the medial surface of the arm.

3. **Posterior Cord** (Fig. 2):

a. SUBSCAPULAR NERVES — usually three in number and termed the upper, middle, and lower. They supply the muscles of the posterior wall of the axilla: the upper innervates the subscapular, the middle (thoracodorsal), the latissimus dorsi, and the lower, the teres major.

b. AXILLARY — extends dorsally and leaves the axilla via the quadrilateral space accompanied by the posterior humeral artery and innervates the deltoid and teres minor muscles.

c. RADIAL NERVE — is a direct continuation of the posterior cord lying behind the axillary artery. It is the largest terminal branch of the brachial plexus.

Long Thoracic Nerve (Fig. 1):

This nerve arises from the anterior primary divisions of C_5, C_6, and C_7. It pierces the middle scalene, then passes behind the brachial plexus into the axilla, where it runs along the medial wall sending branches to the digitations of the serratus anterius.

Axillary Lymph Nodes (Fig. 3):

The axillary nodes may be arbitrarily divided into groups that are related to the four axillary walls, the apex, and the base. They are as follows:

1. **Posterior (Subscapular)** — six or seven in number; along the subscapular vessels and thoracodorsal nerve.

2. **Lateral (Brachial)** — four or five in number; along lower part of axillary vein.

3. **Anterior (Anterior Pectoralis)** — four or five in number; along edge of the pectoralis major.

4. **Medial (Posterior Pectoral)** — three or four; along the lateral thoracic artery and vein.

5. **Central** — three to five; lies at the base of the axilla in the fatty tissue.

6. **Apical (Infraclavicular)** — four or five; at apex of triangle, closely related to axillary vein.

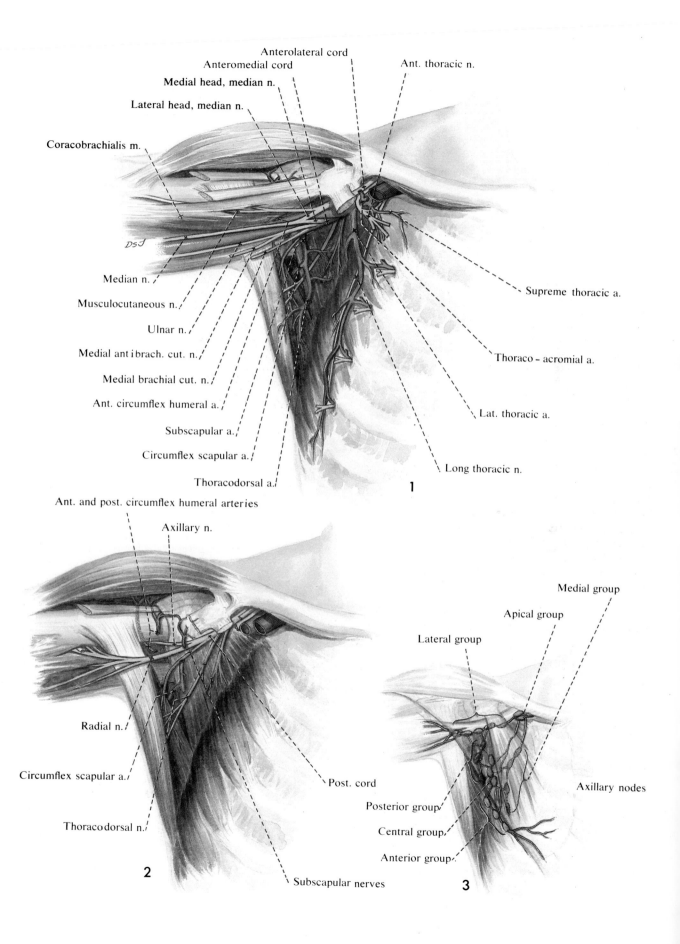

Anterolateral cord

Anteromedial cord

Medial head, median n.

Lateral head, median n.

Ant. thoracic n.

Coracobrachialis m.

Median n.

Musculocutaneous n.

Ulnar n.

Medial ant i brach. cut. n.

Medial brachial cut. n.

Ant. circumflex humeral a.

Subscapular a.

Circumflex scapular a.

Thoracodorsal a.

Supreme thoracic a.

Thoraco - acromial a.

Lat. thoracic a.

Long thoracic n.

1

Ant. and post. circumflex humeral arteries

Axillary n.

Radial n.

Circumflex scapular a.

Thoracodorsal n.

Post. cord

Subscapular nerves

2

Medial group

Apical group

Lateral group

Posterior group

Central group

Anterior group

Axillary nodes

3

CARCINOMA OF THE BREAST:

Anatomic Basis of Physical Signs (Fig. 1):

The classic physical signs of carcinoma of the breast are illustrated in Figure 1.

1. Neoplastic invasion of the retinaculum cutis (ligaments of Cooper), which are fibrous strands extending from the breast lobules to the corium, produces shortening of them with subsequent depression or fixation of the overlying skin (Fig. 1a).

2. Neoplastic involvement of the lactiferous ducts may produce also shortening of these structures and fixation, retraction, or inversion of the nipple (Fig. 1b).

3. When cancer has traversed the *retromammary space* and has become attached to or invaded the deep fascia on the pectoralis major muscle, contraction of the muscle produces an upward movement of the breast, a clinical sign of advanced disease (Fig. 1c).

Lymphatic Vessels of the Breast (Fig. 2; Figs. 4 and 5, page 43):

A dense subareolar plexus receives lymph not only from the skin of the areola and nipple but also from the entire central portion of the gland. From this plexus an inferior and a superior trunk arise to transport lymph to the axilla. The superior trunk receives tributaries from the outer one-half of the breast. The inferior trunk arises from the medial border of the subareolar plexus, passes downward, then laterally to the outer border of the pectoralis major muscle, receiving tributaries from the medial one-half of the breast. Both of these trunks penetrate the deep fascia at the lateral border of this muscle and terminate in axillary nodes.

The two trunks described above constitute the main lymph drainage routes from the breast, but there are two accessory routes to nodes at the apex of the axilla: (1) *transpectoral,* directly from the deep aspect of the breast through the pectoralis major muscle, along the course of the pectoral branch of the thoraco-acromial artery to the apical (Halsted) group of the lymph nodes; (2) *retropectoral,* from the upper and medial portion of the breast to the outer edge of the pectoralis major muscle, upward beneath its surface to the lateral and apical nodes. By these accessory routes the main group of axillary nodes is by-passed. The cutaneous drainage of the breast is discussed on page 42.

Lymph Nodes of the Breast (Fig. 2):

Axillary—the primary pathway of lymphatic drainage from the breast is through the axilla. The axillary lymph nodes lie deep to the axillary fascia in close association with the major blood vessels in the axilla. For descriptive purposes they are customarily divided into six groups:

1. ANTERIOR GROUP (ANTERIOR PECTORAL)—is located on the medial wall of the axilla lying on or in the fascia of the serratus anterior muscle along the lower border of the pectoralis major muscle.

2. POSTERIOR GROUP (SUBSCAPULAR)—nodes in this group lie along the subscapular vessels and the thoracodorsal nerve.

3. CENTRAL NODES (3 TO 5)—are imbedded in the fat of the central axilla.

4. LATERAL GROUP (4 TO 5) (BRACHIAL)—lie on the anterior and inferior aspect of the axillary vein lateral to the pectoral minor muscle.

5. MEDIAL GROUP (3 TO 4)—is located behind the pectoral minor muscle, in reality, a superior extension of the anterior group.

6. APICAL GROUP (INFRACLAVICULAR, HALSTED NODES) (4 TO 5)—in both the anatomical and the functional sense the highest in the axilla, is located medial to the insertion of the pectoral minor on and inferior to the axillary vein. The collecting trunks from all other axillary nodes empty into this group of nodes. From them, efferent vessels pass upward behind the clavicle to (a) join the venous system at the junction of the jugular and subclavian veins, or (b) join the jugular and bronchomediastinal lymph trunk to form a common trunk, or (c) empty into the supraclavicular nodes.

Internal Mammary Nodes—some lymph from the medial hemisphere of the breast passes directly medially to the nodes along the course of the internal mammary vessels on the same side. These nodes vary in size (2 to 6 mm.) and number. An average of four on each side is usual, with one node in each of the first three interspaces and another in the fifth or sixth interspace. Efferent vessels from the group join other lymph vessels in the base of the neck on each side, as described in the preceding paragraph. These nodes and vessels are an important route of metastasis in cancer of the breast, especially for lesions in the medial one-half of the breast.

There is also communication between the lymphatic plexuses of the two breasts by vessels which cross the midline, and lymphatics from the lower medial part of the breast connect with those of the upper abdomen, passing through the upper end of the corresponding sheath of the rectus abdominis muscle.

Routes of Venous Spread from Cancer of the Breast (Fig. 3):

The breast is drained by axillary, internal mammary, and intercostal veins. Direct venous communications exist between the breast and (1) the superior vena cava via the axillary vein, (2) the vertebral venous plexus via the intercostal and azygos system of veins, and (3) the portal venous system via the azygos system, and via vessels in the falciform ligament. These communications can explain the frequent spread of breast cancer to the lungs, liver, and bones of the axial skeleton.

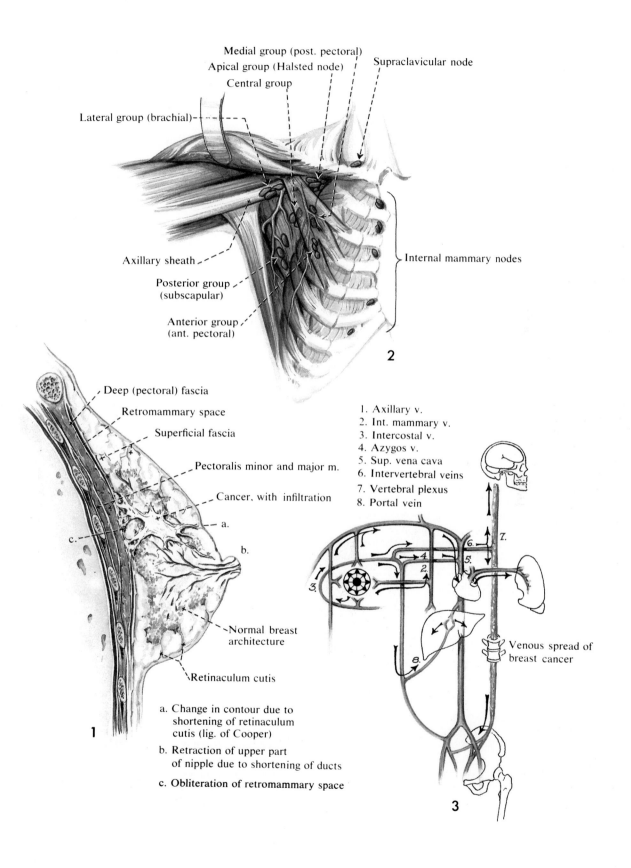

Medial group (post. pectoral)

Apical group (Halsted node)

Central group

Supraclavicular node

Lateral group (brachial)

Axillary sheath

Posterior group
(subscapular)

Anterior group
(ant. pectoral)

Internal mammary nodes

2

Deep (pectoral) fascia

Retromammary space

Superficial fascia

Pectoralis minor and major m.

Cancer, with infiltration

a.

b.

c.

Normal breast
architecture

Retinaculum cutis

1. Axillary v.
2. Int. mammary v.
3. Intercostal v.
4. Azygos v.
5. Sup. vena cava
6. Intervertebral veins
7. Vertebral plexus
8. Portal vein

Venous spread of
breast cancer

a. Change in contour due to
shortening of retinaculum
cutis (lig. of Cooper)

b. Retraction of upper part
of nipple due to shortening of ducts

c. Obliteration of retromammary space

1

3

Radical Mastectomy:

The principles underlying "radical" operation for cancer have been reviewed on page 40. The application of these principles to the breast and axilla is the purpose of this presentation.

Removal "en bloc" of the entire breast containing the tumor, the overlying skin, the underlying muscles and fascia in which invasion and metastases are likely to occur relatively early in the course of the disease, and all of the axillary lymphatics is the immediate goal of the procedure. Muscles and fasciae specifically removed during the operation are: the pectoralis major and minor muscles, the deep fascia over the exposed parts of the serratus anterior and external abdominal oblique muscles, and the upper end of the anterior sheath of the rectus abdominis muscle.

A large variety of skin incisions is used, and the area of skin incised may or may not require skin graft for closure of the incision. Our purpose is not to recommend or to describe a technique but to define the landmarks and show the extent, as well as the contents, of the field of dissection in the usual radical operation for cancer of the breast.

Superiorly, the incision (Fig. 1) must allow exposure of the clavicle and the insertion of the pectoralis major muscle into the humerus. Inferiorly, it must permit removal of the upper part of the anterior sheath of the rectus muscle. In the center, the nipple, areola, and skin over the dome of the breast, including the area of the tumor, must be removed.

The area to be exposed by the reflection of the skin flaps in order that the radical excision may be carried out is shown in Figure 1. *Anteriorly,* the dissection goes 1 cm. or more beyond the midline in order to interrupt and remove any lymphatic vessels going to the opposite side; *inferiorly,* the upper 6 to 8 cm. of the anterior rectus sheath is exposed; *laterally,* the dissection must be carried into the arm to permit section of the tendon of the pectoralis major muscle at its insertion into the bicipital groove of the humerus. Below this point laterally, the dissection is carried past the anterior margin of the latissimus dorsi muscle, and in the inferolateral part of the field, the interdigitating bundles of the serratus anterior and external abdominal oblique muscles are exposed. Superiorly, the limit of the field of dissection is the anterior surface of the clavicle.

Structures to Be Removed:
1. Skin over the tumor and of the dome of the breast
2. All breast tissue
3. Pectoralis major and minor muscles
4. Upper part of anterior sheath of rectus abdominis muscle
5. Nerves to pectoral muscles
6. Intercostobrachial nerve
7. Thoraco-acromial vessels
8. All tributaries to the axillary vein from the breast and axilla (the subscapular vein may be preserved)
9. Axillary lymph glands and vessels with the fat in which they are imbedded

Structures to Be Preserved (Fig. 2):
1. Brachial plexus
2. Axillary artery
3. Axillary vein
4. Cephalic vein
5. Subscapular artery
6. Subscapular nerve
7. Thoracodorsal nerve (nerve to latissimus dorsi)
8. Long thoracic nerve, on medial wall

Structures Exposed in the Complete Field of Operation:
1. Margin and one-half of anterior surface of the sternum
2. Anterior intercostal membranes
3. Costal cartilages (2, 3, 4 and 5)
4. Cut ends of perforating branches of internal mammary vessels
5. Upper part of rectus abdominis muscle
6. External intercostal muscles
7. Anterior surface of medial two-thirds of clavicle
8. Serratus anterior muscle
9. External abdominal oblique muscle
10. Long thoracic nerve
11. Axillary vein from origin to termination
12. Cords and branches of the brachial plexus
13. Axillary artery
14. Cut tendon of insertion of pectoralis minor into coracoid process of scapula
15. Subscapular nerves
16. Thoracodorsal nerve (nerve to latissimus dorsi)
17. Subscapular, teres major, and latissimus dorsi muscles
18. Coracobrachialis and short head of biceps muscles
19. Cephalic vein

Extended Radical Mastectomy—the usual "radical" operation for carcinoma of the breast allows removal of only regional lymph nodes in the axilla. The so-called "extended radical" operation involves the removal of both supraclavicular and internal mammary lymphatics as an extension of the usual procedure. In the "extended" procedure a part of the anterior chest wall and the medial end of the clavicle and first rib may be removed to permit "en bloc" removal of the supraclavicular and internal mammary lymph nodes and vessels.

Modified Radical Mastectomy—has become a most popular form of surgical treatment. It differs from the radical mastectomy in that the pectoralis major and minor muscles are preserved. The preservation of these muscles results in a more functional use of the upper extremities, but it does prevent performance of the classic en-bloc dissection of the axillary lymph nodes. However, adequate samplings of the nodes can be achieved.

Simple Mastectomy—consists of removal of the breast tissue, skin, and nipple, leaving the axillary nodes untouched. This technique is frequently followed by radiation and/or chemotherapy and breast reconstruction.

Excision of the Tumor Mass (Lumpectomy)—is performed for in situ and very small tumors or in the debilitated patient. It is followed by radiation therapy.

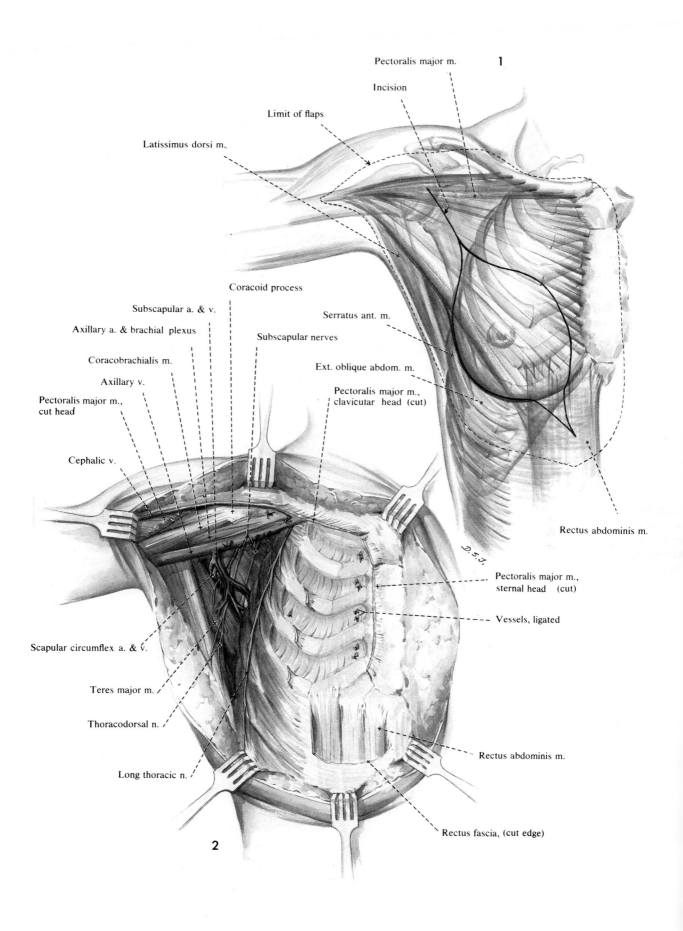

1

Pectoralis major m.

Incision

Limit of flaps

Latissimus dorsi m.

Coracoid process

Subscapular a. & v.

Axillary a. & brachial plexus

Coracobrachialis m.

Axillary v.

Pectoralis major m., cut head

Cephalic v.

Subscapular nerves

Serratus ant. m.

Ext. oblique abdom. m.

Pectoralis major m., clavicular head (cut)

Rectus abdominis m.

Pectoralis major m., sternal head (cut)

Vessels, ligated

Scapular circumflex a. & v.

Teres major m.

Thoracodorsal n.

Long thoracic n.

Rectus abdominis m.

Rectus fascia, (cut edge)

2

The Upper Extremity

THE BRACHIUM (ANTERIOR COMPARTMENT):

The brachium extends from the lower border of the teres major to a line drawn through the medial and lateral epicondyles of the humerus. It contains the extensor and flexor muscles of the brachium, the terminal branches of the brachial plexus, and the brachial artery and veins.

Superficial Fascia (Fig. 1):

Two main venous channels may be seen, one in the lateral bicipital groove, the *cephalic vein,* and the other in the medial bicipital groove, the *basilic.* The former has already been discussed on page 44. The basilic vein arises from the ulnar side of dorsal venous rete of the hand and ascends through the arm in the medial bicipital groove. At the midportion of the arm it pierces the deep brachial fascia, enters the neurovascular bundle, and joins the two brachial veins at the lower border of the teres major to form the axillary vein.

The cutaneous nerves of the arm and forearm are all direct or indirect branches of the cords of the brachial plexus. In addition to the brachial plexus, the lateral cutaneous branch of T_2 *(intercostobrachial)* extends into medial side of the arm. This explains why a brachial plexus block does not produce complete anesthesia of the arm.

Deep Fascia (Fig. 2):

The brachial fascia is a tough circular encasement for the muscles of this area. It is continuous above with the axillary, pectoral, and latissimus dorsi fascial coverings. Below, it is continuous with the antibrachial fascia and attaches to the epicondyles and the olecranon process. It sends septa medially and laterally to the humerus. The septa divide the brachium into two closed compartments, an anterior (flexor) and posterior (extensor), which limit effusions either hemorrhagic or inflammatory.

Muscular Contents (Figs. 3, 4, and 5):

The muscles related to the anterior compartment of the arm may be divided into two groups, an intrinsic group found within the flexor compartment, and an extrinsic group which inserts into the humerus.

Extrinsic Muscles;

1. DELTOID—arises from the clavicle, the acromion process and spine of the scapula and covers the joint, producing the rounded contour of the shoulder. It inserts on a tuberosity on the lateral aspect of the middle of the humeral shaft. It is mainly an abductor of the arm and is innervated by the axillary nerve.

2. SUBSCAPULAR—arises in the subscapular fossa of the scapula and inserts into the lesser tubercle of the humerus and forms part of the "rotator cuff" (page 78). Its chief function is medial rotation.

3. PECTORALIS MAJOR (page 44)—inserts into lateral lip of the bicipital groove of the humerus and acts as a flexor, adductor, and medial rotator of the humerus.

4. LATISSIMUS DORSI (page 44)—inserts into the bicipital groove.

5. TERES MAJOR (page 44)—gains attachment to medial lip of bicipital groove and acts as a medial rotator, adductor, and extensor.

Intrinsic Muscles—lie in the anterior or flexor compartment and are innervated by the musculocutaneous nerve.

1. CORACOBRACHIALIS—arises from the coracoid process of the scapula and inserts at the middle of the medial surface of the shaft of the humerus. It is pierced by the musculocutaneous nerve. This muscle acts as a flexor and adductor of the arm at the shoulder.

2. BICEPS BRACHII—the short head arises from the coracoid process; the long head takes origin from the supraglenoid tuberosity of the scapula. The biceps tendon inserts mainly into the radial tuberosity; however, some of its fibers expand medially and downward to insert in the antibrachial fascia *(lacertus fibrosus)* (Fig. 2). Aside from its function as a flexor of the forearm, it acts as a very strong supinator.

3. BRACHIALIS—takes origin from lower three-fifths of the shaft of the humerus under cover of the biceps and inserts on the coronoid process of the ulna. In addition to its innervation by the musculocutaneous, the lower lateral fibers usually receive a twig from the radial. It serves to flex the arm at the elbow.

Neurovascular Bundle (Fig. 5):

The neurovascular bundle lies in the medial bicipital groove and contains the brachial artery and three terminal branches of the brachial plexus, the musculocutaneous, ulnar, and median nerves.

1. **Musculocutaneous Nerve**—leaves the bundle in the upper arm, pierces the coracobrachialis, then descends between the brachialis and biceps, and continues superficially as the lateral antibrachial cutaneous. It supplies the three intrinsic muscles of the anterior compartment; the coracobrachialis, biceps and brachialis.

2. **Median Nerve**—is formed by medial and lateral heads as described in the axilla (page 46). In the upper arm the nerve lies lateral to the brachial artery, but in its descent through the arm it crosses anterior to the artery and comes to lie on the medial side in the lower arm and cubital region. It gives off no branches in the arm.

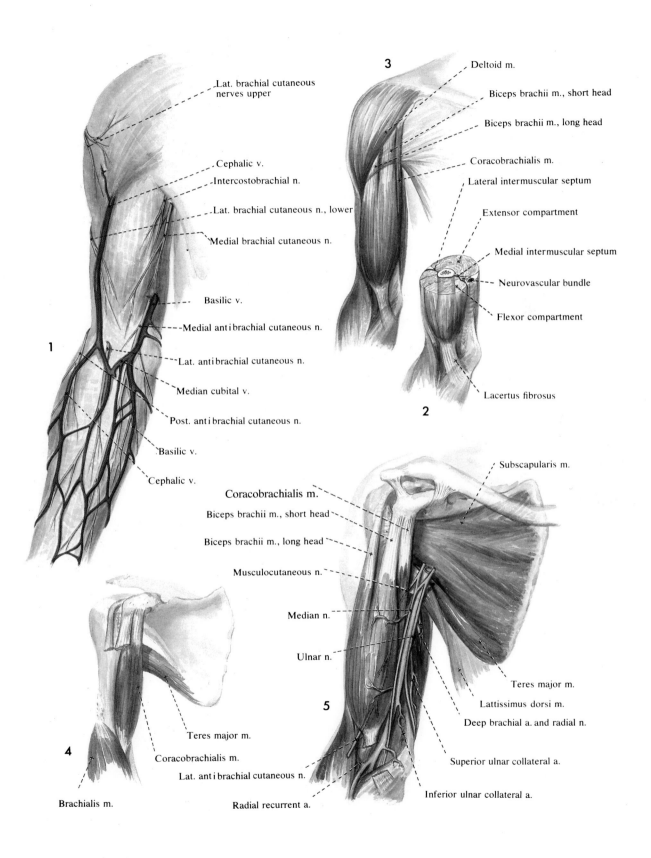

3

Deltoid m.

Biceps brachii m., short head

Biceps brachii m., long head

Coracobrachialis m.

Lateral intermuscular septum

Extensor compartment

Medial intermuscular septum

Neurovascular bundle

Flexor compartment

Lacertus fibrosus

2

Lat. brachial cutaneous nerves upper

Cephalic v.

Intercostobrachial n.

Lat. brachial cutaneous n., lower

Medial brachial cutaneous n.

Basilic v.

Medial antibrachial cutaneous n.

Lat. antibrachial cutaneous n.

Median cubital v.

Post. antibrachial cutaneous n.

Basilic v.

Cephalic v.

1

Subscapularis m.

Coracobrachialis m.

Biceps brachii m., short head

Biceps brachii m., long head

Musculocutaneous n.

Median n.

Ulnar n.

Teres major m.

Lattissimus dorsi m.

Deep brachial a. and radial n.

Superior ulnar collateral a.

Inferior ulnar collateral a.

5

Teres major m.

Coracobrachialis m.

Lat. antibrachial cutaneous n.

Brachialis m.

Radial recurrent a.

4

3. **Ulnar Nerve**—lies along the medial border of the brachial artery in the upper arm. At the insertion of coracobrachialis it pierces the medial intermuscular septum and enters the posterior compartment. It gives off no branches in the arm.

4. **Brachial Artery**—supplies the entire brachium. It begins at the lower border of the teres major as a continuation of the axillary and terminates at the elbow by dividing into a radial and ulnar branch. In addition to its muscular and nutrient branches, its main trunks are as follows:

a. DEEP BRACHIAL (PROFUNDA)—is the largest branch and leaves the bundle in the upper arm to enter the posterior compartment accompanied by the radial nerve.

b. SUPERIOR ULNAR COLLATERAL—arises from the brachial about midarm, pierces the medial intermuscular septum, and accompanies the ulnar nerve into the posterior compartment.

c. INFERIOR ULNAR COLLATERAL—takes origin just above the elbow from the medial side of the brachial descending anterior to the medial epicondyle.

The brachial artery is accompanied by two brachial veins, the *venae comitantes*. At the lower margin of the teres major these two veins join along with the basilic vein to form the axillary vein.

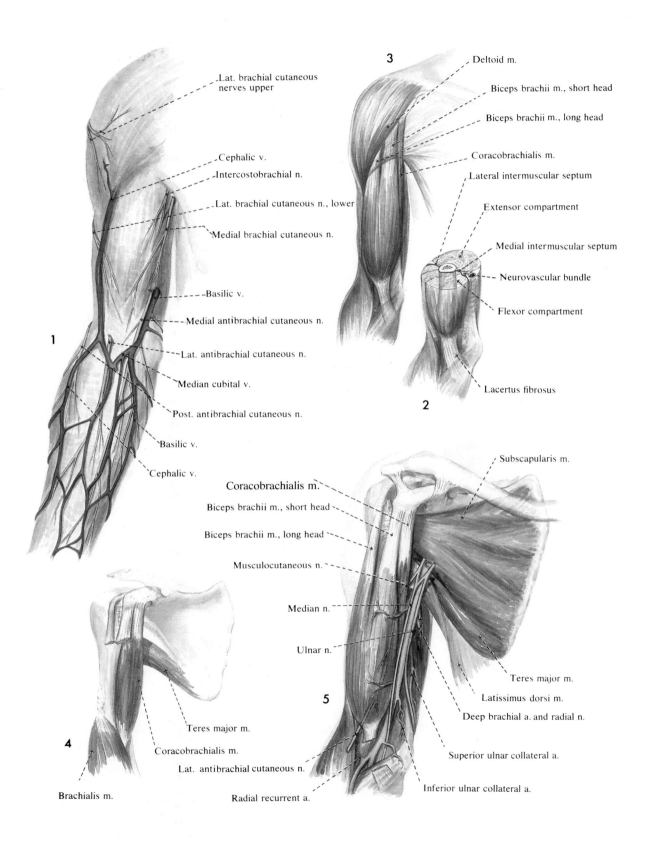

1

Lat. brachial cutaneous nerves upper

Cephalic v.

Intercostobrachial n.

Lat. brachial cutaneous n., lower

Medial brachial cutaneous n.

Basilic v.

Medial antibrachial cutaneous n.

Lat. antibrachial cutaneous n.

Median cubital v.

Post. antibrachial cutaneous n.

Basilic v.

Cephalic v.

3

Deltoid m.

Biceps brachii m., short head

Biceps brachii m., long head

Coracobrachialis m.

Lateral intermuscular septum

Extensor compartment

Medial intermuscular septum

Neurovascular bundle

Flexor compartment

Lacertus fibrosus

2

Subscapularis m.

Coracobrachialis m.

Biceps brachii m., short head

Biceps brachii m., long head

Musculocutaneous n.

Median n.

Ulnar n.

Teres major m.

Latissimus dorsi m.

Deep brachial a. and radial n.

Superior ulnar collateral a.

Inferior ulnar collateral a.

5

Teres major m.

Coracobrachialis m.

Lat. antibrachial cutaneous n.

4

Brachialis m.

Radial recurrent a.

THE BRACHIUM
(POSTERIOR COMPARTMENT):

Contains a single muscle and is of particular importance because of the presence of the radial nerve.

Superficial Fascia (Fig. 1):

The *lateral brachial cutaneous nerve,* a branch of the axillary, winds around the posterior border of the deltoid. Anesthesia in this area may be one of the early signs of injury to the axillary nerve.

Deep Fascia:

The brachial fascia has already been described on page 52. However, it may be noted here that it is more adherent to the muscle of this compartment than in the anterior compartment.

Muscular Contents (Figs. 1 and 2):

As in the anterior compartment, we may describe two groups of muscles associated with the humerus, an intrinsic (the triceps) and an extrinsic group. The latter group is made up of the deltoid and certain of the scapular muscles, the so-called SIT muscles, which insert on the greater tubercle of the humerus: the supraspinatus, infraspinatus, and teres minor. These three muscles are associated with the capsule of the shoulder joint and help form the posterior part of the "rotator cuff" (Fig. 4, page 79).

Extrinsic Muscles:

1. DELTOID — has been described on page 52. With retraction or removal of the posterior fibers, one may see its innervation by the axillary nerve. Accompanying the nerve is the posterior humeral circumflex artery.

2. SUPRASPINATUS — arises from the supraspinatus fossa and inserts into the superior facet of the greater tubercle. It is important in initiating abduction through the first 15 degrees, the deltoid then carrying through to 90 degrees. This muscle is innervated by the suprascapular nerve from the brachial plexus.

3. INFRASPINATUS — takes origin from the infraspinatus fossa and gains attachment to the middle facet of the greater tubercle. It is the main lateral rotator of the humerus and is innervated by the supraspinatus nerve. After removal of the muscle from the fossa, the circumflex scapular may be visualized with its important anastomosis with the transverse scapular forming a collateral channel between the first portion of the subclavian with the third portion of the axillary artery.

4. TERES MINOR — arises from axillary border of the scapula and inserts into the lower facet of the greater tubercle. It, too, is a lateral rotator of the humerus, but is innervated by a branch from the axillary nerve.

Intrinsic Muscles:

TRICEPS BRACHII — is usually divided anatomically into a long, lateral, and medial head. A more practical division is into a superficial and deep head. The *superficial head* consists of the long and lateral heads. The *long head* arises from the infraglenoid tuberosity of the scapula and the lateral head from the posterior surface of the humerus above the radial groove. These two heads fuse in a **V**-shaped manner. The *deep head (medial head)* arises from the posterior surface of the humerus below the radial groove. The heads fuse and insert into the olecranon process of the ulna. This muscle is the extensor of the forearm and, like all extensor muscles of the upper extremity, is innervated by the radial nerve.

Neurovascular Bundle (Fig. 2):

The neurovascular bundle of the posterior compartment lies in the radial groove and consists of the deep brachial artery and the radial nerve with their main branches. It may most adequately be exposed by dividing the two portions of the superficial head, i.e., the long and lateral.

1. **Deep Brachial Artery** — the largest of the three main branches of the brachial enters the posterior compartment between the long and lateral heads of the triceps where it gives rise to an important recurrent branch which anastomoses with the posterior humeral circumflex, forming a collateral channel between the brachial and axillary arteries. It descends laterally in the radial groove between the medial (deep) and lateral heads of the triceps accompanied by the radial nerve. In the groove it divides into a *posterior branch (medial collateral),* which passes behind the lateral epicondyle to enter into the cubital anastomosis. The *anterior branch (radial collateral)* pierces the lateral intermuscular septum and passes in front of the lateral epicondyle and also enters into the cubital anastomosis.

2. **Radial Nerve** — arises from the posterior cord of the brachial plexus in the axilla and enters the posterior compartment in the musculospiral (radial) groove of the humerus between the lateral and medial heads of the triceps. It may be divided into a (1) *common trunk,* (2) *superficial,* and (3) *deep branch.* The two latter branches are discussed on page 62.

COMMON RADIAL — innervates the three heads of the triceps and gives rise to the cutaneous branches to the posterior surface of the arm and forearm. It pierces the lateral intermuscular septum and lies between the brachioradialis and brachialis and here innervates the "lateral mobile wad" of the forearm extensors. Because of the intimate relation of the nerve to the humerus, it is frequently injured in fractures of the humeral shaft.

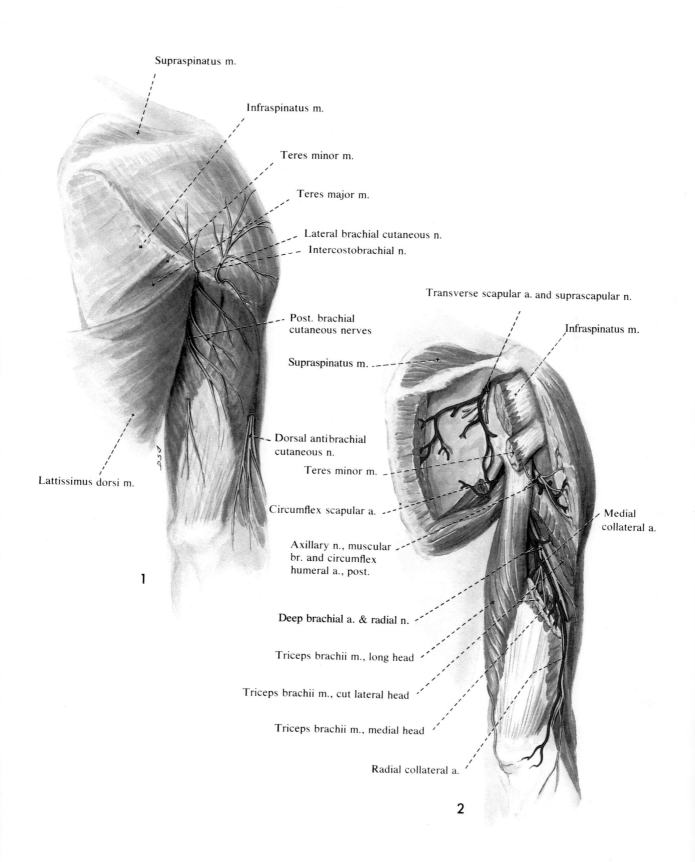

Supraspinatus m.

Infraspinatus m.

Teres minor m.

Teres major m.

Lateral brachial cutaneous n.

Intercostobrachial n.

Post. brachial cutaneous nerves

Supraspinatus m.

Dorsal antibrachial cutaneous n.

Lattissimus dorsi m.

Teres minor m.

Circumflex scapular a.

Axillary n., muscular br. and circumflex humeral a., post.

Transverse scapular a. and suprascapular n.

Infraspinatus m.

Medial collateral a.

Deep brachial a. & radial n.

Triceps brachii m., long head

Triceps brachii m., cut lateral head

Triceps brachii m., medial head

Radial collateral a.

1

2

MUSCLE ATTACHMENTS TO THE HUMERUS:

Since muscle pull plays such a determinant role in the displacement of fractures of the humerus and in their correct management, Figure 1 is devoted to the important muscle attachments to this bone.

1. **Supraspinatus** — is inserted into the superior facet of the greater tubercle of the humerus and the capsule of the shoulder joint.

2. **Subscapularis** — inserts into the lesser tubercle and joint capsule as well as into the humeral shaft for about 1 inch distal to the tubercle.

3. **Pectoralis Major** — gains attachment to the lateral lip of the bicipital groove of the humerus.

4. **Latissimus Dorsi** — attaches to the floor of the bicipital groove.

5. **Teres Major** — inserts into the medial lip of the bicipital groove.

6. **Deltoid** — inserts into the deltoid tuberosity on the middle of the lateral side of the humerus.

7. **Coracobrachialis** — attaches opposite the deltoid on the medial side of the shaft of the humerus.

8. **Biceps Brachii** — although neither arising nor inserting on the humerus, influences bone displacement of fractures of that bone because of the upward pull exerted by its insertion into the tuberosity of the radius.

9. **Brachialis** (Fig. 4, page 53) — arises from the distal three-fifths of the anterior surface of the humerus and inserts on the coronoid process of the ulna.

10. **Infraspinatus and Teres Minor** (Fig. 2, page 57) — insert into the middle and lower facets of the greater tubercle of the humerus, respectively.

FRACTURES OF THE UPPER END OF THE HUMERUS:

These may be grouped as follows: fractures of the anatomic neck, of the tubercles, separation of the epiphysis, and fracture of the surgical neck.

1. **Fractures at the Anatomic Neck** — the anatomic neck is a narrow strip that encircles the margins of the head. The usual cause of fracture is a fall upon the shoulder, and the bony fragments are impacted rather than displaced.

2. **Fractures of the Tubercles** — if the tubercle is separated from the humerus, the arm will be drawn in the direction of pull of the intact muscles. As an example, when the greater tubercle is detached, the supra- and infraspinatus and teres minor muscles pull the detached fragment upward and backward out of control, allowing the arm to be rotated medially by the intact subscapular muscle.

3. **Fracture at the Surgical Neck** (Fig. 2) — the surgical neck is the region immediately distal to the head and tubercles where the proximal end of the humerus and the shaft join. Fractures here usually result from falls on the elbow when the arm is abducted, but the deformity is the result of muscle pull rather than the direction of the injuring force. The fracture line occurs above the insertion of the pectoralis major, teres major, and latissimus dorsi insertions. The abducted proximal fragment is controlled mainly by the supraspinatus which is the most powerful muscle attached to it. The distal fragment is pulled inward by the pectoralis major, teres major, and latissimus dorsi, and upward by the deltoid, biceps, and coracobrachialis muscles.

Reduction is effected by traction on the arm parallel with the body. This makes taut the tendon of the long head of the biceps which rolls the proximal fragment of the humerus into its normal position and holds it there.

4. **Separation of the Upper Epiphysis** — normally the epiphysis fuses by the twenty-first year; consequently, separations occur before that age. Since the epiphysis includes the tubercles, the displacement that occurs with separation is similar to that in fractures through the surgical neck.

FRACTURES OF THE SHAFT OF THE HUMERUS:

The shaft of the humerus extends from the surgical neck to the supracondylar ridges and is usually injured by a direct force resulting in a transverse fracture. Displacement of the fragments varies depending on the relation of the fracture to the insertion of the deltoid muscle. Delayed union or nonunion of fractures of the midshaft is not uncommon. This may be explained in part by the fact that the nutrient artery of the humerus enters the bone near its middle and may be ruptured in fractures in this region. Another frequent complication is radial nerve injury. The possibility of this complication is obvious because of the intimate relationship of the nerve to the humeral shaft (Fig. 2, page 57).

1. **Fracture of the Shaft Above the Deltoid Insertion** (Fig. 3) — results in *adduction* of the *proximal fragment* because of the muscular pull exerted by the pectoralis major, latissimus dorsi, teres major, and supscapularis muscles. The *distal fragment* is *abducted* and pulled *upward* by the powerful deltoid.

2. **Fracture of the Shaft Below the Deltoid Insertion** (Fig. 4) — results in *abduction* of the *proximal fragment* by the deltoid and *elevation* of the *distal fragment* by the upward pull of the triceps, biceps, and coracobrachialis muscles.

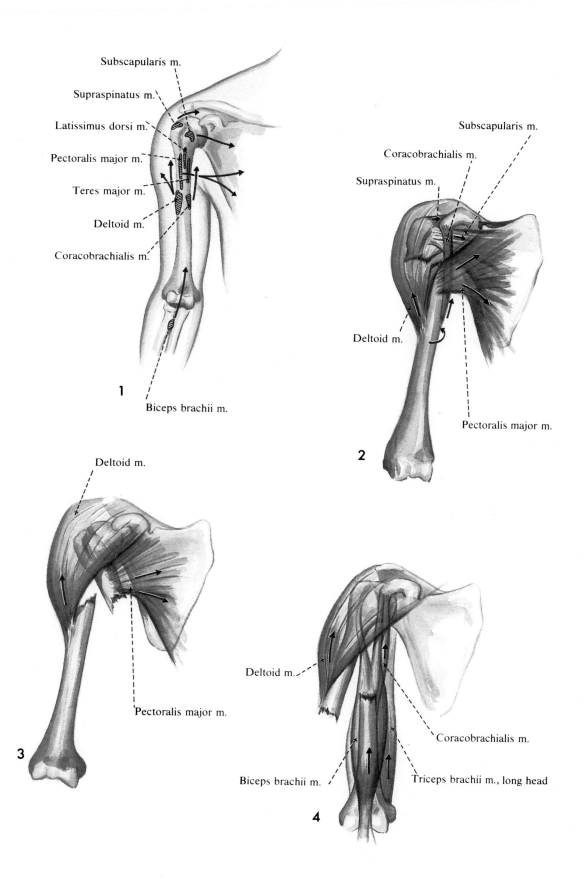

Subscapularis m.

Supraspinatus m.

Latissimus dorsi m.

Pectoralis major m.

Teres major m.

Deltoid m.

Coracobrachialis m.

1

Biceps brachii m.

Subscapularis m.

Coracobrachialis m.

Supraspinatus m.

Deltoid m.

Pectoralis major m.

2

Deltoid m.

Pectoralis major m.

3

Deltoid m.

Coracobrachialis m.

Biceps brachii m.

Triceps brachii m., long head

4

FRACTURES OF THE LOWER END OF THE HUMERUS:

These occur in great variety and in large numbers in childhood and are due principally to falls on the out-stretched hand. The force is transmitted through the bones of the forearm to the wide and flattened end of the humerus, which is weakened by the presence of the olecranon, coronoid, and radial fossae. Also, the superficial position of the epicondyles exposes them to fracture by direct injury.

Fractures in this region include separation of the epiphyses, particularly the medial epiphysis; fracture of the epicondyles; and condylar, intercondylar, and supracondylar fractures. The mechanics of displacement and of neurovascular complications of supracondylar fractures are shown in Figs. 1, 2, and 3.

DISPLACEMENT IN SUPRACONDYLAR FRACTURES:

By far the most common type of supracondylar fracture is the so-called extension type in which the injuring force carries the distal fragment of the humerus posteriorly, and the triceps, brachialis, and biceps muscles produce overriding of the two fragments. Not only is this more frequent than the so-called flexion type of supracondylar fracture, in which the distal fragment is displaced anteriorly, but it accounts for most of the neurovascular complications in association with fractures about the elbow (Fig. 3). The fracture line often extends inferiorly through one of the fossae into the joint resulting in T-shaped or Y-shaped fractures.

PRINCIPLES OF REDUCTION IN SUPRACONDYLAR FRACTURES:

Traction is necessary to achieve reduction, and acute flexion with the tightened triceps tendon serving as a splint is necessary to maintain it.

Because of the break in the continuity of the humerus the strong supinating action of the biceps is lost. In consequence, the elbow joint comes under control of the pronators and is held in full pronation. Attempts to place the forearm in even slight supination results in a varus deformity since the elbow is fixed by the pronators. In the management of these fractures the forearm is placed in full pronation during and after reduction (Figs. 1 and 2).

NEUROVASCULAR COMPLICATIONS IN SUPRACONDYLAR FRACTURES:

The injuring force carries the condyles backward and strips the periosteum away from the posterior surface of the proximal fragment. The anterior edge of the proximal fragment often tears the periosteum and injures the attached soft tissues. Thus, the brachial artery and the median and radial nerves may be damaged with the initial injury, or they may be compressed subsequently by fragments of bone, by blood that infiltrates the anticubital fossa, or by callus formation (Fig. 3).

SURGICAL EXPOSURE OF THE HUMERUS:

Anterior Approach:

Any part of the incision shown in Fig. 4 may be used to expose the underlying humerus. For example, the incision may go from the lower margin of the clavicle near the tip of the coracoid process of the scapula to the deltoid tuberosity if exposure of only the upper one-third of the humerus is needed. Retraction of the deltoid laterally exposes the humerus lateral to the bicipital groove (Fig. 3, page 81).

An extension of this incision distally permits exposure of the midshaft of the humerus. When carried still further, the lower one-third of the shaft can be exposed in the interval between the brachioradialis laterally and the brachial and biceps muscles medially.

Posterior Approach:

The relationship of the *axillary nerve* beneath the deltoid muscle to the posterior aspect of the surgical neck of the humerus, and the relation of the *radial nerve* to the posterior surface of the shaft of the humerus, must be constantly in the mind of the surgeon approaching the humerus from behind (Fig. 2, page 57).

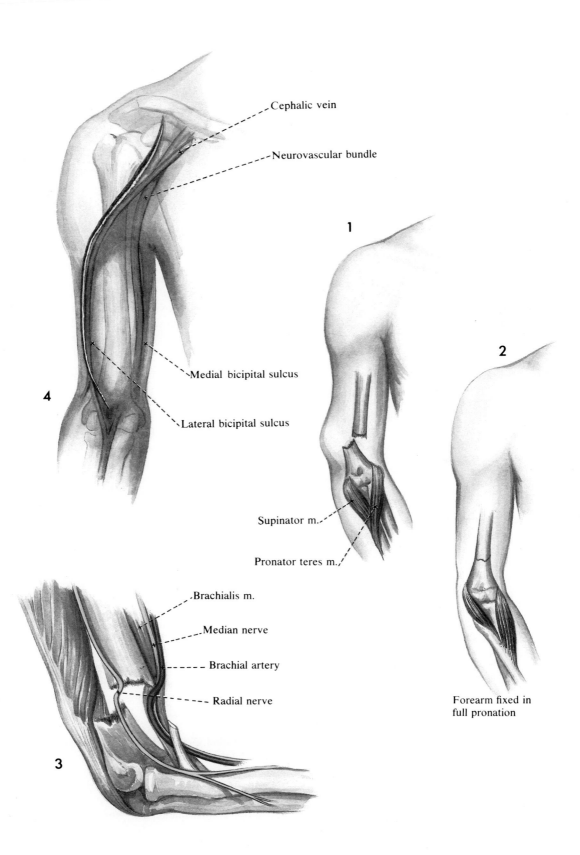

Cephalic vein

Neurovascular bundle

1

2

Medial bicipital sulcus

4

Lateral bicipital sulcus

Supinator m.

Pronator teres m.

Brachialis m.

Median nerve

Brachial artery

Radial nerve

Forearm fixed in
full pronation

3

THE ANTIBRACHIUM
(ANTERIOR COMPARTMENT):

The antibrachium extends from a line drawn between the two humeral epicondyles and terminates at the lower cutaneous fold of the wrist. Like the brachium, it may be divided into an anterior (flexor) and a posterior (extensor) compartment.

Deep Fascia:

The antibrachial fascia is thickened over the anterior surface of the wrist joint to form the *volar carpal ligament* and over its posterior surface to form the *dorsal carpal ligament* (Fig. 1, page 65).

Muscular Contents:

The muscles of the anterior compartment may be divided into four layers. With the exception of one and a half muscles (flexor carpi ulnaris and one-half of the flexor digitorum profundus) they are innervated by the median nerve.

1. **First Layer** — all arise from the medial epicondyle and the ulna (Fig. 1).

a. PRONATOR TERES — inserts into middle third of lateral surface of the radius and is pierced by the median nerve.

b. FLEXOR CARPI RADIALIS — inserts into base of the second and third metacarpals.

c. PALMARIS LONGUS — at its insertion becomes continuous with the palmar aponeurosis.

d. FLEXOR CARPI ULNARIS — gains its main attachment into the pisiform bone. It is pierced and innervated by the ulnar nerve.

2. **Second Layer** — consists of only one muscle with an extensive origin (Fig. 2).

FLEXOR DIGITORUM SUBLIMIS — arises from the humerus, ulna, intermuscular septum, and radius. Between the humeral and septal attachments a tendinous *sublimis tunnel* is formed under which passes the ulnar artery and median nerve. Its four tendons insert into the shafts of the middle phalanges of the second to fifth fingers. The median nerve is adherent to its under surface.

3. **Third Layer** — is made up of two muscles whose tendons extend into the terminal phalanx of all the fingers (Fig. 3).

a. FLEXOR DIGITORUM PROFUNDUS — takes origin from the ulna and adjacent intermuscular septum and inserts on the terminal phalanx of the second to fifth finger. The ulnar half of the muscle is innervated by the ulnar nerve; its radial half is innervated by the median nerve.

b. FLEXOR POLLICIS LONGUS — takes origin from the radius and adjacent intermuscular septum, to insert on the terminal phalanx of the thumb. It is innervated by the median nerve.

4. **Fourth Layer** — made up of one muscle in the distal portion of the forearm (Fig. 4).

PRONATOR QUADRATUS — arises from the volar surface of the ulna and inserts into the volar surface of the radius.

Blood Supply (Figs. 2, 3, and 4):

The blood vessels of the anterior compartment are the terminal branches of the brachial artery. The latter terminates at the level of the neck of the radius by dividing into a radial and ulnar branch.

1. **Radial Artery** — is the smaller of the two terminal branches, lies superficial in position in the forearm, but under cover of the brachioradialis muscle in most of its course. Shortly after its origin, it gives rise to a *radial recurrent* which anastomoses with the anterior branch of the profundus. In addition to muscular branches it gives rise to an important *superficial volar branch* and a *radial volar carpal artery* (Fig. 2, page 71).

2. **Ulnar Artery** — passes through the sublimis tunnel and immediately gives rise to two branches, the *volar* and *dorsal recurrents,* which anastomose with the inferior and superior ulnar collaterals, respectively. It then gives origin to the *common interosseous,* which in turn gives off an *interosseous recurrent* which joins with the posterior (radial) branch of the profunda (Fig. 1, page 65). In addition the common interosseous gives rise to the *volar* and *dorsal interossei* lying on the respective surfaces of the interosseous membrane. It also supplies muscular, nutrient, and carpal branches.

Nerve Supply (Figs. 2 and 3):

The main supply to the anterior compartment is by the median nerve, innervating all but one and one-half muscles.

1. **Median Nerve** — descends into the anticubital fossa between the heads of the pronator teres and becomes adherent to the under surface of the flexor digitorum sublimis muscle. In the lower third of the forearm it lies superficial in position between the tendons of the palmaris longus on the ulnar side and the flexor carpi radialis on the radial side. It continues into the wrist, deep to the transverse carpal ligament. In the anticubital fossa it sends off branches to the pronator teres, flexor carpi radialis, palmaris longus, and flexor digitorum sublimis. At the level of the radial tuberosity, it gives rise to the volar interosseous, which accompanies the artery of the same name, to innervate the muscles of the third and fourth layers.

2. **Ulnar Nerve** — lies in a groove on the posterior aspect of the medial epicondyle at the elbow, then pierces the flexor carpi ulnaris to gain access to the flexor compartment of the forearm. It supplies the flexor carpi ulnaris, and the ulnar half of the profundus. The nerve descends to the wrist where it passes superficial to the transverse carpal ligament but deep to the volar carpal ligament.

3. **Radial Nerve** — the *common radial* appears in the cubital region between the brachialis and brachioradialis and, after innervating the "lateral mobile wad" of muscles of the extensor group, divides into a superficial and deep branch. The *deep radial* passes to the posterior compartment. The *superficial radial,* which is entirely sensory, passes through the anterior compartment under cover of the brachioradialis running parallel with the radial artery. At the lower third of the forearm it pierces the deep fascia and appears on the dorsum of the hand.

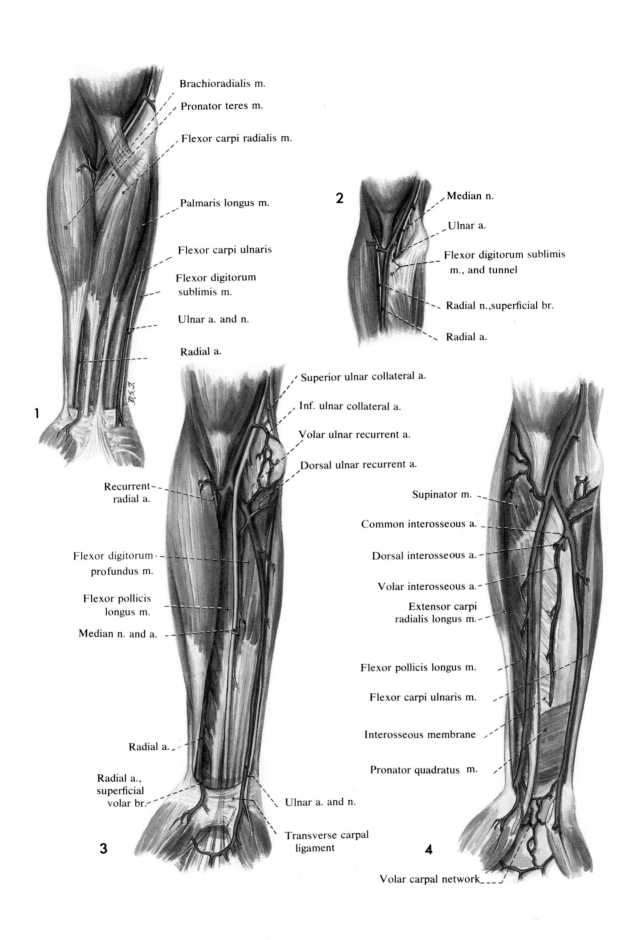

Brachioradialis m.

Pronator teres m.

Flexor carpi radialis m.

2

Median n.

Ulnar a.

Palmaris longus m.

Flexor digitorum sublimis m., and tunnel

Flexor carpi ulnaris

Flexor digitorum sublimis m.

Radial n.,superficial br.

Ulnar a. and n.

Radial a.

Radial a.

1

Superior ulnar collateral a.

Inf. ulnar collateral a.

Volar ulnar recurrent a.

Dorsal ulnar recurrent a.

Recurrent radial a.

Supinator m.

Common interosseous a.

Flexor digitorum profundus m.

Dorsal interosseous a.

Volar interosseous a.

Flexor pollicis longus m.

Extensor carpi radialis longus m.

Median n. and a.

Flexor pollicis longus m.

Flexor carpi ulnaris m.

Interosseous membrane

Radial a.

Pronator quadratus m.

Radial a., superficial volar br.

Ulnar a. and n.

Transverse carpal ligament

3

4

Volar carpal network

THE ANTIBRACHIUM (POSTERIOR COMPARTMENT):

This compartment contains the extensor muscles of the forearm, the deep (posterior interosseous) branch of the radial nerve, and the posterior interosseous branch of the ulnar artery.

Superficial Fascia (Fig. 1, page 53):

Deep Fascia (Fig. 1):

A thickening of this layer of fascia occurs over the dorsum of the wrist and is termed the *dorsal carpal ligament*.

Muscular Contents:

The muscles in this compartment may be divided into two layers, a superficial and deep.

1. **Superficial Layer** (Fig. 1)—of muscles has a closely associated origin extending from the lateral epicondylar ridge of the humerus to the lateral epicondyle. They may be subdivided into three groups: lateral (three muscles), intermediate (two muscles), and medial (one muscle).

a. LATERAL—also described as the "lateral mobile wad" because they may be grasped as a group at the lateral boundary of the cubital space. Topographically, this group may be utilized in the surgical approach to the radial head, the incision being placed along the posterior extension of this muscle mass. Since they are all innervated by the *common* radial nerve, their functional status is important in determining the level of injury of the radial nerve in the upper extremity.

(1) *Brachioradialis*—becomes tendinous at mid-forearm and inserts on the base of the styloid process of the radius. Although included with the extensor muscles and innervated by the radial nerve, it actually acts to flex the elbow. (Fig. 1, Page 63).

(2) *Extensor Carpi Radialis Longus*—extends to the base of the second metacarpal. It functions as an extensor and a radial abductor of the wrist.

(3) *Extensor Carpi Radialis Brevis*—inserts into the base of the third metacarpal and acts in a similar fashion as the extensor longus.

b. INTERMEDIATE—consists of two muscles arising from the lateral epicondyle, extending to the dorsal assembly of the phalanges and innervated by the *deep* radial nerve.

(1) *Extensor Digitorum Communis*—divides above the wrist into four tendons which extend to the fingers as part of the dorsal assembly over the phalanges. They act mainly to extend the metacarpophalangeal joints of the fingers.

(2) *Extensor Digiti Quinti Proprius*—supplies an additional tendon into the dorsal assembly allowing for independent extension of the little finger.

c. MEDIAL—is made up of a single muscle which receives its nerve supply from the *deep* radial nerve.

Extensor Carpi Ulnaris—is inserted into the base of the fifth metacarpal and acts mainly as an ulnar deviator of the wrist and only weakly as an extensor.

2. **Deep Layer** (Fig. 2)—these muscles arise from the radius, interosseous membrane, and ulna and insert mainly on the thumb and index finger. All are innervated by the *deep* radial nerve.

a. SUPINATOR—arises from lateral epicondyle and upper ulna and inserts on the lateral volar surface of upper radius. As the name suggests, it acts as a supinator of the forearm.

b. ABDUCTOR POLLICIS LONGUS—takes rise from the ulna and interosseous membrane to insert on the base of the first metacarpal and acts to abduct the thumb.

c. EXTENSOR POLLICIS BREVIS—originates from the radius and interosseous membrane and inserts on the base of the proximal phalanx of the thumb. It acts to extend the metacarpophalangeal joint.

d. EXTENSOR POLLICIS LONGUS—arises from the ulna and adjacent interosseous membrane to insert on the base of the distal phalanx of the thumb. Its main function is to extend the distal phalanx.

e. EXTENSOR INDICIS PROPRIUS—arises from the ulna and interosseous membrane and extends to the dorsal assembly of the index finger. It adds extensor power to the metacarpophalangeal joint of the index finger.

Anconeus—although located in this compartment, this muscle is morphologically and physiologically a part of the triceps. It arises from the lateral epicondyle and inserts into the olecranon process and adjacent shaft of the ulna. It receives its nerve supply from the radial trunk by a branch arising in the radial groove.

Neurovascular Bundle (Fig. 2):

The neurovascular bundle in the posterior compartment of the forearm appears between the superficial and deep layers of muscles at the lower border of the supinator muscle as it emerges under the *tendinous supinator arc*. It is made up of the dorsal interosseous artery and nerve (deep radial).

1. **Dorsal Interosseous Artery**—arises from the common interosseous branch of the ulnar artery in the anterior compartment. It emerges between the supinator and abductor pollicis longus and supplies the muscles of the compartment. It gives rise to the *interosseous recurrent* artery which enters into the cubital anastomosis (Fig. 1).

2. **Dorsal Interosseous Nerve (Deep Radial)**—takes origin from the common radial in the anterior compartment, pierces the supinator and enters the posterior compartment. It innervates all muscles of the posterior compartment except the lateral superficial group. Injury to this nerve results in the typical "wrist drop."

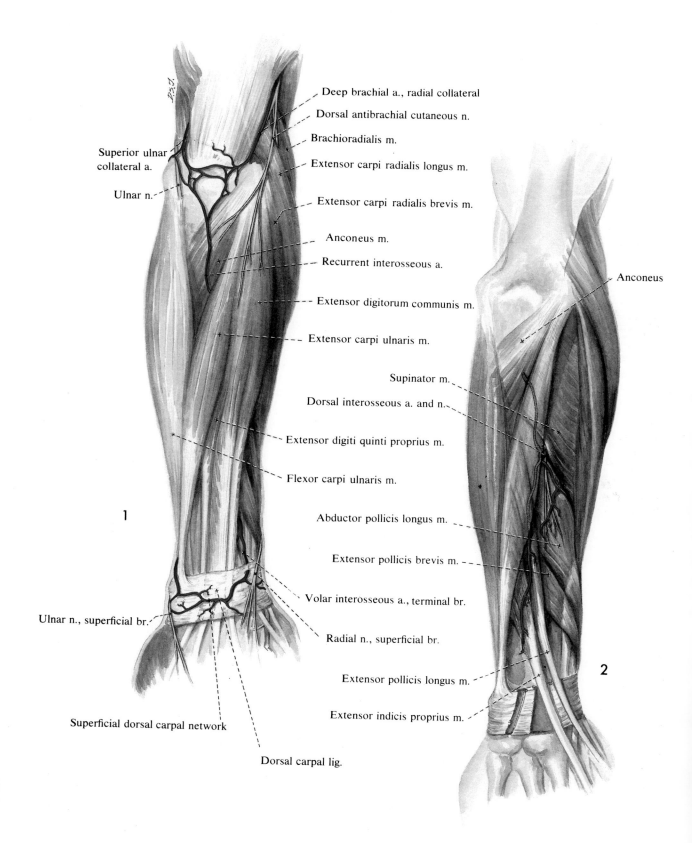

Deep brachial a., radial collateral

Dorsal antibrachial cutaneous n.

Brachioradialis m.

Superior ulnar collateral a.

Extensor carpi radialis longus m.

Ulnar n.

Extensor carpi radialis brevis m.

Anconeus m.

Recurrent interosseous a.

Anconeus

Extensor digitorum communis m.

Extensor carpi ulnaris m.

Supinator m.

Dorsal interosseous a. and n.

Extensor digiti quinti proprius m.

Flexor carpi ulnaris m.

Abductor pollicis longus m.

Extensor pollicis brevis m.

Volar interosseous a., terminal br.

Ulnar n., superficial br.

Radial n., superficial br.

Extensor pollicis longus m.

Superficial dorsal carpal network

Extensor indicis proprius m.

Dorsal carpal lig.

1

2

CLINICAL CONSIDERATIONS OF
THE FOREARM (ANTIBRACHIUM):

The surgical anatomy of the forearm is concerned principally with fractures: the forces that account for displacement, the anatomical facts bearing on their reduction and fixation, and the surgical approach to the bones when open reduction is necessary. Occasionally, in addition, the surgeon must expose one of the bones or other structures in the forearm for the removal of a tumor or repair of an injury other than fracture.

Fractures of the Bones of the Forearm:

From the standpoint of fractures, the shaft of the ulna may be considered a continuation of the humerus, whereas the radius is an upward continuation of the hand. With a fall on the pronated hand, the main force is communicated to the distal end of the radius and passes upward to the humerus. A fracture of the radius alone or of both the radius and ulna may result. When due to such indirect violence, the fractures usually occur at different levels but the fracture of the ulna is usually at the distal end.

The displacement in fractures of the bones of the forearm is usually considerable. The muscles tend to pull the distal fragments proximally. In addition the pronator teres and pronator quadratus pull the two bones toward one another, tending to obliterate the interosseous space.

1. **Isolated Fractures of the Ulna** — are always due to direct violence and tend to be compound because of the subcutaneous position of the posterior border of the bone. The direction of the injuring force plays a major role in displacement of the fragments of this bone.

2. **Fractures of the Shaft of the Radius** — in these, however, displacement depends largely upon the pull of muscles rather than upon the fracturing force. In consequence, displacement varies with the level of the fracture.

a. FRACTURES OF THE SHAFT OF THE RADIUS ABOVE THE INSERTION OF THE PRONATOR TERES (Figs. 1 and 2) — and below the insertion of the supinator result in a rotation deformity due to the pull of the biceps and supinator on the proximal fragment (flexed and supinated) and the now unopposed pull of the pronator teres and pronator quadratus on the distal fragment.

b. FRACTURES OF THE RADIAL SHAFT BELOW THE INSERTION OF THE PRONATOR TERES (Fig. 3) — the proximal fragment is brought anteriorly (flexed) by the biceps and medially by the pronator teres, but it tends to remain in the neutral position as regards rotation because the action of the biceps and supinator opposes that of the pronator teres. The lower fragment is displaced toward the ulna by the pronator quadratus, the brachioradialis, and the extensors and abductors of the thumb. With the ulna and the inferior radioulnar joint intact, there is usually no overriding of fragments.

Surgical Approach to the Long Bones of the Forearm:

1. **Ulna** — may be exposed along its entire length without jeopardy to any important structure by an incision along its posterior margin which lies between the flexor carpi ulnaris and the extensor carpi ulnaris.

2. **Radius** — is more difficult to expose. An anterior or posterior approach may be used. The topographic landmark for either approach is the "lateral mobile wad" of muscles consisting of the brachioradialis and extensor carpi radialis longus and brevis. These three muscles can be moved as a unit across the part of the radius covered by the supinator, independent of the neighboring muscles. The anterior and posterior edges of the "wad" serve as guides for the incision.

For an anterior approach to the entire shaft of the radius, an incision is begun in the antibrachium just lateral to the biceps tendon and extended distally along the anterior border of the brachioradialis as far as the wrist. The deep fascia is divided along the length of the incision. The brachioradialis and extensor carpi radialis longus and brevis are mobilized as a unit by dividing the recurrent radical vessels (Fig. 3, page 63). The supinator muscle is peeled off the radius and retracted laterally. This maneuver exposes the underlying radial shaft and protects the deep radial (dorsal interosseous) nerve which pierces the supinator. The forearm is placed in a pronated position to expose the entire shaft of the radius.

To expose the radius via a posterior approach an incision is made along the posterior edge of the lateral mobile wad of muscles (Fig. 4). The antibrachial fascia is opened and the extensor digitorum communis muscle is identified and carefully separated from the extensor carpi radialis brevis. The two muscles are then retracted to expose the deeper-lying supinator muscle (Fig. 5). Care must be taken to isolate and protect the deep radial nerve as it pierces the supinator muscle. The forearm is then supinated in order to locate the anterior margin of the muscle which is cut to expose the shaft. Additional exposure of the radius is obtained by elevation and retraction of the abductor pollicis longus and the extensor pollicis brevis muscles (Fig. 5).

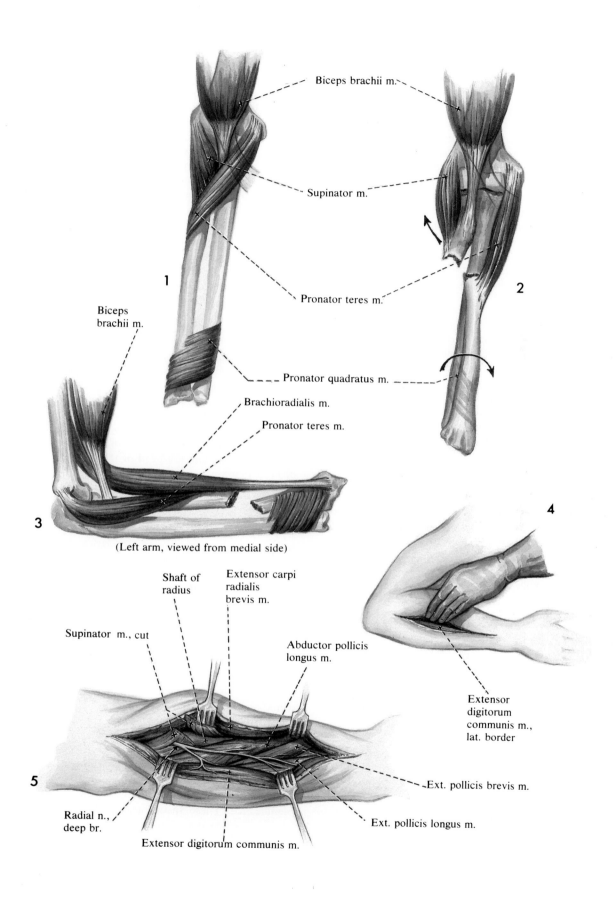

Biceps brachii m.

Supinator m.

Pronator teres m.

1

2

Biceps
brachii m.

Pronator quadratus m.

Brachioradialis m.

Pronator teres m.

3

(Left arm, viewed from medial side)

4

Shaft of
radius

Extensor carpi
radialis
brevis m.

Supinator m., cut

Abductor pollicis
longus m.

Extensor
digitorum
communis m.,
lat. border

5

Ext. pollicis brevis m.

Radial n.,
deep br.

Ext. pollicis longus m.

Extensor digitorum communis m.

THE HAND (PALMAR OR VOLAR SURFACE):

Two major eminences are present on the palmar surface: the *thenar eminence* on the radial side, and the *hypothenar eminence* on the ulnar side. These eminences correspond to the thenar and hypothenar muscular compartments. Smaller eminences are seen in the distal palm between the phalanges, the *monticuli*, beneath which the common digital arteries and nerves divide into their proper digital branches (Fig. 1).

Certain of the skin creases are of topographic importance. The proximal skin crease at the wrist marks the level of the wrist joint, and the distal skin crease (*rasceta*), the proximal border of the transverse carpal ligament. The creases on the phalanges overlie the interphalangeal joints. The remainder of the skin creases are of significance only in that incisions in the palm should not cross these creases.

Superficial Fascia (Fig. 2):

This layer is sparse, particularly over midpalm where the skin is adherent to deep fascia. Three *palmar cutaneous nerves* are present in this layer in its proximal part, arising from the radial, median, and ulnar nerves. A small subcutaneous muscle also is found in this layer, the *palmaris brevis*, which is innervated by the ulnar nerve. This muscle is usually well developed when the palmaris longus is absent.

Deep (Palmar) Fascia (Fig. 2):

The palmar fascia is divided into three parts: the *thenar fascia* covering the muscles of the thenar compartment, the *hypothenar fascia* covering the muscles of the hypothenar compartment, and the *palmar aponeurosis*, a thickened portion of the deep fascia over the middle compartment. The latter fibers radiate from the palmaris longis tendons to the phalanges.

Middle Compartment:

1. **Superficial Neurovascular Structures** (Fig. 3) — with the removal of the palmar fascia the superficial vessels and nerves of the palm are seen.

   a. SUPERFICIAL VOLAR ARCH — is formed mainly by the superficial branch of the ulnar artery. This artery in turn usually joins the superficial volar branch of the radial to complete the arch. Topographically, the arch lies about three fingers' breadth distal to the rasceta. From the arch arise a number of small muscular and skin branches. One of the latter is a *proper digital* to the ulnar side of the little finger. Three *common digitals* also arise from the convexity of the arch, descend through the palm, and supply proper digital branches to all fingers except the radial side of the index finger, which is supplied by the deep arch.

   b. SUPERFICIAL ULNAR NERVE — arises from the volar branch of the ulna at the wrist superficial to the transverse carpal ligament and gives off a ramus to the palmaris brevis and a communicating branch to the median nerve. It then supplies a proper digital branch to the ulnar side of the little finger and a common digital which supplies the adjacent margins of the little and ring fingers.

   c. MEDIAN NERVE — passes from the forearm deep to the transverse carpal ligament, where it divides into a medial and lateral division. The medial division receives a communicating branch from the ulnar and sends two common digital branches which supply adjacent sides of the index and middle and middle and ring fingers, respectively. The lateral division is a common digital nerve dividing into three proper digitals to supply the thumb and radial side of the index finger. An important motor nerve also arises from this lateral division, the *recurrent branch*; this nerve supplies the three thenar muscles: the abductor, flexor, and opponens pollicis. The median nerve in the palm also supplies the two radial lumbricals.

2. **Superficial Musculotendinous Structures** (Fig. 3) — in the middle compartment, deep to the superficial neurovascular structures, lie the long tendons of the phalanges, the *flexor digitorum sublimis* and *profundus*. The sublimis tendons split to attach to the middle phalanges, whereas the profundus tendons insert on the distal phalanges. The tendons enter an osseofibrous tunnel which extends from the head of the metacarpals to the distal phalanx.

   The *fibrous tendon sheath* prevents the tendons from bowstringing during flexion. The sheath is thin over the joints, and the fibers are crossed (*cruciate ligament*), whereas over the phalanges the fibers are strong and transversely arranged (*annular ligament*).

   The *mucous tendon sheaths* lie deep to the fibrous sheath and extend from the neck of the metacarpals to the insertion of the profundus tendon. The sheaths of the thumb and little finger extend to the carpal region as the *radial* and *ulnar bursae* (Fig. 1, page 75).

   The *lumbrical muscles* are four in number, arising from the tendons of the flexor digitorum profundus (Fig. 3). These muscles pass to the radial side of the fingers and insert on the extensor assembly (Fig. 4, page 73). The two lumbricals on the radial side are innervated by the median nerve; the other two are innervated by the deep ulnar nerve. These muscles along with the interossei flex the metacarpophalangeal joints and extend the interphalangeal joints.

3. **Fascial Spaces** — between the long flexor tendons and the deep muscles of the middle compartment are located potential fascial spaces which are of surgical significance. These spaces are considered on page 74.

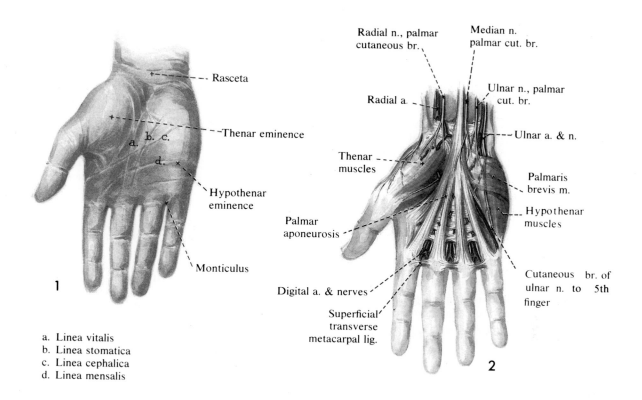

Rasceta

Thenar eminence

a. b. c.

d.

Hypothenar eminence

Monticulus

1

a. Linea vitalis
b. Linea stomatica
c. Linea cephalica
d. Linea mensalis

Radial n., palmar cutaneous br.

Median n. palmar cut. br.

Radial a.

Ulnar n., palmar cut. br.

Thenar muscles

Ulnar a. & n.

Palmar aponeurosis

Palmaris brevis m.

Hypothenar muscles

Digital a. & nerves

Cutaneous br. of ulnar n. to 5th finger

Superficial transverse metacarpal lig.

2

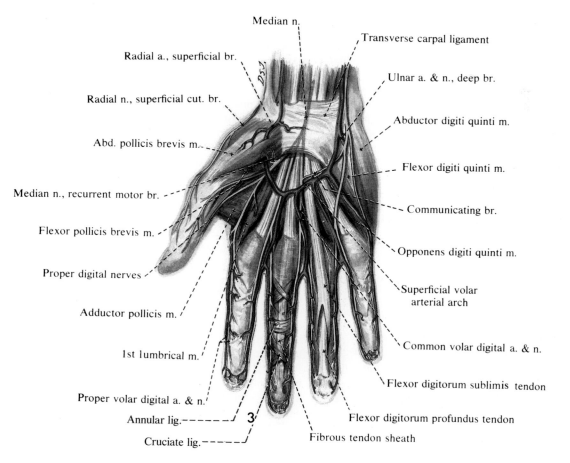

Median n.

Transverse carpal ligament

Radial a., superficial br.

Ulnar a. & n., deep br.

Radial n., superficial cut. br.

Abductor digiti quinti m.

Abd. pollicis brevis m.

Flexor digiti quinti m.

Median n., recurrent motor br.

Communicating br.

Flexor pollicis brevis m.

Opponens digiti quinti m.

Proper digital nerves

Superficial volar arterial arch

Adductor pollicis m.

Common volar digital a. & n.

1st lumbrical m.

Flexor digitorum sublimis tendon

Proper volar digital a. & n.

Flexor digitorum profundus tendon

Annular lig.

3

Cruciate lig.

Fibrous tendon sheath

4. **Deep Muscular Structures** (Figs. 1 and 2):

a. ADDUCTOR POLLICIS—is seen on the radial side of the middle compartment, forming part of the floor of this area. It arises from the third metacarpal (transverse head) and from the carpal area (oblique head) and inserts into the base of the first phalanx. It is innervated by the deep ulnar nerve.

b. THREE VOLAR INTEROSSEI—make up the remainder of the deep muscles of the middle compartment. They arise from the second, fourth, and fifth metacarpal bones, and insert on the extensor assembly. The first is inserted on the ulnar side of the index finger, the second on the radial side of the ring finger, and the third on the radial side of the little finger. These three muscles are innervated by the deep ulnar nerve. Their main function is adduction of the fingers with the middle finger as the axis. However, they also act in conjunction with the lumbricals and dorsal interossei as flexors of the metacarpophalangeal joints and extensors of the interphalangeal joints.

5. **Deep Neurovascular Structures** (Figs. 1 and 2):

a. DEEP VOLAR ARCH—is formed by the radial artery and the deep branch of the ulnar artery. The radial artery enters the palm from the dorsum of the hand between the heads of the first dorsal interosseous muscle and then passes between the oblique and transverse heads of the adductor pollicis, where it joins the deep ulnar artery. Topographically, it lies two fingers' breadth distal to the rasceta. The arch gives rise to the following branches:

(1) *Princeps Pollicis*—is actually a common digital branch to the thumb, dividing into two proper volar digitals. This artery may at times join the superficial ulnar artery to form the superficial volar arch.

(2) *Volar Radial Artery of Index Digit*—passes to the radial side of the index finger. It may in the absence of the superficial volar artery complete the superficial volar arch.

(3) *Volar Metacarpals*—are three in number and descend in the second, third, and fourth interosseous spaces and terminate by anastomosing with the common digitals of the superficial arch.

(4) *Carpal Recurrent Branches*—anastomose at the wrist with the volar radial and ulnar carpals to form the volar carpal network.

b. DEEP ULNAR NERVE—accompanies the deep volar arch through the middle compartment. It is described in more detail in the discussion of the hypothenar compartment.

Thenar Compartment (Figs. 1 and 2):

1. **Musculotendinous Contents**—three muscles form the eminence in this thenar compartment. They are all triangular in shape and are innervated by the recurrent branch of the median nerve.

a. ABDUCTOR POLLICIS BREVIS—arises from the volar surface of the transverse carpal ligament and greater multangular and inserts on the base of proximal phalanx of the thumb.

b. FLEXOR POLLICIS BREVIS—arises from the carpus and inserts on the ulnar side of the proximal phalanx.

c. OPPONENS POLLICIS—takes origin from the transverse carpal ligament and gains attachment to the radial side of the first metacarpal.

Two other muscles related to the thumb in this area are:

d. ADDUCTOR POLLICIS—arises in the middle compartment from the third metacarpal and carpus and attaches to the proximal phalanx of the thumb on its ulnar side. This muscle is innervated by the deep ulnar nerve.

e. FLEXOR POLLICIS LONGUS TENDON—enters the hand deep to transverse carpal ligament and enters the osteofibrous canal of the thumb where it extends to the base of the distal phalanx. Its mucous tendon sheath is termed the *radial bursa* (Fig. 1, page 75).

2. **Neurovascular Contents:**

a. RECURRENT BRANCH OF MEDIAN NERVE—is the motor nerve to this compartment. It arises from the lateral division of the medial nerve after the latter passes under the transverse carpal ligament. Topographically, its position may be located by flexing the ring finger to the thenar eminence.

b. PRINCEPS POLLICIS ARTERY (Fig. 2):

Hypothenar Compartment (Figs. 1 and 2):

1. **Muscular Contents**—form the hypothenar eminence and are innervated by the deep ulnar nerve. The names of these muscles indicate their function.

a. ABDUCTOR DIGITI QUINTI—arises mainly from the pisiform bone and inserts into the ulnar side of the proximal phalanx of the little finger.

b. FLEXOR DIGITI QUINTI—takes origin from the hook of the hamate and transverse carpal ligament and gains attachment to the base of the proximal phalanx.

c. OPPONENS DIGITI QUINTI—has an origin similar to that of the flexor of the little finger. Its insertion is into the fifth metacarpal.

2. **Neurovascular Structures:**

a. ULNAR NERVE—enters the palm deep to the volar carpal but superficial to the transverse carpal ligament at the wrist. As it passes the radial side of the pisiform bone, it divides into a superficial and deep branch. The *superficial ulnar nerve* is described on page 68. The *deep ulnar nerve* pierces the hypothenar compartment and continues into the middle component accompanying the deep volar arch. It innervates the hypothenar muscles, all the interossei, the two ulnar lumbricals, and the adductor pollicis.

b. ULNAR ARTERY—closely accompanies the ulnar nerve and also divided into a superficial and deep branch. The *superficial ulnar artery* has been considered on page 68 and the *deep ulnar artery,* under the deep volar arch described above.

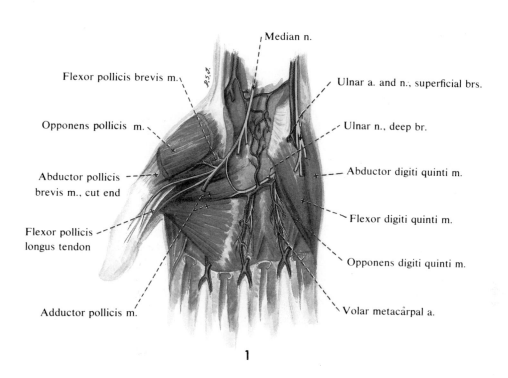

Median n.

Flexor pollicis brevis m.

Ulnar a. and n., superficial brs.

Opponens pollicis m.

Ulnar n., deep br.

Abductor pollicis brevis m., cut end

Abductor digiti quinti m.

Flexor digiti quinti m.

Flexor pollicis longus tendon

Opponens digiti quinti m.

Adductor pollicis m.

Volar metacarpal a.

1

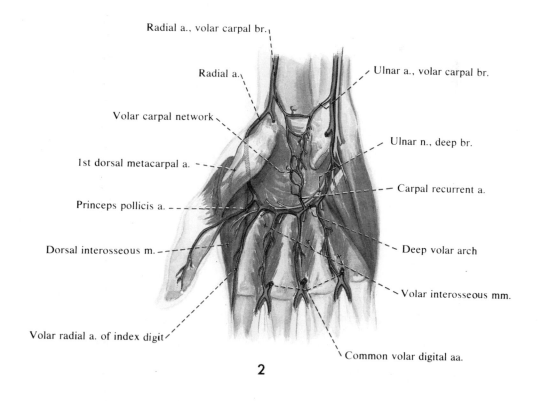

Radial a., volar carpal br.

Radial a.

Ulnar a., volar carpal br.

Volar carpal network

Ulnar n., deep br.

1st dorsal metacarpal a.

Carpal recurrent a.

Princeps pollicis a.

Dorsal interosseous m.

Deep volar arch

Volar interosseous mm.

Volar radial a. of index digit

Common volar digital aa.

2

THE HAND (DORSAL SURFACE) AND WRIST

Skin—the skin over the dorsal surface of the hand is so thin and freely movable that the underlying dorsal venous rete and extensor tendons are visible. The tendons of the thumb form an important topographic landmark, the *snuffbox* or *tabatière*. This is a triangular depression on the dorsal surface of the wrist bounded on the radial side by the tendons of the extensor pollicis brevis and abductor pollicis longus and on the ulnar side by the extensor pollicis longus. In the superficial fascia of this space is the lower portion of the cephalic vein, and in the depth, the radial artery.

Superficial Fascia—in this plane are seen the vessels forming the dorsal venous rete and the superficial nerves.

1. DORSAL VENOUS RETE (Fig. 1)—arises from a longitudinal plexus of veins over the fingers which drain into the dorsal metacarpal veins. Communications between the latter veins form the dorsal venous rete which in turn gives rise to the basilic and cephalic veins.

2. SUPERFICIAL NERVES (Figs. 1 and 2)—are derived from three sources: the dorsal ramus of the ulnar, the superficial branch of the radial, and the posterior antibrachial cutaneous nerve. Note that the dorsal surface of the distal portions of the index, middle, and radial half of the ring finger are innervated by the median nerve.

Extensor Tendons (Fig. 3)—arise in the antibrachium and pass deep to the dorsal carpal ligament in synovial sheaths through specific osseofibrous canals. There are six such canals on the dorsum of the wrist. From radial to ulnar side their contents are:

1. Extensor pollicis brevis and abductor pollicis longus
2. Extensor carpi radialis longus and brevis
3. Extensor pollicis longus
4. Extensor digitorum communis and extensor indicis proprius
5. Extensor digiti quinti proprius
6. Extensor carpi ulnaris

Over the dorsal surface of the hand the extensor tendons are joined by oblique tendinous bands (*juncturae tendinum*) and fascia, forming an aponeurotic extensor tendon sheet.

Dorsal Subaponeurotic Space (Fig. 2, page 75)—is a loose connective tissue layer between the extensor tendon aponeurosis and the underlying interosseous muscles and bones.

Dorsal Interosseous Muscles (Fig. 3)—four such muscles arising from adjacent sides of the metacarpal bones in each interspace. Each muscle inserts on the extensor assembly of the phalanges (Fig. 4). The first dorsal interosseous inserts on the radial side of the index finger, the fourth, on the ulnar side of the ring finger, and the second and third insert on the radial and ulnar sides of the middle finger, respectively. These muscles act as abductors of the fingers and, in association with the lumbricals and volar interossei, as flexors of the metacarpophalangeal joint and extensors of the interphalangeal joints. They are all innervated by the deep ulnar nerve.

Dorsal Metacarpal Arteries (Fig. 3)—the first dorsal metacarpal artery arises directly from the radial; the remaining three vessels arise from the *dorsal carpal rete*. The rete is formed by the dorsal carpal branches of the ulnar and radial arteries. The dorsal metacarpal arteries extend to the level of the metacarpophalangeal joints where they divide into proper dorsal digital branches. At the base of the metacarpal bones, perforating branches anastomose with the branches of the deep palmar arch.

Extensor Assembly—the extensor tendons of the second to fifth digit, as well as the tendons of the lumbricals and interossei, insert onto the phalanges. This rather complex arrangement of fibers is illustrated in Figure 4.

VOLAR ASPECT OF THE WRIST (Fig. 5):

Because of the frequency of lacerations in this area, knowledge of the relational anatomy of the volar surface of the wrist is important. Also of significance clinically is the *carpal tunnel syndrome*, resulting from compression of the median nerve by chronic irritation and inflammation of the transverse carpal ligament.

Transverse Carpal Ligament—is a thick fibrous band extending from the pisiform and hook of the hamate on the ulnar side, to the tubercle of navicular and greater multangular on the radial side. The ligament splits at its radial attachment to form a separate compartment transversed by the flexor carpi radialis tendon and its sheath.

1. STRUCTURES SUPERFICIAL TO THE LIGAMENT (Fig. 5, and Figs. 2 and 3, page 69)—include the following: *palmaris longus tendon* in the midline, the *palmar cutaneous branches of the median and ulnar nerves* on either side of the tendon, and the *ulnar artery and nerve*, which lie in relation to the pisiform bone.

2. STRUCTURES DEEP TO THE LIGAMENT—lie in the carpal tunnel, and from radial to ulnar side are as follows: *Flexor pollicis longus* tendon with its mucous sheath (*radial bursa*), the *median nerve*, and the *flexor digitorum sublimis* and *profundus* tendons and their common mucous sheath (ulnar bursa).

The sublimis tendons of the middle and ring finger are superficial in position, immediately deep to which are the sublimis tendons of the index and little fingers. The profundus tendons of all four fingers are aligned on the deepest level.

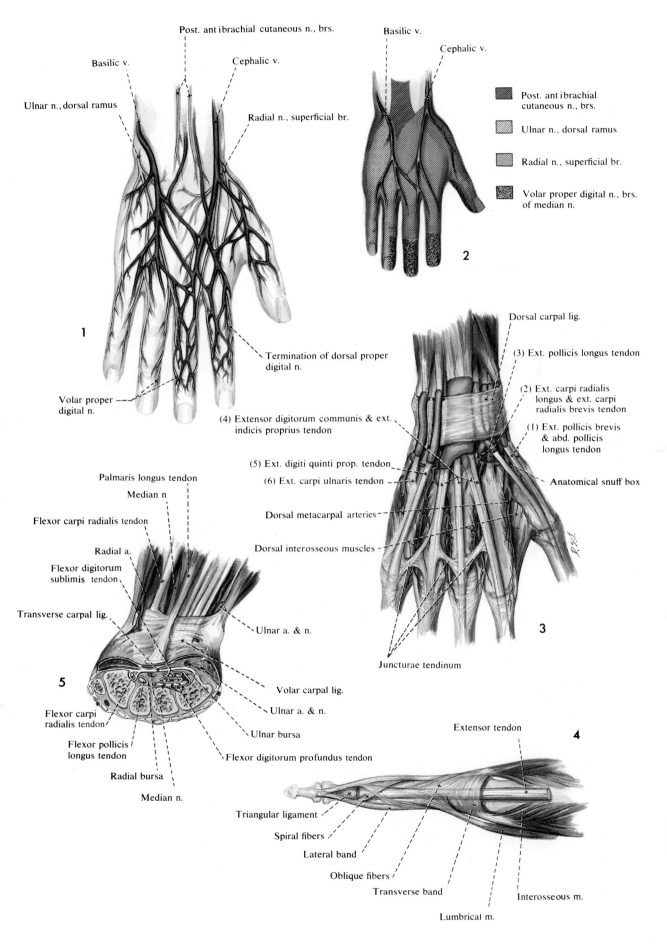

Post. antibrachial cutaneous n., brs.

Basilic v.

Cephalic v.

Ulnar n., dorsal ramus

Radial n., superficial br.

Basilic v.

Cephalic v.

Post. antibrachial cutaneous n., brs.

Ulnar n., dorsal ramus

Radial n., superficial br.

Volar proper digital n., brs. of median n.

1

2

Termination of dorsal proper digital n.

Volar proper digital n.

(4) Extensor digitorum communis & ext. indicis proprius tendon

Dorsal carpal lig.

(3) Ext. pollicis longus tendon

(2) Ext. carpi radialis longus & ext. carpi radialis brevis tendon

(1) Ext. pollicis brevis & abd. pollicis longus tendon

Anatomical snuff box

(5) Ext. digiti quinti prop. tendon

(6) Ext. carpi ulnaris tendon

Dorsal metacarpal arteries

Dorsal interosseous muscles

Juncturae tendinum

3

Palmaris longus tendon

Median n

Flexor carpi radialis tendon

Radial a.

Flexor digitorum sublimis tendon

Transverse carpal lig.

Ulnar a. & n.

Volar carpal lig.

Ulnar a. & n.

Ulnar bursa

Flexor digitorum profundus tendon

5

Flexor carpi radialis tendon

Flexor pollicis longus tendon

Radial bursa

Median n.

Extensor tendon

4

Triangular ligament

Spiral fibers

Lateral band

Oblique fibers

Transverse band

Lumbrical m.

Interosseous m.

THE ANATOMY OF HAND INFECTIONS:

Only correct surgical care of deep infections in the hand can prevent serious destruction of tissue and permanent impairment of functions. Of particular importance are those infections located in the flexor synovial tendon sheaths and palmar fascial spaces. The latter are not spaces in the true sense of the word, but are fascial intervals which distend easily and limit the spread of pus or fluid. Infections of the tendon sheaths commonly spread to the fascial spaces and vice versa.

Mucous (Synovial) Tendon Sheaths (Figs. 1 and 3):

These sheaths are bursal protective elements which envelop the flexor tendons of the fingers.

1. **Proper Digital Mucous Tendon Sheaths** — extend from the neck of the metacarpal bones to the insertion of the long flexor tendons on the distal phalanx of the index, middle, and ring-fingers. Like all mucous sheaths, they consist of a parietal and visceral layer between which is found lubricating synovial fluid. Interrupted mesotendons of the sheath termed *vincula* (longus and brevis) transmit blood vessels to and from the tendon.

2. **Radial Bursa** — is the mucous sheath of the flexor pollicis longus and extends from the insertion of the tendon on the distal phalanx of the thumb to a level in the forearm approximately 2.5 cm. proximal to the transverse carpal ligament.

3. **Ulnar Bursa** — is the common sheath which envelops the tendons of the flexor digitorum sublimis and the flexor digitorum profundus, extending from the distal part of the forearm under the transverse carpal ligament to the middle of the palm, where it teminates along the tendon of the index, middle, and ring fingers, but on the ulnar side continues as the flexor digital sheath of the little finger. Frequently there is a communication between the ulnar and radial bursae at the wrist, which accounts for the so-called *horseshoe abscess*.

Palmar Fascial Spaces:

Between the flexor tendons of the fingers with their mucous sheaths and the accompanying lumbrical muscles anteriorly and the metacarpal bones with the interossei and the adductor pollicis muscles posteriorly, lie the thenar and midpalmar "spaces" (Figs. 1 and 2). They lie in the middle compartment of the palm separated by a fibrous partition at the third metacarpal (Fig. 2). A third "space" of similar character and significance, the adductor space, exists behind the adductor pollicis muscle.

1. **Thenar Space** (Figs. 1 and 2) — is bounded by the flexor tendons of the index finger and the associated first lumbrical muscle on its volar side and the adductor pollicis muscle dorsally. It is limited on the radial side

by the flexor pollicis longus tendon and the radial bursa, and on the ulnar side by a firm anterior-posterior septum extending from the fascia covering the flexor tendons to the third metacarpal bone. The proximal extension of the space is to the distal edge of the transverse carpal ligament and the distal limit at the line of the proximal transverse crease of the palm with an extension along the first lumbrical muscle.

2. **Midpalmar Space** (Figs. 1 and 2) — has the same proximal and distal boundaries as the thenar space. Distally, however, it has extensions related to the second, third, and fourth lumbrical muscles. Its volar boundary is the flexor tendons of the middle, ring, and little fingers and the associated lumbrical muscles. The fascia covering the anterior interosseous muscles and metacarpal bones form the dorsal limits. The space is limited on the ulnar side by the hypothenar muscles and fascia, and on the radial side by the same fascial septum extending to the third metacarpal as described above.

3. **Adductor Space** (Figs. 2 and 4) — is in continuity with the thenar space and lies between the adductor pollicis muscle and the first dorsal interosseous muscle. The two spaces communicate at the distal border of the adductor muscle.

Other Fascial Spaces:

A *subcutaneous* and a *subaponeurotic* space (Fig. 2) are present on the dorsum of the hand. These are of much less importance than the palmar spaces.

Located in the forearm, but of importance because infection may reach it from the bursae in the deep palmar spaces, is the *retrotendinous space of Parona*. It lies in the lower part of the anterior compartment of the forearm between the flexor pollicis longus and flexor digitorum profundus in front and the pronator quadratus behind.

Surgical Incisions (Fig. 3):

Several incisions which may be used for drainage of closed space infections of the hand are shown in Figures 3 and 4. The proper digital sheaths may be opened as shown in Figure 3A. A lateral incision avoids transection of the flexion creases of the fingers. Incision for drainage of the radial bursa is shown in Figure 3B. The incision must not be extended too far into the palm for fear of injury to the recurrent branch of the median nerve. The ulnar bursa may be approached by any of three incisions depending upon the severity of the infection (Fig. 3C, D, E).

The midpalmar space may be approached by an incision parallel to the distal palmar crease (Fig. 3F) or through the web between the ring and middle fingers (Fig. 3G). The thenar space may best be approached through an incision on the dorsal aspect of the web between the thumb and index fingers (Fig. 4). Such an approach also permits drainage of the adductor space.

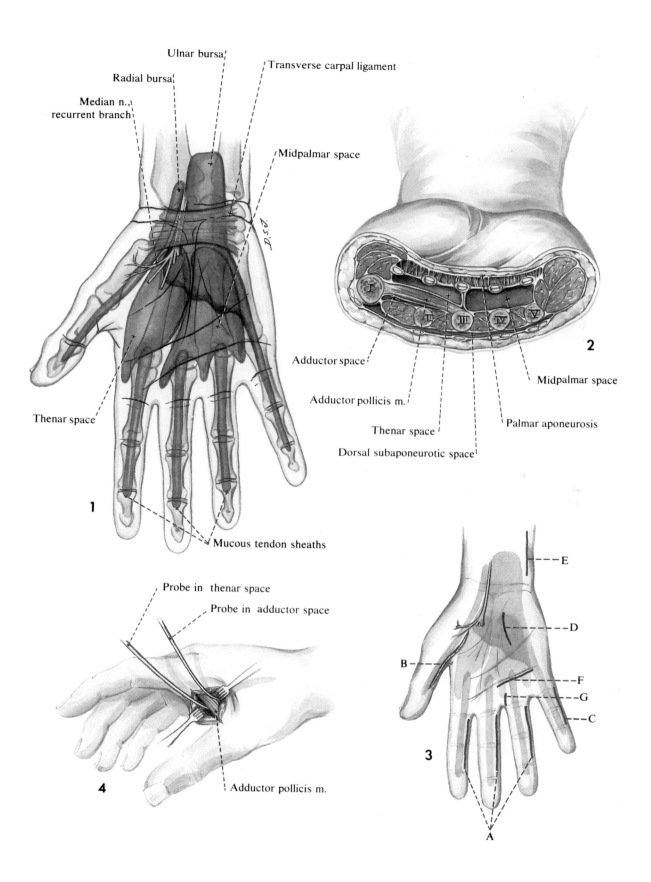

Median n.,
recurrent branch

Radial bursa

Ulnar bursa

Transverse carpal ligament

Midpalmar space

Thenar space

1

Mucous tendon sheaths

Adductor space

Adductor pollicis m.

Thenar space

Dorsal subaponeurotic space

Midpalmar space

Palmar aponeurosis

2

Probe in thenar space

Probe in adductor space

Adductor pollicis m.

4

E

D

B

F

G

C

A

3

INJURIES OF THE FINGERS AND HAND:

Anesthesia in Surgery of the Hand and Fingers:

Major injuries of the hand proper can rarely be managed without regional or general anesthesia. In addition, a tourniquet is needed to provide a bloodless field of dissection for the identification and repair of nerves and tendons. The anatomy of *brachial plexus block* by the supraclavicular approach for such a purpose is illustrated in Figure 1, page 31. The two main shortcomings of brachial plexus block are frequent lack of complete anesthesia and complicating penumothorax. They can be avoided by the use of *axillary block*. In the latter, the anesthetic solution is injected above the neurovascular bundle on the medial side of the arm 2 cm. below the margin of the pectoralis major. At this point, all the nerves to the forearm and hand can be blocked (median, ulnar, radial, musculocutaneous, and medial cutaneous nerves of the forearm).

For the management of surgical lesions in the distal part of the fingers, *digital nerve block* is admirably suited (Figs. 1 and 2). A needle introduced on the medial and lateral aspects of the dorsum of the finger near its base permits the injection of an anesthetic solution about both the volar and digital nerves. Complete anesthesia of the tissues distal to the sites of injection will follow promptly. The surgeon's failure to direct the needle to the position of the dorsal digital nerve is a common cause of incomplete anesthesia.

Incisions for the Exposure of Severed Tendons:

In the hand, it is of paramount importance that scar contractures be avoided by the placement of incisions along flexion creases and parallel with lines of cleavage rather than across them (Fig. 3). In extending a palmar wound or planning an incision to recover and repair a cut nerve or tendon this principle must be observed.

Knowledge of the position of the hand at the time of injury is a helpful guide to the tendon ends and to proper planning of the incision or incisions to expose them. If the tendons in the fingers or palm are divided when the fingers are completely extended, the distal ends remain close to the site of injury but the proximal ends are drawn proximally by the contraction of the flexor muscles. If, however, the fingers are flexed at the moment of section there will be little retreat of the proximal end, but the end of the distal segment may travel a surprisingly great distance when the fingers are extended.

For exposure of a tendon in a finger, the fibrous flexor sheath should be incised close to its attachment to bone rather than in its center.

In extensive repair of nerves and tendons in the palm, an **S**-shaped incision which extends from the radial border of the hand in a curved manner following the midpalmar or proximal palmar crease to the wrist is useful. It may be extended into the forearm in a similar curved manner.

Fractures of the Metacarpals and Phalanges:

These fractures are the most common in the entire skeletal system. Their importance as a cause of disability is self-evident, and a knowledge of the factors that govern the displacement of bony fragments is essential to their proper management. These factors are:

1. The attachment and direction of pull of the tendons

2. The direction of the fracturing force

The complicated arrangement of tendons attachments on the dorsal and volar surfaces of the phalanges is shown in Figure 4.

On the dorsum of the proximal phalanx, by means of an extensor expansion, a common extensor tendon, a lumbrical, and one or more interossei insert into the dorsal aspects of the base of the middle and distal phalanges of each finger. Through the same medium, the middle and distal phalanges of the index and little fingers are attached to the special extensors of these digits.

On the volar side, the tendons of the flexor digitorum sublimis split and insert into the base of the volar aspect of the middle phalanx. Passing through the gap, the tendon of the flexor profundus inserts into the base of the terminal phalanx.

1. **Fracture of the Metacarpal Shaft** (Figs. 5 and 6) — produces a flexion deformity or dorsal angulation owing to the greater strength of the flexor muscles of the hand. Reduction requires traction and extension.

2. **Fracture of the Shaft of the Proximal Phalanx** (Figs. 7 and 8) — produces an extension deformity or palmar angulation owing to the pull of the lumbrical and interosseous muscles through the extensor expansion. Relaxation of these muscles by flexion of the metacarpophalangeal and interphalangeal joints effects reduction.

3. **Fractures of the Middle Phalanx:**

a. PROXIMAL TO THE ATTACHMENT OF THE SUBLIMIS TENDON (Figs. 9 and 10) — results in a flexion deformity. Fixation is by means of an extension splint.

b. DISTAL TO THE ATTACHMENT OF THE SUBLIMIS (Figs. 11 and 12) — results in the opposite or an extensor deformity or volar angulation. Flexion will permit reduction.

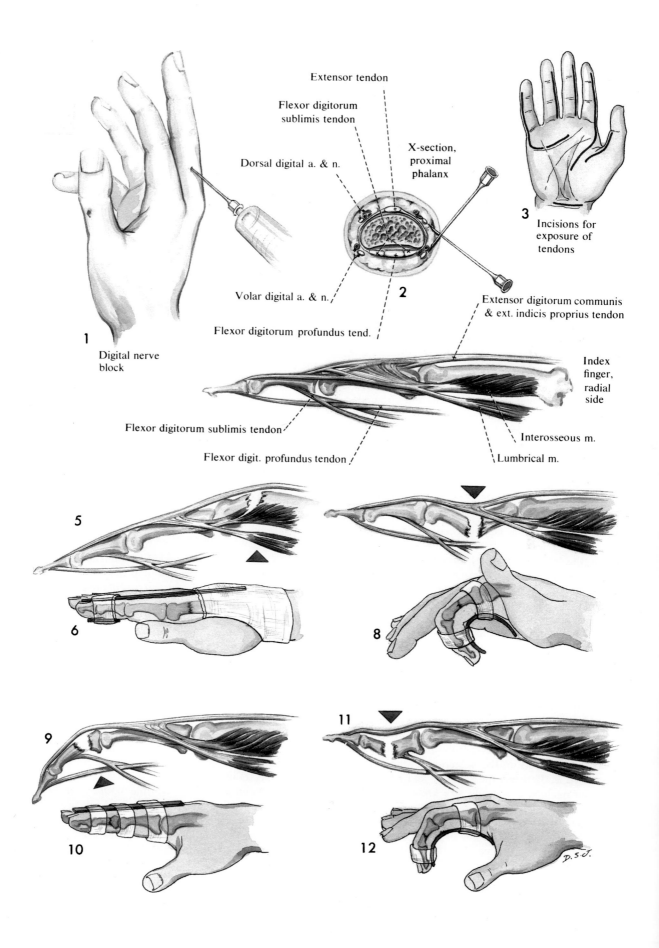

Extensor tendon

Flexor digitorum
sublimis tendon

Dorsal digital a. & n.

X-section,
proximal
phalanx

Volar digital a. & n.

2

Flexor digitorum profundus tend.

3

Incisions for
exposure of
tendons

Extensor digitorum communis
& ext. indicis proprius tendon

1

Digital nerve
block

Index
finger,
radial
side

Flexor digitorum sublimis tendon

Interosseous m.

Flexor digit. profundus tendon

Lumbrical m.

5

6

8

9

10

11

12

D. S. J.

MAJOR JOINTS OF THE UPPER EXTREMITY:

Although many bony articulations in the upper extremity are of clinical significance, only the three major joints will be discussed here: the shoulder, elbow, and wrist joints. Each joint under consideration is a *diarthrodial joint*. This type of articulation has the following characteristics:

1. Consists of two or more bones, each covered by articular hyaline cartilage.

2. The bones are united by a fibrous capsule continuous with the periosteum of the bone.

3. A synovial membrane lines the fibrous capsule and covers all portions of bone enclosed in the capsule and not covered with hyaline cartilage.

A generalization can be made in regard to the innervation of the joints: a joint is innervated by the same nerves that innervate the muscles that cross the joint. This is referred to as *Hilton's law*.

SHOULDER JOINT:

The shoulder joint is a diarthrodial joint of the enarthrodial (ball and socket) type. It is the most mobile of all the joints, permitting flexion, extension, abduction, adduction, medial and lateral rotation, and circumduction. Because of certain of its anatomic features, it is the most frequently dislocated joint in the body (page 80).

1. **Bony Parts** (Figs. 1 and 2)—consist of the shallow, concave glenoid cavity of the scapula and the large convex head of humerus, each covered by articular hyaline cartilage.

2. **Articular Capsule** (Figs. 1 to 5)—is a lax fibrous layer uniting the bony parts. It is attached superiorly to the circumference of the glenoid cavity. The upper parts of the humeral attachment are on the anatomic neck, whereas the lower portion attaches to the shaft about 2 cm. below the articular surface of the head (Figs. 1 and 2). The looseness of the capsule is compensated in part by certain ligamentous reinforcements:

a. CORACOHUMERAL LIGAMENT (Fig. 3)—is a broad band arising from the coracoid process and inserting into the greater tubercle of the humerus. This ligament strengthens the superior portion of the joint capsule.

b. GLENOHUMERAL LIGAMENTS (Fig. 5)—are three ligamentous bands which reinforce the anterior portion of the capsular ligament. These bands can be distinguished by viewing the inner aspect of the capsule, and are described as the *superior, middle,* and *inferior glenohumeral ligaments*. They arise from the rim of the glenoid cavity and insert on the humerus in relation to the lesser tubercle. Between the superior and middle band is seen an opening of varying size known as the *subscapular recess*.

c. GLENOID LABRUM (Fig. 5)—is a rim of dense fibrocartilage along the margin of the glenoid cavity. It deepens the cavity somewhat, thereby affording a better receptive area for the head of the humerus.

d. TRANSVERSE HUMERAL LIGAMENT (Fig. 3)—extends between the lesser and greater tubercle and converts the intertubercular groove into a canal for passage of the tendon of the long head of the biceps.

3. **Synovial Membrane** (Fig. 6)—lies deep to the articular capsule and attaches to the scapular and humeral articular margins. The synovial membrane has two constant extensions: one, as the *subscapular bursa* which extends through the subscapular recess described above; the second, as a prolongation inferiorly as the *synovial sheath of the long tendon of the biceps*. Sometimes the synovial membrane of the joint extends through the posterior wall of the capsule as the *infraspinatus bursa*.

4. **Musculotendinous Relations** (Figs. 3 to 5)—are probably the most important anatomic feature of the shoulder joint, for it depends upon the muscular control for its integrity. Certain muscles are intimately related to the anterior, superior, and posterior surfaces of the capsule. The inferior aspect receives no musculotendinous reinforcement and constitutes the "weak area" of the articular capsule.

a. SUBSCAPULAR—reinforces the anterior portion of the capsule.

b. SUPRASPINATUS—is related to the superior aspect of the joint.

c. INFRASPINATUS AND TERES MINOR—strengthen the joint posteriorly.

d. LONG TENDON OF THE BICEPS—arises from the supraglenoid tuberosity and passes through the joint capsule surrounded by a tubular sheath derived from the synovial membrane. It performs a very important action in maintaining joint stability.

The subscapularis tendon in front, and the supraspinatus, infraspinatus, and teres minor above and behind form what is known clinically as the "rotator cuff."

5. **Other Relations**—include bony, muscular, and neurovascular structures as well as bursae.

a. SUPERIORLY (Fig. 3)—an osseofibrous arch, consisting of the *acromion process* and the *coraco-acromial ligament*, protects the joint. Between this arch and the underlying capsule and supraspinatus tendon is the *subacromial bursa*.

b. ANTERIORLY (Figs. 1 and 2, page 47)—the *axillary vessels* and terminal branches of the *brachial plexus* are separated from the joint by the subscapular muscle and bursa.

c. POSTERIORLY—overlapping the infraspinatus and teres minor muscles is the *deltoid muscle*. This muscle is also related to the superior, anterior, and lateral aspects of the joint, producing the rounded contour to the shoulder.

d. INFERIORLY (Fig. 4)—the *axillary nerve* and *posterior humeral circumflex artery* and *vein* are closely related to the capsule. These vessels, along with the anterior humeral circumflex and transverse scapular vessels, supply and drain the shoulder joint. In this location the *long head of the triceps* may also be seen.

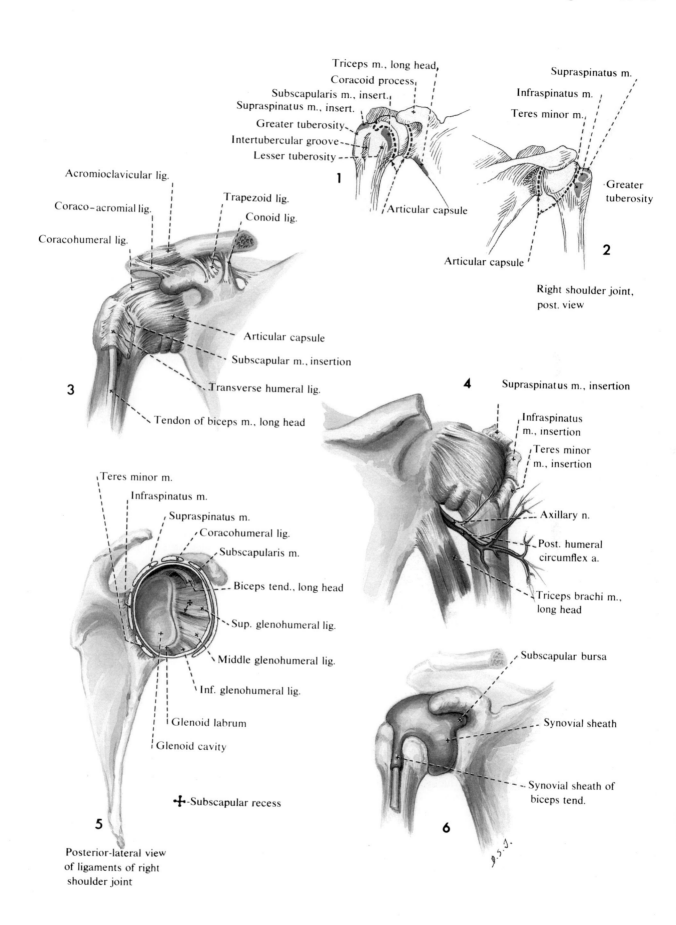

Triceps m., long head,
Coracoid process,
Subscapularis m., insert.
Supraspinatus m., insert.
Greater tuberosity
Intertubercular groove
Lesser tuberosity

Supraspinatus m.
Infraspinatus m.
Teres minor m.

Articular capsule

1

Greater tuberosity

Articular capsule

2

Right shoulder joint,
post. view

Acromioclavicular lig.
Coraco-acromial lig.
Coracohumeral lig.

Trapezoid lig.
Conoid lig.

Articular capsule
Subscapular m., insertion
Transverse humeral lig.
Tendon of biceps m., long head

3

4

Supraspinatus m., insertion
Infraspinatus m., insertion
Teres minor m., insertion
Axillary n.
Post. humeral circumflex a.
Triceps brachi m., long head

Teres minor m.
Infraspinatus m.
Supraspinatus m.
Coracohumeral lig.
Subscapularis m.
Biceps tend., long head
Sup. glenohumeral lig.
Middle glenohumeral lig.
Inf. glenohumeral lig.
Glenoid labrum
Glenoid cavity

✚-Subscapular recess

5

Posterior-lateral view
of ligaments of right
shoulder joint

Subscapular bursa
Synovial sheath
Synovial sheath of biceps tend.

6

CLINICAL CONSIDERATIONS OF THE SHOULDER JOINT:

The Rotator Cuff:

Degenerative changes or rupture of fibers by trauma may produce significant lesions of an acute or chronic nature in the rotator cuff (page 78). *Calcific deposits* may develop in any of the tissues of the cuff (subscapularis, supraspinatus and infraspinatus, and teres minor muscles), but in about half of the affected shoulders it occurs as a single lesion in the supraspinatus portion of the cuff. The clinical term "bursitis" of the shoulder joint is usually a misnomer. Whereas calcium deposits may be present in the two bursa (the subacromial and subcoracoid) of the shoulder area to account for pain and limitation of motion of the joint, they are usually not in these bursae, but in the tissues of the rotator cuff.

Surgical Approaches to the Shoulder:

Aspiration of the shoulder joint may be carried out by inserting a needle just below the tip of the coracoid process and directing it posteriorly and slightly laterally.

Anterior Approach (Figs. 1, 2, and 3) — is useful in exposing: (1) the shoulder joint; (2) the long and short heads of the biceps; (3) the subscapularis muscle and tendon; (4) the glenoid fossa, and (5) the axillary surface of the scapula. Exposure of the latter two structures requires an osteotomy of the coracoid process. This incision is designed to protect the axillary nerve from injury. The position and course of the nerve must be constantly in the surgeon's mind. This approach through the deltopectoral cleft provides these two essentials: good exposure and protection of the axillary nerve. It may be extended superiorly (Fig. 1, dotted line) for better access to the humeral head and inferiorly for the shaft of the humerus.

Posterior Approach — by extension of the anterosuperomedial incision around the lateral and posterior margins of the acromion and the lateral part of the spine of the scapula, the posterior aspect of the shoulder joint may be exposed (Fig. 4, dotted line). However, exposure may be limited to the posterior aspect by an incision along the posterior margin of the deltoid (Fig. 4).

Shoulder Dislocations:

The shoulder is the most frequently dislocated major joint in the body. Several anatomic features of the joint are responsible for this fact:

1. Its unprotected position which makes it vulnerable to trauma
2. The extreme mobility of the joint, which is to be accounted for by:
   a. The disparity in the size of the articular surface of the head of the humerus and the small, shallow glenoid fossa
   b. The laxity of the joint capsule

Dislocating Forces — a fall upon the outstretched hand or upon the elbow when the arm is adducted (Fig. 5), a direct blow upon the shoulder or violent muscle action alone may produce dislocation of the shoulder.

Types of Dislocation — the forces described above will also determine in part the type of dislocation which will occur. Often there is avulsion of the glenoid labrum, the fibrous capsule, and the glenohumeral ligaments from the anteroinferior aspect of the rim of the glenoid fossa, permitting displacement of the humeral head inferiorly (Fig. 6). Dislocations may also occur through a simple rent in the capsule or with an intact but stretched joint capsule.

1. SUBCORACOID (Fig. 7b) — is the most frequent type. The head of the humerus lies below the coracoid process deep to the short head of the biceps and coracobrachialis muscles.

2. SUBGLENOID (Fig. 7c) — is the second most frequent site for the head to lodge in dislocation. Ninety-eight per cent of shoulder dislocations are the subcoracoid or subglenoid types.

3. SUBCLAVICULAR (Fig. 7a) — dislocation occurs should the dislocating force be great enough and properly directed. The head slides further anteriorly beneath the pectoralis minor and clavicle.

4. Subspinous type is a rare posterior displacement in which the humeral head passes backward to lie beneath the spine of the scapula.

Injuries to Associated Structures:

1. **To Musculotendinous Structures of Rotator Cuff** — is a common, if not constant and important factor predisposing to recurrent dislocation. The injury usually involves tearing or stretching of the suprascapular and subscapularis muscles. The tendon of the long head of the biceps may be torn or dislocated.

2. **To Capsule** — in addition to a tear in the inferior part of the capsule other ligamentous reinforcements of the capsule may be disrupted. The most common injury is a detachment of the glenoid labrum (Fig. 6) or disruption of the glenohumeral ligaments.

3. **To Bone** — such as an associated fracture of the glenoid rim or neck of the scapula, or the greater tuberosity of the humerus.

4. **To Nerves** — in 5 per cent of acute dislocations. Usually it is temporary, and involves only the ulnar nerve, but the radial, axillary, and median nerves may be damaged.

5. **To Vessels** — contusion with thrombosis or laceration with severe hemorrhage may occasionally affect the axillary, subscapular, or posterior humeral circumflex arteries.

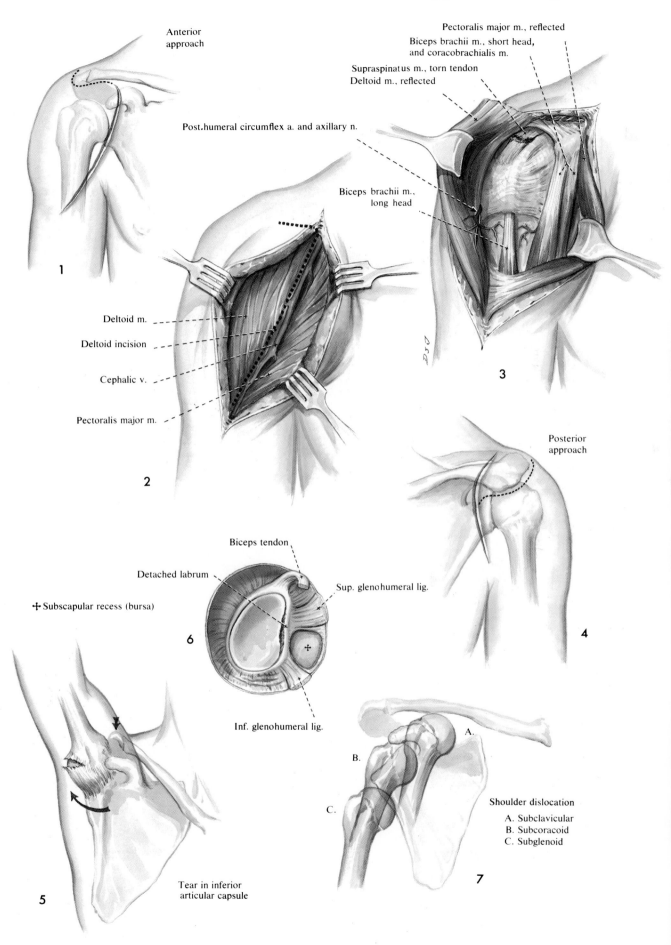

Anterior
approach

1

Post.humeral circumflex a. and axillary n.

Deltoid m.

Deltoid incision

Cephalic v.

Pectoralis major m.

2

Pectoralis major m., reflected
Biceps brachii m., short head,
and coracobrachialis m.
Supraspinatus m., torn tendon
Deltoid m., reflected

Biceps brachii m.,
long head

DSG

3

Posterior
approach

4

Biceps tendon

Detached labrum

Sup. glenohumeral lig.

✛ Subscapular recess (bursa)

6

Inf. glenohumeral lig.

A.

B.

C.

Shoulder dislocation

A. Subclavicular
B. Subcoracoid
C. Subglenoid

7

Tear in inferior
articular capsule

5

ELBOW JOINT:

The elbow actually consists of three separate joints: the *humero-ulnar, humeroradial,* and *proximal radio-ulnar joints.* They are all diarthrodial joints having a common synovial membrane. The humeral joints are the *ginglymus* (hinge-joint) type and are limited to extension and flexion. The radio-ulnar joint is classified as a *trochoidal* type, in which the articular surface of one bone is a disk that glides in a corresponding concave surface of the other bone, resulting in pronation and supination.

1. **Bony Parts** (Figs. 1 and 2)—of the humeroulnar joint consist of the *trochlea of the humerus* and the *semilunar notch of the ulna.* The humeroradial joints join the *capitulum of the humerus* and the *fovea on the head of the radius.* The *medial part of the radial head* and the *radial notch of the ulna* make up the bony parts of the radioulnar articulation.

2. **Articular Capsule** (Figs. 1 and 2)—is attached to the anterior surface of the humerus on ridges extending from the medial and lateral epicondyles to a point above the *radial* and *coronoid fossae.* Below it is attached to the articular margin of the coronoid process of the ulna and the neck of the radius *(anterior capsular ligament).* On the posterior surface of the humerus it attaches to the margins of the olecranon fossa above and to the margins of the olecranon process of the ulna and neck of the radius below *(posterior capsular ligament).* This area is the weakest part of the joint, accounting for the fact that posterior dislocations are most frequent in occurrence. The capsule is reinforced by lateral and medial reinforcements.

a. ULNAR COLLATERAL LIGAMENT (Figs. 3 and 4)—is a triangular thickening in the capsule extending from the medial epicondyle of the humerus to the medial edge of the coronoid process of the ulna.

b. RADIAL COLLATERAL LIGAMENT (Figs. 3 and 4)—extends from the lateral epicondyle and inserts into the neck of the radius and annular ligament.

c. ANNULAR LIGAMENT (Figs. 3 and 4)—encircles the head of the radius, retaining it into the radial notch of the ulna.

3. **Synovial Membrane** (Fig. 5)—extends from the margin of the articular surface of the humerus and lines the fossae of the humerus. It is reflected over the deep surface of the capsule and extends inferiorly as a pouch between the radial notch, annular ligament, and circumference of the head of the radius, the *sacciform recess.*

WRIST JOINT:

Like the elbow joint, the wrist is a compound joint consisting of the *radiocarpal* and the *distal radio-ulnar joint.* The radiocarpal joint is a diarthrodial, *ellipsoidal* type in which a convex surface is held in a concave surface. The actions of this joint are flexion, extension, abduction, adduction, and circumduction. The radio-ulnar is *trochoidal,* permitting pronation and supination.

1. **Bony Parts** (Figs. 6 and 7)—of the radiocarpal joint consist on the proximal side of the concavity formed by the *articular surface of the radius* and the *articular disk* and the distal convex surface of the carpus, which is made up of the *navicular, lunate,* and *triquetral bones.* The radio-ulnar joint articulation joins the *head of the ulna* with the *ulnar notch of the radius.*

2. **Articular Capsule** (Figs. 6 and 7)—extends from the anterior margin of the lower end of the radius and styloid process and the lower end of the ulna. The capsule attaches to the volar surface of the navicular, lunate, and triquetral carpal bones. The capsule is described as having four ligaments:

a. ANTERIOR RADIOCARPAL LIGAMENT (Fig. 8)—is attached to the styloid process and the anterior margin of the lower end of the radius and ulna above and the volar surface of the navicular, lunate, and triquetral below.

b. DORSAL RADIOCARPAL LIGAMENT (Fig. 9)—gains attachment to the dorsal end of the radius and its styloid process and the posterior margin of the articular disk. It passes downward to attach to the first row of carpal bones and the dorsal intercarpal ligament.

c. ULNAR COLLATERAL LIGAMENT (Figs. 8 and 9)—extends from the styloid process of the ulnar and inserts by two divisions: one into the medial side of the triquetrum, the other attaches to the pisiform and transverse carpal ligament.

d. RADIAL COLLATERAL LIGAMENT (Figs. 8 and 9)—is attached to the styloid process of the radius above to the navicular below.

e. ARTICULAR DISK—is a fibrocartilaginous structure radiating from the radius to the base of the styloid process of the ulna. The disk enters into two distinct articulations separating the distal radio-ulnar from the radiocarpal joints.

3. **Synovial Membranes** (Fig. 10)—of the radiocarpal and the distal radio-ulnar joints are distinct from one another. The synovial membrane of the distal radio-ulnar joint is large and lax, extending between the articular surface of the ulna and proximal surface of the articular disk and protruding between the radius and ulnar articular surfaces.

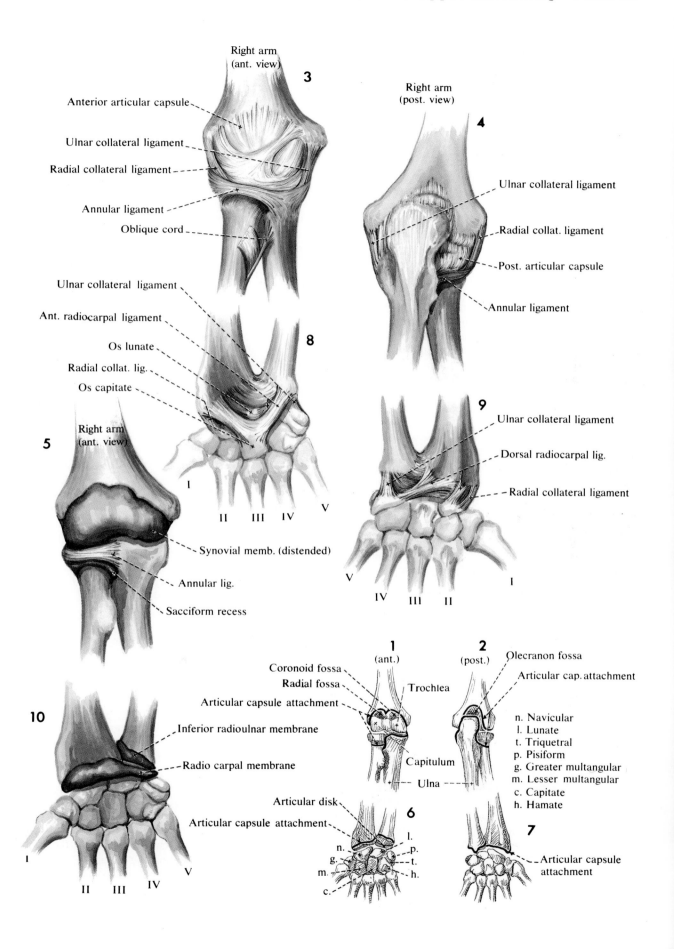

3 Right arm (ant. view)

Anterior articular capsule

Ulnar collateral ligament

Radial collateral ligament

Annular ligament

Oblique cord

4 Right arm (post. view)

Ulnar collateral ligament

Radial collat. ligament

Post. articular capsule

Annular ligament

8

Ulnar collateral ligament

Ant. radiocarpal ligament

Os lunate

Radial collat. lig.

Os capitate

I II III IV V

5 Right arm (ant. view)

Synovial memb. (distended)

Annular lig.

Sacciform recess

9

Ulnar collateral ligament

Dorsal radiocarpal lig.

Radial collateral ligament

V IV III II I

10

Inferior radioulnar membrane

Radio carpal membrane

I II III IV V

1 (ant.) **2** (post.)

Coronoid fossa

Radial fossa

Articular capsule attachment

Trochlea

Capitulum

Ulna

Olecranon fossa

Articular cap. attachment

n. Navicular
l. Lunate
t. Triquetral
p. Pisiform
g. Greater multangular
m. Lesser multangular
c. Capitate
h. Hamate

Articular disk

Articular capsule attachment

6

n.
g.
m.
c.

l.
p.
t.
h.

7

Articular capsule attachment

CLINICAL CONSIDERATIONS OF THE ELBOW AND WRIST:

Of particular clinical interest are the relations of certain muscles, nerves, and vessels which may be injured when the joints or the bones immediately about them are damaged. These same structures must be protected in the operative approach to the joints. Finally, as a result of pathologic changes in the joints, progressive lesions of clinical importance may affect these structures, e.g., delayed ulnar palsy, carpal tunnel syndrome.

1. **Relation of the Ulnar Nerve to the Medial Epicondyle** (Fig. 1) — is a posterior one. The nerve lies in a shallow groove secured and protected by an aponeurosis stretching between the epicondyle and the olecranon. It enters the forearm between the two heads of the flexor carpi ulnaris. In this superficial position behind the medial epicondyle, it is exposed to injury by a direct blow or by pressure. Its liability to damage in fractures of the medial epicondyle is apparent. Furthermore, because it is fixed in position by overlying strong fascia, progressive valgus deformity of the elbow, as may occur after ill-managed fractures of the capitellum, damages the nerve by stretching *(delayed ulnar palsy)*. Release of the nerve and transplantation to a position in front of the medial epicondyle adds effective length to the nerve. This maneuver may be helpful in relieving delayed ulnar palsy or in accomplishing anastomosis of an ulnar nerve which has been divided at this level.

2. **Relation of Radial Nerve to Lateral Epicondyle and to the Supinator Muscle** (Fig. 2) — The nerve lies on the front of the lateral epicondyle of the humerus in the interval between the brachioradialis and brachialis muscles. At this level it divides into its two terminal branches: the superficial (sensory) and deep (motor). The *superficial ramus* passes distally deep to the brachioradialis. The *deep ramus* immediately turns posteriorly to reach the back of the forearm after passing around the lateral aspect of the radius piercing the supinator muscle. Injuries to the radial nerve in fractures of the humerus have already been mentioned (page 58). It may also be injured by anterior dislocation of the head of the radius, and it is an important structure to be protected in the surgical approach to the elbow by the anterolateral route.

3. **Anterolateral Approach to the Elbow** — for open reduction of fractures of the radius and excision of tumors begins in the arm lateral to the biceps and extends distally along the anterior margin of the brachioradialis (Fig. 3). The deep fascia is then opened, the radial nerve is brought into view on the front of the lateral epicondyle between the brachioradialis laterally and the biceps and brachialis muscles medially (Fig. 2). Its superficial (sensory) and deep (motor) branches are identified (see above) and protected. The lateral antibrachial cutaneous nerve (branch of musculocutaneous) appears between the tendon of the biceps and the brachialis muscle and must be protected by retraction medially (Fig. 2). With the hand supinated, the upper end of the radius is exposed and the joint entered by an incision into the periosteum of the radius medial to the attachment of the supinator and lateral to the attachment of the pronator terres.

4. **Exposure of the Ulnar Nerve in the Region of the Elbow Joint through a Posterior Medial Incision** (Fig. 1) — an incision is centered over the groove between the medial epicondyle and the olecranon process. The nerve lies beneath the deep fascia in a groove in the triceps, just behind the medial intermuscular septum. The fascial roof bridging the interval between the epicondyle and the olecranon must be cut to expose and free the nerve as it enters the forearm between the two heads of the flexor carpi ulnaris. Branches of the nerve to this muscle must be preserved.

5. **Carpal Tunnel Syndrome or Median Neuritis at the Wrist** (Fig. 4) — at the wrist, unyielding walls of a tunnel are formed by the carpal bones posteriorly and the strong transverse carpal ligament anteriorly which bridges the interval between the pisiform and hamate bones medially and the navicular and the greater multangulum laterally. Through this closed space pass the flexor tendons with their mucous sheaths and the median nerve (Fig. 5, page 73).

Any lesion which reduces the cross-sectional area of this tunnel, may produce pressure on the median nerve. Distal to the *tunnel*, the median nerve furnishes sensory fibers to the radial three and a half fingers and motor fibers to the muscles of the thenar eminence. Pain and paresthesias, and weakness or paralysis with atrophy of the thenar muscles, are characteristic of the syndrome. A positive Tinel's sign (a tingling sensation in the distal end of the radial three fingers when percussion is made over the medial nerve at the wrist) and a delayed medial nerve conduction time are diagnostic of the syndrome.

Surgical decompression may be necessary. A longitudinal incision is made from the superior to the inferior border of the ligament medial to the median nerve, taking care to avoid its recurrent motor branch.

6. **Fracture of the Navicular** (Fig. 5) — is a common carpal injury. The fracture occurs at the narrow "waist," producing two fragments. Normally, the navicular has a nutrient vessel entering the distal half and another entering the proximal half. Occasionally, both vessels go to the distal half, in which case fracture at the usual site deprives the proximal segment of its blood supply. Delayed union or non-union may result. The latter may require excision of the proximal fragment. A characteristic clinical sign of the fracture is acute tenderness and swelling in the "anatomic snuff box."

7. **Dislocation of the Lunate** (Fig. 6) — is always anterior and the bone comes to lie in the carpal tunnel. Impingement on the median nerve and flexor tendons produces symptoms as described under Carpal Tunnel Syndrome. There is also apparent shortening of the third metacarpal. Open reduction may be required.

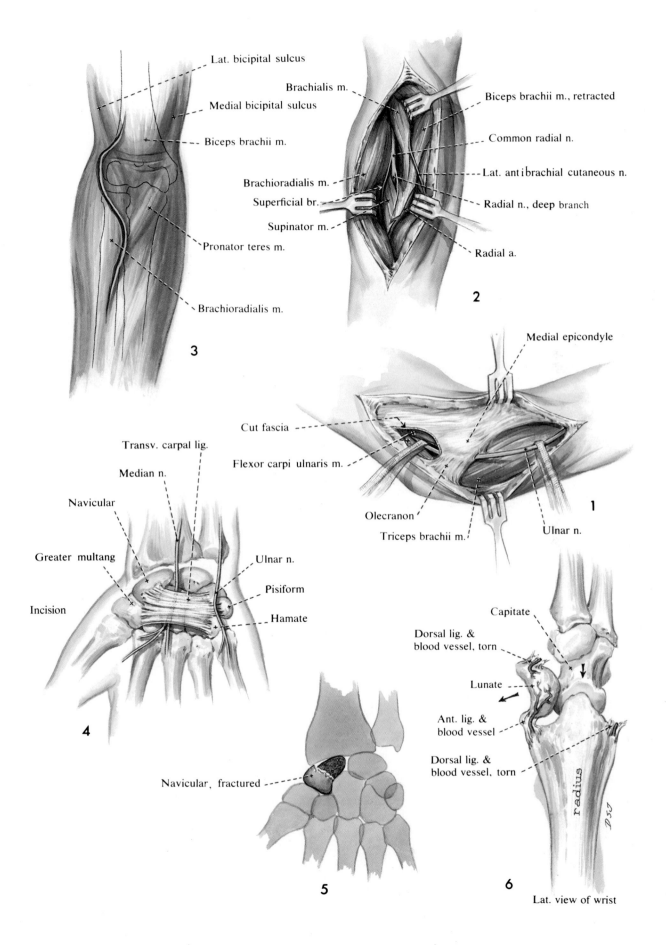

Lat. bicipital sulcus

Brachialis m.

Biceps brachii m., retracted

Medial bicipital sulcus

Common radial n.

Biceps brachii m.

Lat. antibrachial cutaneous n.

Brachioradialis m.

Superficial br.

Radial n., deep branch

Supinator m.

Pronator teres m.

Radial a.

Brachioradialis m.

3

2

Medial epicondyle

Transv. carpal lig.

Median n.

Navicular

Cut fascia

Flexor carpi ulnaris m.

Greater multang

Ulnar n.

Pisiform

Incision

Hamate

Olecranon

Triceps brachii m.

Ulnar n.

1

4

Capitate

Dorsal lig. & blood vessel, torn

Lunate

Ant. lig. & blood vessel

Dorsal lig. & blood vessel, torn

Navicular, fractured

radius

5

6

Lat. view of wrist

The Thorax

BONY THORACIC CAGE (Fig. 1):

The bony cage is conical in shape with an open apex above, the *superior thoracic aperture,* through which pass the esophagus, the trachea, and the great vessels leading to and from the neck and upper extremities. The base, the *inferior thoracic aperture,* is closed by the diaphragm which has foramina allowing passage of important structures to and from the abdominal cavity (page 127). The constituents of the cage are 12 thoracic vertebrae, 12 pairs of ribs, 10 pairs of costal cartilages, and the sternum.

Topography (Fig. 2):

A number of longitudinal topographic lines may be drawn on the thoracic wall which are convenient in describing and localizing certain points on the surface of the chest. Some of these lines are shown in Figure 2. A most important topographic landmark is the transverse protuberance in the midsternal line at the junction of the manubrium and body of the sternum, the *angle of Louis,* which marks the level of the second rib.

Skin and Subcutaneous Tissue (page 43):

Muscles of the Thoracic Wall (Figs. 2 and 3):

The muscles of the thoracic wall may be divided into an extrinsic and intrinsic group.

Extrinsic Muscles — have either their origin or insertion on the bony thorax. Those extrinsic muscles related to the anterior thoracic wall are discussed on page 44. On the posterior wall, the following muscles may be seen (Fig. 3):

1. TRAPEZIUS — arises from the occipital bone, ligamentum nuchae, and supraspinatus ligament from C_7 to T_{12} and inserts on the clavicle, acromion, and spine of the scapula. It is innervated by the spinal accessory and deep cervical plexus.

2. LATISSIMUS DORSI — takes origin from an aponeurosis covering the lumbar and lower portion of thoracic area and iliac crest and inserts into the intertubercular groove of the humerus. It receives nerve fibers from the middle subscapular (thoracodorsal) nerve from the posterior cord of the brachial plexus.

Other extrinsic muscles related to the posterior thoracic wall are illustrated in Figure 3.

Intrinsic Muscles (Fig. 2) — have both their origin and insertion on the thoracic wall and are innervated by thoracic nerves.

1. EXTERNAL LAYER:

External Intercostals — are the main muscles derived from this layer. They extend caudally in an anterior direction and are homologous to the external oblique muscle of the abdominal wall. The fibers extend between the ribs, but between the costal cartilages they are membranous, the *anterior intercostal membrane.*

2. MIDDLE LAYER:

Internal Intercostals — pass caudally in a posterior direction and are homologous to the internal oblique in the abdominal wall. The fibers extend from the sternal border to the angle of the rib where they become membranous, the *posterior intercostal membrane* (Fig. 3).

3. INTERNAL LAYER — is derived from the same muscle sheet that produces the transverse abdominis and consists of two main muscle groups:

a. *Transverse Thoracic* — extends from the third to sixth costal cartilage and inserts into the lower part of the body and xiphoid process of the sternum.

b. *Innermost Intercostals* — are deep to internal intercostal passing from rib to rib in a similar direction. (See Fig. 3, page 89.)

Endothoracic Fascia (Fig. 2):

This is a thin but distinct fascial layer which lines the thoracic cage. It is continuous above with the cervical prevertebral fascia, with Sibson's fascia along the border of the first rib, and behind the sternum with the cervical pretracheal fascia. Below it overlies the diaphragm and is continuous with the fascia lining the abdominal cavity, the *endo-abdominal fascia.* Deep to this fascial plane is the thoracic cavity.

Intercostal Spaces:

There are eleven intercostal spaces. They are wider above than below, and wider anteriorly than posteriorly. Each interspace contains the intrinsic thoracic muscles and the intercostal nerves, arteries and veins.

1. **Intercostal Arteries** — are of two types, anterior and posterior.

a. ANTERIOR INTERCOSTALS (Fig. 4) — arise from the internal mammary artery from the first portion of the subclavian artery (page 22). As the artery descends through the thorax it gives rise to two anterior intercostals in each interspace, a *superior* and *inferior.* At the level of the sixth costochondral junction it divides into a *superior epigastric* artery, which passes into the abdomen, and the *musculophrenic.* The latter gives rise to the anterior intercostals of the sixth to ninth interspace. The lower two spaces contain no anterior arteries. Needles inserted into the anterior chest wall should be placed in the midportion of the space to avoid the superior and inferior branches of the internal mammary artery.

b. POSTERIOR INTERCOSTALS (Figs. 3 and 4) — arise from two sources. The costocervical trunk of the second portion of the subclavian (page 26) gives rise to the posterior branches of the first and second interspace via the *superior intercostal.* The remaining branches, one in each interspace, arise from the descending thoracic aorta. In relation to the posterior thoracic wall they lie in the middle of the interspace, but as they pass laterally to anastomose with the anterior intercostals, the main branches lie in the subcostal groove at the upper portion of the interspace (see Fig. 3, page 89). These relations should be kept in mind during surgical incisions or paracentesis of the thoracic wall.

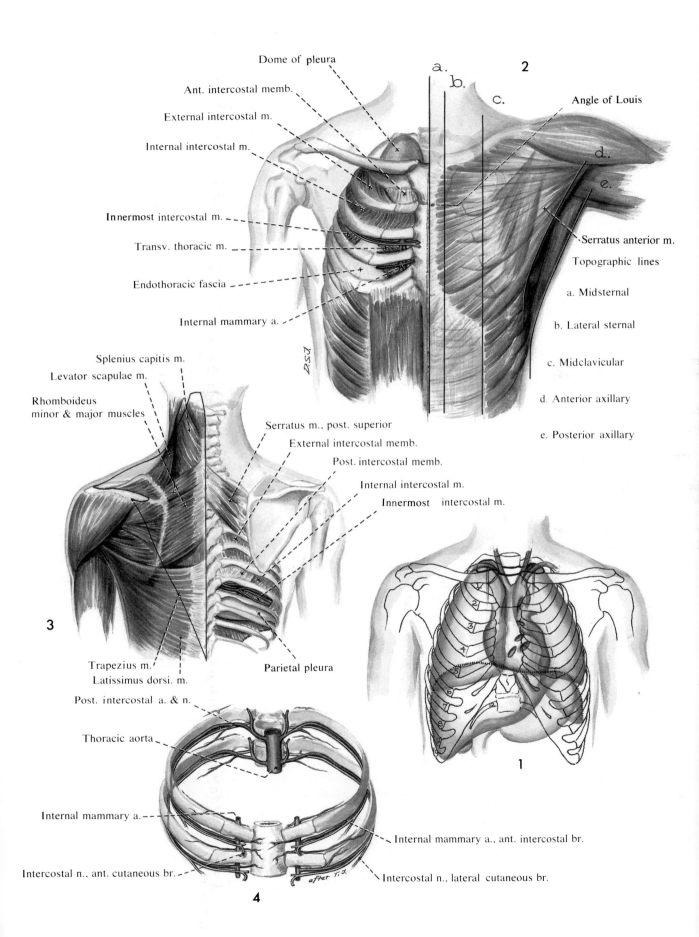

Dome of pleura

Ant. intercostal memb.

External intercostal m.

Internal intercostal m.

Innermost intercostal m.

Transv. thoracic m.

Endothoracic fascia

Internal mammary a.

2

a.   b.   c.

Angle of Louis

d.

e.

Serratus anterior m.

Topographic lines

a. Midsternal

b. Lateral sternal

c. Midclavicular

d. Anterior axillary

e. Posterior axillary

Splenius capitis m.

Levator scapulae m.

Rhomboideus
minor & major muscles

Serratus m., post. superior

External intercostal memb.

Post. intercostal memb.

Internal intercostal m.

Innermost intercostal m.

3

Trapezius m.

Latissimus dorsi. m.

Parietal pleura

Post. intercostal a. & n.

Thoracic aorta

Internal mammary a.

Intercostal n., ant. cutaneous br.

Internal mammary a., ant. intercostal br.

Intercostal n., lateral cutaneous br.

1

4

after T.J.

TYPICAL THORACIC NERVES (Fig. 1):

The midthoracic nerves may be considered as typical spinal nerves. There are 31 pairs of segmentally arranged spinal nerves—8 cervical, 12 thoracic, 5 lumbar, 5 sacral, and 1 coccygeal. Each nerve arises from the cord by two roots, a *dorsal* or *sensory root* and a *ventral* or *motor root*. On each dorsal root is a collection of nerve cell bodies called a *spinal ganglion*. (A *ganglion* is a collection of nerve cell bodies outside the central nervous system.) The ventral root fibers arise from accumulation of nerve cell bodies within the central nervous system called *nuclei*. These fibers consist of somatic motor impulses to striated musculature and, in the thoracic, upper lumbar, and some sacral roots, visceral motor (autonomic) fibers. The two roots pierce the dura and join at the intervertebral foramina to form a mixed spinal nerve. This mixed nerve divides into four branches:

1. **Meningeal Ramus**—is a small branch which re-enters the intervertebral foramen to supply the meninges and vertebral column.

2. **Posterior Primary Division**—supplies the autochthonous (true) muscles and skin of the back.

3. **Rami Communicantes**—consists of fibers going to and from the sympathetic ganglia and is made up of a *white* and *gray ramus*. The former contains myelinated (white) preganglionic fibers from cord to ganglia; the latter, the unmyelinated (gray) fibers which join the anterior primary divisions, to be distributed to the body wall. *All* spinal nerves possess a gray ramus, but only the thoracic and upper lumbar nerves have a white ramus. These fibers constitute the thoracolumbar sympathetic outflow.

4. **Anterior Primary Divisions**—of the cervical, lumbar, sacral, and coccygeal nerves unite to form *plexuses*. The anterior divisions of the thoracic nerves, with the exception of the first and last, divide in a typical manner. They radiate to the anterior thoracic and abdominal walls between the middle and internal muscular layers, giving rise to muscular and cutaneous branches. In the thorax, the 12 pairs of anterior divisions are referred to as *intercostal* nerves; however, the twelfth is actually *subcostal*. The first thoracic nerve enters mainly into the brachial plexus (page 24), whereas the twelfth aids in the formation of the lumbar plexus. The second to the sixth nerves run purely an intercostal course, but the seventh to twelfth extend to the abdominal wall.

The anterior primary divisions of the second to twelfth thoracic nerves give off cutaneous branches which are important in neurologic diagnosis as to the level of spinal cord injury. The first thoracic nerve enters almost wholly into the brachial plexus, and its cutaneous area is supplied by the supraclavicular branches of the superficial cervical plexus.

a. LATERAL CUTANEOUS BRANCHES—arise in line with the midaxillary line of either side and divide into anterior and posterior rami. An exception is that of the second thoracic, which extends into the brachium as the intercostal *brachial nerve* (Figs. 2 and 3, page 45).

b. ANTERIOR CUTANEOUS BRANCHES—enter the subcutaneous tissue in line with parasternal line and divide into medial and lateral branches.

CUTANEOUS INNERVATION OF VENTROLATERAL ABDOMINAL AND THORACIC WALL (Fig. 2):

1. **Supraclavicular Nerves** (C_3 and C_4)—from the superficial cervical plexus supply the first intercostal space.

2. T_2 **to** T_6—supply the thoracic wall.

3. T_7 **to** T_9—supply the abdominal wall above the umbilicus.

4. T_{10}—supplies the umbilical region.

5. T_{11} **to** T_{12}—supply the region from below the umbilicus to an area two-thirds the distance between umbilicus and pubis.

INTERCOSTAL NERVE BLOCK (Fig. 3):

The intercostal nerves are located in the posterolateral thoracic wall in the subcostal groove below the intercostal vein and artery in each interspace. A skin wheal is made over the lower aspect of the ribs in the anterior axillary line. The needle is inserted until the bone is encountered (Fig. 3-1). It is then withdrawn slightly and reinserted so as to pass just below the lower edge of the rib (Fig. 3-2).

SENSORY INNERVATION OF THE DIAPHRAGM (Figs. 4 and 5):

The nerve supply to the diaphragm is of importance in the diagnosis of certain intrathoracic and intra-abdominal pathologic processes. This is a dual innervation; the peripheral rim of the diaphragm and related pleura are innervated by branches of the intercostal nerves, and pain in this area is referred to the lower thoracic and upper abdominal areas (Fig. 5). The central portion of the diaphragm is innervated by the phrenic nerve, and irritation in this area refers pain to the neck and shoulder, which are supplied by nerves from the same spinal segments as the phrenic nerve (Fig. 5).

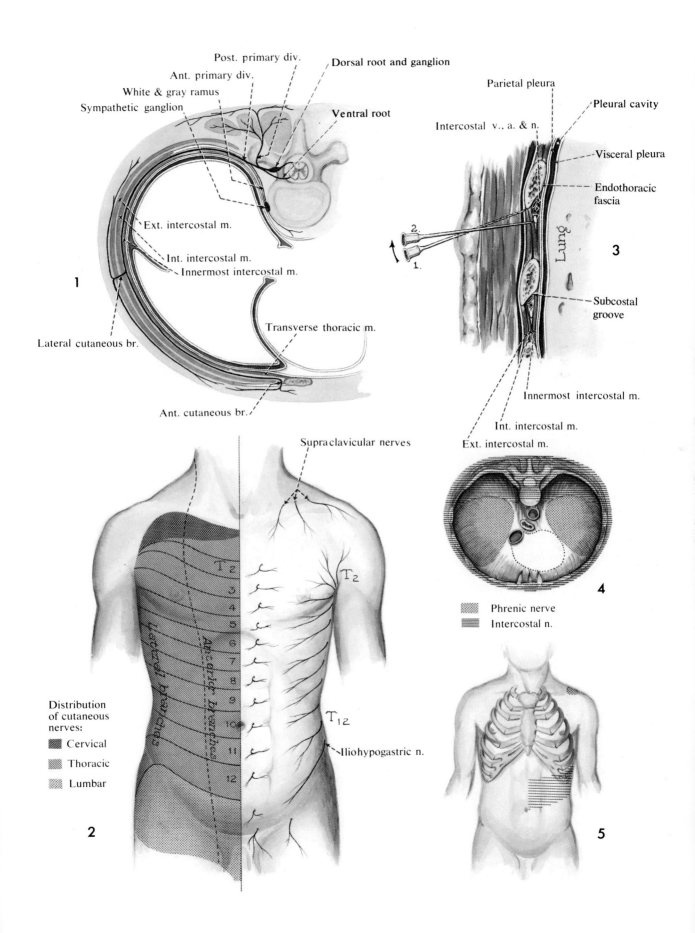

Post. primary div.

Ant. primary div.

Dorsal root and ganglion

White & gray ramus

Parietal pleura

Sympathetic ganglion

Ventral root

Pleural cavity

Intercostal v., a. & n.

Visceral pleura

Endothoracic fascia

Ext. intercostal m.

1

Int. intercostal m.

Innermost intercostal m.

3

Lung

Subcostal groove

Transverse thoracic m.

Lateral cutaneous br.

Innermost intercostal m.

Ant. cutaneous br.

Int. intercostal m.

Ext. intercostal m.

Supraclavicular nerves

4

Phrenic nerve

Intercostal n.

T 2

T₂

Distribution of cutaneous nerves:

Cervical

Thoracic

Lumbar

T₁₂

Iliohypogastric n.

2

5

CHEST WALL INCISIONS:

The position of the patient on the operating table will vary with the surgical approach. It may be supine, lateral, or prone. In general, the lateral approach is the most satisfactory for the hilum of the lung, the posterior mediastinum, and the diaphragm. Its chief disadvantage is the possibility of spillover of bronchial secretions into the dependent lung. The supine position is free from this objection but it affords much more limited exposure of structures in the posterior part of the chest. The prone position is not frequently used and is usually reserved for those patients with excessive tracheobronchial secretions in whom spillage to the opposite lung is an especial hazard during the operative procedure.

Exposure of the anterior and middle parts of the mediastinum may be obtained through a median or transverse sternotomy. Also a thoraco-abdominal incision which crosses the costal arch is useful in the management of combined thoracic and abdominal wounds and, less often, in the repair of a diaphragmatic hernia, gastric resection (cardia), and partial hepatectomy.

Anterior Incision (Fig. 1):

This approach affords only limited exposure, but it is frequently used for an open biopsy of the lung or, with decreasing frequency, for open cardiac resuscitation. With the patient in a supine position, an incision is made in the skin and subcutaneous tissue over the anterior part of the fourth intercostal space from the lateral margin of the sternum, inferior to the breast, to the anterior or mid-axillary line. It is then carried through the fibers of the pectoralis major and minor muscles. In making the incision through the intercostal muscles of the fourth interspace, the anterior end of the cut stops about 1.5 cm. lateral to the sternal border in order to avoid section of the internal mammary vessels. The lung is exposed when the parietal pleura is opened.

This incision may be extended to the posterior axillary line at the skin level and to the neck of the ribs at the level of the intercostal muscles to give wide exposure for a major intrathoracic procedure such as division of a patent ductus arteriosus, a pulmonary-aortic anastomosis, or pulmonary resection. When it is extended posteriorly in this manner the latissimus dorsi muscle with the thoracodorsal nerve and subcapsular vessels can be retracted laterally and be kept intact.

Lateral Incision:

This approach, or a modification of it, is the basic standard incision through which most procedures on the lung, the esophagus, the mediastinum, and the diaphragm are performed.

Figure 2 shows the position of the patient on the operating table and the topography of a right posterolateral incision. In Figures 3 and 4, the successive structures which must be cut as the chest cavity is entered through the bed of the sixth rib are shown; Figure 5 illustrates the extent of exposure of intrathoracic structures which may be obtained with this approach.

An incision through the bed of the sixth rib, or through the sixth interspace, may be made beginning at a point at the level of the angle of the scapula about midway between the vertebral border of the scapula and the posterior midline (Fig. 2). As the incision is carried forward, it passes downward just caudal to the angle of the scapula and may be extended to the midclavicular line. In the posterior angle the lower fibers of the trapezius muscle and the underlying rhomboid major are cut. Anteriorly the fibers of the latissimus dorsi must be cut across the entire belly of the muscle. Deep to the latissimus and extending to the anterior axillary line is the serratus anterior with the long thoracic nerve lying on its surface. These must be cut in the line of the incision. The cut edges of these structures are shown as slightly separated in Figure 3.

In Figure 4, the margins of the wound are retracted, the periosteum of the sixth rib has been incised and a long segment of the rib has been removed subperiosteally. An incision in the periosteum of the bed of the rib and the underlying parietal pleura opens the pleural cavity (Fig. 5). The lung is shown partially collapsed and the upper lobe retracted inferiorly. The accessibility of the anterior, superior, and posterior mediastinal structures and the root of the lung is well shown.

Median Sternotomy:

The sternal splitting incision is sometimes used to approach the anterior or superior mediastinum, in removal of the thymus or a tumor of the thymus, or for exploration of the mediastinum in the search for a functioning parathyroid adenoma when none has been found in the neck.

An incision is made in the midline through skin and subcutaneous tissue from the upper border of the manubrium to the xiphoid. With a sternal splitting knife or saw, the sternum is split through parts or the whole of its length. As this is done, care must be taken to avoid injury to the left innominate veins and the pericardium.

The Transverse Sternotomy:

This incision is used to approach the heart and the middle mediastinal structures. A long transverse incision is made below the breasts over the fourth intercostal space. The sternum is divided, the fibers of the pectoralis major muscle on each side are cut to expose the anterior intercostal membrane and external intercostal muscles. The internal mammary vessels must be ligated and divided as the incision is carried through the soft tissue of the intercostal spaces about 1 cm. lateral to the margins of the sternum. When the margins of this incision are spread widely, excellent exposure of the heart and great vessels is provided. This incision may be made in an interspace higher or lower, depending upon the need.

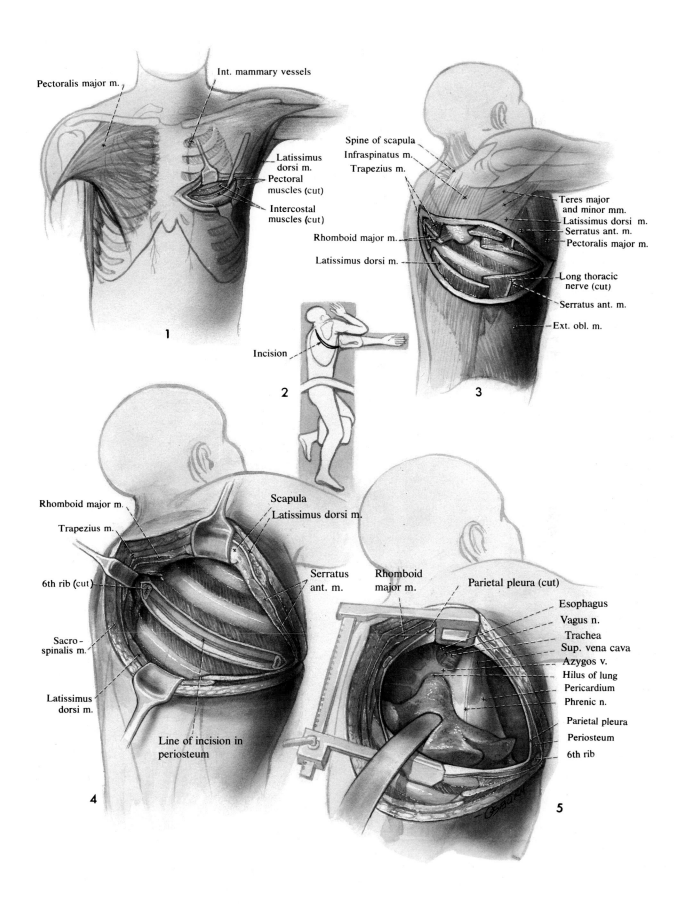

Pectoralis major m.

Int. mammary vessels

Latissimus dorsi m.
Pectoral muscles (cut)
Intercostal muscles (cut)

1

Spine of scapula
Infraspinatus m.
Trapezius m.

Teres major and minor mm.
Latissimus dorsi m.
Serratus ant. m.
Pectoralis major m.

Rhomboid major m.

Latissimus dorsi m.

Long thoracic nerve (cut)
Serratus ant. m.
Ext. obl. m.

3

Incision

2

Rhomboid major m.
Trapezius m.

Scapula
Latissimus dorsi m.

6th rib (cut)

Serratus ant. m.

Rhomboid major m.

Parietal pleura (cut)

Esophagus
Vagus n.
Trachea
Sup. vena cava
Azygos v.
Hilus of lung
Pericardium
Phrenic n.

Parietal pleura
Periosteum
6th rib

Sacro-spinalis m.

Latissimus dorsi m.

Line of incision in periosteum

4

5

The Thorax

COMPRESSION INJURIES OF THE CHEST:

Automobile collisions account for most compression injuries of the chest today, though falls from considerable heights, the passage of a wheel over the chest, and other such crushing forces produce some of these injuries. Understandably, they may be, and often are, associated with serious trauma to other regions of the body. Since the driver of a car is more likely to receive a compression injury of the chest than are other passengers, and since the mechanism of injury is clear, we have used this situation for illustration in Figures 1 and 2.

The crushed chest results from the severe thrust of the anterior chest wall against the upper end of the steering column. Not only are several ribs fractured, but each is broken in two or more places and, in addition, the sternum may be detached from the costal cartilages on one or both sides. Rarely the sternum itself is fractured. The gravity of the injury depends upon the number of ribs fractured, whether those on one or both sides are involved, and on the injuries to intrathoracic organs. Because of the remarkable elasticity of the ribs and chest cage in children, compression may produce injury within the chest in the absence of rib fracture or significant damage to the chest wall. A number of young children have sustained rupture of the trachea or a major bronchus without injury to the chest cage. But a crushed chest wall which allows serious paradoxical motion of the chest wall will in itself produce severe respiratory embarrassment. Some means of stabilization, either by external traction, or by internal splinting with the use of a mechanical respirator is commonly necessary to correct the ventilatory deficiency. The common intrathoracic injuries and complications associated with this type of severe compression injury to the chest are listed on page 91 and shown in Figure 3.

A sharp, bony fragment of rib may produce serious hemorrhage into the pleural space by tearing an intercostal vessel or the parenchyma of the lung or both. In the crushed chest, blood loss sufficient to produce hypovolemic shock is common. Bleeding into the pleural space under these conditions is usually self-limiting, and continued hemorrhage requiring thoracotomy for its control is most unusual.

Laceration of the lung accounts not only for hemorrhage into the pleural cavity, but for the escape of air. The volume of blood and air which accumulates determines the extent of pulmonary collapse. If this accumulation is sufficient to produce a positive pressure on the side of injury, a shift on the mobile mediastinum toward the uninjured side may interfere with ventilation enough to threaten life. This is the "tension pneumothorax" which demands immediate relief.

By way of the torn parietal pleura which opens the tissue planes of the chest wall to intrapleural air, and by way of the perivascular and peribronchial planes of loose areolar tissue in the lung, air can make its way from the torn lung into the subcutaneous tissues of the chest wall and into the mediastinum and by way of the latter to the neck. The presence of air beneath the skin is manifest by swelling, which may be slight or alarming in appearance, and by crepitation. Small amounts which may not be evident clinically can be detected on the roentgenogram.

Occasionally the injuring force produces a tear in a major bronchus or the intrathoracic portion of the trachea either by a shearing action or by bursting pressure when the glottis is closed at the moment of injury. Blood in the tracheobronchial tree as a result of such a tear or following any injury to the lung parenchyma may produce serious obstruction.

Blood in the bronchi and trachea accounts in part for the wet-lung syndrome. The term is a clinical one, indicating the presence of blood, mucus, serum, or fluid in the lung, bronchi, and trachea. In all major wounds of the chest, the lung tissue reacts to produce more than the normal amount of interstitial and intra-alveolar fluid, the quantity depending upon the type and severity of the injury. The factors responsible for this accumulation of fluid are (1) pulmonary trauma, (2) increased respiratory effort, (3) tracheal obstruction, (4) anoxia, and (5) an ineffective cough.

Because it permits frequent removal of blood and secretions from the airway, tracheostomy has attained an important place in the management of these patients. The procedure also reduces resistance to air flow and reduces dead space.

With involvement of the lower part of the chest cage by the forces of compression, injury to the heart may be produced. This may be contusion of the myocardium or, rarely, a tear in the pericardium which results in hemorrhage and cardiac tamponade. With compression of the lower chest, injuries below the diaphragm, such as lacerations of the liver or spleen, may also occur.

Intrathoracic complications may be expected in two-thirds of all cases of multiple rib fractures. The physician must be prepared to expect and to recognize them promptly and to respond with appropriate therapeutic measures.

RIB
  1. fracture
PLEURA
  2. laceration
  3. subcutaneous emphysema
  4. pneumothorax
  5. mediastinal deviation
LUNG
  6. laceration
  7. hemothorax
TRACHEA
  8. laceration of bronchus
  9. blood in trachea
LIVER
  10. laceration
SPLEEN
  11. laceration

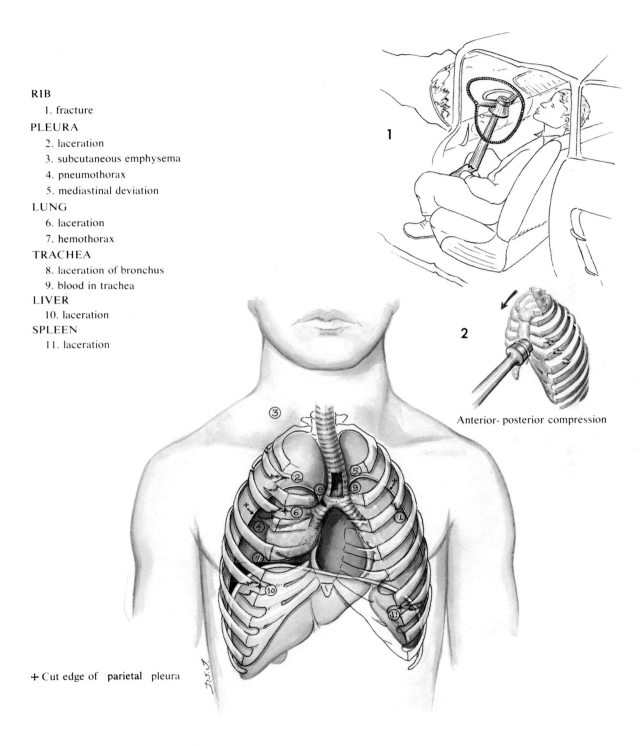

1

2   Anterior- posterior compression

+ Cut edge of parietal pleura

3   **Compression Injuries of the Chest**

MEDIASTINUM:

The mediastinum is that portion of the thoracic cavity included between the thoracic spine behind, the sternum in front, and the two pleural cavities laterally. It is limited superiorly by the superior thoracic aperture and inferiorly by the diaphragm. This area is arbitrarily divided into certain subdivisions which have no anatomic, physiologic, or surgical significance aside from assisting in the didactic approach to this region (Fig. 1). This space cannot be anatomically divided, for it is ever changing in size and shape with respiration and cardiac activity. Surgically considered, the mediastinum has an anatomic continuity from the neck to the abdomen. A line drawn from the lower border of the fourth thoracic vertebra to the junction of the body (gladiolus) and manubrium of the sternum (*angle of Louis*) arbitrarily divides the mediastinum into a *superior* and *inferior* compartment. The pericardial sac further subdivides the inferior compartment into three divisions. Anterior to the sac is the *anterior mediastinum;* the area behind, the *posterior mediastinum*, whereas the pericardial sac, its contents and laterally related structures constitute the *middle mediastinum* (Fig. 1).

The approach in many surgical procedures involving mediastinal structures is through the pleural cavity. The relational anatomy of these mediastinal structures to the pleura bounding this compartment *(mediastinal pleura)* is therefore important to the surgeon. It will be seen that in relation to the right mediastinal pleura they are *primarily* venous structures, whereas on the left, arterial.

1. Right Mediastinum (Fig. 2):

a. **Anterior to the Right Lung Root:**

(1) RIGHT ATRIUM — and right surface of the pericardial sac produce the largest impression on the mediastinal wall.

(2) INFERIOR VENA CAVA — produces a small eminence between the right atrium and diaphragm.

(3) SUPERIOR VENA CAVA AND RIGHT INNOMINATE VEIN — extends superiorly from the right atrium to the superior thoracic aperture.

(4) RIGHT PHRENIC NERVE AND PERICARDIACOPHRENIC VESSELS — adhere to the pericardial sac

and descend in alignment with the venous channels mentioned above.

b. **Posterior to the Right Lung Root:**

(1) AZYGOS VEIN — ascends behind the lung root and arches over the root to empty into the superior vena cava.

(2) ESOPHAGUS — is related to the right mediastinal pleura in the upper two-thirds of the thorax lying on the vertebral column.

(3) TRACHEA — in its thoracic portion is deviated to the right and bifurcates into its major bronchi at the lower border of T_4.

(4) RIGHT VAGUS NERVE — adheres to the lateral side of the trachea in the upper thorax, then passes behind the root of the lung and is related to the esophagus in the lower chest.

2. Left Mediastinum (Fig. 3):

a. **Anterior to the Left Lung Root:**

(1) LEFT VENTRICLE, ATRIUM — and left surface of the pericardial sac produce the largest eminence as viewed from the left pleural cavity.

(2) LEFT PHRENIC NERVE AND PERICARDIACOPHRENIC VESSELS — descend along the pericardial sac to the diaphragm.

b. **Posterior to the Left Lung Root:**

(1) DESCENDING THORACIC AORTA — forms a prominent impression of the mediastinal pleura behind the lung root and the *aortic arch,* an impression over the root. (Note the comparison with the azygos vein on the right side.)

(2) LEFT COMMON CAROTID AND SUBCLAVIAN ARTERIES — extend upward from the aortic arch to the superior aperture.

(3) LEFT VAGUS NERVE — crosses the aortic arch and passes behind the root of the lung, where it adheres to the lateral wall of the esophagus.

(4) LEFT SUPERIOR INTERCOSTAL VEIN — passes from posterior to anterior superfically over the upper portion of the arch.

(5) ESOPHAGUS — may be seen in the lower thorax in the *esophageal triangle.* Its boundaries are the pericardial sac in front, the descending aorta behind, and the diaphragm below.

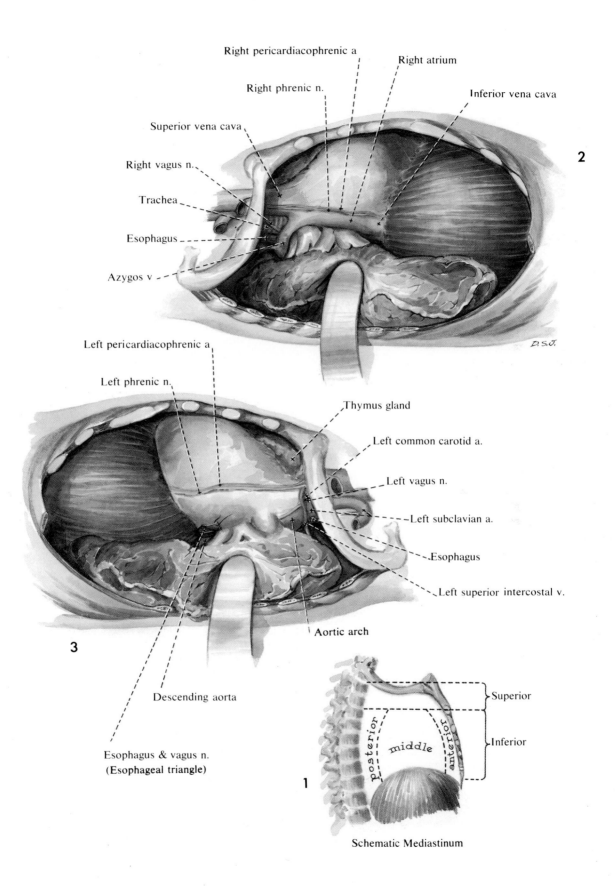

Right pericardiacophrenic a

Right phrenic n.

Right atrium

Inferior vena cava

Superior vena cava

Right vagus n.

Trachea

Esophagus

Azygos v

2

Left pericardiacophrenic a

Left phrenic n.

Thymus gland

Left common carotid a.

Left vagus n.

Left subclavian a.

Esophagus

Left superior intercostal v.

Aortic arch

3

Descending aorta

Esophagus & vagus n.
(Esophageal triangle)

posterior

middle

anterior

Superior

Inferior

1

Schematic Mediastinum

The Thorax

SUPERIOR MEDIASTINUM:

This anatomic space lies between the mediastinal pleura in an area between the superior thoracic aperture and a line drawn between the angle of Louis and lower border of T_4. The key structure in this area is the *aortic arch*. As it passes posteriorly and to the left it gives rise to three branches (Figs. 1 and 2).

1. **Innominate Artery** — is the first and largest branch and arises at the level of the upper border of the second right costal cartilage. It ascends obliquely to the right of the sternoclavicular joint, where it divides into right common carotid and right subclavian arteries.

2. **Left Common Carotid Artery** — ascends from the arch through the superior aperture and continues into the cervical area.

3. **Left Subclavian Artery** — also exits through the superior aperture to the root of the neck.

Other structures in this area are all related to the aortic arch, either in front, behind, or below.

1. **Anterior to the Right** (Figs. 1 and 2) — these structures are described to the right because of the curvature of the arch to the left.

a. THYMUS — is a bilobed organ which reaches its greatest size at adolescence; thereafter, it undergoes involution. It may extend into the neck above or the anterior mediastinum below. The arterial supply is mainly by the internal mammary vessels (Fig. 1). Its venous drainage is into the left innominate or internal mammary veins.

b. INTERNAL MAMMARY ARTERY — arises from the first portion of the subclavian artery. It descends through the thorax lying on the pleura to the level of the third costal cartilage. Below this level the transverse thoracic muscle intervenes between the artery and pleura. It is accompanied by venae comitantes.

c. INNOMINATE VEINS — both right and left arise at the junction of the subclavian and internal jugular veins and join to form the superior vena cava.

d. SUPERIOR VENA CAVA — in its extrapericardial part lies in the superior mediastinum and receives the azygos vein (Fig. 2, page 95).

e. RIGHT PHRENIC NERVE — enters the mediastinum between the right subclavian vein and artery and descends along the lateral surface of the right innominate and superior vena cava.

2. **Anterior to the Left** (Figs. 2 and 3):

a. LEFT SUPERIOR INTERCOSTAL VEIN — is a remnant of the left superior vena cava. It drains the upper three interspaces of the left chest and empties into the left innominate vein.

b. LEFT PHRENIC NERVE — enters the thorax deep to the left innominate vein and between the left common carotid and left subclavian arteries. It is the most anterior of the nerves crossing the aortic arch, and passes anterior to the root of the lung.

c. LEFT VAGUS NERVE — is the most posterior nerve crossing the aortic arch. At the thoracic inlet it is crossed by the phrenic nerve, then passes over the arch and proceeds through the inferior mediastinal compartment behind the lung root.

d. LEFT INFERIOR CERVICAL VAGAL CARDIAC BRANCH (not shown) — takes origin from the vagus in the neck and passes to the superficial cardiac plexus beneath the aortic arch (*ganglion of Wrisberg*).

e. LEFT SUPERIOR CERVICAL SYMPATHETIC CARDIAC BRANCH (not shown) — arises from the left superior cervical sympathetic ganglion and crosses the arch just anterior to the left vagus nerve to terminate in the superficial cardiac plexus.

3. **Posterior to the Arch on the Right Side** (Fig. 3):

a. ESOPHAGUS — rests on the vertebral column and is deviated to the right by the aortic arch.

b. TRACHEA — is just anterior to the esophagus and is also deviated to the right by the arch of the aorta.

c. RIGHT VAGUS NERVE — extends along the lateral wall of the trachea in the superior mediastinum, then passes posterior to the lung root.

d. LEFT RECURRENT LARYNGEAL NERVE — lies in the left tracheo-esophageal groove after arising from the main left vagus trunk under the aortic arch.

e. THORACIC DUCT — ascends through the posterior mediastinum on the right side of the chest but crosses behind the esophagus between T_6 and T_4 to the left of the midline. It extends upward through the superior aperture to the root of the neck.

4. **Below the Aortic Arch** (Fig. 3):

a. BIFURCATION OF PULMONARY ARTERY — occurs in the concavity of the aortic arch. The left pulmonary artery is seen extending into the left hilum. The right pulmonary artery extends posterior to the ascending aorta and superior vena cava to supply the right lung (Fig. 2, page 113).

b. LIGAMENTUM ARTERIOSUM — is a fibrous cord remnant of the *ductus arteriosus* (Botalli) in the fetus. It extends from the region of the pulmonary artery bifurcation to the under surface of the arch of the aorta, usually opposite the origin of the left subclavian artery (Fig. 2).

c. LEFT RECURRENT LARYNGEAL NERVE — arises from the left vagus as the latter nerve crosses the aortic arch and winds around the concavity of the arch under the ligamentum arteriosum. Posterior to the arch it lies in the tracheo-esophageal groove.

d. LEFT MAIN STEM BRONCHUS — takes origin from the tracheal bifurcation at the lower border of T_4 and extends beneath the aortic arch and left pulmonary artery to reach the left lung hilus.

e. SUPERFICIAL CARDIAC PLEXUS (not shown) — receives the two cardiac branches which pass over the arch of the aorta: the left cervical inferior vagal cardiac, and the left superior cervical sympathetic cardiac branch. The ganglion associated with this plexus (the *ganglion of Wrisberg*) is located under the arch to the right of the ligamentum arteriosum. All other cardiac branches from the vagus and cervical sympathetic ganglia go to the *deep cardiac plexus* located under the bifurcation of the trachea.

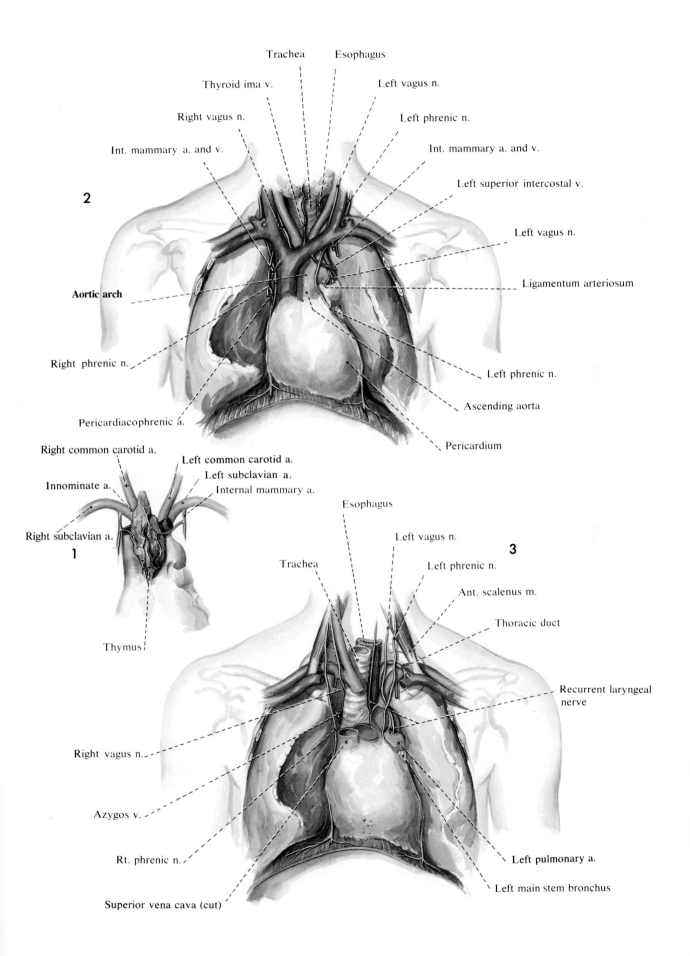

Trachea

Esophagus

Thyroid ima v.

Left vagus n.

Right vagus n.

Left phrenic n.

Int. mammary a. and v.

Int. mammary a. and v.

Left superior intercostal v.

2

Left vagus n.

Aortic arch

Ligamentum arteriosum

Right phrenic n.

Left phrenic n.

Ascending aorta

Pericardiacophrenic a.

Pericardium

Right common carotid a.

Left common carotid a.

Left subclavian a.

Innominate a.

Internal mammary a.

3

Esophagus

Left vagus n.

Right subclavian a.

Left phrenic n.

1

Trachea

Ant. scalenus m.

Thoracic duct

Thymus

Recurrent laryngeal nerve

Right vagus n.

Azygos v.

Left pulmonary a.

Rt. phrenic n.

Left main stem bronchus

Superior vena cava (cut)

POSTERIOR MEDIASTINUM:

This space is bounded posteriorly by the vertebral bodies (T_5 to T_{12}), anteriorly by the pericardial sac, laterally by the mediastinal pleura, and inferiorly by the diaphragm. The superior boundary, a line drawn from the angle of Louis to the lower border of T_4, is in continuity with the superior mediastinum, whose key structure, the aortic arch, extends posteriorly and descends through the posterior mediastinum.

1. **Descending Thoracic Aorta** (Figs. 1 and 2) — extends from the lower border of T_4 to the lower border of T_{12}. In its upper part it lies to the left side of the vertebral bodies, but during its descent through the thorax it comes to lie in the midline. Parietal (a to d) and visceral (e to g) branches arise from this portion of the aorta.

a. POSTERIOR INTERCOSTALS — are discussed on page 86. Nine such branches arise directly from the aorta.

b. SUPERIOR PHRENICS — arise just above the diaphragm and are distributed to the superior surface of that structure (Fig. 1, page 127).

c. MEDIASTINAL BRANCHES — supply lymph nodes and areolar tissue in the area.

d. ARTERIA ABERRANS — is a small twig which passes upward to the right behind the esophagus. It is a remnant of the right dorsal aortic arch.

e. PERICARDIAL BRANCHES — are two to three small twigs extending to the posterior surface of pericardial sac.

f. BRONCHIAL ARTERIES (Fig. 4, page 113) — are usually three in number, one right and two left. The *upper left branch* arises from the aorta just below the tracheal bifurcation; the *lower left branch* arises from the aorta just below the level of the left bronchus. The *right bronchial artery* usually arises from the first right upper aortic intercostal artery.

g. ESOPHAGEAL ARTERIES — see below.

2. **Esophagus** (Figs. 1 and 2) — descends into the superior mediastinum and is deviated slightly to the right by the aortic arch. It lies in direct contact with the right mediastinal pleura (Fig. 2, page 95). The arch may produce an impression on the esophagus, as is evidenced by radiographic and esophagoscopic examination. A second impression may be visualized by the endoscopist just below the arch caused by the left main bronchus crossing anteriorly. Below this level the esophagus curves to the left behind the pericardial sac. Enlargement of the left atrium may produce a visible defect in the esophageal lumen as seen during a barium swallow. In the lower one-third of the thoracic cavity the esophagus crosses anterior to the aorta and to the left. Here it may be identified in the *esophageal triangle* (see Fig. 3, page 95).

a. INNERVATION (Fig. 1) — of the thoracic esophagus is by the autonomic nervous system; the parasympathetic fibers arising from the vagus, and the sympathetic fibers from the thoracic sympathetic ganglionic chain. In the upper thorax these fibers arise from the right vagus trunk, left recurrent nerve, and upper thoracic sympathetic ganglia. In the posterior mediastinum the vagal branches form an *esophageal plexus*, which is joined by branches of the lower thoracic sympathetic ganglia. The visceral sensory fibers from this structure have not been definitely established.

b. BLOOD SUPPLY (Fig. 2) — to the cervical and upper thoracic portions of the esophagus is by the inferior thyroid arteries (Fig. 1, page 23) and from an upper intercostal artery. The area related to the tracheal bifurcation is supplied by branches of the right and left bronchial arteries. Usually two esophageal branches arise from the aorta to supply the lower part of the esophagus; however, ascending branches from the left gastric artery also supply this portion.

The esophageal veins are small and numerous. In the upper portion of the esophagus they drain into deep veins of the neck, mainly the inferior thyroid, and into the upper intercostal veins. The remaining vessels are tributaries of the azygos on the right and hemiazygos on the left. The lowermost of these veins communicate with the left gastric (coronary) vein which drains the abdominal esophagus. This is an important connection between portal and systemic venous system, as is evidenced by the development of *esophageal varices* associated with portal hypertension.

3. **Azygos System of Veins** (Fig. 3) — consists of three major longitudinal venous channels.

a. HEMIAZYGOS VEIN — arises in the lumbar region of the abdomen, pierces the left crus of the diaphragm (Fig. 1, page 121), and ascends into the thorax lying behind the aorta. At the level of T_8 it crosses to the right side to empty into the azygos vein. It receives the lower five intercostal veins, as well as esophageal, mediastinal vessels, and accessory azygos vein.

b. ACCESSORY AZYGOS VEIN — descends along the left side of the vertebral column draining the fifth to seventh interspace and empties into the hemiazygos.

c. AZYGOS VEIN — takes origin in the abdomen, pierces the diaphragm (Fig. 1, page 127), and ascends through the mediastinum to the right of the vertebral bodies to the level of T_4. Here it arches over the root of the right lung to empty into the superior vena cava. It receives all intercostal veins of the right side as well as bronchial, esophageal, and mediastinal vessels.

4. **Thoracic Duct** (Fig. 3) — begins in the abdomen and ascends through the posterior mediastinum between the azygos vein and descending thoracic aorta to the level of T_6 to T_4, where it crosses to the left side and extends into the root of the neck (Fig. 1, page 23).

5. **Sympathetic Trunk** (Fig. 3) — is actually beyond the limits of the posterior mediastinum, since it lies on the heads of the ribs and is covered by the costal portion of parietal pleura. Twelve *vertebral ganglia* are usually present, but the first may fuse with the inferior cervical sympathetic ganglion to form the *stellate ganglion*. Each of these ganglia has white and gray rami communicantes (page 86). Some preganglionic (white) fibers do not synapse in the ganglionic cord but pass through to *paravertebral* ganglia. These fibers are called *splanchnic nerves*, of which there are three: the *greater splanchnic nerve* (T_5 to T_9), the *lesser splanchnic nerve* (T_{10} to T_{11}), and the *least splanchnic nerve* (T_{12}). These fibers carry vasomotor impulses to the abdominal blood vessels and carry sensory impulses from certain abdominal organs.

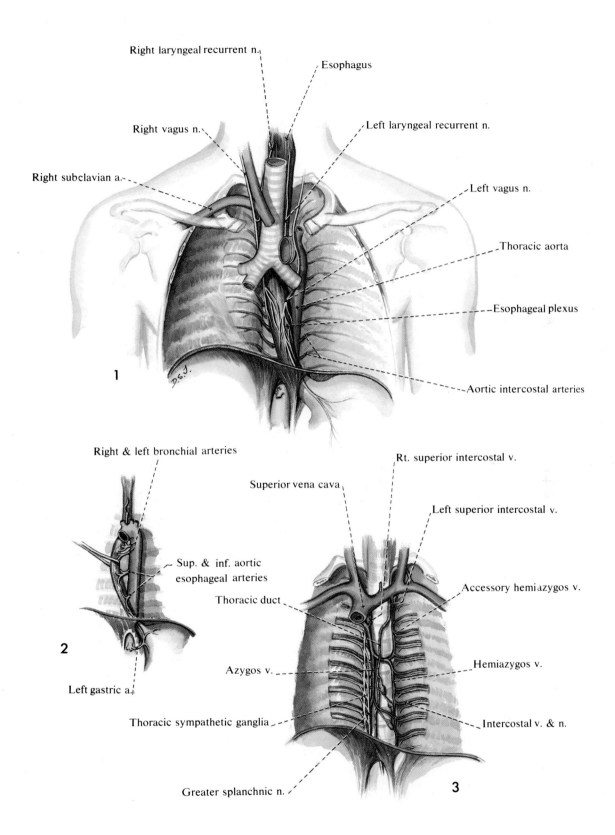

Right laryngeal recurrent n.

Esophagus

Right vagus n.

Left laryngeal recurrent n.

Right subclavian a.

Left vagus n.

Thoracic aorta

Esophageal plexus

1

Aortic intercostal arteries

Right & left bronchial arteries

Rt. superior intercostal v.

Superior vena cava

Left superior intercostal v.

Sup. & inf. aortic
esophageal arteries

Accessory hemiazygos v.

Thoracic duct

2

Azygos v.

Hemiazygos v.

Left gastric a.

Intercostal v. & n.

Thoracic sympathetic ganglia

Greater splanchnic n.

3

The Thorax

MEDIASTINAL TUMORS:

The mediastinum is the site of a great variety of abnormal masses. Tumors so classified in radiologic and surgical literature are not always within the strict anatomical boundaries of the mediastinum, nor are they always neoplasms. A good example is a neurogenic tumor of the "mediastinum" which usually occurs posteriorly in a location external to the pleura and in contact with the vertebral bodies and ribs. On a roentgenogram it appears to extend from the mediastinum, but in fact it may arise and lie beyond the strict confines of the mediastinum.

Recognizing the fact that the boundaries of the mediastinum and of its subdivisions are artificial and arbitrary, there are still several clinically useful generalizations which may be made about the correlation of tumor type and location. In this, the following table has some usefulness and four examples of the most common lesions producing masses in the mediastinum have been chosen for illustration on the accompanying plate.

Tumors of Thymus — occur in the superior or anterior part of the inferior mediastinum (Figs. 1 and 2). The majority are situated anterior to the arch of the aorta and the base of the heart, but a few approach the level of the diaphragm. Behind the thymus lies the pericardium covering the base of the heart, the ascending aorta, the main pulmonary artery, the superior vena cava, and the left innominate vein. (Rarely one or both lobes of the thymus lie posterior to the left innominate vein). A sternal splitting incision gives good access to the gland and to its blood supply. Laterally, the lobes of the thymus (and the sides of a thymoma) are in contact with the mediastinal pleura. By this account of the relations of the thymus, the nonresectability of most malignant (invasive) thymomas is easy to understand. Invasion of the pleurae, pericardium, superior vena cava, and left innominate vein occurs often and early. Malignant thymomas are a cause of obstruction in the superior vena cava or left innominate vein second in frequency only to that caused by the mediastinal metastases from bronchogenic carcinoma.

Mediastinal Goiter — thyroid tissue extending from the lower pole of the thyroid gland in the neck may present as an anterior mediastinal tumor (*substernal goiter*). Less commonly a thyroid mass descends from the neck along a plane posterior to the innominate veins and the superior vena cava to occupy a place in the posterior mediastinum as shown in Figure 3. In the more common anterior position, surgical removal can be done easily through a cervical approach, but when the thyroid mass is large and occupies a posterior position, an approach through the right chest is preferable. The important relations of the thyroid mass in the mediastinum are as follows: inferiorly, the right main bronchus in the root of the lung; laterally, the mediastinal pleura; anteriorly, the superior vena cava; medially, the right vagus nerve, the trachea, and the ascending aorta. It is most important to recall that the blood supply of the tumor is from the neck: the inferior thyroid artery and veins.

Neurogenic Tumors — are the most common primary tumors in the mediastinum. Nearly all are posterior and arise from the sympathetic chain or the posterior portions of the intercostal nerves (Fig. 4). Rarely, one of these tumors may have its origin in the neck and extend through the thoracic inlet into the superior mediastinum. Neurogenic tumors arising near an intervertebral foramen may extend both into the posterior mediastinum and into the spinal canal. These are the so-called dumbbell tumors which may produce serious compression of the spinal cord (Fig. 5).

Several features of neurogenic tumors lying in or near the intervertebral foramen are of interest. A tumor in this position may often be revealed by the roentgen appearance of an enlargement of the foramen by pressure from the expanding tumor and by narrowing of the neck of the adjacent rib. The surgeon who removes the tumor must recall that an extension of the arachnoid through the foramen into the chest cavity is common and a subarachnoidpleural fistula may result from surgical injury.

A fourth class of mediastinal "tumor" is not a neoplasm, but an *aortic aneurysm* (Fig. 6). It is an important lesion to consider from both the diagnostic and therapeutic points of view. The position and relation of an aneurysm depend upon the parts of the aorta involved. Understandably, the mass may occupy the superior, anterior, or posterior parts of the mediastinum or a combination of any or all of these. The relationship of the recurrent laryngeal nerve to the aortic arch can account for several signs of such an aneurysm, like the brassy cough and voice changes which may accompany it.

Location of Tumors and Cysts in the Mediastinum

Superior Mediastinum	Inferior Mediastinum		
	Anterior	*Middle*	*Posterior*
Lymphoma	Lymphoma	Lymphoma	—
Goiter	Goiter	—	Goiter
Thymoma	Thymoma	—	Neurogenic tumors
Parathyroid adenoma	Parathyroid adenoma	—	Meningocele
Bronchogenic cyst	—	Bronchogenic cyst	Gastroenteric cyst
Aneurysms:			
Aortic arch	Teratoma and dermoids		Diaphragmatic hernia
Innominate artery			

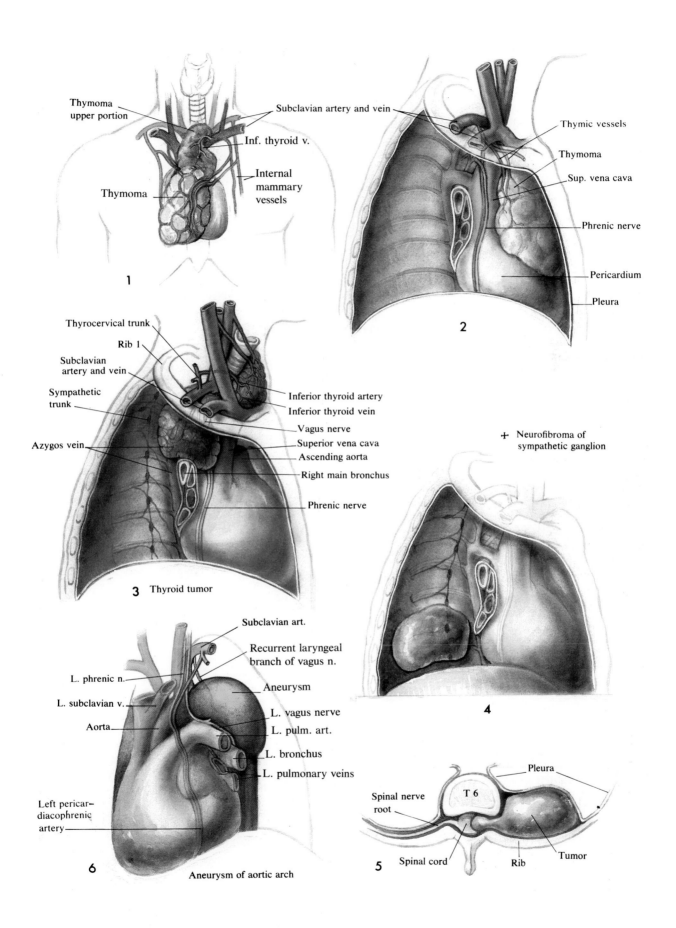

1

Thymoma upper portion
Subclavian artery and vein
Inf. thyroid v.
Internal mammary vessels
Thymoma

Thymic vessels
Thymoma
Sup. vena cava
Phrenic nerve
Pericardium
Pleura

2

Thyrocervical trunk
Rib 1
Subclavian artery and vein
Sympathetic trunk
Azygos vein
Inferior thyroid artery
Inferior thyroid vein
Vagus nerve
Superior vena cava
Ascending aorta
Right main bronchus
Phrenic nerve

3 Thyroid tumor

+ Neurofibroma of sympathetic ganglion

4

Subclavian art.
Recurrent laryngeal branch of vagus n.
Aneurysm
L. phrenic n.
L. subclavian v.
Aorta
L. vagus nerve
L. pulm. art.
L. bronchus
L. pulmonary veins
Left pericardiacophrenic artery

6

Aneurysm of aortic arch

Pleura
Spinal nerve root
T 6
Spinal cord
Rib
Tumor

5

CLINICAL ANATOMY OF THE ESOPHAGUS AND THE VAGUS NERVES:

The length of the esophagus, which is of considerable interest to the endoscopist, is approximately as follows: from teeth to cricoid, 15 cm.; from cricoid to stomach, 25 cm. Of clinical importance are three distinct constrictions; one located at its beginning in the neck, another where it is crossed by the left main bronchus, and the third where it passes through the diaphragm. These three sites of narrowing account for the lodgement of swallowed foreign bodies, for the peculiar susceptibility of these areas to caustics, and for the localization of perforations.

The pleural relations are described on pages 94 and 98. Knowing them, one readily understands why perforations of the thoracic esophagus may enter not only the planes of the mediastinum, but also one or both pleural spaces. Mediastinitis and empyema are the usual sequel to perforation.

The relation of the esophagus to the heart whose left atrium lies in contact with its anterior surface are useful to the fluoroscopist. Enlargement of the left atrium may produce a recognizable deformity of the adjacent esophagus.

Tracheo-esophageal Fistula:

The relation of the esophagus to the trachea is an intimate one anatomically as well as developmentally. Embryological defects may result in persistent communication between the trachea and esophagus. For an explanation of such a congenital fistula, the reader can refer to almost any embryology textbook.

Acquired tracheo-esophageal fistulas are usually due to malignant disease or, less often, to infection, trauma, or a traction diverticulum such as shown in Figure 1. The malignancy may be primary in the upper thoracic esophagus or in the left main bronchus, but it may also be secondary in the subcarinal or lateral tracheal lymph nodes from a primary source elsewhere.

Esophageal Cancer:

Numerous lymph nodes of the posterior mediastinum lie in contact with the esophagus and receive their lymph from it. They are also in immediate contact with the important structures related to the esophagus. Resection of a wide margin of normal tissue about these nodes in operations for cancer is impossible. Further complicating the problem of adequate surgery for carcinoma of the esophagus is the lymph drainage into the inferior cervical nodes from the upper thoracic esophagus and into the left gastric nodes not only from the lower esophagus but from the entire tube below the level of the aortic arch.

Vascular Anomalies:

At least two vascular anomalies in the mediastinum may account for compression of the esophagus. An anomalous right subclavian artery is shown in Figure 2. The right subclavian, instead of arising in the normal way from the innominate artery, comes from the left side of the aortic arch. In order to reach its normal exit from the thoracic inlet, it passes upward and to the right across the midline. Usually it lies posterior to the esophagus about the level of the third thoracic vertebra. Although such an arrangement does not necessarily produce symptoms, and indeed it usually does not, it may cause pressure on the esophagus sufficient to interfere with swallowing. The radiologist can detect the presence of this anomaly with accuracy. If symptoms warrant, they may be relieved safely and without embarrassment to the circulation of the extremity by the division of the artery close to its origin.

The second major vascular anomaly associated with compression of the esophagus is that of the double aortic arch (Fig. 4, page 111). With this defect, the symptoms due to compression of the trachea may obscure those due to constriction of the esophagus.

Vagus Nerves (Figs. 3, 4, and 5):

The course and distribution of the *vagus nerves* and their branches in the chest have been described on pages 96 and 98. The origin of the left recurrent laryngeal nerve from the left vagus at the inferior margin of the arch of the aorta has three relations of clinical importance. One is to the persistent ductus arteriosus, in the surgical dissection of which the nerve may be injured. The second is to the lymph nodes at the root of the left lung (Fig. 3). Bronchogenic carcinoma arising in the left lung and metastasizing to these nodes is a common cause of left recurrent nerve palsy. And finally, fixed beneath the aortic arch the continuity of the left recurrent nerve may be interrupted by pressure of an expanding aneurysm of the arch, by enlarging lymph nodes, or by a greatly enlarged and tense left atrium. Below the lung roots, the vagi reach the wall of the esophagus where numerous branches of each anastomose to form the esophageal plexus. Near the lower end of the thorax the right vagus emerges as a single trunk on the posterior aspect of the esophagus. The left vagus becomes a single trunk on the anterior surface of the esophagus, and both nerves then enter the abdomen through the esophageal hiatus.

The number and placement of vagal nerve trunks immediately above and at the hiatus are not constant. From the many studies bearing on these patterns, a few generalizations are helpful. The anterior (left) vagus and the posterior (right) vagus are each represented by a single trunk at this level in approximately 80 per cent of people. In 10 per cent or more, there is an additional branch lying near and running a parallel course. With the esophagus held under tension, these nerves are more readily felt than seen lying on or near the esophagus. In 90 to 95 per cent of cases, complete vagotomy. can be effected by section of such trunks as can be found in this manner, either just above or just below the diaphragm (Figs. 4 and 5).

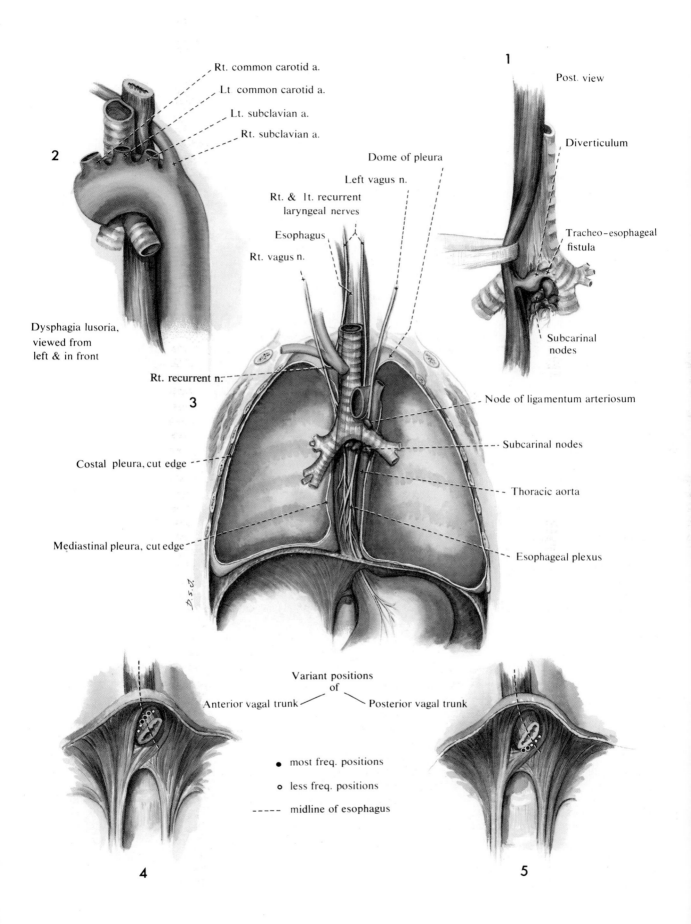

1 Post. view

Diverticulum

Tracheo-esophageal fistula

Subcarinal nodes

2

Rt. common carotid a.

Lt. common carotid a.

Lt. subclavian a.

Rt. subclavian a.

Dysphagia lusoria, viewed from left & in front

Dome of pleura

Left vagus n.

Rt. & lt. recurrent laryngeal nerves

Esophagus

Rt. vagus n.

Rt. recurrent n.

3

Costal pleura, cut edge

Mediastinal pleura, cut edge

Node of ligamentum arteriosum

Subcarinal nodes

Thoracic aorta

Esophageal plexus

Variant positions of

Anterior vagal trunk — Posterior vagal trunk

● most freq. positions

○ less freq. positions

----- midline of esophagus

4

5

The Thorax

MIDDLE MEDIASTINUM:

The middle mediastinum consists of the pericardial sac, its contents, and the laterally related structures, the phrenic nerves and pericardiacophrenic artery and veins. The latter are branches and tributaries of the internal mammary vessels.

1. **Pericardium**—consists of two layers, a *fibrous* and a *serous* layer. The *fibrous* layer is continuous with the middle layer of deep cervical fascia above, with the adventitial coverings of the pulmonary vessels laterally, and with the central tendon of the diaphragm below. The *serous* pericardium includes an outer *parietal* layer adherent to the under surfaces of the fibrous pericardium, which at the arterial and venous attachments of the heart is reflected back upon the great vessels and heart as the *visceral* layer of serous pericardium. That portion covering the heart is referred to as the *epicardium*. The potential space between the two layers of serous pericardium is termed the *pericardial cavity*, which contains a small amount of serous fluid.

Two major pericardial sinuses can be identified:

a. TRANSVERSE SINUS (Fig. 1)—is a posterior communication between the right and left sides of the pericardial cavity. It is bounded anteriorly by the aorta and pulmonary artery and posteriorly the left atrium, right pulmonary artery, and superior vena cava. When there is insufficient length of the right pulmonary artery extrapericardially, this vessel may be ligated in this sinus where it is readily accessible.

b. OBLIQUE SINUS (Fig. 2)—is bounded anteriorly by the left atrium, posteriorly by the parietal serous pericardium, cephalad and to the left by the left pulmonary veins, and caudally to the right by the inferior vena cava.

2. **Topography of the Heart** (Fig. 3)—may be outlined on the chest wall by surface lines drawn between the following four points:

a. Third right costal cartilage, 1/2 inch from right sternal border.

b. Third left costal cartilage, 1 inch from left sternal border.

c. Sixth right chondrosternal junction.

d. Fifth interspace, 3½ inches from left sternal border.

The anatomic locations of the cardiac valves and the areas of maximum audibility are illustrated in Figure 3.

3. **External Anatomy of the Heart**—may be best described as consisting of an apex, base, and two surfaces in the fixed specimen. The *apex* is directed to the left anteriorly, and caudally. It is located in the fifth left interspace, 3½ inches from the left sternal border. The *base* corresponds to the area occupied by the roots of the great vessels and extends from the fifth to the ninth vertebral level and directed posteriorly to the right and cranialward. The two surfaces are the *anterior (sternocostal)* and *posterior (diaphragmatic)*.

Sulci may be seen on the surfaces of the heart which contain the main cardiac blood vessels and adipose tissue and are important in the topography of the heart chambers (Fig. 1). A *coronary (atrioventricular) sulcus*

encircles the heart, separating the atria above the sulcus from the ventricles below. The *longitudinal (interventricular) sulcus* marks the separation of the right and left ventricles on the anterior and posterior surfaces and is distinguished as the *anterior* and *posterior longitudinal sulci*.

4. **Blood Supply of the Heart** (Fig. 4)—consists of major arteries and veins which lie in the above-mentioned sulci. The arterial supply is by the two main coronary arteries arising from the base of the ascending aorta.

a. RIGHT CORONARY ARTERY—arises in the right sinus of Valsalva and swings laterally in the coronary sulcus. In its course over the anterior surface it sends branches to the right atrium, right ventricle, and a *right marginal branch* along the margo acutus. It extends on to the posterior surface in the coronary sulcus to anastomose with the left coronary artery and gives rise to the *posterior descending artery*, which descends through the posterior longitudinal (interventricular) sulcus to anastomose with the descending branch of the left coronary artery.

b. LEFT CORONARY ARTERY—takes origin from the left aortic sinus, passes to the left between the pulmonary artery and left atrium, and divides into two main branches. The *anterior descending artery* extends over the anterior wall to the interventricular sulcus and anastomoses with the posterior descending branch of the right coronary. This branch is most frequently involved in coronary occlusion. The *circumflex branch* extends to the posterior surface of the heart in the coronary sulcus to anastomose with the corresponding branch of the right coronary.

5. **Venous Drainage of the Heart** (Fig. 5)—is by the cardiac and Thebesian veins. The cardiac veins accompany the coronary arteries and with but one exception, anterior cardiac veins, drain into the *coronary sinus*, which lies in the coronary sulcus on the posterior surface of the heart. It receives the following cardiac veins and empties into the right atrium (Fig. 1, page 107).

a. GREAT CARDIAC VEIN—lies in the anterior longitudinal sulcus and passes to the left side of the heart in the coronary sulcus to terminate in the coronary sinus.

b. MIDDLE CARDIAC VEIN—ascends in the posterior longitudinal sulcus and empties into the coronary sinus.

c. SMALL CARDIAC VEIN—follows the marginal branch of the right coronary artery to the coronary sulcus and terminates in the right portion of the coronary sinus.

d. OBLIQUE VEIN OF THE LEFT ATRIUM—lies on the posterior surface of that chamber and descends into the coronary sinus. It is a remnant of the left superior vena cava and may extend into the *pulmonary fold of Marshall* (Fig. 2).

e. ANTERIOR CARDIAC VEINS—are several small branches which drain the anterior surface of the right ventricle and usually empty directly into the right atrium.

f. LEAST CARDIAC (THEBESIAN) VEINS—are small vessels within the muscular walls of the heart and open directly into the heart chambers. They are most numerous in relation to the right atrium.

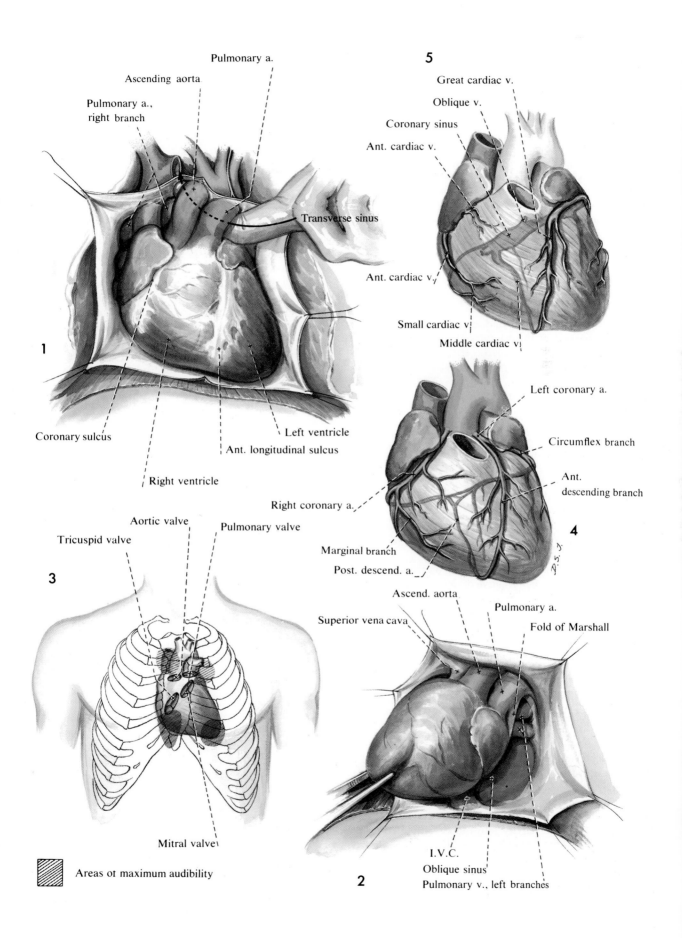

1

Pulmonary a.

Ascending aorta

Pulmonary a.,
right branch

Transverse sinus

Coronary sulcus

Left ventricle

Ant. longitudinal sulcus

Right ventricle

5

Great cardiac v.

Oblique v.

Coronary sinus

Ant. cardiac v.

Ant. cardiac v.

Small cardiac v.

Middle cardiac v.

Left coronary a.

Circumflex branch

Ant.
descending branch

Right coronary a.

Marginal branch

Post. descend. a.

4

3

Tricuspid valve

Aortic valve

Pulmonary valve

Mitral valve

Areas of maximum audibility

Ascend. aorta

Pulmonary a.

Superior vena cava

Fold of Marshall

I.V.C.

Oblique sinus

Pulmonary v., left branches

2

INTERNAL ANATOMY OF THE HEART CHAMBERS:

The heart arises as a primitive tube which at its caudal end receives the great veins in a chamber termed the *sinus venosus*. From this chamber blood is propelled into the *primitive atrium*, thence to the primitive *ventricle*, and consequently to the *truncus arteriosus,* which is in continuity with the aortic roots. A partitioning occurs in the region of the primitive atrium and ventricle, converting this tube into a four-chambered heart. The sinus venosus, truncus arteriosus, and embryonic pulmonary veins are absorbed in part into these chambers to give rise to the adult derivatives of the heart.

1. **Right Atrium** (Fig. 1)—exhibits a roughened and smooth area separated on the anterior wall by the *crista terminalis*. The roughened anterior wall is the *right auricle,* a derivative of the primitive atrium. It is thrown into folds due to the underlying *pectinate muscles*. The smoother portion consists of two parts, one derived from the absorbed portion of the sinus venosus into which the venous channels enter, and an area on the posterior wall which is part of the interatrial septum. In the area derived from the sinus venosus, certain orifices may be seen:

a. SUPERIOR VENA CAVA ORIFICE—is located at the cephalic end of the right atrium.

b. INFERIOR VENA CAVA ORIFICE—is partially guarded by the *Eustachian valve*.

c. CORONARY SINUS ORIFICE—opens medial to the inferior vena cava orifice and is guarded by the *Thebesian valve*.

d. FORAMINA VENARUM MINIMARUM—transmit the Thebesian veins and smallest cardiac veins into the right atrium.

The smooth areas derived from the *interatrial septum* make up the posterior wall of the atrium. Certain important structures are seen in this area:

a. FOSSA OVALIS—is a depression on the posterior right atrial wall and is a derivative of the *septum primum.*

b. LIMBUS FOSSAE OVALIS—is derived from the *septum secundum,* which fuses with the septum primum to seal off the right and left atrial chambers. In some 20 per cent of people this fusion may be incomplete, resulting in an anatomic but not necessarily a physiologic communication between the right and left side of the heart.

RIGHT ATRIOVENTRICULAR ORIFICE—is a communication leading from the front of the atrium downward and to the left to the right ventricle. The tricuspid valve guards this orifice on its ventricular side.

2. **Right Ventricle** (Fig. 1)—also consists of a roughened and smooth area, the two areas being demarcated grossly by the muscular ridge termed the *crista supraventricularis*. The roughened area is that portion derived from the primitive ventricle. Here myocardial bundles throw the ventricular cavity into ridges termed *trabeculae carneae*. Three specific muscles, the *papillary muscles,* are related to right ventricular cavity and connect with the cusps of the tricuspid valves by *chordae tendineae*. These muscles serve as tensors of the tricuspid valve. An *anterior papillary muscle* extends from the anterior ventricular wall to the anterior and posterior cusps, a *posterior papillary muscle* between the posterior and medial cusps, and the *papillary muscle of the conus (Luschka)* to the anterior and medial cusp from the septal wall. In the smooth area derived from the truncus arteriosus is located the pulmonary orifice:

PULMONARY ORIFICE—arises in the region of the *conus arteriosus,* an absorbed portion of the original *truncus arteriosus*. Three semilunar valves are located here: the right, left, and anterior. They are hemispherical in shape, the concavity being directed away from the ventricle so that back pressure within the great vessels brings the three valves into apposition, thereby preventing reflux of blood into the ventricle during diastole.

3. **Left Atrium** (Fig. 2)—like the right atrium, presents a roughened and smooth surface. The roughened portion is the *left auricle,* derived from the primitive atrium in which are located the *pectinate muscles*. The smooth area is derived from the absorption of the pulmonary veins and the interatrial septum. The pulmonary veins arise independent of the older venous channels emptying into the sinus venosus. They drain the branches of the lung buds and converge as a common trunk entering the left atrium. As the heart increases in size, this single trunk is absorbed into the left atrial wall until four of the pulmonary veins enter this chamber on its dorsal surface. The orifices in this part of the chamber are:

a. PULMONARY VEIN OSTIA—are four in number, two right and two left.

b. LEFT ATRIOVENTRICULAR ORIFICE—is an opening from the anterior part of the atrium, forward, downward, and to the left into the left ventricle, guarded by the *bicuspid* or *mitral valve* on the ventricular side.

4. **Left Ventricle** (Fig. 3)—consists of two embryologic parts. That derived from the primitive ventricle is a thick muscular wall in which are seen the *tuberculae carneae*. In addition, an *anterior* and *posterior papillary muscle* are located in this chamber, extending from the ventricular walls and attaching to the cusps of the mitral valve by *chordae tendineae*. Separating the right and left ventricle is the muscular portion of the *interventricular septum*.

In this part of the chamber a single orifice is found:

a. LEFT ATRIOVENTRICULAR ORIFICE AND VALVE (MITRAL)—has two cusps, an *anterior* and a *posterior cusp,* connected by chordae tendineae with the papillary muscles of this chamber.

An upper smooth portion of the chamber is derived from the absorbed truncus arteriosus and the intermembranous portion of the interventricular septum. In this area is the exit from this ventricular chamber:

b. AORTIC ORIFICE AND VALVES (SEMILUNAR)—is similar to the pulmonary orifice. Three semilunar valves are present: right, left, and posterior valves. Each valve is directed away from the ventricle, and in the middle of the free leaf is a fibrocartilaginous nodule, *nodule of Arantius,* on either side of which is a thin crescentic fold called the *lunula*. Opposite the aortic valves are three dilatations in the aortic wall, the *aortic sinuses of Valsalva*. From the right and left sinus the right and left coronary arteries arise.

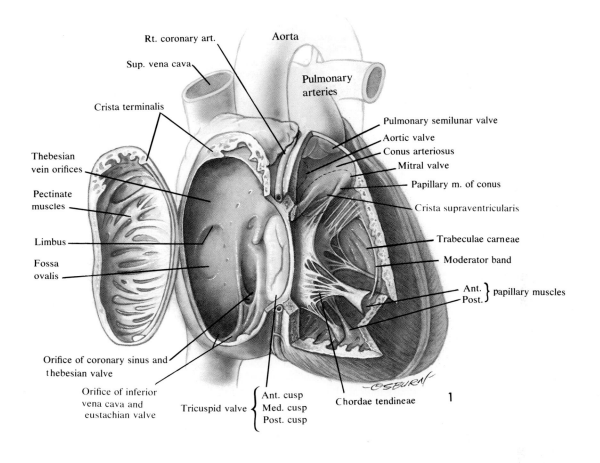

Rt. coronary art.
Aorta
Sup. vena cava
Pulmonary arteries
Crista terminalis
Pulmonary semilunar valve
Aortic valve
Conus arteriosus
Mitral valve
Thebesian vein orifices
Papillary m. of conus
Crista supraventricularis
Pectinate muscles
Trabeculae carneae
Moderator band
Limbus
Fossa ovalis
Ant. } papillary muscles
Post.
Orifice of coronary sinus and thebesian valve
Orifice of inferior vena cava and eustachian valve
Tricuspid valve { Ant. cusp
Med. cusp
Post. cusp
Chordae tendineae
1

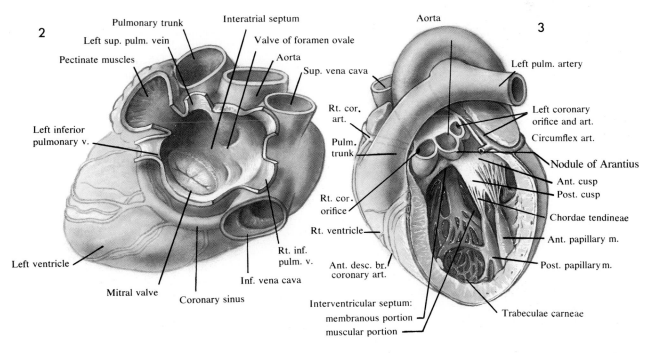

2
Pulmonary trunk
Left sup. pulm. vein
Pectinate muscles
Interatrial septum
Valve of foramen ovale
Aorta
Sup. vena cava
Aorta
3
Left pulm. artery
Rt. cor. art.
Left inferior pulmonary v.
Pulm. trunk
Left coronary orifice and art.
Circumflex art.
Nodule of Arantius
Ant. cusp
Post. cusp
Chordae tendineae
Ant. papillary m.
Post. papillary m.
Rt. cor. orifice
Rt. ventricle
Left ventricle
Rt. inf. pulm. v.
Ant. desc. br. coronary art.
Mitral valve
Coronary sinus
Inf. vena cava
Interventricular septum:
membranous portion
muscular portion
Trabeculae carneae

SURGICAL ANATOMY OF THE HEART:

The development of the artificial heart-lung machine (cardiopulmonary pump oxygenator, cardiopulmonary by-pass) by John H. Gibbon, Jr., M.D., has revolutionized modern heart surgery. The extracorporeal pumps have become more sophisticated, compact, and refined. They now permit the performance of cardiac surgery for coronary artery disease, repair of interatrial and interventricular septal defects, replacement of aortic, mitral, and tricuspid valves, correction of aortic defects and the tetralogy of Fallot, and heart transplants.

1. **Coronary Artery Disease** — is the most common indication for cardiac surgical intervention today. Coronary artery arteriosclerosis is the most common disease affecting the heart. It is estimated that 500,000 to 750,000 deaths occur yearly from coronary occlusion and that each year over 5 million individuals are diagnosed as having coronary artery disease. The cost of caring for the patients exceeds 7 to 8 billion dollars annually. Over the years, many surgical procedures have been attempted. They include resection of the cervical sympathetic cardiac nerves, epicardial abrasive techniques, implantation of various body tissues (e.g., omentum, pectoral muscle) directly to the wall of heart, implantation of the internal mammary artery in the left ventricular wall, and coronary endarterectomy. All of these techniques have fallen into disrepute. Newer procedures include the following:

a. CORONARY BY-PASS (Fig. 1) — is the most common cardiac surgery performed today; it is done almost daily, even in community hospitals. It is particularly indicated in those individuals who have had a myocardial infarction with persistent angina despite optimal medical treatment, in patients with angina and congestive failure, or in those individuals who have had a previous infarction and who are now asymptomatic but who show severe coronary stenosis on coronary angiograms. Coronary angiography is a requisite before any by-pass is contemplated, for it is the only diagnostic procedure that can anatomically orient the surgeon as to the location and extent of obstruction of blood flow to the myocardium. Frequently, the obstruction may be multiple, requiring a two- to eight-vessel by-pass.

The grafts used may be venous or arterial. The most popular venous homograft is the great saphenous vein (Fig. 1, page 277), although the cephalic vein may also be used. The arterial graft is the internal mammary artery related to the ventral wall of the thorax after arising from the first portion of the subclavian artery (Fig. 3, page 43). The proximal end of the venous graft is anastomosed to the ascending aorta and the distal end into the affected coronary artery just distal to the obstructed site. It is most important that the veins be in reversed anatomical position because of their valvular arrangements. With the internal mammary graft, the vessel's origin is kept intact from the subclavian artery and, after being freed from the anterior thoracic wall, its distal end is also anastomosed into the coronary artery distal to the obstruction. It is imperative that the distal anastomosis in both types of grafts be made in an area devoid of arteriosclerotic changes in the adjacent myocardium. Meticulous surgical technique is required at the anastomotic sites in order to preserve patency and to prevent kinking. The reader is advised to refer to a text on cardiac surgery for such information on the technical aspects of anastomosis.

b. CORONARY ANGIOPLASTY (Fig. 2) — or as it is frequently referred to, percutaneous transluminal coronary angioplasty (PTCA), has become increasingly popular since it was introduced in 1977. Advocates of this procedure point out certain advantages over coronary by-pass. They include the fact that it is done under local anesthesia, requires no chest incision or cardiopulmonary by-pass, necessitates only a short hospital stay, and allows a return to normal activities in a week's time. All this results in a great financial saving to the patient.

However, it has been shown that best results are in those patients with a short (less than one year) history of angina not relieved by the usual medical regimen. The plaques are not as old and hard and therefore are more likely to respond to compression. The procedure is also safest in those patients who have obstruction of a single coronary artery. Relief of the angina is usually obtained in 60 per cent of the patients, although some centers claim an 85 to 90 per cent success rate.

A catheter is introduced through either the brachial or femoral artery under direct fluoroscopy and advanced into the ascending aorta and thence into the affected coronary artery. When the tip of the catheter reaches the point of obstruction, a tiny sausage-shaped balloon is inflated by a hydraulically powered inflation device. The balloon compresses the atheromatous plaque, thereby increasing the size of the lumen and resulting in an increased coronary flow.

(Text continued on page 109A)

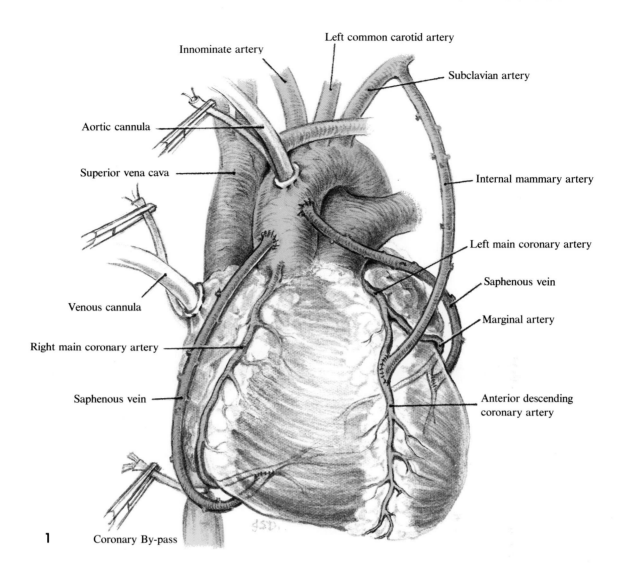

Innominate artery

Left common carotid artery

Subclavian artery

Aortic cannula

Superior vena cava

Internal mammary artery

Left main coronary artery

Saphenous vein

Marginal artery

Venous cannula

Right main coronary artery

Saphenous vein

Anterior descending coronary artery

1   Coronary By-pass

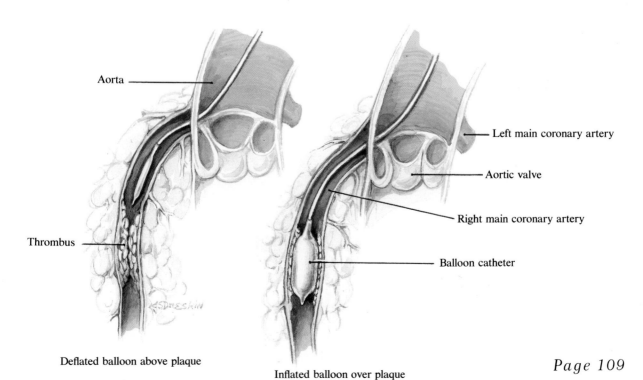

Aorta

Left main coronary artery

Aortic valve

Right main coronary artery

Balloon catheter

Thrombus

Deflated balloon above plaque

Inflated balloon over plaque

2   Coronary Angioplasty

c. HEART TRANSPLANTATION (Fig. 3) — was first successfully performed on a human in December 1967 by Christiaan Barnard. Although the patient survived only 17 days, this achievement created a worldwide interest among cardiac surgeons to duplicate such surgery. The one-year survival rate in 1968 was reported to be 22 per cent. By the mid-1980s, the one-year survival rate had increased to 88 per cent. This increase in survival was due to several factors, including improved methods of procurement and storage of donor organs, tissue typing, and most important, the development of immunosuppressive drugs, especially cyclosporine.

Heart transplants are performed only in patients with terminal heart disease. Donor organs should be received from a relatively young individual with irreversible brain damage but whose heart is still functional.

We will limit our discussion to the anatomical structures involved in heart transplants.

(1) *Preparation of the Recipient Heart* — the heart must first be isolated from the general circulation. This is achieved by passing a catheter into the upper portion of the superior vena cava. A second venous catheter is inserted into the proximal portion of the superior vena cava and passed through the right atrium into the inferior vena cava. Both catheters are fixed in position by caval tapes. Another catheter is placed in the ascending aorta, and the aorta is cross clamped. The pump oxygenator now sustains the general circulation and the recipient heart is isolated. The recipient's heart is removed by cutting both right and left atria just behind the auricular appendages. This maneuver leaves a portion of the recipient right atrium with the caval openings intact and the part of the left atrium with the pulmonary venous ostia remaining.

(2) *Preparation of Donor Heart* — the left atrium is opened by resecting that portion of the posterior wall receiving the pulmonary veins. An incision is made along the lateral wall of the right atrium from the inferior vena caval orifice upward short of the superior vena caval orifice, and the superior vena cava is ligated.

(3) *Implantation of the Donor Heart* — the aorta and pulmonary arterial trunks are transected just above their semilunar valves. The left atrial walls are anastomosed, followed by anastomosis of the right atrial wall. This is followed by suturing the ends of the donor and recipient aortas, removing the aortic cross clamp, and completing anastomosis of the pulmonary artery stumps. The by-pass cannulae are then removed and a temporary pacing wire is inserted to the right ventricle.

d. HEART-LUNG TRANSPLANTATION — is one of the latest attempts at organ transplantation. Such attempts are still in the experimental stage, as evidenced by an estimated 25 per cent operative mortality and a 50 to 60 per cent one-year survival rate. Many problems exist, including adequate selection of the recipient (pulmonary fibrosis being the primary choice), donor inadequacy, rejection, sepsis, and bronchial dehiscence. Single and double lung transplants have been attempted (see page 124), and although they are somewhat more successful than heart-lung transplants, similar complications persist.

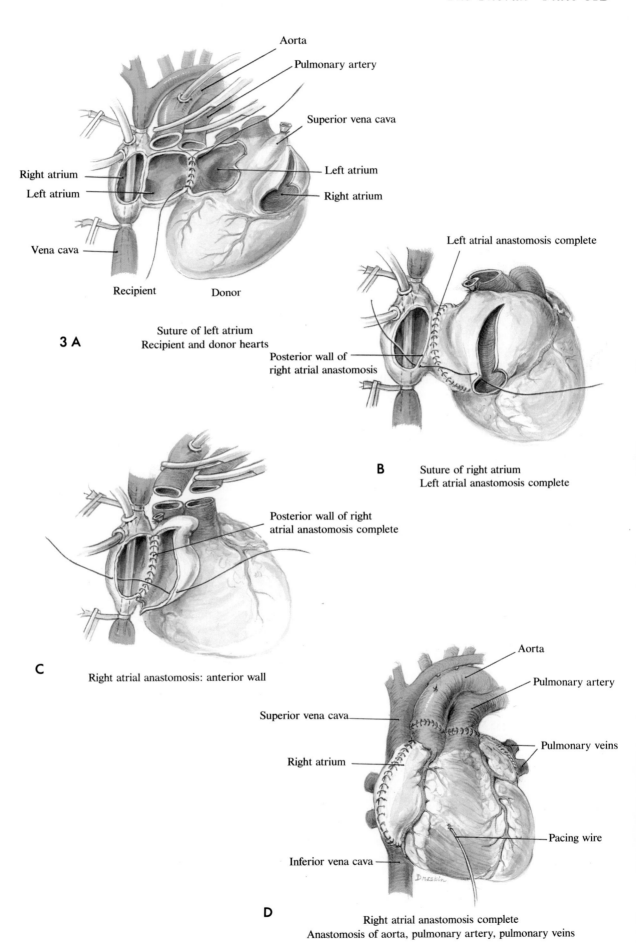

Aorta

Pulmonary artery

Superior vena cava

Right atrium

Left atrium

Left atrium

Right atrium

Vena cava

Recipient   Donor

3 A   Suture of left atrium
Recipient and donor hearts

Left atrial anastomosis complete

Posterior wall of
right atrial anastomosis

B   Suture of right atrium
Left atrial anastomosis complete

Posterior wall of right
atrial anastomosis complete

C   Right atrial anastomosis: anterior wall

Aorta

Pulmonary artery

Superior vena cava

Pulmonary veins

Right atrium

Pacing wire

Inferior vena cava

D   Right atrial anastomosis complete
Anastomosis of aorta, pulmonary artery, pulmonary veins

AORTIC ARCHES: DERIVATIVES AND DEFECTS:

The development of the aortic arch with its branches and of the pulmonary arteries is shown schematically in Figures 1 and 2. The complicated adult arterial pattern (Fig. 2) is derived from the primordium of a truncus arteriosus forming the arterial outlet of the heart, pairs of branchial arch arteries lying in the mesoderm of the pharyngeal arches, and the paired dorsal aorta, distributing blood to the embryonic body, and to the yolk sac and chorion.

The original paired, symmetrical system of vessels is much altered during development by the fusion, hypertrophy, or atrophy of its various components. The final result is the normal pattern as shown in Figure 2, or one of many variations, four of the more common of which are shown in Figures 3 to 6.

The recurrent branches of the vagus in the embryo are related to the sixth arch. On the right side with the degeneration of the distal part of the sixth and the complete degeneration of the fifth arch, the recurrent branch is related to the fourth arch. This explains the relationship of the right recurrent branch of the vagus to the right subclavian artery. On the left side, the distal part of the sixth arch persists as the *ligamentum arteriosum*. The left vagus nerve therefore sends its recurrent branch under the ligament (Fig. 2).

1. **Patent Ductus Arteriosus** (Fig. 3) — is a result of the failure of the fetal ductus to obliterate soon after birth. When the patency occurs in combination with an intracardiac malformation or an anomaly of the aortic arch system, it may have a beneficial effect upon the circulation, but as an isolated lesion it always imposes an increased burden on the heart.

The patent ductus is located between the pulmonary artery near its bifurcation and the aorta immediately below the origin of the left subclavian artery. During surgical closure, the left recurrent laryngeal nerve, which passes beneath it, must be retracted and protected from injury.

2. **Persistence of the Right Dorsal Aortic Arch** (Fig. 4) — occurs when the embryonic right dorsal aorta below the sixth aortic arch fails to obliterate. If the corresponding vessel on the left disappears, then a *right aortic arch* results. However, rarely, the embryonic dorsal aorta immediately below the sixth branchial arch persists bilaterally, in which case a *double aortic arch* results. Either arrangement may be present without symptoms. On the other hand, both may be responsible for compression of the trachea with respiratory distress, or of the esophagus and trachea with respiratory distress and dysphagia.

In the case of a right aortic arch, compression of the lower trachea may be produced by the fixation of the pulmonary artery to the aortic arch by the ductus arteriosus or ligamentum. Surgical section of this structure can relieve the compression.

In a *double aortic arch* the two arches, left (anterior) and right (posterior), encircle both the esophagus and trachea, or only the trachea, and join to form the descending aorta. In some instances, the left (anterior)

arch is obliterated in part or entirely, leaving a fibrous cord. In most instances both of the limbs are patent. Rarely the two arches are of equal size. Usually the left (anterior) arch is somewhat smaller than the right (posterior) one. The presence of symptoms depends upon compression of the trachea or the esophagus and trachea by this "vascular ring."

3. **Coarctation of the Aorta** (Figs. 5 and 6) — is a localized constriction of the aorta which usually occurs just proximal to the point of entrance of the ductus arteriosus. The anatomy of coarctation varies greatly in the location, extent, and degree on constriction. The degree of stenosis and the extent of collateral circulation are features of great importance in determining the abnormal hemodynamic and clinical changes.

Whereas it is usual to distinguish between an "infantile" and an "adult" type of coarctation, these terms are quite inadequate and even misleading, since the "infantile" type may be present in the adult, and vice versa. A more meaningful classification has been suggested as follows:

(1) Coarctation with closed ductus arteriosus (90 per cent)
    a. Coarctation in the vicinity of the ligamentum arteriosum
    b. Coarctation in unusual location
    c. Coarctation with stenosis of the right or left subclavian artery
(2) Coarctation with patent ductus arteriosus (10 per cent
    a. Coarctation distal to the aortic mouth of the ductus
    b. Coarctation proximal to the aortic mouth of the ductus
      i. without systemic collaterals
      ii. with systemic collaterals

This classification, based on anatomic findings, is adequate to explain the variations in the hemodynamic and clinical features. The ductus is often so narrow that no shunt can be demonstrated even if the opening of the ductus is proximal to the coarctation. The direction of a shunt through a ductus situated distal to the coarctation is determined by the development of the collateral circulation. If it is extensive, the shunt may go from the aorta to the pulmonary artery, but if the collaterals are lacking and the coarctation is severe, the blood is shunted from the pulmonary artery to the aorta.

The coarctation usually appears to the surgeon as an obviously narrow segment of the aorta, but occasionally the obstruction may be the result of a "diaphragm," whose position is not so evident on external inspection (Fig. 6).

4. **Other Anomalies: Anomalous Right Subclavian Artery** — instead of arising from the innominate artery, as is usually the case, the right subclavian artery may arise from the left side of the aortic arch. The vessel must then pass upward and to the right, crossing the midline, and behind the esophagus to reach its normal exit on the right side of the thoracic cage. Pressure on the esophagus may be sufficient to interfere with swallowing (Fig. 2, page 103).

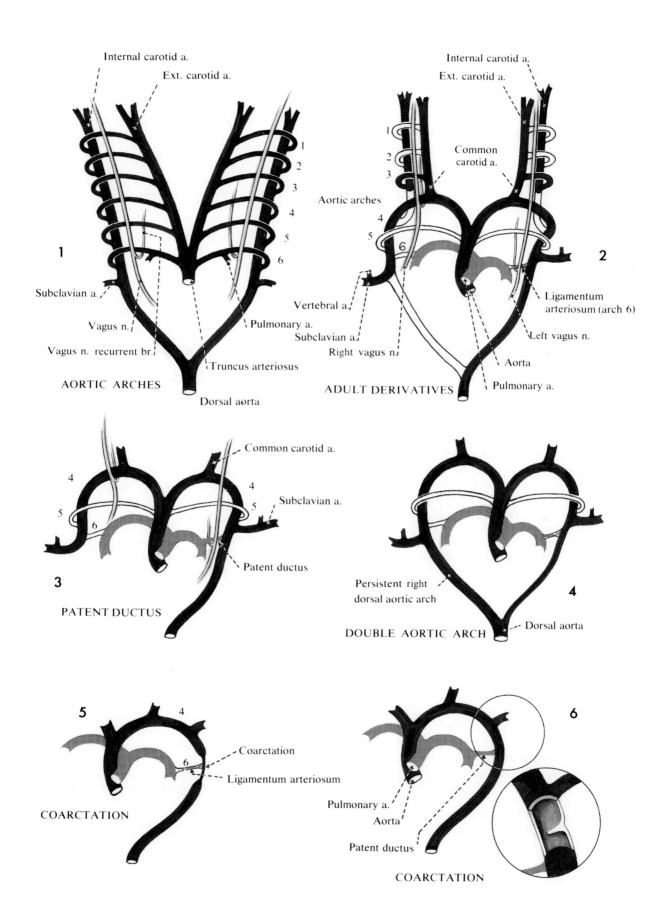

1 — AORTIC ARCHES

Internal carotid a.
Ext. carotid a.
Subclavian a.
Vagus n.
Vagus n. recurrent br.
Pulmonary a.
Truncus arteriosus
Dorsal aorta

2 — ADULT DERIVATIVES

Internal carotid a.
Ext. carotid a.
Common carotid a.
Aortic arches
Vertebral a.
Subclavian a.
Right vagus n.
Ligamentum arteriosum (arch 6)
Left vagus n.
Aorta
Pulmonary a.

3 — PATENT DUCTUS

Common carotid a.
Subclavian a.
Patent ductus

4 — DOUBLE AORTIC ARCH

Persistent right dorsal aortic arch
Dorsal aorta

5 — COARCTATION

Coarctation
Ligamentum arteriosum

6 — COARCTATION

Pulmonary a.
Aorta
Patent ductus

LUNG ROOTS:

The lung root or hilus contains structures that connect the lung with the heart and mediastinal structures. Its main anatomic constituents are the main bronchi and pulmonary arteries and veins (Fig. 1). The bronchial vessels, nerves, and lymph nodes are also seen in this area. In general, the bronchi lie posterior in position in this location, and the pulmonary veins inferior. The position of the pulmonary artery differs on the two sides. On the left side it is anterior and superior to the bronchus, whereas on the right it is slightly anterior and inferior to the bronchus. The hilar structures are encased in a pleural investment *(isthmus)* reflecting from the mediastinal portion of the parietal pleura to visceral pleura. Below the hilar structures, the anterior and posterior pleural reflections come into apposition to form the *pulmonary ligament.* Although this structure is usually avascular, an aberrant pulmonary artery arising from the descending thoracic aorta may be located within the ligament. On the right an important venous channel, the azygos vein and its arch, is related to the root, whereas on the left side an arterial channel consisting of the aortic arch and descending thoracic aorta is related to the root. The phrenic nerve lies anterior to the hilus on either side, and the vagus nerve lies posterior (Figs. 2 and 3, page 95).

1. **Pulmonary Artery** (Fig. 2) – differs from other arteries in that it carries venous blood. It arises from the right ventricle and ascends within the pericardial sac for a distance of approximately 4 cm. It bifurcates into a right and left branch under the aortic arch.

a. LEFT PULMONARY ARTERY – runs a short intrapericardial course in which 57 per cent of the circumference of the vessel protrudes into the pericardial sac. It extends into the hilus cephalad to the left main stem bronchus and gives rise to its segmental branches.

b. RIGHT PULMONARY ARTERY – is longer than the left branch and passes behind the aorta and superior vena cava in the transverse sinus of the pericardial sac. Here 72 per cent of the circumference is accessible within the sac. It then extends into the right hilus where it divides into a superior and inferior division. From these divisions segmental branches arise.

2. **Pulmonary Veins** (Fig. 3) – return oxygenated blood from the lungs to left atrium. There are usually four such veins, two on the right side and two on the left. Frequently on the left side (25 per cent) a *common pulmonary vein* may enter the left atrium, and occasionally (3 per cent) on the right side there may be three separate veins.

a. LEFT SUPERIOR PULMONARY VEIN – lies below the left pulmonary artery and anterior to the left bronchus at the hilus. It receives the veins from the left upper lobe. Extending between the left superior pulmonary vein and left pulmonary artery is the *vestigial fold of Marshall* (Fig. 2, page 105). In this fold may be located a *persistent left superior vena cava.*

b. LEFT INFERIOR PULMONARY VEIN – is located in the ilus just below the left main stem bronchus. It receives tributaries from the left lower lobe of the lung.

c. RIGHT SUPERIOR PULMONARY VEIN – lies in the lung root anterior to and below the right pulmonary artery and anterior to and above the inferior vein. This vein drains the upper and middle lobes of the right lung.

d. RIGHT INFERIOR PULMONARY VEIN – is below and posterior to the right superior vein. It is the most inaccessible vein from an intrapericardial approach because of its posterior-anterior direction of entrance into the left atrium. It receives all branches of the right lower lobe.

3. **Main Bronchi** (Fig. 4) – arise at the tracheal bifurcation at the lower border of T_4. These main bronchi diverge in an oblique course to the hilus of the lung.

a. LEFT MAIN BRONCHUS – arises from the trachea in about a 45 degree angle with the median plane. It is smaller in diameter and has a course approximately twice as long as the right bronchus. It passes below the aortic arch and anterior to the descending thoracic aorta.

b. RIGHT MAIN BRONCHUS – is more aligned with the trachea, its angle with the median plane being 25 degrees. This accounts for the more frequent aspiration of foreign bodies into the right lung. Its course is shorter than that of the left, and it is wider in diameter. Its relation at the hilus is shown in Figure 1.

4. **Bronchial Arteries** (Fig. 4) – are located on the posterior surface of the main bronchi in the hilus; usually one on the right side and two on the left. The *right bronchial artery* most frequently arises from the first right aortic intercostal artery. It may, however, arise in common with the left upper bronchial artery from the thoracic aorta. The left bronchial arteries arise directly from the aorta. The *upper branch* takes origin from the front of the aorta just below the tracheal bifurcation, and the lower branch just below the level of the left bronchus.

5. **Bronchial Veins** (not shown) – are found only at the hilus arising from tributaries draining the segmental and subsegmental divisions of the bronchi. They do not correspond entirely to branches of the bronchial artery, since the tributaries unite to form a right and left trunk which receive tracheal and postmediastinal veins. The right trunk enters the azygos vein, and the left, the accessory azygos.

6. **Pulmonary Plexuses** (not shown) – are continuous with the cardiac plexuses (page 96). Anterior and posterior pulmonary branches of the vagus are joined by rami from the second, third, and fourth thoracic sympathetic trunk ganglia, dorsal to the tracheal bifurcation. These branches form anterior and posterior plexuses on either side which extend into the lungs along the pulmonary artery.

7. **Lymphatics** – of this and other parts of the thorax are discussed on page 130.

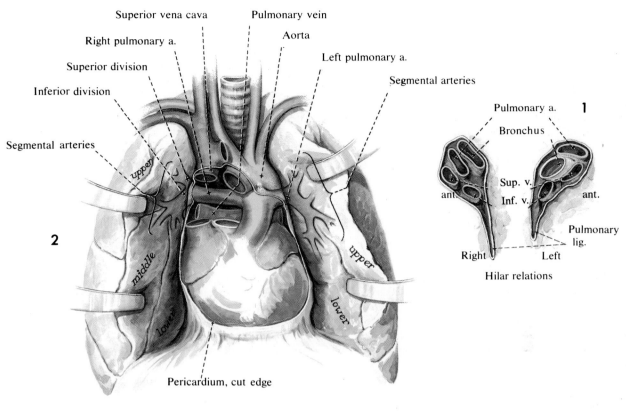

Superior vena cava
Right pulmonary a.
Superior division
Inferior division
Pulmonary vein
Aorta
Left pulmonary a.
Segmental arteries
Segmental arteries

upper
middle
lower
upper
lower

2

Pericardium, cut edge

1
Pulmonary a.
Bronchus
Sup. v.
ant.
Inf. v.
ant.
Pulmonary lig.
Right
Left

Hilar relations

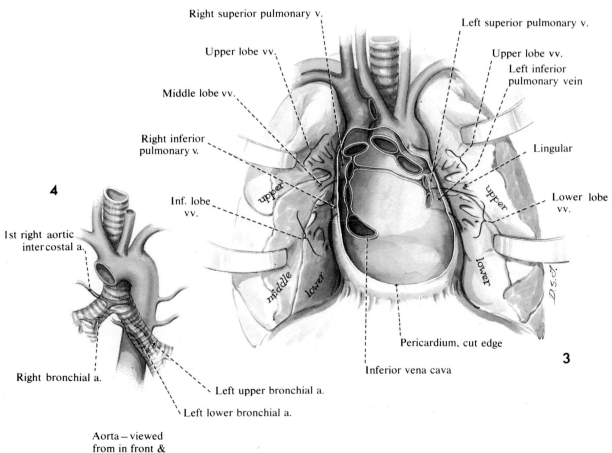

Right superior pulmonary v.
Left superior pulmonary v.
Upper lobe vv.
Upper lobe vv.
Left inferior pulmonary vein
Middle lobe vv.
Right inferior pulmonary v.
Lingular
Inf. lobe vv.
Lower lobe vv.

upper
upper
middle
lower
lower

4

1st right aortic intercostal a.

Right bronchial a.
Left upper bronchial a.
Left lower bronchial a.

Pericardium, cut edge
Inferior vena cava

3

Aorta—viewed from in front & to the left

THE PLEURAL CAVITY AND LUNGS:

The lungs are each encased in a serous sac, the *pleura*. The two sacs are separated by the mediastinum. Like other serous sacs in the body, they consist of a *parietal* and a *visceral* layer, between which is a potential capillary space, the *pleural cavity,* containing a small amount of serous fluid.

1. **Parietal Pleura** (Fig. 1) — is related to the thoracic wall, diaphragm, and mediastinum, and extends above the first rib into the neck.

a. COSTAL — layer of parietal pleura lines the anterior, lateral, and posterior thoracic walls deep to the endothoracic fascia.

b. DIAPHRAGMATIC — layer is continuous with the costal layer as a reflection from the anterior, lateral, and posterior thoracic walls on to the diaphragm.

c. MEDIASTINAL — layer is a reflection of the costal pleura anteriorly and posteriorly, and cervical pleura superiorly. In addition, a reflection upon the mediastinal structures from the diaphragmatic pleura below completes this layer. The anatomic relations to this layer of pleura are extremely important in understanding the anatomy of the mediastinal structures (page 94).

d. CERVICAL (CUPOLA) PLEURA — is that portion of the parietal pleura that covers the apex of the lung. It extends into the root of the neck 1½ inches above the sternal attachment of the first rib. It is protected at this site by a thickening of deep cervical fascia, *Sibson's fascia.*

2. **Isthmus (Mesopneumonium)** (Fig. 1) — is the reflection of mediastinal parietal pleura over the root of the lung, where it becomes visceral pleura. The upper portion of this pleural reflection is occupied by structures going to and from the lung and mediastinum (Fig. 1, page 113). The lower portion is unoccupied, thus forming a double layer of pleura, the *pulmonary ligament.*

3. **Visceral Pleura** — is adherent to the lung; its topography is, therefore, identical to the topography of the lungs proper (Figs. 2, 3, and 4).

4. **Pleura Recesses** (Fig. 1) — are those parts of the pleural cavity that are occupied by the lung (visceral pleura) only during full inspiration.

a. COSTOMEDIASTINAL RECESS — is related to the anterior thoracic wall at the reflection of the costal to mediastinal parietal pleura behind the sternum. This reflection varies on either side.

b. COSTODIAPHRAGMATIC (COSTOPHRENIC) RECESS — is of great value in roentgen diagnosis of pleural effusion.

The topography of the pleural reflections related to the costosternal and costodiaphragmatic recesses are illustrated in Figures 2, 3, and 4.

The lungs arise as a ventral outpouching from the foregut, which divides into right and left buds which form the right and left lungs. The lungs are separated by the mediastinum and covered by visceral pleura.

1. **Shape** — of this organ is irregularly conical, thereby presenting an apex and base. The *apex* extends above the level of the first rib into the root of the neck. Three surfaces of the lung may be described. The *costal surface* is related to the ventral, lateral, and dorsal thoracic wall. The *mediastinal surface* presents two important relationships: one, the *hilus,* is a depression in which the structures leaving and entering the lung are located; the other, the *cardiac fossa,* is an impression produced by the adjacent heart. The left fossa is the more prominent. The *diaphragmatic surface (base)* is concave, adapting itself to the dome of the diaphragm.

Three borders may be defined on each lung. An *anterior border* projects into the costosternal recess of the pleural cavity. On the left side this border presents a *notch (cardiac)* produced by the impingement of pericardial sac to the ventral wall of the thorax. The *inferior border* extends into the costophrenic recesses during respiratory excursions. The *posterior border* is broad and rounded and fits into the concavity on either side of the vertebral column.

2. **Topography** (Figs. 2, 3, and 4) — of the anterior border of the lungs is identical to the anterior pleural reflections. The inferior border, however, is located two ribs higher than the costodiaphragmatic reflection of pleura.

3. **Fissures** (Figs. 3 and 4) — are present in each lung, dividing it into lobes. These fissures are:

a. OBLIQUE FISSURE — divides the lung into an upper and lower lobe. Topographically, it is somewhat lower on the right side, beginning at the angle of the fifth rib, following that rib to midaxillary line, thence to the sixth costochondral junction at the midclavicular line. On the left side it begins at the fourth interspace at the rib angle and descends more vertically, crossing the sixth rib at midaxillary line.

b. HORIZONTAL FISSURE — found only in the right lung, may be topographically represented by a line drawn from the fourth costal cartilage anteriorly, extending posteriorly to the junction with the oblique fissure to the midaxillary line at the level of the fifth rib. This fissure may be absent in from 10 to 20 per cent of right lungs. When present, it divides the superior portion of the right lung into an upper and middle lobe.

4. **Lobes** — of the lung are classically described as an upper, middle, and lower lobe in the right, and an upper and lower lobe in the left. Since the aforementioned fissures may be absent, especially in the right, the number of lobes may be decreased. On the other hand, additional fissures may be present other than those described, producing "accessory" lobes. These are fissures between the segments of the lobes. One of the most common is shown in Figure 5. Occasionally the azygos vein arches over the apex of the right lung, rather than the right hilus, partly isolating the medial portion of the apex as the so-called *azygos lobe* (Fig. 6).

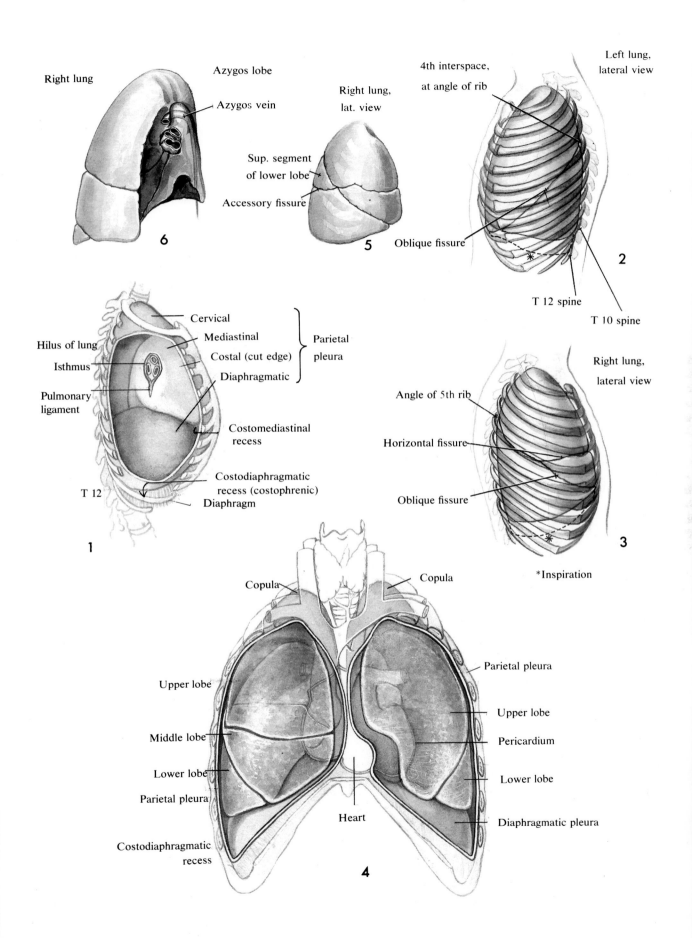

Right lung

Azygos lobe

— Azygos vein

6

Right lung,
lat. view

Sup. segment
of lower lobe

Accessory fissure

5

4th interspace,
at angle of rib

Left lung,
lateral view

Oblique fissure

2

T 12 spine

T 10 spine

Cervical

Mediastinal

Parietal
pleura

Costal (cut edge)

Diaphragmatic

Hilus of lung

Isthmus

Pulmonary
ligament

Costomediastinal
recess

T 12

Costodiaphragmatic
recess (costophrenic)

Diaphragm

1

Angle of 5th rib

Right lung,
lateral view

Horizontal fissure

Oblique fissure

3

*Inspiration

Copula

Copula

Upper lobe

Parietal pleura

Middle lobe

Upper lobe

Lower lobe

Pericardium

Parietal pleura

Lower lobe

Heart

Diaphragmatic pleura

Costodiaphragmatic
recess

4

TRACHEOBRONCHIAL TREE

For those who manage patients with pulmonary disease, an accurate knowledge of the structure of the tracheobronchial tree is essential, (1) for understanding the localization of lung abscesses, (2) for interpreting roentgenograms of the lungs, both the standard projections and bronchograms, (3) for the systematic examination through the bronchoscope of the tracheobronchial tree in search for tumors, foreign bodies, and inflammatory lesions, and (4) for the preservation, by the surgeon removing localized pulmonary lesions, of the adjacent normal bronchopulmonary segments.

The concept of the bronchopulmonary segment as a basic anatomic, pathologic, and surgical unit of the lung is fundamental to many of our current ideas and practices. Just as the lobes constitute major division of the lung with their own bronchial, arterial, and venous supply, so do the bronchopulmonary segments represent units of the lobes. Beyond the hilum of the lobe, the segmental bronchi arise, branch, and rebranch to supply smaller and smaller segments of tissue. The parts supplied by the chief branches of the segmental bronchi are subsegments and each of these in turn is composed of still smaller units down to the lobule.

At the hilum of the lobe, the segmental bronchi are generally accompanied by an artery and vein. The arteries are more variable than the bronchi, however, and the veins vary still more. In addition, the peripheral tributaries of the veins do not accompany the peripheral bronchi and arteries, but, instead, lie either subpleurally or in the plane between bronchopulmonary segments. One of these veins, therefore, drains more than one segment, and each segment is drained by several veins. The intersegmental position of the veins is of considerable usefulness as a guide to the surgeon in defining the limits of the segment to be removed.

Thus, the bronchopulmonary segment should be regarded as the zone of distribution of a segmental bronchus which may or may not be entered by arteries from adjacent segments and which is drained peripherally by veins occupying intersegmental planes. This description emphasizes both the intersegmental position of the veins and that there are arterial branches which cross between segments. In other words, the plane of division between segments is not completely avascular. It also emphasizes the fact that the bronchus rather than the more variable arteries and veins is the more important guide in segmental resections.

On the accompanying plate, the bronchoscopic landmarks and features are illustrated together with projections of the bronchi on the surface of the two lungs. Reference to pages 114 and 118 will also be helpful to the reader in correlation of the many aspects of this bronchopulmonary design.

1. **Trachea and Carina** — the trachea commences in the neck at the lower border of the cricoid cartilage opposite the sixth cervical vertebra, and it ends below by dividing into right and left main stem bronchi, at the level of the sternal angle in line with the lower border of the fourth thoracic vertebra. It lies in the midline except at its bifurcation, where it is slightly to the right.

Within the trachea, the horseshoe-shaped tracheal cartilages are seen beneath the mucosa, and the circular outline of the trachea is flattened posteriorly where those cartilages are deficient. At the lower end of the trachea, the orifices of the two primary bronchi are separated by a sharp margin known as the *carina* (Gr. keel) (Fig. 1).

2. **Right Main Stem Bronchi** — only a slight deflection (20 to 25 degrees) of the distal end of the bronchoscope to the right is required for a view down the right bronchus. It is more directly in line with the trachea than is the left bronchus. The orifice of the right upper lobe bronchus (Fig. 1b) is visible on the lateral wall of the right bronchus immediately below the level of the carina. The use of the right-angled telescope makes possible the examination of the short (1 cm.) stem of the right upper lobe bronchus and the orifice of the three segmental divisions: the apical, anterior, and posterior.

A centimeter or more below the upper lobe orifice, the opening of the middle lobe bronchus can be seen on the anterior lateral wall. Distal to the origin of the middle lobe bronchus, all the bronchi are destined for segments of the lower lobe. The bronchus to its superior segment comes off posteriorly and runs directly backward. The relationship of the origin of this bronchus to that of the middle lobe is surgically important. Though it usually arises just distal to the middle lobe bronchus, it may be exactly opposite or even a little proximal. In performing a right lower lobectomy and preserving the right middle lobe in these circumstances, the surgeon must deal with the bronchus to the superior division of the right lower lobe and the main bronchus below the orign of the middle lobe separately (Fig. 3). Distal to the origin of the superior segmental bronchus, the main bronchus terminates in four bronchi to the basal segments, the medial, anterior, lateral, and posterior, whose orifices are clearly visible.

3. **Left Main Stem Bronchus** (Fig. 1a) — the left primary bronchus is longer than the right and less vertical. About 5 cm. from the carina the left upper lobe bronchus arises from its left lateral wall. Usually with the aid of the telescope, but occasionally without it, the orifices of the upper and lower (lingular) divisions are visible. The first branch of the bronchus to the left lower lobe is to the superior segment. It lies posteriorly about 1 cm. below the upper lobe orifice. Immediately below are the bronchi to the three basal segments, anteromedial, lateral, and posterior.

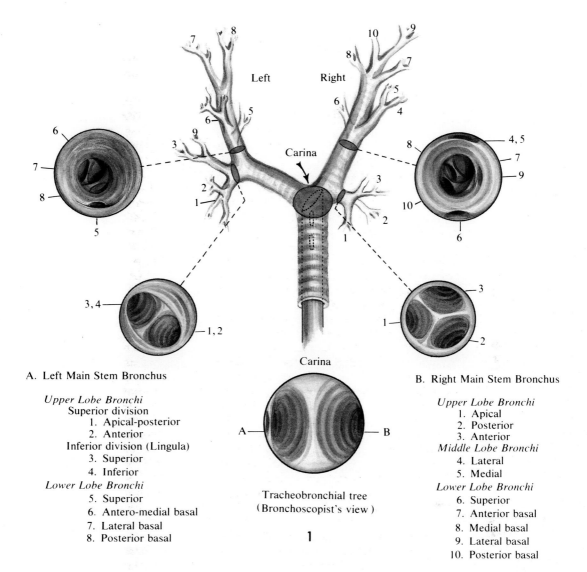

Carina

Tracheobronchial tree
(Bronchoscopist's view)

1

A. Left Main Stem Bronchus

Upper Lobe Bronchi
  Superior division
    1. Apical-posterior
    2. Anterior
  Inferior division (Lingula)
    3. Superior
    4. Inferior
Lower Lobe Bronchi
    5. Superior
    6. Antero-medial basal
    7. Lateral basal
    8. Posterior basal

B. Right Main Stem Bronchus

Upper Lobe Bronchi
    1. Apical
    2. Posterior
    3. Anterior
Middle Lobe Bronchi
    4. Lateral
    5. Medial
Lower Lobe Bronchi
    6. Superior
    7. Anterior basal
    8. Medial basal
    9. Lateral basal
   10. Posterior basal

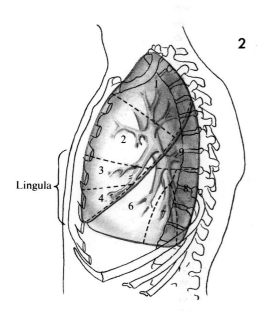

2

Lingula

Left lung

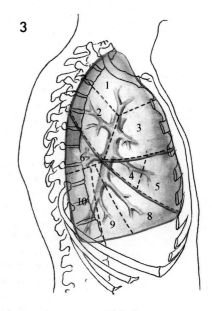

3

Right lung

ROENTGEN ANATOMY OF THE LUNGS: LOBAR AND SEGMENTAL LOCALIZATION:

Familiarity with the pattern of the bronchopulmonary segments presented in preceding pages makes relatively easy the identification of these same segments on roentgenograms of the chest, when they have been made opaque by collapse or consolidation. The shadows produced by these changes are shown in semidiagramatic form on the accompanying plate.

1. **Right Upper Lobe** (Fig. 1):

a. APICAL SEGMENT—PA: An area bounded by the apex of the pleura and the mediastinum, and laterally by an outward concave border extending from the hilum at the level of third interspace anteriorly to the periphery at the level of the first or second rib.

Lateral: a v-shaped area with its apex at the hilum is often difficult to see because of the superimposed shadow of the shoulder.

b. ANTERIOR SEGMENT—PA: A dense, homogeneous opacity roughly quadrilateral and extending from the hilum to the periphery. The lower border is the horizontal fissure and appears as a sharp horizontal line about the level of the fourth costal cartilage. The upper limit is variable, usually convex and sloping from hilum upward and laterally to the periphery at the second rib.

Lateral: A wedge-shaped opacity above the lesser (horizontal) fissure pointing toward the hilum. The base of the wedge extends to the anterior chest wall.

c. POSTERIOR SEGMENT—PA: A shadow similar to that produced by the consolidated anterior segment, but smaller, distinctly quadrilateral, less homogeneous, and with a less sharply defined lower border. Also there is often a clear area between the border of the shadow and the mediastinum.

Lateral: A density situated posteriorly is homogeneous and roughly quadrilateral in shape; the lower border formed by the oblique fissure is clear cut and slopes upward and backward from the hilum to reach the level of T_6.

2. **Right Middle Lobe** (Fig. 1)—PA: A dense triangular opacity extending outward from the right border of the heart to a point about halfway across the lung field. The upper margin, formed by the horizontal fissure, lies at about the level of the fourth costal cartilages; the lower border, formed by the oblique fissure, usually overlaps the diaphragm.

Lateral: A triangular shadow with the apex at the hilum and the base extending to the lower end of the sternum from the fourth costal cartilage to the diaphragm.

3. **Left Upper Lobe** (Fig. 2):

a. APICOPOSTERIOR SEGMENT—PA: A dense homogeneous shadow with a sharp inferolateral margin formed by the oblique fissure extending from the hilum to the first rib. Medially, the opacity blends with that of the mediastinum and superiorly it extends to the dome of the pleura.

Lateral: A wedge similar to, but broader than, that formed by the apical segment of the right upper lobe.

b. ANTERIOR SEGMENT—PA: An oval density whose medial border lies about midway between the hilum and the chest wall. Superiorly, it extends to the first rib, inferiorly to the fourth costal cartilage, and laterally to the chest wall.

c. LINGULAR SEGMENT—PA: A wedge-shaped opacity extending out into the left lung from the border of the left ventricle and cardiophrenic angle. It is usually at the levels of the anterior ends of the sixth or seventh ribs.

4. **The Lower Lobes** (Figs. 3 and 4)—the lower lobes are so similar that they may be considered together. The chief difference between them is the presence of an independent medial basal segment in the right lower lobe.

a. SUPERIOR SEGMENTS—PA: A rather wide band of opacity in the middle zone of the lung extending from hilum to lateral chest wall. The upper border lies at the level of the fifth or sixth ribs posteriorly, and the lower border is at the level of the ninth or tenth ribs posteriorly.

Lateral: A triangular opacity with the base on the posterior chest wall from the fifth to the ninth or tenth vertebra and the apex at the hilum about the level of the fifth rib anteriorly.

When the superior segment is collapsed the size of the shadow in the posterior-anterior view is greatly reduced and does not extend to the lateral chest wall. It is more likely to appear as a small opacity extending laterally from the mediastinum at the level of the seventh or eighth rib posteriorly. In the lateral view, the shadow of the collapsed superior segment is a narrow, wedge-shaped density and the upper, posterior end of the oblique fissure may be displaced inferiorly into a more horizontal position.

b. POSTERIOR BASAL SEGMENTS—PA: An opacity extending out from the lower part of the heart shadow obliterating the cardiophrenic angle. On the left it is often hidden behind the heart.

Lateral: A well defined, triangular shadow with its apex at the hilum and its base at the posterior costophrenic sulcus extending superiorly to the ninth or tenth thoracic vertebra. Collapse of the segment reduces the area of opacity without changing significantly its position.

c. LATERAL BASAL SEGMENTS—PA: A wedge-shaped, obliquely placed opacity with its base upon the lateral part of the diaphragm and adjoining chest wall, obliterating the costophrenic sinus. Its apex is at the hilum. The cardiophrenic angle remains clear.

Lateral: A wedge-shaped opacity behind the midaxillary line with its base on the diaphragm and its apex at the hilum.

d. ANTERIOR BASAL SEGMENTS—PA: Shadow similar to that of the lateral basal segments.

Lateral: A homogeneous wedge-like shadow extending inferiorly and anteriorly from the hilum to the diaphragm in front of the midaxillary line. The anterior border is sharply defined (being formed by the oblique fissure). When the segment is collapsed it may appear as such a narrow band in the lateral view as to be mistaken for thickening of the oblique fissure.

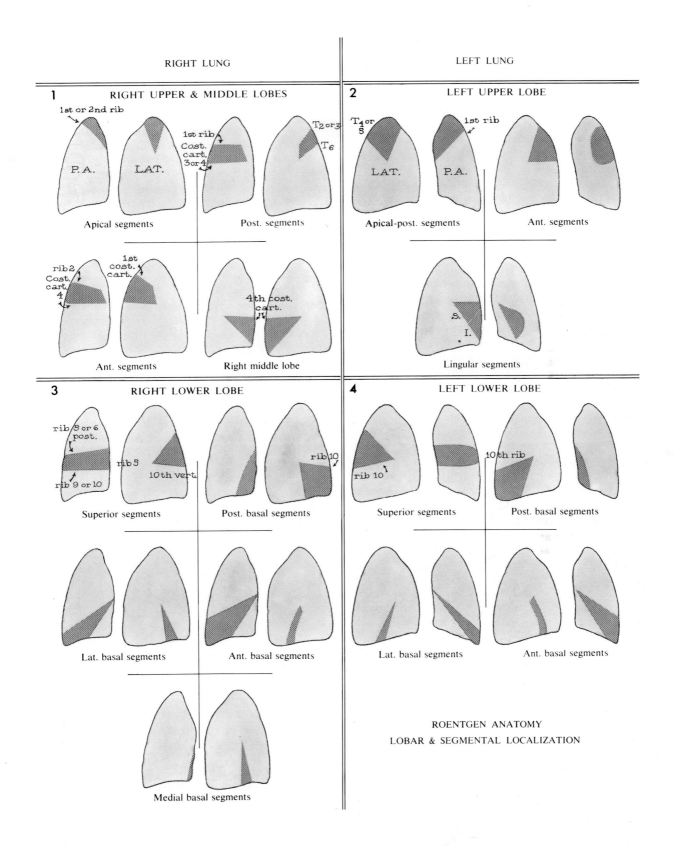

RIGHT LUNG

LEFT LUNG

1 RIGHT UPPER & MIDDLE LOBES

1st or 2nd rib

1st rib
Cost. cart.
3 or 4

T2 or 3
T6

P.A. LAT.

Apical segments

Post. segments

rib 2
Cost. cart.
4

1st cost. cart.

4th cost. cart.

Ant. segments

Right middle lobe

2 LEFT UPPER LOBE

T4 or 5

1st rib

LAT. P.A.

Apical-post. segments

Ant. segments

S.
I.

Lingular segments

3 RIGHT LOWER LOBE

rib 5 or 6 post.
rib 5
rib 9 or 10
10th vert.

rib 10

Superior segments

Post. basal segments

Lat. basal segments

Ant. basal segments

Medial basal segments

4 LEFT LOWER LOBE

rib 10

10th rib

Superior segments

Post. basal segments

Lat. basal segments

Ant. basal segments

ROENTGEN ANATOMY
LOBAR & SEGMENTAL LOCALIZATION

e. MEDIAL BASAL SEGMENT (RIGHT LOWER LOBE)—
PA: A small area of opacity filling the right cardio-phrenic angle.

Lateral: A small triangular shadow based on the diaphragm slightly posterior to its center, with its apex at the hilum. When the segment is collapsed, the shadow may be hidden behind the heart in the posterior-anterior view.

CLINICAL ANATOMY OF THE LUNG ROOTS:

The surgeon operating upon the lung must be prepared to remove the entire lung, a lobe, or a bronchopulmonary segment or segments depending upon the location and the extent of the disease. The lesser the resection, the greater the demand for knowledge of bronchopulmonary and vascular anatomy, because, in removing a diseased segment, the bronchial supply and the blood supply of the adjacent lung segments must be preserved.

On pages 121 and 123 the structures in the hila of the lungs and lobes are shown as the surgeon exposes them through an anterior or lateral approach. Because of the complexities of segmental anatomy due to the many variations in bronchovascular arrangements sufficient space is not available here to illustrate even the common patterns at the hilum of the various segments. The chief technical problems in segmental resection are the identification of bronchial, arterial, and venous elements supplying the segment, and the dissection in the intersegmental planes without injury to adjacent segments. This identification must be accomplished by the isolation of several or all of the arteries entering a lobe so as to identify the branch or branches entering the segment to be removed. If doubt still exists, temporary occlusion of the bronchus with the use of alternate expansion and collapse of the surrounding lung is helpful in fixing the boundaries of the segment. When the proper bronchus has been identified and sectioned, traction on its distal end with simultaneous dissection peripherally permits the isolation of the segmental arteries and veins as they become evident. The great number of variations in vascular patterns, particularly in the left upper lobe, make this approach the only reliable one.

1. **Right Hilum, Anterior Approach** (Fig. 1)—the close relation of the pericardium, phrenic nerve, azygos vein, and superior vena cava to the hilum explains the frequency of involvement of these structures by bronchogenic carcinoma. The relationship of the pericardium to the pulmonary veins is of special importance, since the complete removal of a tumor involving the veins of the hilum may make necessary removal of a part of the pericardium and the ligation of vessels within the pericardial sac.

When the chest has been entered through an anterior or posterolateral incision, dissection of the hilum for an upper lobectomy, a middle lobectomy, or a pneumonectomy is usually commenced on the anterior aspect of a lung root. An incision through the pleura exposes the superior pulmonary vein which is the most anterior structure in the hilum. Its upper division lies in front of the superior branch (truncus anterius) of the right pulmonary artery. In other words, the pulmonary artery lies slightly superior and posterior to the superior vein. Posterior to the artery is the bronchus. The bronchus to the upper lobe may be exposed anteriorly by first dividing the vessels to the right upper lobe. If the middle lobe is to be preserved, care must be taken to leave the trunk of the superior vein and its tributary from the middle lobe. Occasionally, the vein from the middle lobe drains directly into the left atrium and rarely into the inferior pulmonary vein.

At the point of division of the right pulmonary artery into the superior (truncus anterius) and inferior (pars interlobaris) divisions a well defined band of fibrous connective tissue extends from the adventitia of the artery to the pericardium over the lower end of the superior vena cava. Cutting this band allows the surgeon ready access to the trunk of the right pulmonary artery.

Bronchial lymph nodes lie in the angles between tributaries of the pulmonary vein and branches of the artery of the hilum. When they have been made large and more vascular or calcified and fixed by inflammation, hilar dissection may be tedious and difficult. Extensive involvement of these nodes by metastasis is common in bronchogenic carcinoma.

2. **Right Hilum, Interlobar Approach** (Fig. 2)—dissection in the oblique fissure is the easiest approach to one or more branches of the pulmonary artery supplying the posterior segment of the right upper lobe (so-called ascending branches). It is obviously the most direct and simple approach to the structures in the hilum of the middle and lower lobes. The artery or arteries to the middle lobe are anterior branches of the inferior division of the pulmonary artery. The artery to the superior division of the lower lobe is a posterior branch of the same vessel arising at the same or slightly higher level. Division of these branches allows for easy exposure of the corresponding lobar segmental bronchi. Bronchial lymph nodes are also prominent in this approach.

3. **Right Hilum, Posterior Approach** (Fig. 3)—bronchogenic carcinoma involving the hilum or metastasis in bronchial lymph nodes of the hilum, which have broken through the capsules of the nodes, quickly becomes attached to or invades the azygos vein, the pericardium at the entrance of the inferior pulmonary vein, or the esophagus. Isolation and division of the inferior pulmonary vein or its tributaries and the right main bronchus or its upper lobe and lower lobe divisions is usually accomplished by an approach through the pleura covering the posterior face of the lung root. This also exposes the bronchial artery on the posterior membranous part of the main bronchus. Posterior bronchial and inferior tracheobronchial (subcarinal) lymph nodes are most accessible to the surgeon from this aspect of the hilum.

4. **Arterial Supply to Right Lung** (Figs. 1 and 2)—the *right pulmonary artery* enters the lung roots and divides into superior and inferior divisions. The *superior division (truncus anterius)* supplies all three segments of the right upper lobe. In about one third of the cases, however, the posterior segment of the upper lobe may receive its entire or a supplement supply via a *recurrent branch* or branches from the inferior division (Fig. 2). These latter vessels are often small and may be torn by excessive traction on the lobe.

The *inferior division* passes spirally over the middle lobe bronchus and then descends behind the lower lobe bronchus and lies in the interlobar (oblique) fissure (Fig. 2). It usually gives off a single artery to the middle lobe which in turn divides into the medial

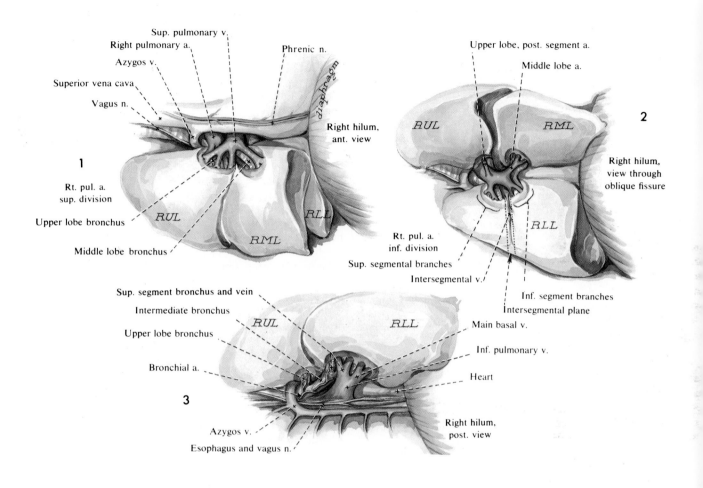

and lateral segment arteries. At times, these segment branches will arise separately. From the interlobar part of the inferior division rises a branch to the superior segment and usually one to the medial basal segment. They come off in successive manner at close interval branches to the anterior, lateral, and posterior basal segments. Frequently, there is not a separate artery for each segment, but several basal segments may be supplied by common trunks in an alternating fashion.

5. **Venous Drainage of the Right Lung**—the pulmonary veins differ from the arteries and bronchi in that they are not segmentally arranged, but emerge subplurally from interlobar and intersegmental fissures (Fig. 2). The *right superior pulmonary vein* is anterior in position at the hilum and drains the entire upper lobe and in most cases the middle lobe (Fig. 1). The *right inferior pulmonary vein* is the most posterior and inferior structure at the hilum and drains the inferior lobe (Fig. 3). The *middle lobe vein* which usually empties into the superior trunk may at times enter the inferior branch or empty separately into the left atrium.

6. **Bronchial Architecture of the Right Lung**—this is discussed on page 116.

SURGICAL ANATOMY OF THE LUNG ROOTS (continued):

1. **Left Hilum, Anterior Approach** (Fig. 1) – the arch of the aorta, the ligamentum arteriosum (ductus arteriosus), and the left recurrent laryngeal nerve, though not strictly anterior relations of the structures in the root of the lung, are seen best from the anterior view of the hilum. When the lung is retracted laterally and posteriorly, the phrenic and vagus nerves are seen in their course in the mediastinum (pages 95 and 97). The vagus disappears as it passes across the arch of the aorta and behind the root of the lung. It is at the inferior margin of the arch that the recurrent laryngeal branch arises and turns medially, posterior to the ligamentum arteriosum. It is at this area too, that a bronchial lymph node is usually located (page 131). Bronchogenic carcinoma in the hilum of the left lung often interrupts the recurrent nerve by direct invasion or, more often, by pressure from an expanding metastasis in this lymph node lying in contact with the nerve. Sudden hoarseness due to paralysis of the left vocal cord should arouse immediately the suspicion that cancer of the left lung may be present.

Incision through the pleura on the root of the lung anteriorly reveals the superior pulmonary vein and the left pulmonary artery in the same relative positions as they occupy the right; i.e., the vein is slightly anterior and inferior to the artery. The superior vein is shown with three tributaries which drain all the bronchopulmonary segments of the left upper lobe.

2. **Left Hilum, Interlobar Approach** (Fig. 2) – when the fissure is opened by retraction of the upper lobe forward, the trunk of the left pulmonary artery with its branches to the segments of both upper and lower lobes can be exposed. The anterior segmental branch often arises anteriorly as shown in Figure 2. The apical or apical-posterior branch usually comes from the superior margin of the artery as shown in Figure 2. The branches to the upper lobe vary in number from two to eight. In this figure, three segmental branches, an anterior, an apical-posterior, and a lingular, are shown. The greater variability of the arteries to the left upper lobe makes identification more difficult than on the right and require somewhat more dissection.

The artery to the superior segment of the left lower lobe commonly arises from the same level as the branch to the lingula. If a lower lobectomy is to be done, the artery to the superior segment and the trunk of the basal segments will need to be ligated separately. The arterial trunk to the lower lobe is posterolateral to the bronchus. The inferior vein, which is inferior and medial, is not easily seen from this aspect nor is it shown here by the artist.

3. **Left Hilum, Posterior Approach** (Fig. 3) – the descending aorta, the vagus nerve, and the esophagus are intimately related to the structures in the lung root. Moreover, the inferior pulmonary ligament is readily exposed and divided by the surgeon approaching the lung root from its posterior surface.

The inferior pulmonary vein, which drains only the left lower lobe, is usually approached posteriorly. The main trunk of the vein is shown with two divisions: one from the superior segment and the second, and larger, from the basal segments.

After arching over the left upper lobe bronchus, the pulmonary artery enters the interlobar fissure behind this bronchus. In performing a left upper lobectomy the surgeon must ligate the branches of the artery to the upper lobe and retract the trunk of the vessel posteriorly in order to expose the upper lobe bronchus at its origin.

The interlobar part of the left main bronchus shown between the inferior vein and the artery lies on a plane slightly anterior to both. On its posterior membranous aspect, the bronchial arteries are evident. In chronic suppurative disease of the lungs and in congenital pulmonary artery atresia, the bronchial arteries are greatly enlarged.

Successful resection of the diseased segments and preservation of adjoining healthy lung segments depends upon an accurate knowledge of the bronchopulmonary segments. The procedure is made difficult (1) by the variations in the patterns of the bronchial and vascular trees, and (2) by the important fact that the diseased segments to be removed are greatly shrunken and distorted, making positive identification of segmental vessels difficult and hazardous. In order to avoid errors in vessel identification, the bronchus of segment to be removed should be found and divided first. In exposing the bronchus and its divisions, it may be necessary to isolate several branches of the artery to the lobe before the proper bronchus is selected. Then, when positive identification of the segmental bronchus has been made, gentle traction upon it facilitates selection of the correct segmental arteries to be divided. Finally, the emerging veins may be isolated and divided as they leave the hilum of the segment or lobe. There is no other way for the surgeon to identify these vessels with certainty during the course of the operation.

4. **Arterial Supply to Left Lung** (Figs. 1, 2, and 3) – the first portion of the *left pulmonary artery* arches over the left upper lobe bronchus and then descends behind the bronchus in the interlobar fissure. Unlike the right pulmonary artery, there is no division of the main trunk; the segment arteries arise directly. From the anterior surface of the *pulmonary arch*, an anterior segment artery may arise (70 per cent). This is the only branch arising in front of the bronchus. Less frequently, it comes off the *interlobar portion* of the main trunk. The remaining branches to the upper lobe arise from the interlobar portion; apical and posterior segment branches may arise separately or as a common trunk. In about two-thirds of the cases, the artery to the lingula arises from the pars interlobaris as a common trunk which divides into superior and inferior segment branches (Fig. 2). Not infrequently the lingular branch takes origin from the anterior surface of the arch of the right pulmonary artery, separately or in common with the anterior segment artery.

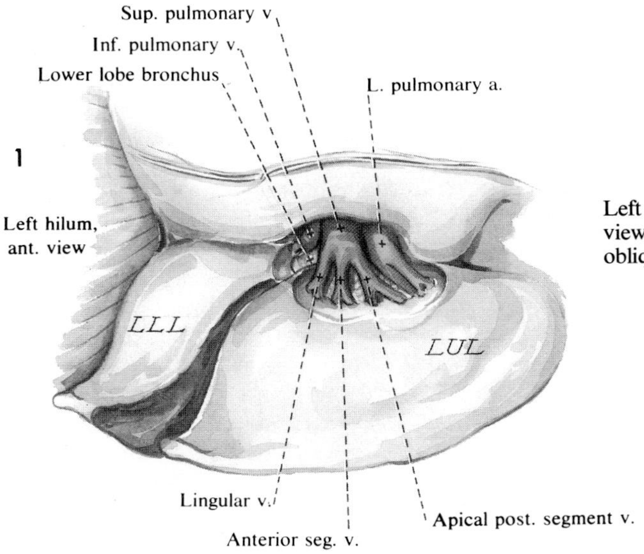
Sup. pulmonary v.
Inf. pulmonary v.
Lower lobe bronchus
L. pulmonary a.
1
Left hilum, ant. view
LLL
LUL
Lingular v.
Anterior seg. v.
Apical post. segment v.

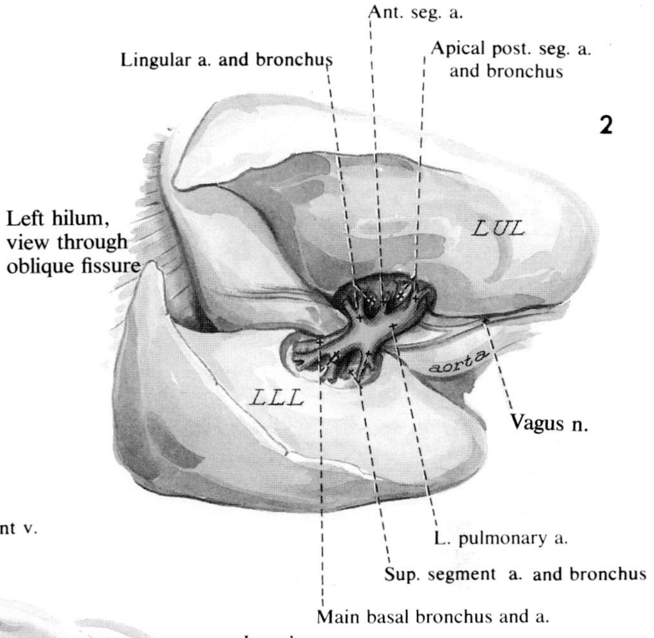
Ant. seg. a.
Lingular a. and bronchus
Apical post. seg. a. and bronchus
2
LUL
Left hilum, view through oblique fissure
aorta
LLL
Vagus n.
L. pulmonary a.
Sup. segment a. and bronchus
Main basal bronchus and a.

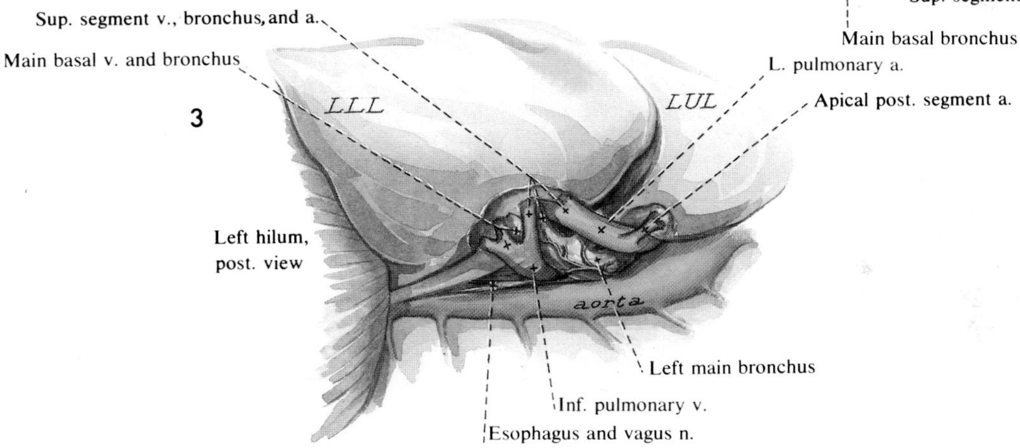
Sup. segment v., bronchus, and a.
Main basal v. and bronchus
L. pulmonary a.
Apical post. segment a.
3
LLL
LUL
Left hilum, post. view
aorta
Left main bronchus
Inf. pulmonary v.
Esophagus and vagus n.

The first artery to the lower lobe is the superior segment branch which arises from the posterior aspect pars interlobaris at a level slightly above the origin of the lingular artery (Fig. 2). The remainder of the left pulmonary artery branches are distributed to the anteromedial, lateral, and posterior basal segments.

Lungs made up wholly of prevailing patterns of arterial branchings are seldom encountered. A variation in pattern in even one segment necessarily modifies the vascular development in adjacent segments. Variations are particularly frequent in the left upper lobe.

5. **Venous Drainage of the Left Lung**—the *left superior pulmonary vein* as on the right side is anterior in position and slightly below the artery at the hilum (Fig. 1). It receives tributaries from all parts of the left upper lobe. The *left inferior pulmonary vein* (Fig. 3) drains the entire lower lobe and may at times (10 per cent) receive a vein from the lingula. These two vessels usually enter the left atrium separately but occasionally join to form a left common pulmonary vein.

6. **Bronchial Architecture of the Left Lung**—is discussed on page 116.

The Thorax

LUNG TRANSPLANTATION:

Lung transplantation is primarily indicated in patients with end-stage lung disease, i.e., pulmonary emphysema, bilateral lung disease with cystic fibrosis, or bronchiectasis. The chest radiograph must be clear, the PaO_2 greater than 300 mm. Hg, and positive end-expiratory pressure 5 cm. of water. Donor and recipient blood types must be compatible.

The types of transplants are single, double, and a combination heart and lung transplant. Single lung transplant is for patients with pulmonary fibrosis. Double lung transplant is better for patients with pulmonary emphysema and those with septic lung disease. The heart-lung transplant is indicated in patients with right-sided heart failure, incident to a parenchymal or vascular disease.

1. **Single Lung Transplant** – preoperatively the patient should have a radial artery catheter and Swan-Ganz catheter inserted. An upper midline incision is made, the omentum is mobilized and tunneled substernally, and the abdomen is closed.

Next, a posterior lateral thoractomy through the fifth rib is done. The main pulmonary artery is encircled with tapes and temporarily occluded. If the patient's ventilatory status and hemodynamics are unaltered, the procedure is done without cardiopulmonary by-pass.

The recipient lung is then removed, leaving a good length of the recipient's pulmonary artery and veins. The bronchus is divided at the lobar orifice level. The left atrium is clamped and opened and the pulmonary veins are anastomosed with polypropylene sutures. The pulmonary artery of the recipient is then anastomosed to the pulmonary artery of the donor, and the donor bronchus is joined end to end to the recipient bronchus. The omentum is then removed from the anterior mediastinum and wrapped around the bronchial anastomosis.

2. **Heart and Lung Transplant** – with the patient on cardiopulmonary by-pass after median sternotomy, the entire heart is extirpated, leaving the right atrium, interatrial septum, and the left posterior atrial wall. Each lung is removed lateral to the pericardium, and the trachea is divided proximal to the carina. Lateral pleural pericardial windows are made and the donor heart and lungs are passed through these openings. The trachea is anastomosed. The donor right atrium is then opened and is anastomosed to the recipient right atrium. Finally, the donor and recipient aortas are joined end to end.

3. **Double Lung Transplants** – first, median sternotomy and cardiopulmonary by-pass are initiated and omentum is retrieved as described under Single Lung Transplant. The donor-lung graft is passed through the pleuro-pericardial windows posterior to the right atrium and vena cava and posterior to the left phrenic nerve. The donor trachea is then anastomosed to the recipient trachea. The aorta is clamped, and after a cardioplegic is inserted and the heart arrested, the left atrium and pulmonary artery are anastomosed. Finally, the omentum is wrapped around the tracheal anastomosis.

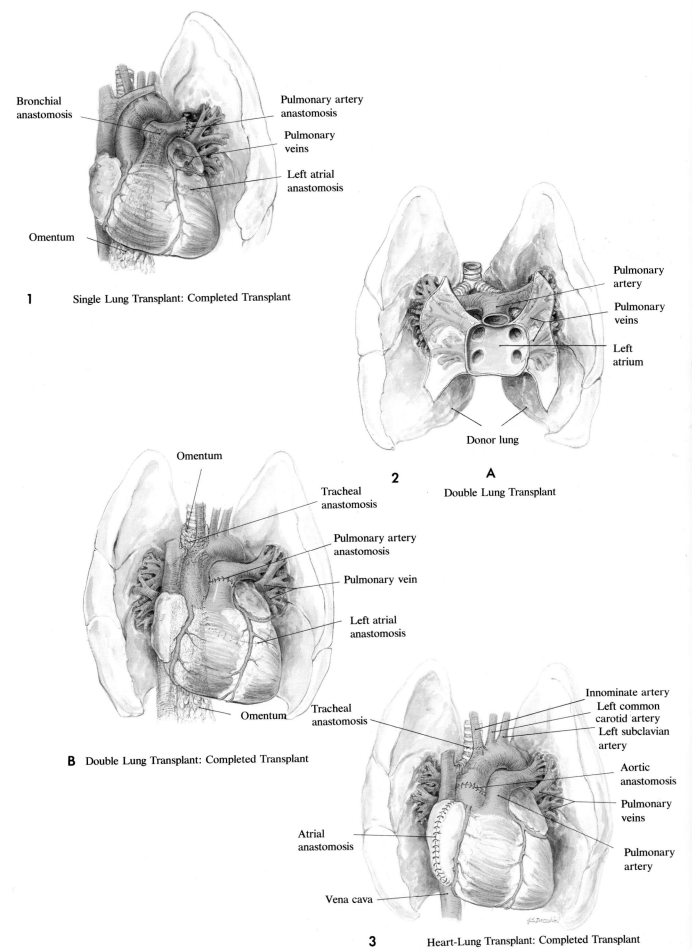

Bronchial
anastomosis

Pulmonary artery
anastomosis

Pulmonary
veins

Left atrial
anastomosis

Omentum

1 Single Lung Transplant: Completed Transplant

Pulmonary
artery

Pulmonary
veins

Left
atrium

Donor lung

2 **A** Double Lung Transplant

Omentum

Tracheal
anastomosis

Pulmonary artery
anastomosis

Pulmonary vein

Left atrial
anastomosis

Omentum

Tracheal
anastomosis

B Double Lung Transplant: Completed Transplant

Innominate artery
Left common
carotid artery
Left subclavian
artery

Aortic
anastomosis

Pulmonary
veins

Pulmonary
artery

Atrial
anastomosis

Vena cava

3 Heart-Lung Transplant: Completed Transplant

THE DIAPHRAGM:

The diaphragm is a musculomembranous partition between the thoracic and abdominal cavities. The muscular portion arises from the thoracic wall and lumbar vertebrae of either side and inserts into the membranous portion, the *central tendon*. It is the main respiratory muscle. With its contraction, the diaphragm descends and enlarges the thoracic cavity, thus aiding in inspiration.

1. **Topography**—of the diaphragm varies with the body build, being lower in slender persons and higher in the broad, stocky type. The position of the body alters the level of the diaphragm. In the supine position the diaphragm is approximately 3 cm. higher than in the standing position. Respiratory movements also alter the topography. In quiet respiration the range of movement is approximately 1 cm.

In the average subject in the erect position at neutral respiratory position, the right leaf is on a level with the tenth thoracic vertebra and the fifth costal cartilage. The left dome is 1 to 1½ cm. lower than the right in the normal subject.

2. **Origin**—of the muscular fibers is from sternal, costal, and lumbar components of either side.

a. STERNAL—slips arise from the xiphoid process and pass upward and backward to insert in the central tendon.

b. COSTAL—fibers arise from the internal surface of the costal cartilages of the seventh and eighth ribs and osseous portions of the last four ribs. These fibers terminate in the anterior and lateral border of the central tendon.

c. LUMBAR—origin is more complex and consists of two crura and four fibrous arches, two on the right and two on the left. The *right crus* arises from the upper three or four lumbar vertebral bodies and intervertebral disks, whereas the *left crus* arises from the upper two lumbar vertebrae. The two fibrous arches on either side are the *medial lumbocostal arch,* which extends from the body of the second lumbar vertebra to the transverse process of the same vertebra. The medial arch overlies the psoas major mucles of the posterior abdominal wall. The *lateral lumbocostal arch* is a fibrous thickening over the quadratus lumborum muscle extending from the transverse process of L_2 to the twelfth rib (Fig. 2).

3. **Insertion**—of the muscular fibers is into the *central tendon* of the diaphragm, which blends with the fibrous layer of pericardium.

4. **Orifices**—in the diaphragm transmit important structures to and from the abdominal cavity; the major

ones are caval, aortic, and esophageal orifices. Other smaller orifices allow passage of other vessels, nerves, and lymphatics.

a. INFERIOR VENA CAVA ORIFICE—is located in the central tendon at the level of T_8, about 1 inch to the right of the midline. The right phrenic nerve also exits from the thorax through this opening.

b. ESOPHAGEAL ORIFICE—lies posterior to the caval orifice and slightly to the left of the midline at the tenth thoracic level. In addition to the esophagus, the orifice transmits the vagus nerves and lower esophageal blood vessels. For detailed description of this opening, see page 129.

c. AORTIC ORIFICE—is bounded by the interconnecting fibers of the right and left crura. This orifice is located at the level of T_{12} and transmits the aorta, thoracic duct, and azygos vein.

d. STERNOCOSTAL TRIANGLE (FORAMEN OF MORGAGNI)—transmits the superior epigastric vessels between the sternal and costal origins on either side (Fig. 1). This may be the site of a diaphragmatic hernia.

5. **Other Structures Passing through the Diaphragm:**

a. BRANCHES FROM T_{12}—behind the lateral lumbocostal arch.

b. THE SYMPATHETIC TRUNK—behind the medial arch.

c. THE GREATER, LEAST, AND LESSER SPLANCHNIC NERVES—through the crura.

d. THE HEMIAZYGOS VEIN—through the left crus.

e. THE MUSCULOPHRENIC VESSELS—between the slips from the seventh and eighth cartilages.

f. THE LOWER FIVE INTERCOSTAL VESSELS AND NERVES—between each of the remaining slips.

6. **Lumbocostal Trigone (Foramen of Bochdalek)**—lies just above the lateral lumbocostal arch (Fig. 2). In this area, owing to a poorly developed costal portion of the muscle, the diaphragm may be closed only by connective tissue. On the left side, this area may be the site of a (congenital) diaphragmatic hernia.

7. **Blood Supply**—of the diaphragm is mainly by the *inferior phrenic arteries,* branches from the abdominal aorta. *Superior phrenic arteries* from the thoracic aorta supply the vertebral portion of the diaphragm on its upper surface. In addition, branches from the superior epigastric, musculophrenics, and lower intercostals—all vessels penetrating this structure—aid in its blood supply.

The venous drainage of the diaphragm is mainly by the inferior phrenic veins, but the exact mode of drainage has not been fully ascertained. Three major inferior phrenic veins are usually present, a left, right, and posterior, which empty into the inferior vena cava.

8. **Nerve Supply**—See page 88.

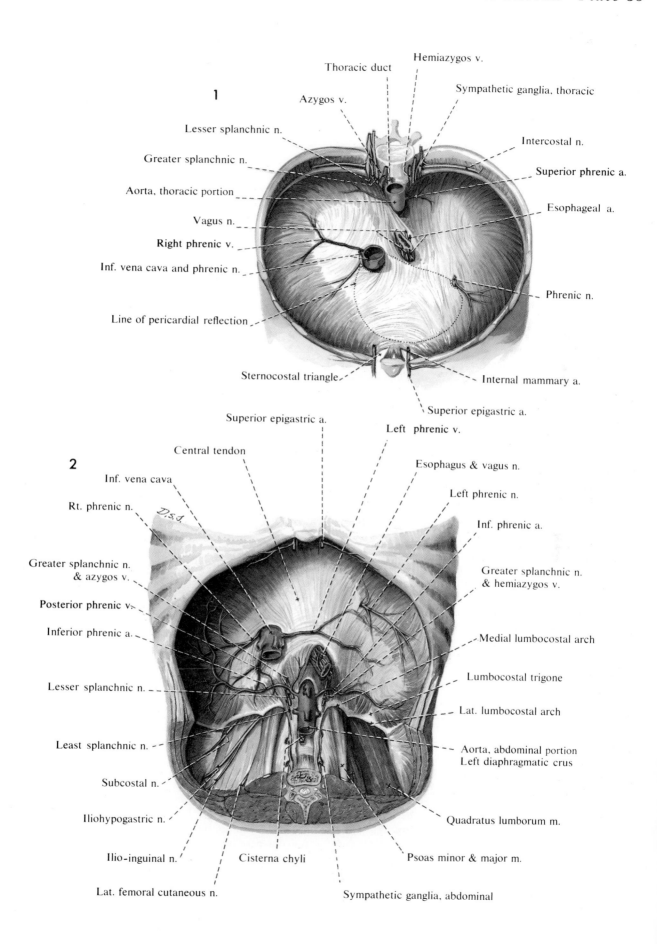

1

Thoracic duct

Hemiazygos v.

Azygos v.

Sympathetic ganglia, thoracic

Lesser splanchnic n.

Intercostal n.

Greater splanchnic n.

Superior phrenic a.

Aorta, thoracic portion

Esophageal a.

Vagus n.

Right phrenic v.

Inf. vena cava and phrenic n.

Phrenic n.

Line of pericardial reflection

Sternocostal triangle

Internal mammary a.

Superior epigastric a.

Superior epigastric a.

Left phrenic v.

Central tendon

Esophagus & vagus n.

2

Inf. vena cava

Left phrenic n.

Rt. phrenic n.

Inf. phrenic a.

Greater splanchnic n.
& azygos v.

Greater splanchnic n.
& hemiazygos v.

Posterior phrenic v.

Medial lumbocostal arch

Inferior phrenic a.

Lumbocostal trigone

Lesser splanchnic n.

Lat. lumbocostal arch

Least splanchnic n.

Aorta, abdominal portion
Left diaphragmatic crus

Subcostal n.

Quadratus lumborum m.

Iliohypogastric n.

Ilio-inguinal n.

Cisterna chyli

Psoas minor & major m.

Lat. femoral cutaneous n.

Sympathetic ganglia, abdominal

CLINICAL ANATOMY OF THE DIAPHRAGM:

The surgeon's interest in the diaphragm is focused mainly on the problem of hernias related to this structure. These hernias occur in areas of congenital or acquired weakness. Diaphragmatic hernias are most frequently acquired in the sense that they appear in the middle of life rather than at its beginning. By far the most common hernial site is through the esophageal hiatus.

1. **Congenital Hernias** — the diaphragm, pericardium, and heart develop in the neck. In migrating to their ultimate destinations they carry their nerve supply with them, which explains the innervation of these structures by cervical cord fibers. Several structures enter into the formation of the diaphragm. They are: (a) *the septum transversum* from which arises the anterior portion of the diaphragm, including the central tendon, (b) two posterior portions, the *pleuroperitoneal folds*, and (c) lateral ingrowths from the body wall which go to form that part of the diaphragm attached to the ribs. During development, an interval exists between the posterior pleuroperitoneal folds and the lateral wall ingrowth on either side and are known as the *pleuroperitoneal canals*. These communications between pleural and peritoneal cavities exist for a time, but normally are closed by a double-layered membrane made up of pleura and peritoneum. Between these layers striated muscles develop to complete and strengthen the diaphragm.

The persistence of a *pleuroperitoneal canal* accounts for most diaphragmatic hernias in infancy and childhood. They usually occur on the left side and if arrest of development of the diaphragm occurs very early, the defect is complete and the hernia has no sac (90 per cent). The defect (*foramen of Bochdalek*) is situated at the periphery of the diaphragm in the region of its attachment to the tenth and eleventh ribs (Fig. 3).

A less frequent type of congenital hernia may occur anteriorly through the diaphragm between the attachment to the posterior surface of the xyphoid and the attachment to the lower costal cartilages (Fig. 1). This small *sternocostal trigone* normally transmits the superior epigastric artery. It is also referred to as the *foramen of Morgagni* or *space of Larrey*. A hernia through this space on the left is uncommon because of the pericardial attachment.

2. **Acquired Hernias** — esophageal hiatal hernia is the most common of this type exceeding by far the frequency of traumatic hernias (Fig. 2). The anatomy at the esophageal hiatus is of great interest (a) in its relation to the cardiac valvular mechanism and, (b) to the fixation of the cardiac end of the stomach.

The esophageal hiatus is a gap between fibers of the right crus of the diaphragm (Fig. 4). When the fibers of the hiatal margin (*esophageal sling*) contract the action on the esophagus is twofold, first the walls of the esophagus are compressed, and second, the angulation of the lower esophagus is increased. It is believed that these actions are most important in maintaining the competence of the cardia (Figs. 5 and 6).

Although no intrinsic sphincter at the cardia can be demonstrated anatomically, many physiologic observations point to the presence of an intrinsic sphincter mechanism in the last 2 to 5 cm. of esophagus. When swallowing is not occurring, the "sphincter" is in a state of tonic contraction with its walls tightly opposed. Within 1.5 to 2.5 seconds after swallowing, the "sphincter" relaxes; this inhibition requiring intact vagi and Auerbach plexuses. After peristaltic contraction reaches this region, the sphincter closes and undergoes a strong, prolonged aftercontraction. This prevents regurgitation of food, gastric juice, and air. Excessive intragastric pressure, however, may overcome this resistance.

Another anatomic factor claimed by many as important in the fixation of the cardia is the peritoneal reflections. The peritoneum is reflected from the diaphragm to the abdominal esophagus and stomach on their anterior and lateral surfaces. Posteriorly, however, the reflection occurs lower so that a posterior bare area covered only by retroperitoneal fatty tissue is in continuity with that of the esophageal hiatus. Excessive accumulation of fat in this area may contribute to enlargement of the hiatus and predisposition of the hernia.

If the peritoneum may act as a "ligament" of the cardia, so may the connective tissue in the area. The fascia on the under surface of the diaphragm becomes continuous at the cardia with the fascia propria of the esophagus. This connective tissue layer is known as the *phreno-esophageal ligament*, a structure whose role in the pathogenesis and repair of hiatal hernia has received considerable attention (Fig. 7).

a. SLIDING HERNIA (Fig. 8) — this is the most common type of hiatal hernia. In this type of hernia the acute angle between the esophagus and stomach disappears and the cardia slides up into the mediastinum taking the elongated tissues of the phreno-esophageal ligament and peritoneum with it. The stomach hangs like a bell from the esophagus which, in roentgenograms, appears somewhat tortuous and redundant unless it has been shortened by chronic esophagitis. When shortening has occurred, the hernia is no longer reducible. Symptoms suggesting the presence of esophagitis should prompt surgical correction of the hernia before damage to the esophagus has become irreversible.

b. PARAESOPHAGEAL (ROLLING) HERNIA (Fig. 9) — this type of esophageal hernia resembles in many ways an indirect inguinal hernia. During development, a protrusion of the peritoneal sac may remain in the hiatus in some persons in much the same way as it may remain in the inguinal canal. Since, during development, the stomach rotates forward from the retroperitoneal space behind in the region of the cardia, the latter remains bare on its posterior surface and any peritoneal sac must protrude into the mediastinum anterior to the esophagus. For similar reasons, an inguinal sac must always be anterior to the spermatic cord. This "preformed" hernial pre-esophageal sac may remain empty during the lifetime of a person, or, at any age, a part of

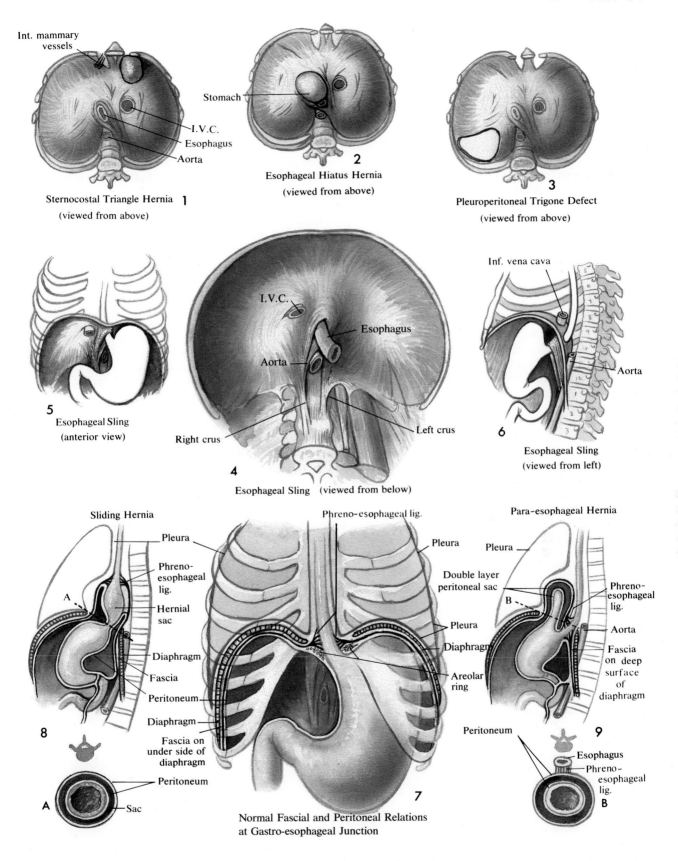

Sternocostal Triangle Hernia **1**
(viewed from above)

- Int. mammary vessels
- I.V.C.
- Esophagus
- Aorta

Esophageal Hiatus Hernia **2**
(viewed from above)

- Stomach

Pleuroperitoneal Trigone Defect **3**
(viewed from above)

5 Esophageal Sling
(anterior view)

4 Esophageal Sling (viewed from below)

- I.V.C.
- Esophagus
- Aorta
- Right crus
- Left crus

Esophageal Sling **6**
(viewed from left)

- Inf. vena cava
- Aorta

Sliding Hernia

- Pleura
- Phreno-esophageal lig.
- Hernial sac
- Diaphragm
- Fascia
- Peritoneum
- Diaphragm
- Fascia on under side of diaphragm
- Peritoneum
- Sac

8
A

Phreno-esophageal lig.

- Pleura
- Pleura
- Diaphragm
- Areolar ring

7
Normal Fascial and Peritoneal Relations at Gastro-esophageal Junction

Para-esophageal Hernia

- Pleura
- Double layer peritoneal sac
- Phreno-esophageal lig.
- Aorta
- Fascia on deep surface of diaphragm
- Peritoneum
- Esophagus
- Phreno-esophageal lig.

9
B

the anterior wall of the stomach may protrude into the hernial sac. Only the anterior wall of the stomach can find its way into the sàc by "*rolling*" upward. In extreme examples, the stomach may be found upside down within the herniated peritoneal sac. In spite of this displacement, the esophagus still enters the stomach at an acute angle and the cardia usually lies within the abdomen.

Page 129

LYMPHATICS OF THE THORAX:

The lymphatics of the thorax are divided into a superficial and deep set of vessels.

Superficial Lymphatic Vessels:

These vessels drain the ventral, lateral, and posterior chest walls and have no intermediate nodes. The vessels draining the lateral wall drain into the medial axillary (posterior pectoral) nodes and those draining the posterior wall empty into the posterior axillary (subscapular) nodes. Of great clinical significance are the vessels related to the ventral wall which are described on page 48.

Deep Lymphatic Vessels:

These vessels are interrupted by intermediate nodes and drain the inner wall of the thorax and the visceral structures of the thoracic cavity. The nodal groups may, therefore, be divided into *parietal* and *visceral* and consist of five sets of *paired* longitudinal chains in the right and left chest cavity (Fig. 1). The parietal nodes consisting of the internal mammary (sternal) and posterior intercostal chains lie anterior and posterior, respectively, in position on each side of the chest. The three longitudinal visceral chains are the anterior mediastinal, tracheobronchial, and posterior mediastinal. Both the anterior and posterior mediastinal chains extend upward into the anatomically designated superior mediastinum.

1. **Parietal Nodes:**

a. INTERNAL MAMMARY (STERNAL) CHAIN—has previously been described on page 48 in regard to its role in the lymphatic drainage of the breast. In addition, this chain receives vessels from the upper abdominal wall and diaphragm.

b. INTERCOSTAL CHAIN—consists of one or two nodes in each interspace near the rib head and receives vessels from the inner portion of the posterior chest wall and costal pleura. Efferent vessels from these nodes enter the thoracic duct either directly or indirectly by passing through the posterior mediastinal chain (Fig. 4).

2. **Visceral Nodes:**

a. ANTERIOR MEDIASTINAL NODES—are divided into a superior and inferior group.

(1) *Inferior (Diaphragmatic) Group* (Fig. 1)—consists of several small nodes lying on the upper surface of the diaphragm and are subdivided into anterior and lateral nodes. The *anterior nodes* lie in relation to the sternocostal triangle of the diaphragm; the *lateral nodes* are related to the phrenic nerve at the diaphragm. In addition to receiving afferents from the diaphragm and pleura, they receive lymph vessels draining the upper abdominal viscera. Their efferent vessel pathways are shown in Figure 4.

(2) *Superior Group*—is located in the superior mediastinum in relation to the great veins and aortic arch. This group is subdivided into three sets of nodes; a *right, left,* and *transverse* (Fig. 2).

The *right set* consists of a few nodes paralleling the course of the phrenic nerve in relation to the superior vena cava and right innominate veins. The *left set* lie in relation to the aortic arch. The lowest of the nodes is constant and located anterior to the ligmentum anteriosum *(node of the duct of Botalli);* the uppermost node lies in relation to the left common carotid artery. Connecting the right and left set are two or three nodes which constitute the *transverse set.* These nodes are related to the left innominate vein; one is fairly constant lying in the innominate angle, *the node of Bartels.* Their prevailing afferent and efferent communications are shown diagrammatically in Figure 4.

b. TRACHEOBRONCHIAL NODES—extend along the respiratory airway from the uppermost portion of the thoracic trachea to the pulmonary hilus (Fig. 3). A few nodes lie in relation to the segmental bronchi within the lung and are referred to as *pulmonary* nodes, and those related to the lobar bronchi as *bronchial* nodes. The afferent vessels from these nodes draining the lung and visceral pleura extend upward to the *tracheobronchial* nodes, of which there are two groups; the *lateral tracheobronchial* nodes lying at the tracheobronchial angle on either side and the *inferior tracheobronchial* (subcarinal) nodes which lie below the bifurcation of the trachea.

Finally, there are other nodes scattered along the trachea in superior mediastinum. These are the *tracheal* or *paratracheal* nodes. Efferent vessels from the tracheobronchial chain mainly join the anterior mediastinal nodes to form the *bronchomediastinal trunk* (Fig. 4).

c. POSTERIOR MEDIASTINAL CHAIN—consists of a few nodes located either in a para-esophageal or para-aortic position (Fig. 1). They receive lymph vessels from the esophagus and mediastinal tissue, and may receive some channels from the lower lobes of the lung. Their efferent vessels empty into the thoracic duct.

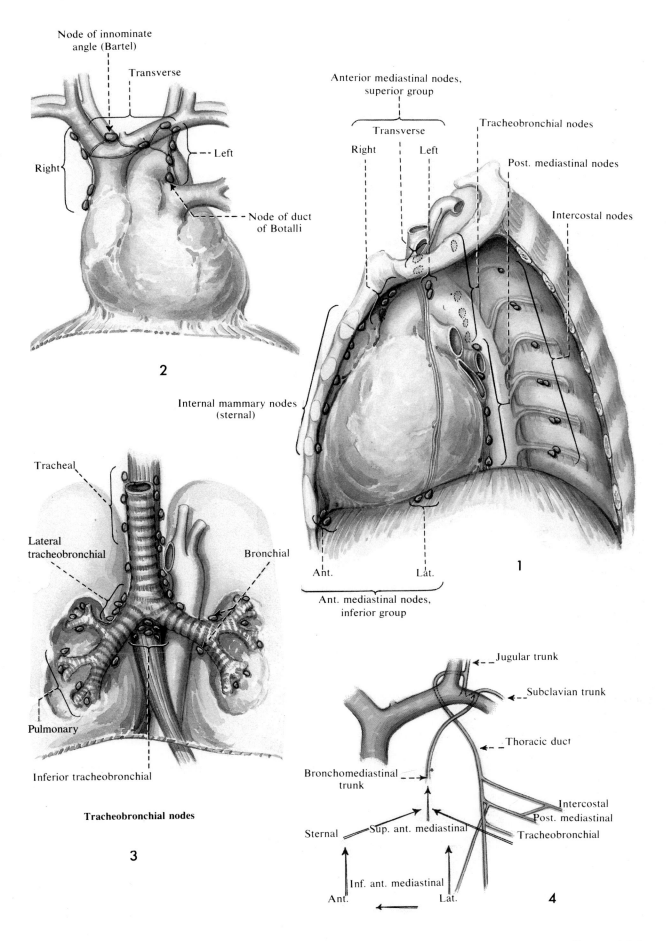

Node of innominate
angle (Bartel)

Transverse

Right

Left

Node of duct
of Botalli

2

Anterior mediastinal nodes,
superior group

Transverse

Right   Left

Tracheobronchial nodes

Post. mediastinal nodes

Intercostal nodes

Internal mammary nodes
(sternal)

Ant.   Lat.

1

Ant. mediastinal nodes,
inferior group

Tracheal

Lateral
tracheobronchial

Bronchial

Pulmonary

Inferior tracheobronchial

Tracheobronchial nodes

3

Jugular trunk

Subclavian trunk

Thoracic duct

Bronchomediastinal
trunk

Intercostal
Post. mediastinal
Tracheobronchial

Sternal   Sup. ant. mediastinal

Inf. ant. mediastinal

Ant.   Lat.

4

The Abdomen

VENTROLATERAL ABDOMINAL WALL:

The ventrolateral abdominal wall is an area bounded above by the xiphoid process of the sternum and the costal margin (cartilages of ribs 7 to 10), and posteriorly by the lateral border of the erector spinae muscle mass. Its lower boundary, from lateral to medial, is the crest of the ilium, the anterior superior iliac spine, the inguinal ligament, the pubic tubercle, and the superior ramus of the os pubis (Fig. 1).

1. **Topographic Lines** — for descriptive purposes certain topographic lines may be drawn on the abdominal wall in order to divide the wall into smaller descriptive areas. The simplest method is to draw a perpendicular and transverse line through the umbilicus and divide the abdominal wall into an *upper* and *lower quadrant* on either side of the midline (Fig. 1, dotted lines). A more elaborate system divides the abdominal wall into nine areas. This division is made by drawing two perpendicular lines on each side of the body bisecting the inguinal ligaments *(midinguinal lines)*. Two transverse lines are made; one at the level of the tenth costal cartilage *(subcostal line)* and the other between the tubercles of the iliac crest *(the intertubercular line)*. The three central areas thus defined are, from above: the *epigastrium*, the *umbilical area*, and the *hypogastrium*. The lateral areas on each side are designated as the *hypochondrium*, the *lumbar area*, and the *iliac area* (Fig. 1).

2. **Landmarks** (Figs. 2 and 3) — several natural topographic landmarks are present on the abdominal wall, the most important of which are:

a. LINEA ALBA — is a linear furrow in the midline extending from the xiphoid to the symphysis. This line marks the medial border of the rectus abdominis muscles. It is more marked in the supraumbilical area.

b. LINEA SEMILUNARIS — is a muscular impression on the abdominal wall along the lateral border of the rectus abdominis.

c. LINEAE TRANSVERSAE — are located at the level of the tendinous inscriptions of the rectus abdominis muscles. They are located at the level of the xiphoid, at the umbilicus, and midway between the latter two structures. Rarely is there an inscription below the umbilicus. This fact explains the greater retraction of the severed ends of the rectus in transverse incisions below the umbilicus.

3. **Contour** — the contour of the abdomen is normally flat from above downward and evenly rounded from side to side in the adolescent and muscular adult. In wasting diseases, however, the abdomen becomes depressed or scaphoid in shape. Protuberance of the abdominal wall, which is normal in the infant, is much more common in the adult due to either *fat, fetus, feces, flatus,* or *fluid*.

4. **Superficial Fascia** — the superficial fascia of the abdominal wall is continuous with that of the thorax;

however, below the umbilicus this layer splits into a superficial and deep layer. The superficial fatty layer is termed *Camper's fascia* and continues as the superficial fascia of the thigh. The deep layer is referred to as *Scarpa's fascia*. This layer extends into the thigh and inserts into the fascia lata one finger's breadth below the inguinal ligament (Fig. 3). Medial to the pubic tubercle, Camper's and Scarpa's fasciae fuse and extend into the penis as the *penile fascia*. This same fused layer extends into the scrotum as the *dartos fascia* and into the perineum where it is termed *Colles' fascia* (Fig. 3).

a. NERVE SUPPLY — of the ventrolateral abdominal wall is by the cutaneous rami of the lower six thoracic and the first lumbar nerves. The major trunks of these nerves traverse the abdominal wall between the internal oblique and transverse abdominis muscles; their anterior cutaneous rami pierce the rectus sheath and supply the skin of the anterior abdomen. The anterior cutaneous ramus of T_{10} innervates the skin at the level of the umbilicus, T_7, T_8, and T_9 supply the supra-umbilical area, and T_{11}, T_{12} and L_1 supply the infra-umbilical area (Fig. 2).

Lateral cutaneous rami are also given off from these nerve trunks to supply the lateral abdominal wall. The lateral cutaneous rami of T_7, T_8, and T_9 also supply a portion of the thoracic wall, and the lateral rami of T_{12} and L_1 extend into the gluteal region.

b. ARTERIAL SUPPLY — of the subcutaneous tissue of the supra-umbilical portion of the abdominal wall is mainly by the internal mammary artery via twigs from its terminal branches, the *superior epigastric* and *musculophrenic arteries*. The *lower intercostal* arteries also supply this part. The infra-umbilical portion is supplied by three small branches of the femoral artery: the *superficial epigastric, superficial circumflex iliac,* and *superficial external pudendal* (Fig. 2).

c. VENOUS DRAINAGE — like the arterial supply, may be divided into supra- and infra-umbilical pathways. The infra-umbilical area is drained by veins which accompany the three above-mentioned arteries. These veins are given the same name as their corresponding arteries and drain into the *great saphenous vein* (Fig. 2). The veins above the umbilicus are tributaries of the internal mammary, intercostal, and lateral thoracic veins and drain, therefore, indirectly into the superior caval system. A communicating channel connects the supra- and infra-umbilical vessels (the *thoraco-epigastric vein*) and forms an important collateral channel between the inferior and superior caval systems. This is particularly important in obstruction of the abdominal vena cava. In the region of the umbilicus, there is also an anastomosis with the portal system via the para-umbilical vein.

d. LYMPHATIC DRAINAGE — of the anterior abdominal wall above the umbilicus is into the *axillary nodes;* whereas below the umbilicus the lymph channels terminate in the *subinguinal nodes* of the thigh. There is also lymphatic connections between those of the anterior abdominal wall and intra-abdominal lymph channels in the region of the umbilicus (Fig. 3).

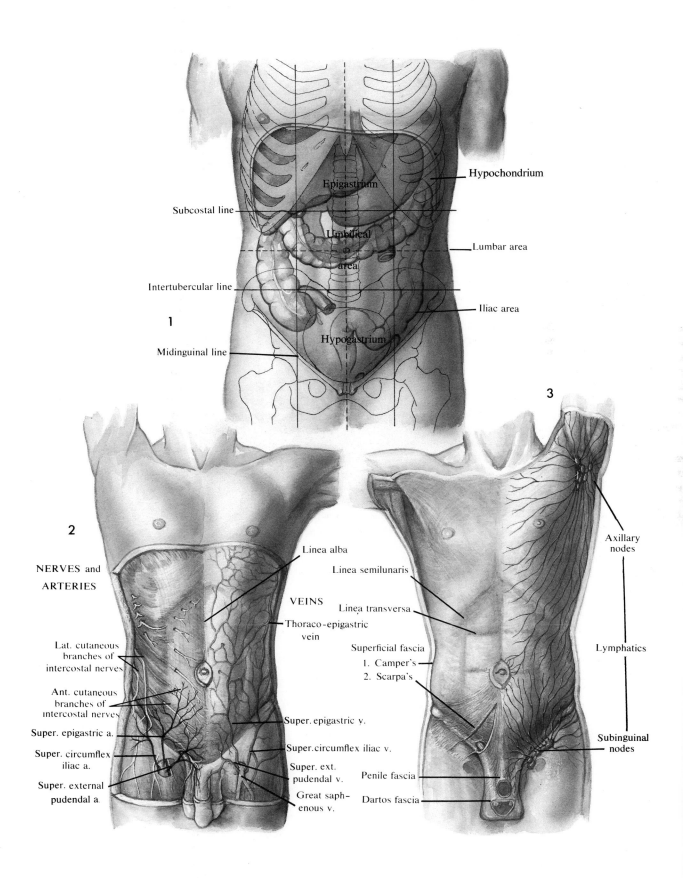

Subcostal line

Epigastrium

Hypochondrium

Umbilical area

Lumbar area

Intertubercular line

Iliac area

Hypogastrium

Midinguinal line

1

2

NERVES and
ARTERIES

Lat. cutaneous
branches of
intercostal nerves

Ant. cutaneous
branches of
intercostal nerves

Super. epigastric a.

Super. circumflex
iliac a.

Super. external
pudendal a.

Linea alba

VEINS

Thoraco-epigastric
vein

Super. epigastric v.

Super. circumflex iliac v.

Super. ext.
pudendal v.

Great saph-
enous v.

3

Linea semilunaris

Linea transversa

Superficial fascia
1. Camper's
2. Scarpa's

Penile fascia

Dartos fascia

Axillary
nodes

Lymphatics

Subinguinal
nodes

5. **Deep Fascia and Muscles** – the flat muscles of the abdominal wall are derived from the same embryonic muscle sheets as are the intercostal muscles of the thorax (page 86). Because of this common origin, their innervation is similar, i.e., intercostal nerves. Likewise, three muscle layers are present on the abdominal wall, each covered by its own layer of deep fascia. In addition, vertically directed muscles are present on either side of the midline incorporated by a special deep fascial sheath.

a. FASCIA OF THE EXTERNAL OBLIQUE – is a deep fascial layer which is thickened in the region of the symphysis pubis to form the *suspensory ligament of the penis*. As the testis descends through the abdominal wall (see page 138) it carries a part of this fascial layer into the scrotum where it is termed the *external spermatic fascia*.

b. EXTERNAL OBLIQUE MUSCLE (Fig. 1) – has a broad origin from the lower eight ribs and its fibers fan out in a downward and forward direction. The posterior fibers descend in an almost vertical direction and attach to the external lip of the iliac crest. The anteriormost fibers extend medially passing in front of the rectus to insert in a median raphe, the *linea alba*. The intermediate fibers are more complex in the areas of insertion and will be considered in the discussion of the inguinal region (page 136).

c. FASCIA OF THE INTERNAL OBLIQUE – lies in the internal between the exterior and interior oblique muscles. In this fascial plane two branches of the lumbar plexus may be identified: the *iliohypogastric* and *ilioinguinal* nerves (Fig. 1, p. 137). The former supplies the hypogastric region and the skin around the symphysis pubis. The ilioinguinal nerve becomes superficial through the subcutaneous inguinal ring and is distributed to the upper inner thigh and scrotum (or labia). This fascial layer is carried into the scrotum by the descent of the testis and forms the *middle spermatic fascia*.

d. INTERNAL OBLIQUE MUSCLE FIBERS (Figs. 1 and 2) – arise from below and are directed upward and forward. Posterior fibers arise from the lumbodorsal fascia, the intermediate fibers from the intermediate lip of the iliac crest, and the anterior fibers from the lateral one-half of the inguinal ligament. The posterior fibers insert in the lower four ribs, whereas the intermediate fibers terminate in the linea alba. In the upper two-thirds of the abdominal wall the fibers inserting into the linea alba split around the rectus muscle, whereas in the lower one-third all the aponeurotic fibers of the internal oblique pass in front of the rectus (Figs. 2 to 5). The insertion of the fibers arising from the inguinal ligament is discussed on page 136.

e. FASCIA OF TRANSVERSE ABDOMINIS – is practically nonexistent in the inguinal region. In the upper two-thirds of the abdominal wall, one finds in this plane the segmental nerves T_7 to T_{12} which extend medially to enter the rectus sheath (Fig. 2). In the lower abdomen in this plane runs the *deep circumflex iliac* branch of the external iliac artery (Fig. 2, p. 137).

f. TRANSVERSE ABDOMINIS MUSCLE (Fig. 2) – arises from the same sites as both the external and internal oblique muscles; specifically, the lower six costal cartilages, the lumbodorsal fascia, the internal lip of the iliac crest, and the lateral one-fourth of the inguinal ligament. The greater part of its fibers insert into the linea alba; those of the upper two-thirds of the abdomen pass behind and those of the lower one-third in front of the rectus abdominis (Figs. 2 to 5). Its inguinal fiber insertion will be considered on page 136.

g. RECTUS ABDOMINIS MUSCLE FIBERS – have their origin from the costal cartilages of T_5 to T_7 and the xiphoid process, and descend vertically on each side of the midline to insert on the pubic crest. The fibers are interrupted by three transverse tendinous bonds: one at the level of the umbilicus, one at the level of the xiphoid (T_7), and the third between the other two (Fig. 2). Occasionally, a fourth may be present below the umbilicus.

h. PYRAMIDALIS MUSCLE – is a rudimentary structure located in front of the lower portion of the rectus arising from the superior pubic ramus and inserting into the linea alba (Fig. 2).

i. RECTUS SHEATH (Figs. 3 to 5) – envelops the rectus and pyramidalis muscles and consists, therefore, of an anterior and posterior lamella which differ in composition on the upper two-thirds and lower one-third of the abdominal wall.

(1) *Anterior Lamella* – in the upper two-thirds of the sheath, is made up of the aponeurosis of the external oblique and the anterior leaf of the internal oblique (Figs. 3, 4, and 5). In the lower one-third of the abdomen all the aponeurotic layers of the flat muscles pass anterior to the rectus.

(2) *Posterior Lamella* – is made up of the posterior leaf of the internal oblique and transverse abdominis muscles and transversalis fascia in the upper abdomen, whereas only the transversalis fascia is present in the lower abdomen. The point of transition of the internal oblique and transverse abdominis muscles to an anterior position is marked on the posterior lamella as the *linea semicircularis* or *line of Douglas* (Fig. 2). It is at this point that the inferior epigastric artery enters the rectus sheath, and an internal hernia (Spigelian) may present itself at the line of transition.

(3) *Contents* – in addition to the rectus and pyramidalis muscles, the sheath contains the superior and inferior epigastric vessels and the termination of nerves T_7 to T_{12} (Fig. 2).

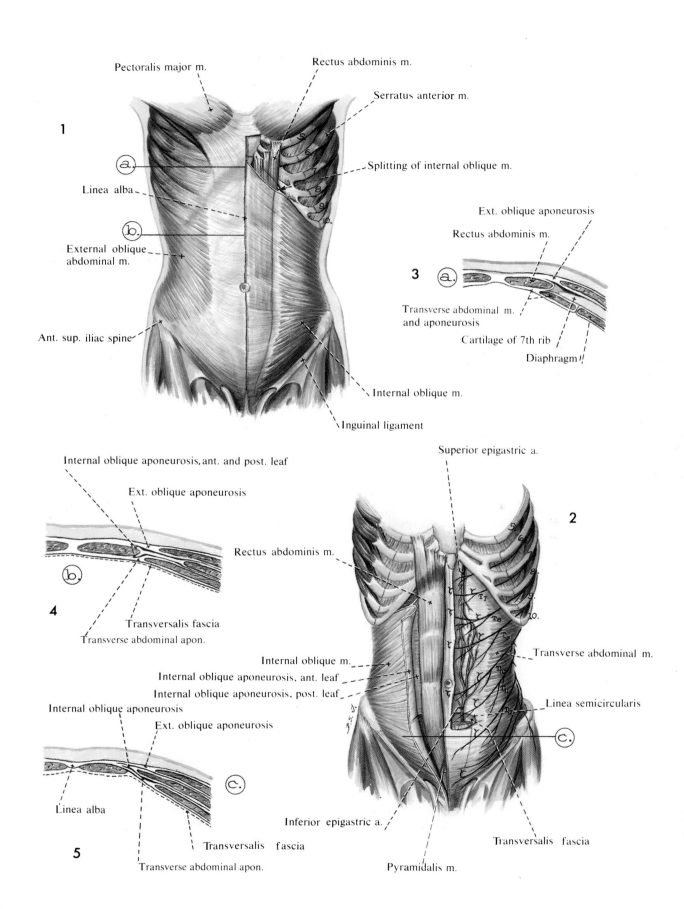

1

Pectoralis major m.

Rectus abdominis m.

Serratus anterior m.

Splitting of internal oblique m.

ⓐ

Linea alba

ⓑ

External oblique abdominal m.

Ant. sup. iliac spine

Internal oblique m.

Inguinal ligament

3 ⓐ

Ext. oblique aponeurosis

Rectus abdominis m.

Transverse abdominal m. and aponeurosis

Cartilage of 7th rib

Diaphragm

Internal oblique aponeurosis, ant. and post. leaf

Ext. oblique aponeurosis

Rectus abdominis m.

ⓑ

4

Transversalis fascia

Transverse abdominal apon.

Superior epigastric a.

2

Internal oblique aponeurosis

Ext. oblique aponeurosis

ⓒ

Internal oblique m.

Internal oblique aponeurosis, ant. leaf

Internal oblique aponeurosis, post. leaf

Transverse abdominal m.

Linea semicircularis

ⓒ

Linea alba

Transversalis fascia

5

Transverse abdominal apon.

Inferior epigastric a.

Pyramidalis m.

Transversalis fascia

j. ENDO-ABDOMINAL FASCIA—is a continuous fascial lining of the entire abdominal cavity much as the endothoracic and endopelvic fasciae line their respective cavities. Where this fascial layer lies in relation to certain muscles of the abdominal wall it is given a specific name: for example, where it covers the psoas muscles, *psoas fascia*, and quadratus lumborum muscle, *quadratus fascia*; on the ventrolateral abdominal wall where it lies deep to the transverse abdominis muscle, it is termed the *transversalis fascia* (Fig. 2). It helps form the posterior lamella of the rectus sheath and in the inguinal region has certain thickenings which will be considered below. The transversalis fascia, like other fascial layers of the abdominal wall is drawn into the scrotum by the descent of the testis to form the *internal spermatic fascia*.

6. **Extraperitoneal Fatty Tissue** (Fig. 3)—this abdominal wall layer lies deep to the transversalis fascia and contains five important structures related to the lower abdominal wall.

a. INFERIOR EPIGASTRIC VESSELS—artery and vein on either side, arise from the external iliac artery and drain into the external iliac vein just above the inguinal ligament. The vessels enter the rectus sheath at the level of the linea semicircularis.

b. OBLITERATED UMBILICAL ARTERIES—arise from the internal iliac artery and extend toward the umbilicus from either side. The proximal pelvic portions of these fetal vessels remain patent as the *superior vesical arteries*.

c. URACHUS—is a midline fibrous cord which extends from the apex of the bladder to the umbilicus. This represents the remains of the embryonic allantoic stalk.

7. **Peritoneum**—the parietal layer of peritoneum is the deepest layer of the abdominal wall and is thrown into folds over structures laying in the extraperitoneal fatty layer. In the upper abdomen, a fold of peritoneum over the obliterated left umbilical vein forms the *falciform ligament* and *ligamentum teres hepatis*. In the infra-umbilical area a fold of peritoneum over the urachus is termed the *medial umbilical plica*. The fold over the underlying obliterated umbilical arteries forms the *lateral umbilicus plicae* and the fold over the inferior epigastric arteries, the *plicae epigastrica* (Fig. 3). Between these peritoneal folds are recesses called fovea. The fovea between the medial and lateral umbilical plicae is the *supravesical fovea* (Fig. 3-1), between the lateral umbilical plica and the plica epigastrica is the *medial inguinal fovea* (Fig. 3-2), and lateral to the plica epigastrica is the *lateral inguinal fovea* (Fig. 3-3).

8. **Inguinal Region**—the complex insertion of the flat muscles of the abdominal wall into the pubis will be considered here.

a. EXTERNAL OBLIQUE APONEUROSIS—intermediate fibers fold inward upon themselves between the anterior superior iliac spine and the pubic tubercle to form the *inguinal (Poupart's) ligament*. The more anterior fibers split, some fibers inserting in the pubic tubercle and others in the front of the symphysis pubis. Those fibers inserting in the tubercle form the *inferior (lateral, external) crus* while those fibers inserting in front of the symphysis form the *superior (medial, internal) crus*. Some aponeurotic fibers extend between the crura and are termed the *intracrural fibers* (Fig. 1).

(1) *Lacunar (Gimbernat's, Triangular) Ligament*—is formed by fibers of the inferior crus which pass backward and medially to attach to the pecten ossis pubis of the *same* side.

(2) *Reflexed (Colles') Ligament*—is formed by fibers of the superior crus which cross the midline to attach to the tubercle and pecten ossis pubis of the *opposite* side.

b. INTERNAL OBLIQUE FIBERS—arising from the lateral half of the inguinal ligament arch forward and insert in the front of the os pubis between the tubercle and symphysis. These arching fibers are termed the *falx inguinalis* (Fig. 1).

c. TRANSVERSE ABDOMINIS FIBERS—arising from the inguinal ligament likewise arch forward to insert in the os pubis. Some of the arching fibers join those of the internal oblique to form the *conjoined tendon* (Fig. 2). Some muscle fibers of the internal oblique and transverse abdominis are pulled into the scrotum as the testis descends to form the *cremasteric muscle* of the spermatic cord. A few isolated transverse abdominal arching muscle fibers attach to the inguinal ligament just medial to the epigastric vessels as the *interfoveolar muscle*.

d. TRANSVERSALIS FASCIA (Figs. 2 and 3)—presents certain thickenings which according to various investigators may lend strength to the posterior wall of the inguinal canal. They include:

(1) *Interfoveolar (Hesselbach's) Ligament*—is a vertical thickening of the transversalis fascia which extends from the level of the arching fibers of the transverse abdominis muscle and inserts into the superior ramus of the pubis just medial to the epigastric vessels in relation to the above-mentioned interfoveolar muscle.

(2) *Henle's Ligament*—is described both as a thickening of the transversalis fascia and a lateral expansion of the rectus sheath. It extends vertically along the lower lateral border of the rectus to attach to the pubis behind the conjoined tendon (Fig. 3-4).

(3) *Iliopubic Tract*—is a thickened transverse band extending from the anterior superior iliac spine to the pubic tubercle.

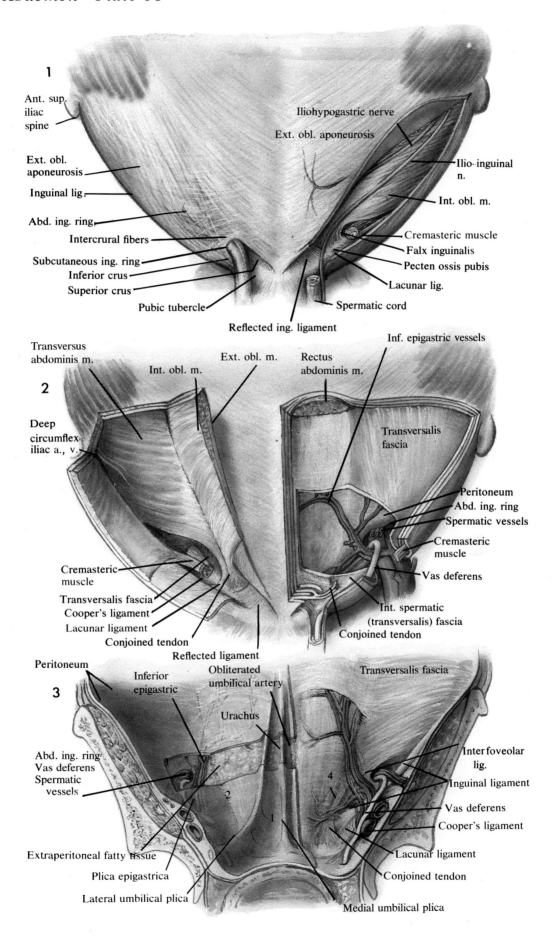

1

Ant. sup. iliac spine

Ext. obl. aponeurosis

Inguinal lig.

Abd. ing. ring

Intercrural fibers

Subcutaneous ing. ring

Inferior crus

Superior crus

Pubic tubercle

Iliohypogastric nerve

Ext. obl. aponeurosis

Ilio-inguinal n.

Int. obl. m.

Cremasteric muscle

Falx inguinalis

Pecten ossis pubis

Lacunar lig.

Spermatic cord

Reflected ing. ligament

2

Transversus abdominis m.

Int. obl. m.

Ext. obl. m.

Rectus abdominis m.

Inf. epigastric vessels

Deep circumflex iliac a., v.

Transversalis fascia

Peritoneum

Abd. ing. ring

Spermatic vessels

Cremasteric muscle

Vas deferens

Cremasteric muscle

Transversalis fascia

Cooper's ligament

Lacunar ligament

Conjoined tendon

Int. spermatic (transversalis) fascia

Conjoined tendon

Reflected ligament

3

Peritoneum

Inferior epigastric

Obliterated umbilical artery

Urachus

Transversalis fascia

Abd. ing. ring

Vas deferens

Spermatic vessels

Interfoveolar lig.

Inguinal ligament

Vas deferens

Cooper's ligament

Lacunar ligament

Conjoined tendon

Extraperitoneal fatty tissue

Plica epigastrica

Lateral umbilical plica

Medial umbilical plica

9. **Descent of the Testis**—the mechanism of descent of the testis is not clearly understood; it descends from its embryonic retroperitoneal abdominal position to its adult scrotal position, passing through the abdominal wall of either side and bringing with it layers of abdominal wall as well as its blood and nerve supply and ductal connections. That portion of the abdominal wall through which it descends is designated as the inguinal canal in the adult. The layers of the wall drawn down to form the scrotum and spermatic cord are outlined below (Figs. 1 to 4).

Key to Figure 4

Abdominal Wall Layers	Scrotum Layers
1. Skin	1. Skin
2. Superficial fascia (Camper's and Scarpa's)	2. Dartos fascia and muscle
3. Fascia of external oblique	3. External spermatic fascia
4. External oblique	4. (Testis passes between crura)
5. Fascia of internal oblique	5. Middle spermatic fascia
6. Internal oblique	6. ⎫
7. Transverse abdominis	7. ⎬ Cremasteric muscle
8. Transversalis fascia	8. Internal spermatic fascia
9. Extraperitoneal fat	9. Extraperitoneal fat
10. Peritoneum	10. Tunica vaginalis testis

A.R. = abdominal inguinal ring	*P.V.* = processus vaginalis (funicular portion)
S.R. = subcutaneous inguinal ring	*V.* = vas deferens
	E. = epididymis

10. **Inguinal Canal**—the inguinal canal represents the passage of the testis and spermatic cord (or round ligament of uterus) through the lower abdominal wall. One can describe an anterior and posterior wall, a roof, and a floor, as well as an abdominal and subcutaneous ring. It is a slit in the ventro-abdominal wall approximately 1½ inches in length which passes downward and forward and lies parallel to and immediately above the inguinal ligament. In the living, it is not truly a canal because the anterior and posterior walls are in apposition because of intra-abdominal pressure, and it is occupied by the spermatic cord.

a. Subcutaneous (superficial) inguinal ring— lies just above and medial to the pubic tubercle. It is actually bounded by the superior and inferior crura of the external oblique aponeurosis (Fig. 1, page 137).

b. Abdominal (deep) inguinal ring—is topographically located ½ inch above the midinguinal point and is bounded below by the inguinal ligament, medially by the inferior epigastric vessels (interfoveolar ligament), and laterally and above by the arching fibers of the transverse abdominis muscles (Fig. 2, page 137).

c. Anterior wall—is formed by the aponeurosis of the external oblique and the medial inguinal fibers of the internal oblique (Fig. 1, page 137).

d. Floor—is made up of the inguinal ligament laterally and the lacunar ligament medially (Fig. 1, page 137).

e. Roof—comprises the arching fibers of the transverse abdominis and internal oblique muscles (Figs. 1 and 2, page 137).

f. Posterior wall—is formed mainly by the transversalis fascia, but medially the conjoined tendon and reflexed ligaments reinforce the wall (Figs. 2 and 3, page 137).

11. **Spermatic Cord** (Figs. 5 and 6)—this structure is made up of vessels, nerves, and lymphatics supplying the testis. Since the testis developed in the lumbar area, the origin or termination of these structures will be in the same area. The testis is connected to the genital system through the vas deferens; hence its vascular and nerve supply will be related to the pelvic cavity. In essence, the spermatic cord comprises the following:

a. Fascia (three layers)—consists of the *external* (from external oblique fascia), the *middle* (from internal oblique fascia) and the *internal spermatic fascia* (from transversalis fascia). Incorporated with the middle layer are fibers of the *cremasteric muscle* derived from internal oblique and transverse abdominis muscle.

b. Arteries (three)—are the *internal spermatic (testicular)* from the aorta supplying the testis, the *external spermatic (cremasteric)* from the inferior epigastric supplying the covering of the cord, and the *artery of the vas* from the internal iliac which supplies the vas deferens.

c. Nerves (three)—consist of the *genitofemoral* from the lumbar plexus whose genital branch supplies the cremasteric muscle. In addition, the *ilioinguinal nerve* traverses the cord, exits through the subcutaneous inguinal ring, and supplies the skin of the scrotum. *Sympathetic fibers* to the vas arise from the hypogastric plexus while those to the testis arise in the aortic plexus.

d. Veins (three)—the *internal spermatic veins,* draining the testis, form a plexus in the cord, the *pampiniform plexus*. These veins finally merge into a single trunk which drains into the inferior vena cava on the right and the renal vein on the left. The *deferential vein* which drains the vas empties into the pelvic plexus, whereas the *external spermatic veins,* draining the covering of the cord, empty into the inferior epigastric veins.

e. Lymphatics—of the testicle terminate in the lumbar nodes while those of the vas drain into the external iliac nodes.

f. Vas (ductus) deferens—extends from the ductus epididymis through the spermatic cord and at the abdominal inguinal ring leaves the other constituents of the cord, loops over the inferior epigastric artery and passes into the pelvis along its lateral wall.

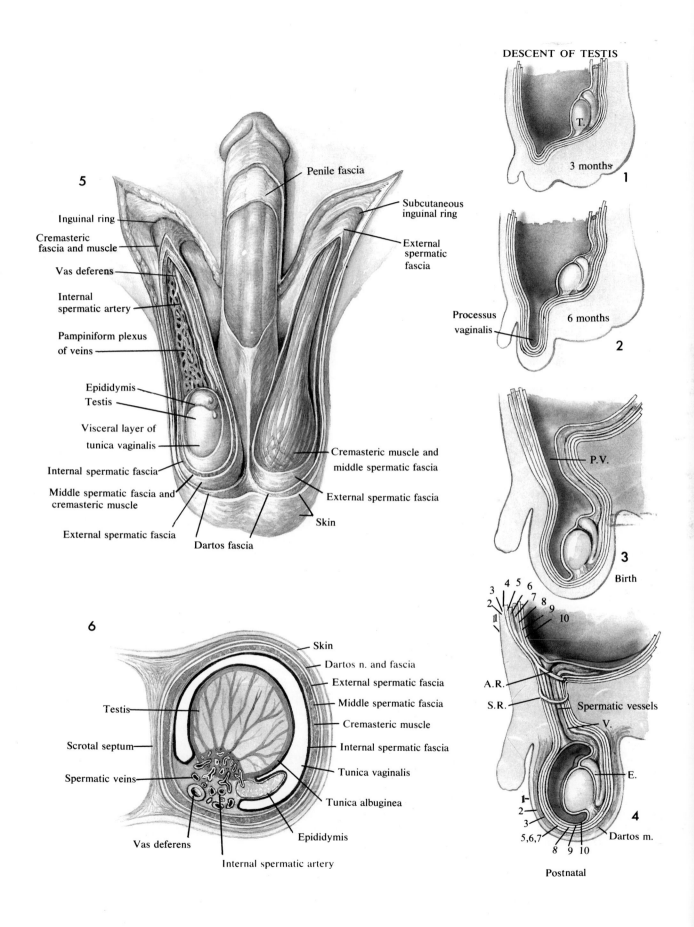

DESCENT OF TESTIS

T.

3 months

1

Processus vaginalis

6 months

2

P.V.

3

Birth

3 4 5 6
2 7 8 9
1 10

A.R.

S.R.

Spermatic vessels

V.

E.

1
2
3
5,6,7
8 9 10

Dartos m.

4

Postnatal

5

Penile fascia

Subcutaneous inguinal ring

External spermatic fascia

Inguinal ring

Cremasteric fascia and muscle

Vas deferens

Internal spermatic artery

Pampiniform plexus of veins

Epididymis

Testis

Visceral layer of tunica vaginalis

Internal spermatic fascia

Middle spermatic fascia and cremasteric muscle

External spermatic fascia

Dartos fascia

Skin

External spermatic fascia

Cremasteric muscle and middle spermatic fascia

6

Skin

Dartos n. and fascia

External spermatic fascia

Middle spermatic fascia

Cremasteric muscle

Internal spermatic fascia

Tunica vaginalis

Tunica albuginea

Epididymis

Testis

Scrotal septum

Spermatic veins

Vas deferens

Internal spermatic artery

CLINICAL ANATOMY OF INGUINAL HERNIA:

Halsted in 1892 said, "There is perhaps no operation which has had so much of vital interest to both physician and surgeon as herniotomy and there is no operation which, by the profession at large, would be more appreciated than a perfectly safe and sure cure for rupture." The ideal of a "perfectly safe" procedure has been nearly attained; that of a "sure cure" escapes us yet. However, our present-day success in inguinal hernia repairs rewards the effort of the surgeon and the confidence of the patient much more often than when Halsted's words were written.

The resourcefulness which will enable the surgeon to meet the demands of each operation can come only from an accurate knowledge of the anatomy of the inguinal region. Armed with a clear knowledge of the structure of the inguinal area and the fundamental needs for correction of the abnormality presented by hernia, the modern surgeon can achieve a high degree of success measured in terms of safety and permanency. Even though the operative procedures we have today are neither perfectly safe nor sure of cure, they are remarkably safe and effective when correctly used.

Inguinal hernias are classified as *indirect* or *direct,* based upon the relation of the neck of the sac to the deep inferior epigastric vessels.

1. **Indirect (Oblique)**—the neck of the hernia sac is at the deep (abdominal) ring, lateral to the deep inferior epigastric vessels. It is most common in young individuals in whom two main varieties are found:

a. CONGENITAL—is a form due to the persistence of the processus vaginalis and failure of the funicular portion to obliterate (Fig. 3, page 139).

b. INFANTILE (FUNICULAR)—type results when the tunica vaginalis testis forms normally, but the processus vaginalis persists in the inguinal canal.

The herniated sac in indirect hernias at the subcutaneous (superficial) inguinal ring has the following covers: (1) skin and subcutaneous tissue, (2) external spermatic fascia, (3) cremasteric muscle and middle spermatic fascia, and (4) internal spermatic (transversalis) fascia.

Surgical correction of an indirect hernia may be approached by an oblique inguinal incision (Fig. 1). The anterior wall of the inguinal canal is opened by incising the external oblique aponeurosis. The cord is then elevated from its bed and an incision through the cremasteric and internal spermatic fascia exposes the peritoneal sac of the indirect hernia in the cord (Fig. 2). The sac is excised after its intestinal contents is reduced and the neck of the sac is closed at the abdominal inguinal ring. Sutures are placed to close the cremasteric fascia, followed by the placement of sutures to bring the lower margin of the conjoined tendon and the internal oblique muscle to the shelving edge of the inguinal ligament (Fig. 3).

2. **Direct**—the neck of this hernial sac lies medial to the deep inferior epigastric vessels in the inguinal (Hesselbach's) triangle. This type of hernia is almost always acquired and although it does not traverse the inguinal canal, it does present through the subcutaneous inguinal ring. Its coverings are: (1) skin and subcutaneous tissue, (2) external spermatic fascia, and (3) internal spermatic (transversalis fascia).

3. **Inguinal (Hesselbach's) Triangle**—this triangle, the site of direct inguinal hernia, is bounded laterally by the deep inferior epigastric vessels, medially by the lateral border of the rectus abdominis muscle, and inferiorly by the inguinal ligament (Fig. 3, page 137). The triangle lies just posterior to the subcutaneous inguinal ring and marks the area of the posterior wall of the inguinal canal formed only by the transversalis fascia. This obviously weak area is a frequent site of hernia in the adult. In order to repair surgically a direct hernia, an incision similar to that used in indirect hernia repair is used (Fig. 1). The direct hernia presents itself as a bulge through the posterior wall of the inguinal canal medial to the inferior epigastric vessels in Hesselbach's triangle (Fig. 4). An incision is made through the transversalis fascia to expose the hernia sac which is reduced and maintained in position by plication sutures placed in the transversalis fascia. The conjoined tendon is then sutured to the shelving edge of the inguinal ligament behind the cord. Additional sutures may be placed lateral to the deep abdominal ring to strengthen the posterior wall (Fig. 5).

4. **Dangers and Safeguards in Inguinal Herniorrhaphy**—attention should be especially directed to the avoidance of injury to the following structures during the course of operation for inguinal hernia: the iliohypogastric and ilioinguinal nerves; the structures in the spermatic cord (vas deferens, internal spermatic artery, spermatic veins); the bowel if it lies in the hernial sac; the deep inferior epigastric vessels; the external iliac vessels; and the urinary bladder.

The nerves may be readily identified and protected. The iliohypogastric nerve lies beneath the aponeurosis of the external abdominal oblique and passes through it into the subcutaneous fat a centimeter above the subcutaneous ring. The ilioinguinal nerve lies along the anterior surface of the spermatic cord in the canal and exits at the external ring. The vas deferens lies posteriorly in the spermatic cord and is in contact with the posterior wall of an indirect sac. Because it is so small in infants and young boys, it is not only easily injured but, if injured, it is almost impossible to repair.

Injuries to the external iliac artery and vein and to the deep inferior epigastric vessels are uncommon, but the relation of the deep (abdominal) ring to these vessels makes them liable to injury by a stitch that is too deeply placed either medial or inferior to the ring. Should such an injury occur, it must be recognized and repaired promptly. The deep inferior epigastric vessels may be ligated without adverse effects, but serious extraperitoneal bleeding may be the result of an unrecognized tear of the vessels. While ligation of the deep inferior epigastric vessel will have no adverse effect, injury to the external iliac artery is a threat to the life of the lower limb. Likewise, injury to the external iliac vein has serious, though rarely desperate, consequences and must be carefully avoided. It is particularly exposed to injury when sutures are being placed in Cooper's liga-

INDIRECT INGUINAL HERNIA

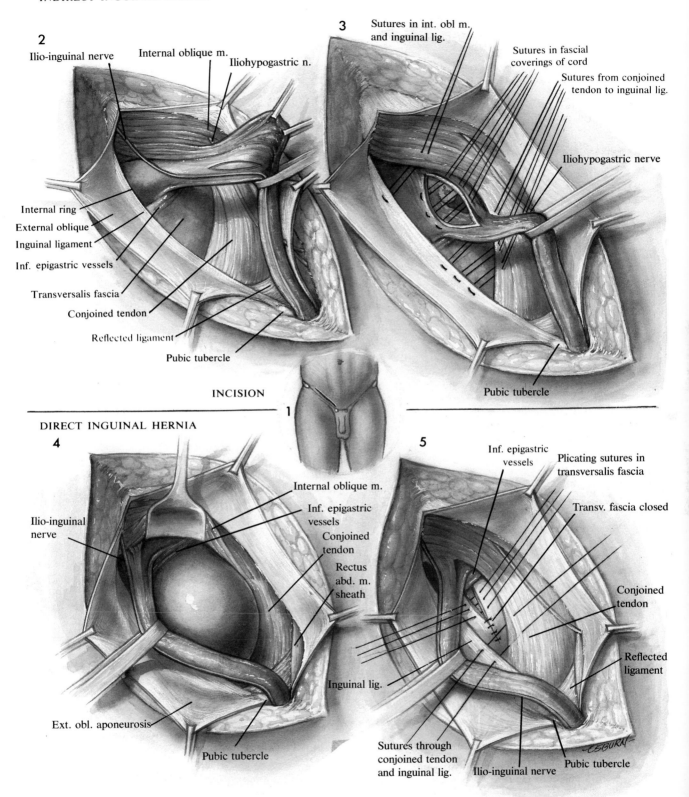

2

Ilio-inguinal nerve

Internal oblique m.

Iliohypogastric n.

3

Sutures in int. obl m. and inguinal lig.

Sutures in fascial coverings of cord

Sutures from conjoined tendon to inguinal lig.

Iliohypogastric nerve

Internal ring

External oblique

Inguinal ligament

Inf. epigastric vessels

Transversalis fascia

Conjoined tendon

Reflected ligament

Pubic tubercle

Pubic tubercle

INCISION

1

DIRECT INGUINAL HERNIA

4

Ilio-inguinal nerve

Internal oblique m.

Inf. epigastric vessels

Conjoined tendon

Rectus abd. m. sheath

5

Inf. epigastric vessels

Plicating sutures in transversalis fascia

Transv. fascia closed

Conjoined tendon

Reflected ligament

Inguinal lig.

Ext. obl. aponeurosis

Pubic tubercle

Sutures through conjoined tendon and inguinal lig.

Ilio-inguinal nerve

Pubic tubercle

ment during the repair of an inguinal or femoral hernia. Good exposure and consciousness of the danger will enable the surgeon to avoid this complication. In dissection within the cord, the pampiniform veins and the internal spermatic artery should be carefully handled so that the circulation of the testis is not impaired.

Two precautionary points should be made in procedures involving the hernial sac. In large direct hernias, the bladder may form a part of the medial wall of the sac and may be injured if the surgeon attempts to excise the sac; and in closing the neck of an indirect sac, the surgeon must avoid injury to the bowel.

5. **Sliding Hernia**—for all practical purposes a sliding hernia may be considered as a form of indirect inguinal hernia, although in rare instances it may occur as a direct hernia. This type of hernia usually involves the cecum on the right side or the sigmoid colon on the left. A peritoneal sac herniates through the abdominal inguinal ring bringing with it the *extraperitoneal* portion of the large bowel previously mentioned which is attached to the posterior wall of the herniated sac. The posterior wall of the sac is therefore formed by the visceral peritoneum covering the anterior and lateral surfaces of the herniated viscus.

The surgical anatomy may best be understood by comparing the sliding hernia with a congenital indirect hernia. In the latter, a loop of small bowel descends through the inguinal canal into the scrotum in a preformed peritoneal sac; it is completely surrounded by the parietal peritoneal sac as shown in Figure 1 on sagittal section and in Figure 1*A* on cross-section. In a sliding hernia, the peritoneal sac lies anterior in position as viewed on sagittal section and the bowel herniates in a retroperitoneal plane—usually a prolapse of the viscus (Figs. 2 and 2*B*).

Such an anatomic arrangement makes the technique of repair of a sliding hernia much more complex than the usual inguinal hernia for it particularly predisposes the blood supply of the involved segment of bowel to injury. There is no peritoneal layer behind the herniated bowel, but it is here that the vascular supply to this bowel segment is located. If dissection is carried out in the plane posterior to the herniated bowel on the surgeon's mistaken belief that he is cutting adhesions between the bowel and posterior wall of the sac, the blood vessels to the bowel may be injured, resulting in its devascularization.

Although the anatomy of sliding hernia described above is the prevailing pattern, it must be kept in mind that the peritoneal sac which lies anterior to the sliding hernia may also contain a herniated loop of small bowel, and on rare occasions the bowel prolapse may be completely extraperitoneal so that there is no accompanying peritoneal sac, in which case the bowel itself may be mistaken for a peritoneal sac and opened during repair.

A long-standing hernia is the most common predisposing factor in the formation of a sliding hernia. Since complete reduction of the contents, high ligation of the sac, and repair of the inguinal canal by the usual methods of inguinal herniorrhaphy are impossible in a sliding hernia, other methods must be employed. Suffice it to say that in the average case an extraperitoneal inguinal approach may be utilized as shown in Figure 3. In this illustration, the external oblique aponeurosis and peritoneal sac is opened, exposing the herniated cecum. The spermatic cord lies posterior to the cecum. Not infrequently a combined extraperitoneal inguinal and an intra-abdominal approach (La Roque) must be utilized to effect complete reduction. Whatever the method employed, the defect of the abdominal inguinal ring must be closed by the strongest possible means

since this type of inguinal hernia is associated with a higher incidence of recurrence than any other type.

6. **Inguinal-Femoral Region**—although the ligamentous attachments of the abdominal musculature to the pelvis at this junctional area has already been discussed on page 136 and will be discussed in part on page 284 in regard to femoral hernia, a résumé of these structures, so important to the surgeon, seems appropriate at this point.

a. Inguinal ligament (Figs. 4 and 5)—is formed as a thickening of the lower border of the external oblique aponeurosis which presents a rounded surface toward the thigh and a grooved surface toward the abdomen. It extends from the anterior superior iliac spine laterally to the pubic tubercle medially and forms in part the floor of the inguinal canal.

b. Lacunar ligament (Figs. 4 and 5)—is a triangular aponeurotic membrane which arises from the fibers of the inferior crus of the external oblique aponeurosis and gains an expanded insertion on the os pubis. Its apex is fixed to the pubic tubercle. The anterior edge is in continuity with the medial end of the inguinal ligament and its posterior edge is inserted into the pubic portion of the iliopectineal line (pecten ossis pubis). Its base is a free edge directed lateralward and forming the medial boundary of the femoral ring.

c. Pectineal ligament (Figs. 4 and 5)—extends parallel to the iliopectineal line from the free edge of the lacunar ligament to the iliopectineal eminence. Although it is a definitive anatomic structure, much controversy exists in regard to this ligament. It is regarded by some investigators as an extension of the aponeurotic fibers of the lacunar ligament, by others as a fascial thickening at the junction of the pectineal muscle fascia and iliopectineal ligament (see below), or as a thickening of periosteum along the iliopectineal line. It is of importance to the surgeon repairing large indirect and all direct inguinal hernias by the McVay procedure. In this repair the inferior margin of the transverse abdominis and internal oblique aponeurosis is sutured to the pectineal ligament rather than to the inguinal ligament. This same procedure is used for closure of the upper end of the femoral canal when a femoral hernia is repaired by an inguinal approach.

d. Iliopectineal ligament (Fig. 5)—is a fascial thickening extending between the inguinal ligament and the iliopectineal eminence. Although it is not utilized in inguinal herniorrhaphy, it does divide the subinguinal area into a medial vascular lacuna and a lateral muscular lacuna as discussed on page 276.

e. Iliopubic tract—is a thickening of the transversalis fascia extending from the anterior superior spine to the pubic tubercle. It is attached to, but is separate from, the more anterior inguinal ligament. In the intra-abdominal extraperitoneal approach for the repair of direct inguinal hernia, it has been designated as an important anatomic structure. However, the strength and significance of the iliopubic tract is disputed by many surgeons.

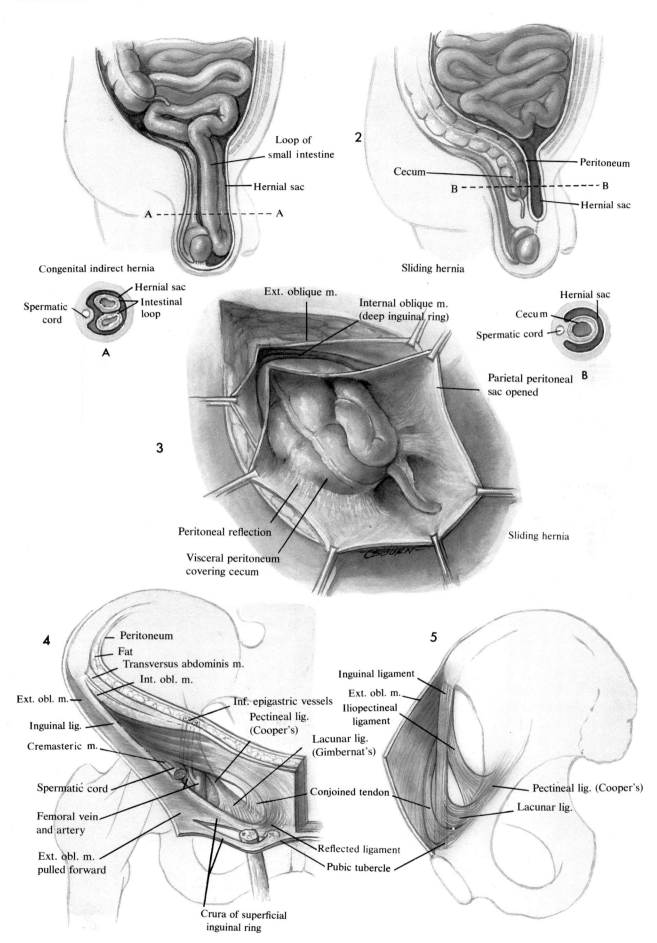

1

Loop of
small intestine

Hernial sac

A ---------- A

Congenital indirect hernia

Spermatic
cord

Hernial sac
Intestinal
loop

A

2

Cecum

Peritoneum

B ---------- B

Hernial sac

Sliding hernia

Hernial sac
Cecum

Spermatic cord

Parietal peritoneal
sac opened

B

3

Ext. oblique m.

Internal oblique m.
(deep inguinal ring)

Peritoneal reflection

Visceral peritoneum
covering cecum

Sliding hernia

4

Peritoneum
Fat
Transversus abdominis m.
Int. obl. m.

Ext. obl. m.

Inguinal lig.

Cremasteric m.

Spermatic cord

Femoral vein
and artery

Ext. obl. m.
pulled forward

Inf. epigastric vessels
Pectineal lig.
(Cooper's)
Lacunar lig.
(Gimbernat's)

Conjoined tendon

Reflected ligament
Pubic tubercle

Crura of superficial
inguinal ring

5

Inguinal ligament

Ext. obl. m.
Iliopectineal
ligament

Pectineal lig. (Cooper's)

Lacunar lig.

POSTEROLATERAL ABDOMINAL WALL:

The posterolateral abdominal wall is a quadrangular area bounded by the lower ribs above, the iliac crest below, the vertebral column medially, and a vertical line extending through the iliac tubercles laterally. A knowledge of the muscular relations in this area is important in surgical approaches to the retroperitoneal structures of the abdominal cavity, particularly the kidney.

1. **Superficial Fascia** — this fatty subcutaneous layer contains posterior cutaneous rami of the thoracic and lumbar nerves as well as small blood vessels and nerves, all of which are surgically insignificant.

2. **Deep Fascia** — the deep fascia of the low back is termed the *lumbodorsal fascia*. It arises from the spinous processes and splits around the erector spinae group of muscles, and then fuses at the lateral border of this same muscle mass. Two layers may therefore be distinguished: an *anterior* and *posterior layer* as related to the erector spinae (Fig. 1).

3. **Muscles** — the muscles of the posterolateral abdominal wall are arranged in three layers:

a. SUPERFICIAL LAYER — is made up of the *latissimus dorsi* and the external oblique muscles. The former arises in part from the bones of the pelvis and the posterior layer of lumbodorsal fascia. Its insertion is described on page 44. The external oblique is discussed on page 134. A triangular interval may exist between the anterior margin of the latissimus dorsi and posterior margin of the external oblique, the base being the iliac crest and the floor, the internal oblique. This muscular weakness in the abdominal wall is termed the *inferior lumbar (Petit's) triangle;* it may be the site of an abdominal hernia (Fig. 1).

b. MIDDLE LAYER — consists of the erector spinae, inferior posterior serratus, and internal oblique muscles (Fig. 1). The *erector spinae (sacrospinalis)* muscles are a part of the intrinsic (autochthonous) muscles of the back. In the lumbar region they are encased between the two layers of lumbodorsal fascia and are innervated by the *posterior* primary divisions of the spinal nerves. The *inferior posterior serratus* muscles arise from the posterior layer of lumbodorsal fascia and insert in the last four ribs. They are actually displaced fibers of the external oblique muscle. The posterior fibers of the *internal oblique* muscle arise from the lumbodorsal fascia on its fused area at the lateral border of the erec-

tor spinae. Its fibers have already been described on page 134. A *superior lumbar triangle (Grynfeltt)* is related to this muscle layer. It has as its base the twelfth rib above and is bounded posteriorly by the erector spinae and laterally by the posterior border of the internal oblique. In the floor of the triangle is the transverse abdominis aponeurosis and it is covered by the latissimus dorsi. All incisions used in approach to the kidney pass through this area and it may be a rare site of hernia (Fig. 1). Upon removal of the erector spinae muscle the anterior layer of lumbodorsal fascia is exposed. This layer, in its upper part, is thickened as the *posterior lumbocostal (Henle's) ligament* which extends from the transverse processes of L_1 and L_2 to the twelfth rib (Fig. 2).

c. DEEP LAYER — of posterolateral abdominal muscles include the transverse abdominis, quadratus lumborum, and psoas major and minor (Figs. 2 and 3). The transverse abdominis arises from the fused anterior and posterior layers of lumbodorsal fascia and is considered on page 134. The *quadratus lumborum* arises from the iliac crest and iliolumbar ligament and inserts on the twelfth rib. From slips arising from T_{12} and all lumbar vertebrae, the *psoas major* muscle takes origin. Although located on the posterior abdominal wall, it must be considered functionally with the hip joint since it inserts in the lesser trochanter of the femur. Muscular fascicles arising from T_{12} and L_1 and inserting in the iliopectineal eminence constitute the *psoas minor*. In man, its function is negligible.

4. **Topography** — certain palpable bony landmarks are present in the posterolateral wall of the abdominal cavity and are important to the surgeon when he is planning injections through the wall for such purposes as direct aortography by the translumbar route, renal aspiration biopsy, or spinal anesthesia. It is important that the physician also envision the topography of the abdominal and thoracic viscera which are related to the wall when he is carrying out such injections as mentioned above or performing an extraperitoneal lumbar approach to the renal or perirenal area.

a. BONY LANDMARKS — are usually easily palpable. The *twelfth rib*, which forms the upper border of this region, is the most difficult to palpate because of its variable length and the presence of the overlying erector spinae muscle mass. No examination of the patient with acute abdominal pain is complete without palpation of this region of the body, particularly in the angle between

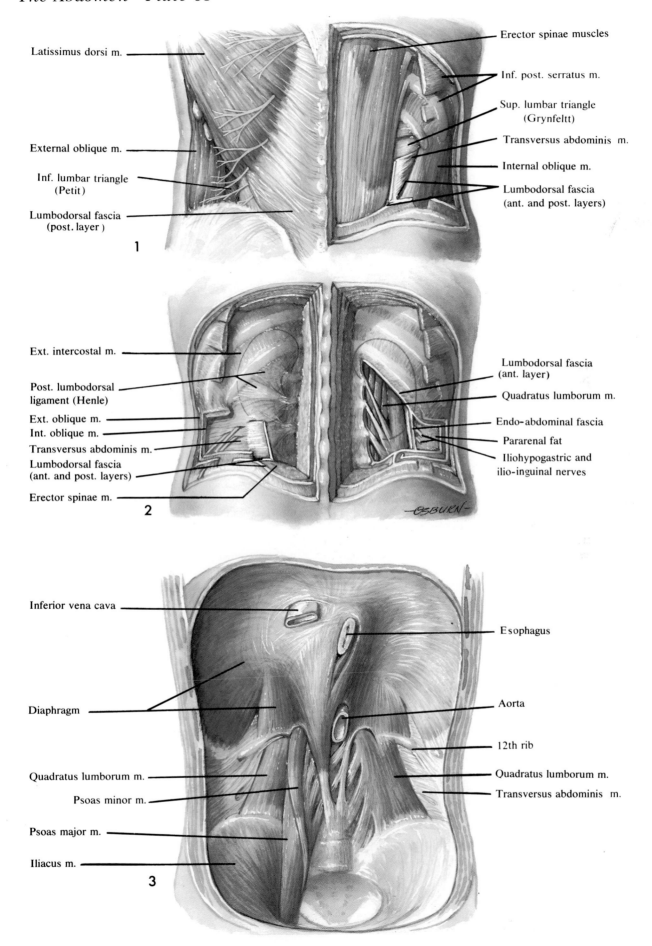

Latissimus dorsi m.

External oblique m.

Inf. lumbar triangle (Petit)

Lumbodorsal fascia (post. layer)

Erector spinae muscles

Inf. post. serratus m.

Sup. lumbar triangle (Grynfeltt)

Transversus abdominis m.

Internal oblique m.

Lumbodorsal fascia (ant. and post. layers)

1

Ext. intercostal m.

Post. lumbodorsal ligament (Henle)

Ext. oblique m.
Int. oblique m.
Transversus abdominis m.
Lumbodorsal fascia (ant. and post. layers)

Erector spinae m.

Lumbodorsal fascia (ant. layer)

Quadratus lumborum m.

Endo-abdominal fascia

Pararenal fat

Iliohypogastric and ilio-inguinal nerves

2

ESBURN

Inferior vena cava

Diaphragm

Quadratus lumborum m.

Psoas minor m.

Psoas major m.

Iliacus m.

Esophagus

Aorta

12th rib

Quadratus lumborum m.

Transversus abdominis m.

3

the twelfth rib and vertebral column *(costovertebral angle)*. Tenderness localized in this area is almost always diagnostic of an inflammatory process in the kidney (Fig. 1).

The five *lumbar spines* are palpable in the midline of the posterior abdominal wall. The first lumbar spine topographically marks the level of origin of the superior mesenteric artery, the pelvis of the kidneys, and the transpyloric plane. At the upper level of the second lumbar spine, the spinal cord ends. At this same level is the duodenojejunal flexure, the cisterna chyli, and the lower pole of the left kidney. At the level of the third lumbar spine is the lower pole of the right kidney, and between the third and fourth spine is the umbilical level. The fourth spinous process of the lumbar spine marks the topographic level for the bifurcation of the aorta and the summit of the iliac crest, and at the fifth spinous level the inferior vena cava begins.

The *iliac crest* is palpable through the skin for its entire length. It terminates posteriorly as the posterior superior spine of ilium which marks the level of the second sacral posterior foramen. This landmark is used in injections for sacral anesthesia (Fig. 4, page 271). A transverse line drawn through the summit of each crest passes through the fourth lumbar interspace, the site most frequently utilized in subarachnoid injections (Fig. 1, page 269).

b. Visceral topography—of both thoracic and abdominal structures is important in the posterolateral abdominal wall (Fig. 1). Of the thoracic viscera, the *parietal pleura* is in jeopardy during incisions or injections in the upper regions of the posterior abdominal wall. The posterior line of costodiaphragmatic pleural reflection of each side extends from the level of the tenth rib in the midaxillary line, to the lower border of the tenth rib, thence to the level of the lower border of T_{12}. The pleura actually descends below the twelfth rib margin at its medial extremity and may be accidentally opened in making surgical incisions to expose the kidney or to drain a subphrenic abscess. Such an injury is even more likely in those individuals possessing only a rudimentary twelfth rib. The *lung* is less likely to be injured for in its neutral position its lower border reaches only to the tenth rib adjacent to the vertebral column. However, should overinflation of the lung occur at the same time the pleural cavity is inadvertently opened, it too is liable to injury.

Of the abdominal viscera, the *kidney* is most intimately related to the posterior muscular wall. To indicate its surface markings, the *parallelogram of Morris* may be used; two vertical lines are drawn, one 2.5 cm. and the other 9.5 cm. from the midline. Two horizontal lines are drawn to complete the parallelogram—the upper at the level of the spine of T_{11} and the lower line at the level of the spinous process of L_3. The hilum of the kidney is at the level of the first lumbar spinous process about 5 cm. from the midline. The long axis of the kidney is slightly oblique so that the upper pole is slightly more medial than the lower pole. It should also be recalled that the right kidney is approximately 1 cm. lower than the left one. Although the topographic markings described above are predominate, individual variations in position may exist as well as variations during deep respirations and change of body position.

The course of the abdominal portion of the *ureter* may be drawn on the back as a line extending from the renal hilum, which is 5 cm. from the midline at the level of the first lumbar spine, downward to the posterior superior iliac spine.

The topography of the abdominal *aorta* on the posterior wall is important to the surgeon performing translumbar aortography. This structure lies to the left of the midline extending from the level of the transpyloric plane at the spine of the first lumbar, vertically downward to its bifurcation at the level of the fourth lumbar spine. The branches of the abdominal aorta are more fully discussed on page 206. The vertebral levels of origin of its main branches are important for accurate roentgen interpretation. The three unpaired visceral branches arise from the anterior surface of the aorta; the celiac axis at the upper border of L_1, the superior mesenteric at the lower border of L_1, and the inferior mesenteric at the lower border of L_3. The important paired renal arteries arise at the level of the upper border of L_2. These renal vessels are commonly multiple—as many as three on one side may be present.

5. **Translumbar Aortography**—the aorta may be visualized roentgenographically by a variety of techniques, each of which has its advantages, disadvantages, and specific indications, and depends largely upon the suspected underlying disease. Thus in aorto-iliac sclerotic disease, a translumbar aortography is definitely the procedure of choice over the retrograde femoral approach. The level of aortic puncture may be from the level of L_1 to L_3. It is more accurately performed at the higher level because of the constancy of the position of the aorta in this subdiaphragmatic location.

a. Skin puncture—is made 1 cm. below the twelfth rib, 8 cm. (approximately 8 fingers' breadth) to the *left* of the midline (Fig. 2).

b. Needle direction—is upward, medially, and forward at about a 60 degree angle to the sagittal plane. The needle is advanced until it contacts the vertebral body. It is then partially withdrawn and redirected at a lesser angle to the same depth and advanced for another 1 to 2 cm. at which point contact with the aorta is made (Fig. 2). Figure 3 is an aortogram performed by the translumbar approach.

6. **Percutaneous Renal Biopsy**—during the past several years, interest has been shown in the use of a needle biopsy in those cases of diffuse kidney disease in which the diagnosis is not clearly established. Because of the accuracy required and the variability in the position of the kidney, the distance of its lateral border from the spinous processes is measured either by pyelogram or by isotope scanning. This lateral measurement is outlined on the back of the patient, who is usually placed in a supine position. The site of puncture is dependent on the x-ray or scan but usually is 2.5 cm. medial to the lateral line and 1.5 cm. below the twelfth rib. When the kidney is entered, the needle swings characteristically with each respiratory movement.

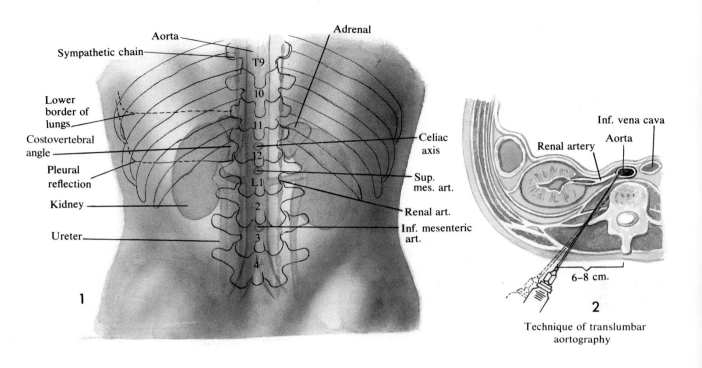

Aorta

Sympathetic chain

Adrenal

T9

10

11

12

L1

2

3

4

Lower border of lungs

Costovertebral angle

Pleural reflection

Kidney

Ureter

Celiac axis

Sup. mes. art.

Renal art.

Inf. mesenteric art.

1

Inf. vena cava

Renal artery

Aorta

6–8 cm.

2

Technique of translumbar aortography

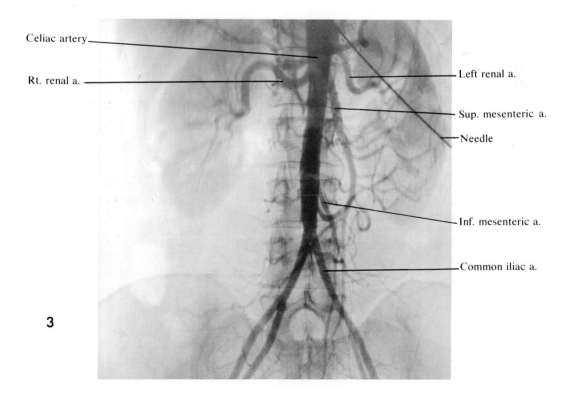

Celiac artery

Rt. renal a.

Left renal a.

Sup. mesenteric a.

Needle

Inf. mesenteric a.

Common iliac a.

3

ROTATION OF THE FOREGUT:

In order to appreciate the normal relationships of the abdominal viscera and the congenital malformations which may occur, a knowledge of the mechanism of the rotation of the gut is imperative. Although embryologic changes take place simultaneously during the development of the embryo, we have chosen, for didactic purposes, to separate these developmental alterations into those of the foregut and midgut at this point and will discuss the embryologic alterations of the hindgut in the discussion of the anorectal canal (page 228). The embryonic gut is a simple tubular structure suspended from ventral and dorsal walls by the double-layered primary ventral and dorsal mesenteries. The caudal portion of the ventral mesentery disintegrates rapidly in the embryo so that the right and left portion of the abdominal cavity intercommunicate. It is the persistent cranial portion of the ventral mesentery and the dorsal mesentery that we will concern ourselves with here.

1. **Ventral Mesentery** (Figs. 1 to 3) — the liver develops into the persisting ventral mesentery. The portion of the ventral mesentery' between the liver and the ventral abdominal wall becomes the *falciform ligament,* the lower free edge of which contains the obliterated left umbilical vein and is termed the *ligamentum teres hepatis.* The ventral mesentery between the liver and developing stomach becomes the *gastrohepatic ligament (lesser omentum),* the lower free border of which extends to the duodenum and contains the common bile duct, hepatic artery, and portal vein. This part is designated as the *hepatoduodenal ligament.*

2. **Dorsal Mesentery** — the portion of original dorsal mesentery suspending the stomach is referred to as *mesogastrium,* the duodenum as *mesoduodenum,* and the colon as *mesocolon.* Only that part related to the jejunum and ileum retain the term *dorsal mesentery.* In the cranial portion of the abdominal dorsal mesentery the spleen develops from an accumulation of mesenchymal cells. The vascular supply to the structures of the foregut which take origin from the celiac axis and lie between the two layers of dorsal mesentery must supply the liver *(hepatic artery),* the stomach *(left gastric),* and the spleen *(splenic artery)* (Fig. 1). That portion of the dorsal mesentery between stomach and spleen becomes the *gastrosplenic ligament* and that between the spleen and midline retroperitoneal aorta, the *spleno-aortic ligament* (Fig. 2).

3. **Mechanism of Rotation of the Foregut** — the rotation of the foregut first takes place as a 90 degree rotation to the right about the *longitudinal axis* of the stomach. In so doing, the dorsal border of the stomach (greater omentum) and the spleen are thrown to the left. A part of the original spleno-aortic ligament is now forced against the posterior parietal peritoneum where the peritoneal layers fuse from aortal to the left kidney. The remaining portion of the spleno-aortic ligament is now termed the *splenorenal (lienorenal) ligament* (Figs. 2 and 3). A second phase of rotation of the foregut is in relation to the *horizonal axis* of the stomach which results from the unequal expansion of the slowly growing ventral mesentery and the rapidly expanding dorsal mesentery. The ventral mesentery fixes the lesser curvature of the stomach while the greater curvature expands. This brings the distal end of the stomach (pylorus) upward and to the right. The original mesoduodenum fuses to the posterior parietal wall to further fix the pylorus (Figs. 2, 3, 4 page 161), and the dorsal mesogastrium is thrown into a large sac posterior and to the left of the stomach, termed the *omental bursa.* The dorsal mesentery is now termed the greater omentum (Figs. 4 and 5).

4. **Omental Bursa** — the bursa, or *lesser peritoneal sac,* becomes isolated from the greater peritoneal cavity except for a small opening, the *epiploic foramen (Winslow)* which is related to the caudal end of the stomach. It is bounded above by the liver (caudate lobe), below by the duodenum, in front by the hepatoduodenal ligament, and behind by the inferior vena cava (Figs. 5 and 6). The bursa expands downward in front of the transverse colon (Fig. 7). Practical consideration of the omental bursa will be given in the ensuing pages dealing with the supramesocolic organs.

5. **Greater Omentum** — this portion of the original dorsal mesentery is the result of a folding and therefore is made up of four peritoneal layers (two anterior and two posterior) (Fig. 7). The inner layers usually fuse, however, and the lowermost portion of the sac is obliterated (Fig. 8). Originally the posterior layer attaches directly to the posterior wall cranial to the attachment of the transverse mesocolon. During later development, however, the posterior layer fuses with the transverse colon and mesocolon to form the definitive *transverse mesocolon* (Fig. 8). Developmentally, therefore, the latter consists of four peritoneal layers. The portion of the anterior layer of greater omentum above the transverse colon is termed the *gastrocolic ligament* and is continuous with the gastrosplenic ligament to the left.

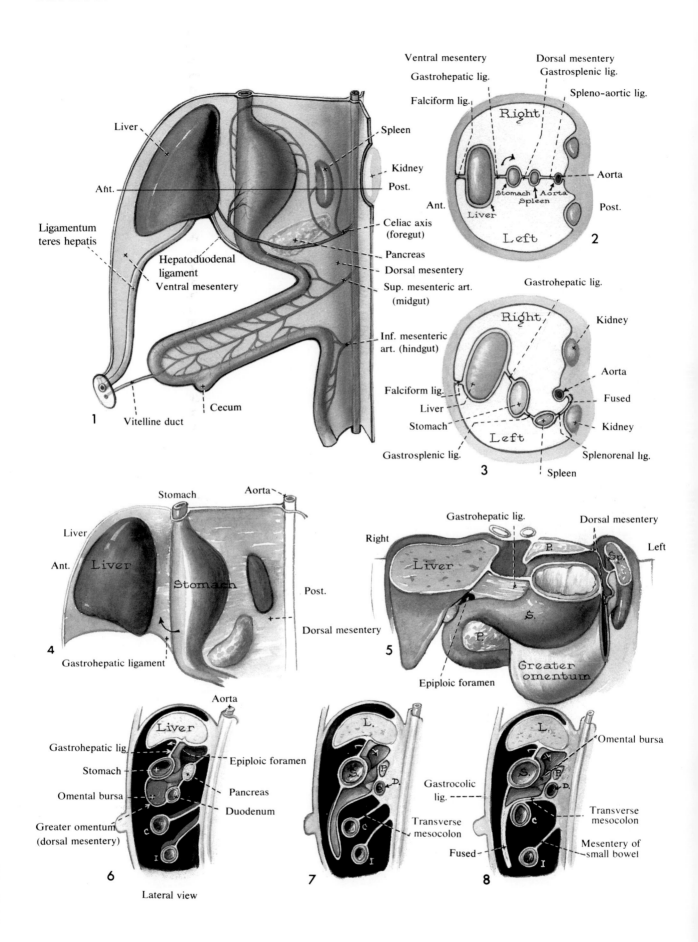

1

Liver
Ant.
Ligamentum teres hepatis
Hepatoduodenal ligament
Ventral mesentery
Vitelline duct
Cecum
Spleen
Kidney
Post.
Celiac axis (foregut)
Pancreas
Dorsal mesentery
Sup. mesenteric art. (midgut)
Inf. mesenteric art. (hindgut)

2

Ventral mesentery
Gastrohepatic lig.
Falciform lig.
Dorsal mesentery
Gastrosplenic lig.
Spleno-aortic lig.
Right
Ant.
Liver
Stomach
Spleen
Aorta
Aorta
Post.
Left

3

Gastrohepatic lig.
Right
Kidney
Aorta
Fused
Kidney
Falciform lig.
Liver
Stomach
Left
Gastrosplenic lig.
Splenorenal lig.
Spleen

4

Stomach
Aorta
Liver
Ant.
Liver
Stomach
Post.
Dorsal mesentery
Gastrohepatic ligament

5

Gastrohepatic lig.
Right
Dorsal mesentery
Left
P.
Sp.
Liver
S.
P.
Greater omentum
Epiploic foramen

6

Aorta
Liver
Gastrohepatic lig.
Stomach
Omental bursa
Greater omentum (dorsal mesentery)
Epiploic foramen
Pancreas
Duodenum
Lateral view

7

L.
S.
P.
D.
C
I
Transverse mesocolon

8

L.
Omental bursa
Gastrocolic lig.
S.
P.
D.
Transverse mesocolon
Fused
Mesentery of small bowel
C
I

ROTATION OF THE MIDGUT:

As noted in the discussion of the foregut, the ventral mesentery caudal to that portion of the embryonic alimentary tract disappears so that the primitive tubular structure of the midgut is suspended only by a dorsal mesentery of visceral peritoneum. The two layers of dorsal mesentery split over the retroperitoneal aorta and continue on the posterior abdominal wall as parietal peritoneum. The midgut is described as that part of the intestinal tract extending from the duodenojejunal junction to the midtransverse colon and is supplied by the *omphalomesenteric* (superior mesenteric) artery which proceeds forward between the two layers of dorsal mesentery and into the yolk sac as the *vitelline artery*. It is the superior mesenteric artery that serves as the axis of rotation of the midgut (Fig. 1).

1. **Mechanism of Rotation** — the three stages of rotation may best be regarded by the surgeon in much the same manner as he would regard a herniated bowel, for indeed, this is what it really is. First is the stage of herniation, although here it is physiologic. Second is the reduction of the hernia, and the final step, its fixation. In each of these stages, a certain amount of rotation and mobilization of the intestinal tract occurs.

a. STAGE OF PHYSIOLOGIC HERNIA — the midgut elongates very rapidly in the early weeks of intrauterine life to the point where it can no longer be accommodated in the primitive coelomic cavity. Because of its attachment to the yolk stalk, it herniates through the umbilical orifice into the primitive umbilical cord as a physiologic hernia. The superior mesenteric artery is the midstructure of this simple loop hernia. That portion of the loop above the artery is referred to as the *cranial (prearterial) loop* (Fig. 1A) and that part below as the *caudal (postarterial) loop* (Fig. 1B). During the first stage a 90 degree counterclockwise rotation takes place which throws the cranial loop to the right (Fig. 2A) and the caudal loop to the left (Fig. 2B).

b. STAGE OF REDUCTION — this stage is the most important in intestinal rotation, for here a further rotation of 180 degrees in counterclockwise rotation occurs. The proximal part of the cranial loop (Fig. 3A) is reduced first, passing *under* the superior mesenteric artery which remains as the axis of rotation. Reduction continues in orderly fashion, the caudal loop (Fig. 3B') being the last to re-enter the abdominal cavity after a 180 degree rotation. At the end of this stage the distal portion of the caudal loop (cecum and proximal colon) are located in the right upper quadrant of the abdomen (Fig. 4B''). This completes the actual rotation of the midgut, so that a total of 270 degrees rotation has taken place in the two stages.

c. STAGE OF FIXATION — during this stage, the cecum descends from its subhepatic position in the right upper quadrant to its normal position (Fig. 4B'' and B'''). Following this descent the dorsal mesentery of the cecum and ascending colon become fixed to the parietal peritoneum of the right flank. The extent of fixation is somewhat triangular in shape, its base extending from ileocecal junction to the right colic flexure and its apex at the duodenojejunal junction. The upper border of the triangle forms the attachment of the right half of transverse mesocolon and the lower border the attachment of the mesentery of the small bowel (Fig. 5). The original mesocolon of the descending colon likewise fuses with the posterior parietal peritoneum but in the form of a quadrangle. The upper border of the quadrangular fusion extends from duodenojejunal junction to the left half of the transverse mesocolon. The lower border extends from the junction of the descending colon and sigmoid to the rectum to form the attachment of the mesosigmoid. The remaining portion of the mesocolon from its original midline attachment to the descending colon fuses with the posterior parietal peritoneum (Fig. 5). The fused visceral and parietal peritoneal layers related to both ascending and descending colons is referred to as *Toldt's fascia* (Fig. 5, page 195). In mobilization of either colon, the surgeon simply reconstructs the original dorsal mesentery by bluntly dissecting in this avascular fascial plane.

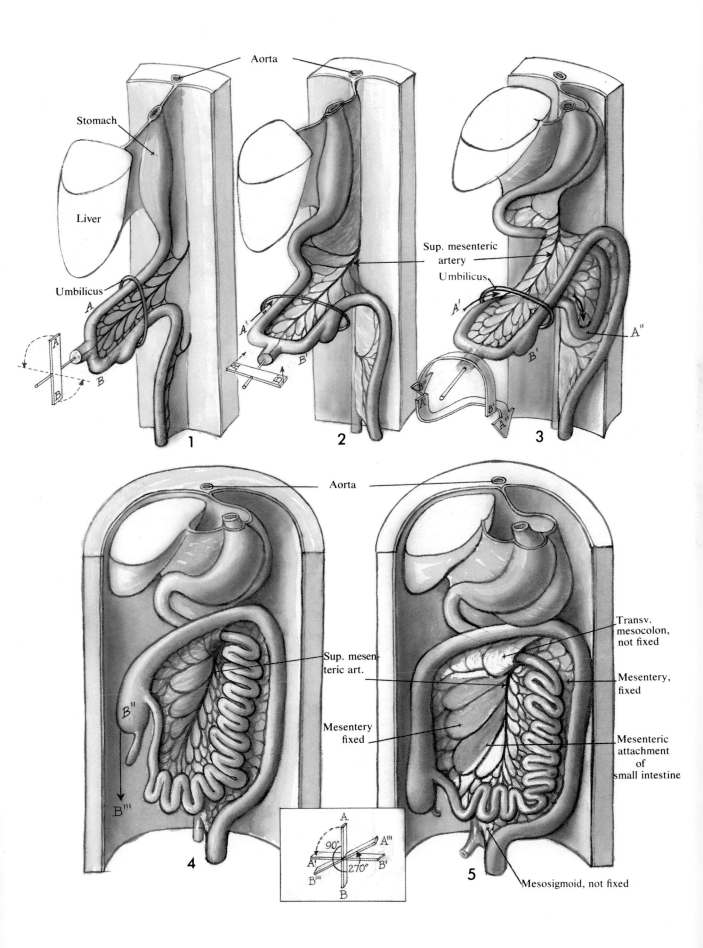

Aorta

Stomach

Liver

Umbilicus

A

B

1

Aorta

A'

B'

2

Sup. mesenteric artery

Umbilicus

A'

B'

A"

3

Aorta

Sup. mesenteric art.

B"

B'''

Mesentery fixed

4

A
90°
A'''
A'
270°
B'''
B'
B

Transv. mesocolon, not fixed

Mesentery, fixed

Mesenteric attachment of small intestine

Mesosigmoid, not fixed

5

ANOMALIES OF INTESTINAL ROTATION:

Congenital malformations resulting from abnormal patterns of rotation, particularly of the midgut, are not uncommon. A knowledge of the normal process of rotation as described on page 150 is therefore important if the surgeon is to understand and correct the unusual disposition of the abdominal viscera encountered in these abnormal conditions. Some of the important anomalies which occur during the three stages are discussed below.

1. **Stage of Physiologic Hernia:**

OMPHALOCELE (EXOMPHALOS) (Fig. 1)—results when rotation fails to continue beyond the first stage (Fig. 2, page 151) and is present at birth. The hernia may consist of a single loop of bowel or may contain the entire intestinal tract, liver, spleen, and pancreas. The covering of the sac is the delicate translucent amnion of the umbilical cord.

2. **Stage of Reduction:**

a. NONROTATION (Fig. 2)—although reduction of the physiologic hernia occurs, further rotation beyond the 90 degree turn which took place in the first stage does not occur. This results in the cranial limb of the embryonic midgut being reduced into the right side of the peritoneal cavity and the caudal limb into the left side. In the fetus, therefore, the small intestine is entirely in the right side of the abdomen and the cecum and remainder of the large bowel on the left side. This anomaly may be completely asymptomatic. Clinically, it is referred to as *"left-sided colon"* and is of significance when diseases of the appendix or ascending colon occur in this aberrant position.

b. REVERSED ROTATION (Fig. 3)—this rare anomaly of stage II is a result of a clockwise rather than the normal counterclockwise rotation of 180 degrees during reduction around the superior mesenteric artery axis. The duodenum comes to lie anterior to the artery, and the transverse colon comes behind the artery. With the fixation of the root of mesentery, obstruction of the transverse colon by the superior mesenteric artery may occur.

c. VOLVULUS (L., to turn; Fig. 4)—if intestinal rotation stops at the end of stage II, that is, without fixation of the mesentery, the entire midgut loop hangs free from a narrow pedicle formed by the superior mesenteric vessels. Such a condition predisposes to a twisting of the bowel over the superior mesenteric vessels, resulting in symptoms of mesenteric vascular occlusion. More frequently, however, the presenting symptoms are those of partial or complete duodenal obstruction dating from birth.

d. INTERNAL HERNIA (Fig. 5)—during the reduction of the cranial loop of the midgut from the umbilical orifice, instead of rotating into the general peritoneal cavity, the loop rotates into the mesentery of the caudal loop which later becomes the mesentery of the large bowel. With subsequent fixation of the mesentery loop, the bowel may become imprisoned beneath the mesentery. The most common type is the *paraduodenal hernia* as illustrated.

e. MALROTATION—the possibilities of irregularities of rotation and fixation of the midgut are unlimited and are grouped together under the term malrotation. The true nature of the anomaly is usually recognized only at operation and if the normal stages of intestinal rotation are kept in mind by the surgeon they are not difficult to understand and repair.

3. **Stage of Fixation:**

a. SUBHEPATIC CECUM (APPENDIX) (Fig. 6)—should rotation stop at the end of stage II, the cecum fails to descend from the right upper to the right lower quadrant, resulting in its location in a subhepatic position. The most significant surgical consideration is in those individuals who have such an anomaly and develop appendicitis.

b. RETROCECAL APPENDIX (Fig. 7)—this condition is probably the most common anomaly of intestinal rotation. During the descent of the cecum into the right lower quadrant, the appendix may be thrown under the cecum and become fixed in that position during the normal process of fixation of the cecum and ascending colon.

c. MOBILE CECUM—if the visceral peritoneum of the cecum fails to fuse to the posterior parietal peritoneum a mobile cecum results. It is of surgical significance because of possible variations in the location of the appendix or the possibility of the twisting or volvulus of the cecum.

4. **Meckel's Diverticulum**—is one of the most common anomalies of the intestines and is due to the partial persistence of the yolk stalk (page 192).

5. **Intussusception** (Fig. 8)—although this condition is not a result of abnormal intestinal rotation, it is considered here because, like many of the congenital deformities, symptoms occur most frequently in the first year of life. It is one of the most common causes of intestinal obstruction in infants and usually is an invagination of the ilium into the cecum. The invaginated bowel is referred to as the *intussusceptum* and the receiving portion of the bowel, the *intussuscipiens*. Obstruction occurs partly because peristalsis is interrupted and partly because the mesentery of the invaginated bowel becomes compressed, causing both venous and arterial obstruction which results in edema, congestion, and subsequent necrosis.

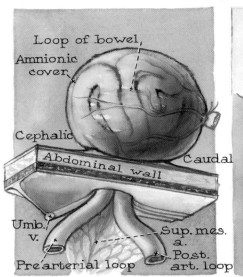

1 Omphalocele

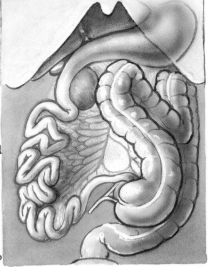

2 Nonrotation

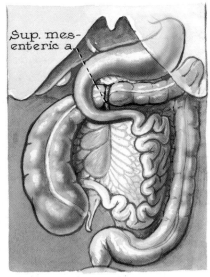

3 Reversed rotation

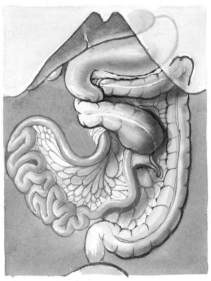

4 Volvulus

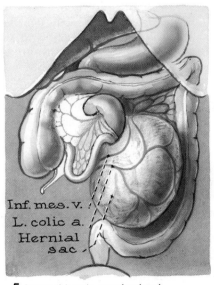

5 Internal hernia paraduodenal

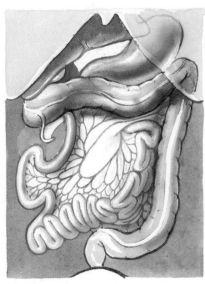

6 Subhepatic appendix

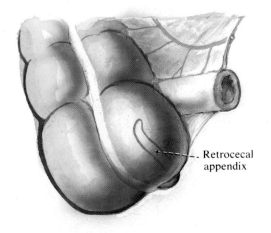

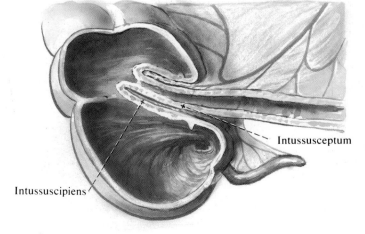

8 Intussusception

THE STOMACH:

The development and peritoneal relations to the stomach have already been considered on page 148. Although there is a great deal of disparity in regard to the subdivision of the stomach, it is generally regarded as having two orifices, two surfaces, two curvatures, and two incisurae.

1. **Structure** — the esophagus, after piercing the diaphragm, takes a very short (2 cm.) abdominal course before entering the stomach.

a. ORIFICES — the *cardiac orifice* (Fig. 1) is located at the level of T_{10} approximately 1 inch to the left of the midline. The *pyloric orifice* (Fig. 1) is situated 1 inch to the right of the midline at the transpyloric plane at the level of the lower border of L_1.

b. SURFACES — *both anterior and posterior surfaces* and their parietal and visceral relations are shown on page 157.

c. CURVATURES — the *lesser and greater* curvatures and their peritoneal relations are discussed on page 148 and 156.

d. INCISURAE (Fig. 1) — are two; the *cardiac incisura* is located at the junction of the abdominal esophagus and greater curvature, while the *angular incisura* is located on the lesser curvature. Arbitrary lines may be drawn from the incisurae to the greater curvature to subdivide the stomach into its various parts.

2. **Parts** (Fig. 1) — by the aforementioned arbitrary lines the stomach is divided into the three major parts:

a. FUNDUS — is that portion located above a horizontal line drawn from the cardiac incisura to the greater curvature.

b. BODY — of the stomach comprises that part of the organ from the above-described line to a vertical line drawn from the angular incisura to the greater curvature.

c. PYLORIC PORTION — consists of the remaining portion of the distal end of the stomach. A line passing from a small indentation on the greater curvature (sulcus intermedius) to the lesser curvature subdivides the pyloric end into a larger proximal *pyloric antrum* and a more tubular *pyloric canal*. The sphincteric area palpable by the surgeon between the stomach and duodenum is termed the *pylorus.*

d. MUSCULAR WALL (Fig. 1) — in addition to the outer serosal (peritoneal) layer and the inner mucosal and submucosal layers, the wall of the stomach consists of three muscular layers. They are an outer *longitudinal,* a middle *circular,* and an incomplete inner *oblique* layer.

3. **Arterial Supply** (Fig. 2) — as a derivative of the foregut, the stomach is supplied entirely by the celiac axis which arises from the abdominal aorta. The main branches are located on the gastric curvatures.

a. LEFT GASTRIC — is usually a direct branch of the celiac axis, running upward and to the left in the posterior wall of the omental bursa where it produces a peritoneal fold (gastrophrenic fold) (Fig. 3, page 157). After sending off esophageal arteries and frequently an aberrant hepatic artery, it descends along the lesser curvature sending anterior and posterior branches to the fundus and body.

b. SPLENIC ARTERY — also traverses the posterior wall of the omental bursa and at the tail of the pancreas it gives rise to the left *gastro-epiploic artery.* This branch runs through the gastrosplenic ligament and descends along the greater curvature. Also arising from the splenic are multiple *short gastric* arteries which serve primarily to supply the posterior surface of the fundus.

c. HEPATIC ARTERY — enters the supply of the stomach via a small branch, the *right gastric artery.* This branch courses along the lesser curvature where it anastomoses with the left gastric. A terminal branch from the gastroduodenal artery, the *right gastro-epiploic artery* turns to the left and runs in the greater omentum paralleling the greater curvature to anastomose with the left gastro-epiploic artery. All arterial branches supplying the stomach penetrate the muscular coats and form a very extensive arterial network in the submucosa.

4. **Venous Drainage** (Fig. 3) — in their peripheral distribution the veins of the stomach follow the arterial branches along the curvatures. All these veins drain directly or indirectly into the portal vein.

a. LEFT GASTRIC (CORONARY) VEIN — empties directly into the portal and communicates above with the azygos system (Fig. 1, page 183).

b. RIGHT GASTRIC VEIN — also drains directly into the portal. An important tributary is the *prepyloric vein of Mayo* which surgeons use as a guide to the gastroduodenal junction.

c. RIGHT GASTRO-EPIPLOIC VEIN — most frequently empties into the superior mesenteric or, as shown in Figure 3, into the middle colic vein.

d. LEFT GASTRO-EPIPLOIC VEIN AND THE SHORT GASTRIC VEINS — drain into the splenic vein directly.

5. **Gastric Nerves** (Fig. 4) — owing to the rotation of the foregut (page 148) the left vagus nerve becomes the *anterior gastric* and the right vagus the *posterior gastric.* Both nerves run close to the lesser curvature and distribute branches to the anterior and posterior surfaces as far as the antrum. The anterior branch also sends a branch in the lesser omentum to the liver and pyloric end of the stomach.

6. **Lymphatics** (Fig. 5) — although numerous anastomoses of the stomach lymphatics must be present, the collecting channels may, for didactic purposes, be divided into four zones, each with its specific associated regional lymph nodes.

a. Zone I — comprises the collecting channels from most of the lesser curvature including the cardia. It is the largest area of drainage and enters the *paracardiac nodes* and *superior gastric nodes* located along the left gastric artery, thence to the celiac nodes.

b. ZONE II — drains the left upper portion of the greater curvature including the fundus and upper part of the body. The lymph channels accompany the short gastric and left gastro-epiploic arteries. The associated nodes are located in the hilum of the spleen and along the splenic artery and are termed the *pancreaticolienal nodes;* they in turn drain into the celiac nodes.

c. ZONE III — lymph channels drain the lower portion of the greater curvature and accompany the right

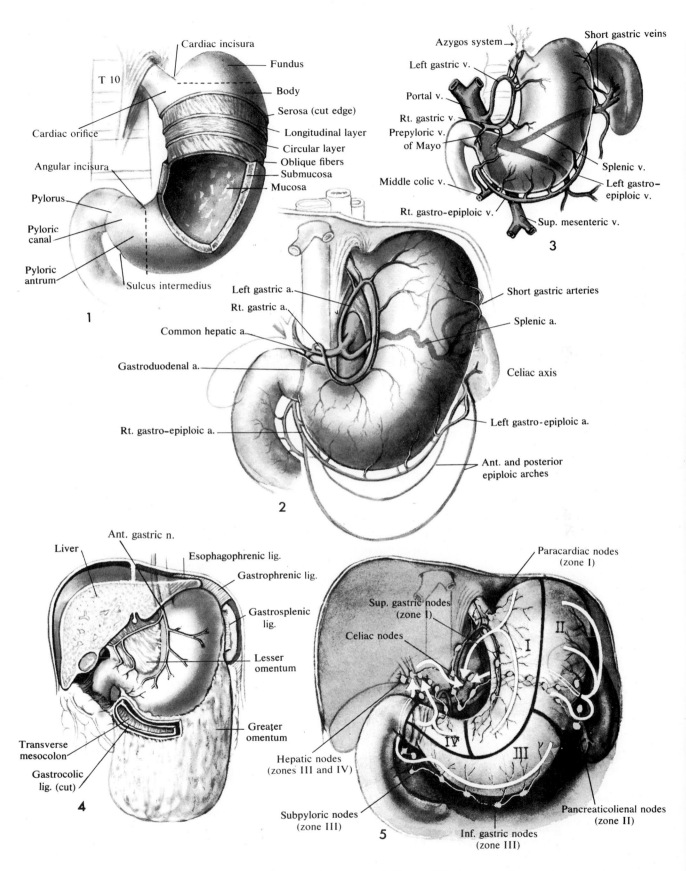

1

T 10

Cardiac incisura

Fundus

Body

Serosa (cut edge)

Longitudinal layer

Circular layer

Oblique fibers

Submucosa

Mucosa

Cardiac orifice

Angular incisura

Pylorus

Pyloric canal

Pyloric antrum

Sulcus intermedius

2

Left gastric a.

Rt. gastric a.

Common hepatic a.

Gastroduodenal a.

Rt. gastro-epiploic a.

Short gastric arteries

Splenic a.

Celiac axis

Left gastro-epiploic a.

Ant. and posterior epiploic arches

3

Azygos system

Short gastric veins

Left gastric v.

Portal v.

Rt. gastric v.

Prepyloric v. of Mayo

Middle colic v.

Rt. gastro-epiploic v.

Splenic v.

Left gastro-epiploic v.

Sup. mesenteric v.

4

Liver

Ant. gastric n.

Esophagophrenic lig.

Gastrophrenic lig.

Gastrosplenic lig.

Lesser omentum

Greater omentum

Transverse mesocolon

Gastrocolic lig. (cut)

5

Paracardiac nodes (zone I)

Sup. gastric nodes (zone I)

Celiac nodes

Hepatic nodes (zones III and IV)

Subpyloric nodes (zone III)

Inf. gastric nodes (zone III)

Pancreaticolienal nodes (zone II)

gastro-epiploic artery. The associated nodes are the *inferior gastric* and *subpyloric nodes*. Here again efferent channels drain into the hepatic and celiac nodes.

d. ZONE IV—is a small area draining the upper portion of the pylorus and the channels enter the hepatic nodes before ultimately draining into the celiac nodes.

6. **Topography**—of the supramesocolic organs the stomach is the most variable in regard to surface topography, since it is a mobile organ with no fixed position, as determined by roentgen studies. The cardiac orifice is the most fixed part of this organ and may be marked on the anterior abdominal wall opposite the tip of the eighth costal cartilage behind the left costal margin. The pyloric orifice is very mobile but in the recumbent position with the patient anesthetized and the stomach emptied, it is usually located at the transpyloric plane (level L_1) just to the right of the midline. The position of the greater curvature is extremely variable and may be as high as the level of T_{12} or as low as the true pelvis.

7. **Relational Anatomy**—anteriorly, the stomach is related to the diaphragm in the left hypocondrium and to the true left lobe (lateral and medial segments) of the liver in the region of the epigastrium. A large portion of the anterior surface of the stomach is directly related to the parietal peritoneum of the anterior abdominal wall without any intervening abdominal viscera (Fig. 1). This latter anatomic relationship is utilized in performing a *gastrostomy,* or a creation of an artificial fistula or stoma between the abdominal wall and stomach for the administration of nutrient liquids in patients who are unable to take food by mouth. The anterior surface of the stomach is in direct relationship with the general peritoneal cavity.

The posterior surface of the stomach is related directly to the lesser peritoneal cavity (omental bursa) (Fig. 2). The visceral peritoneum covering the posterior surface of the stomach forms, in part, the anterior wall of this peritoneal sac. With the omental bursa intervening, the dorsal surface of the stomach is related to the pancreas, cranial to which is the left kidney and left suprarenal, the spleen, splenic vessels, and diaphragm. The transverse mesocolon and transverse colon are related to the stomach caudal to the pancreas. These anatomic structures make up the so-called *"stomach bed."*

8. **Peritoneal Attachments** (Fig. 3)—the stomach is ensheathed by peritoneum, which forms the external or serosal coat of the stomach wall. An understanding of these peritoneal relationships can only be obtained through the knowledge of the embryological development of this organ in relation to the original ventral and dorsal mesenteries of the gastrointestinal tract (page 148). The peritoneum covering the ventral and dorsal surfaces fuse at the lesser curvature to form the *gastrohepatic ligament (lesser omentum)*, a derivative of the ventral mesentery. Within this fused peritoneal layer are located the right and left gastric vessels.

The peritoneum covering the ventral and dorsal surfaces of the stomach also join at the greater curvature to form the greater omentum—a derivative of the embryonic dorsal mesentery. Superiorly, the two peritoneal layers join just to the left of the abdominal esophagus and pass to the diaphragm forming the *gastrophrenic ligament.* This fused peritoneal layer next gains attachment to the hilus of the spleen and is termed the *gastrosplenic ligament.* Between these fused peritoneal layers are located the left gastro-epiploic artery and the short gastric arteries to the stomach. The remainder of the greater omentum extends from the greater curvature of the stomach and fuses with the anterior surface of the transverse colon. That portion of the greater omentum between the greater curvature of the stomach and the transverse colon is now referred to as the *gastrocolic ligament.* Between the anterior and posterior leaflets of the greater omentum, at its attachments to the greater curvature of the stomach, are located the right and left gastroepiploic arteries and veins.

9. **Anatomic Approaches**—the stomach may be approached for diagnostic or therapeutic purposes either via the peroral or abdominal route. The peroral route is utilized either for analysis of gastric secretions, lavage, or gastroscopic examination. Surgical procedures upon the stomach may best be performed by an abdominal approach. Because of the variability of the upper and lower limits of the stomach, an upper midline or a left paramedian incision is utilized in the surgical approach to this organ. In those cases requiring a total gastrectomy, a thoraco-abdominal approach may be required.

10. **Identification**—in the customary exposure for partial or total gastrectomy there is little doubt as to the anatomic site of the stomach. In small incisions used for gastrostomy procedures, the anatomic variability of the location of the stomach may create a problem, for not infrequently the transverse colon is mistakenly entered. The attachment of the greater omentum, however, may serve as an infallible guide in such procedures.

11. **Gastric Resection**—the indications and techniques of the many varieties of gastric resections are available in many surgical texts. Certain fundamental anatomic principles must be adhered to no matter which technique is deemed advisable in any particular situation, one of which is adequate exposure. In all gastric resections it is most important to free the posterior gastric surface from the stomach bed in the omental bursa. This may be accomplished by incising the gastrocolic ligament thereby gaining entrance to the lesser peritoneal sac (omental bursa). Any adhesions between the posterior surface of the stomach and the stomach bed may then be lysed. Next, the transverse mesocolon containing the middle colic artery (Fig. 3) must be separated from the greater omentum and displaced caudalward by packing to prevent injury to this artery which usually results in deprivation of the blood supply to the transverse colon. Other than these two steps, gastric resection is the practical application of the knowledge of the vascular supply and peritoneal fixation of the stomach.

12. **Reconstruction Procedures**—regardless of whether partial or total gastrectomy is performed for the correction of the underlying pathology, anatomic continuity of the gastrointestinal tract must be re-established. Figures 4 and 5 illustrate such an anatomic restoration following a partial gastrectomy. For modifications of these and other reconstructive procedures following gastric resection, the reader is referred to the numerous surgical textbooks related to this subject.

Anterior Relations of Stomach

Posterior Relations of Stomach

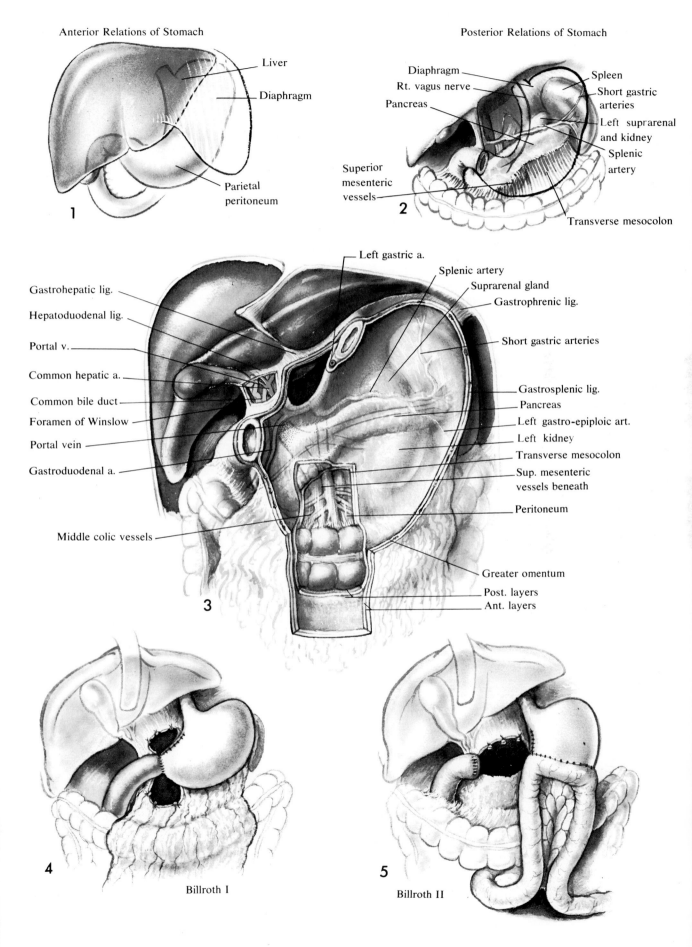

Liver

Diaphragm

Parietal peritoneum

1

Diaphragm

Rt. vagus nerve

Pancreas

Spleen

Short gastric arteries

Left suprarenal and kidney

Splenic artery

Superior mesenteric vessels

2

Transverse mesocolon

Left gastric a.

Splenic artery

Suprarenal gland

Gastrophrenic lig.

Gastrohepatic lig.

Hepatoduodenal lig.

Portal v.

Common hepatic a.

Common bile duct

Foramen of Winslow

Portal vein

Gastroduodenal a.

Short gastric arteries

Gastrosplenic lig.

Pancreas

Left gastro-epiploic art.

Left kidney

Transverse mesocolon

Sup. mesenteric vessels beneath

Peritoneum

Middle colic vessels

Greater omentum

Post. layers

Ant. layers

3

Billroth I

4

Billroth II

5

13. **Vagotomy** – with the introduction of new drugs, such as cimetidine and others, it is possible to inhibit gastric acid secretion rather than simply combat gastric hyperactivity by the use of antacids. Since the advent of such drugs, the indications for operating on peptic, duodenal, and gastric ulcerations have been greatly diminished. However, when surgery is indicated, the procedure of choice is vagotomy and a drainage procedure or vagotomy and antrectomy, depending on the complications of duodenal or gastric ulcerations that are present.

Vagotomy eliminates the cephalic phase of gastric secretion, and the gastrin hormonal phase of secretion is eliminated by antrectomy. Vagotomy decreases gastric motility and tonicity, thereby delaying emptying of the stomach. To enhance drainage following such a procedure, pyloroplasty or enterostomy may be performed.

As described on page 102 and illustrated on Plate 49, Figures 4 and 5, the vagus nerves in their descent through the esophageal hiatus of the diaphragm are extremely variable, which accounts for many of the failures when the technique of vagotomy was first introduced. Techniques have been developed subsequently which have improved the surgical effectiveness of the procedure. Three such procedures have been advocated, each of which has its pros and cons: truncal vagotomy, selective gastric vagotomy, and proximal gastric vagotomy.

a. Proximal gastric vagotomy (Fig. 1) – is achieved by first identifying the anterior vagus nerve and denervating those branches to the body of the stomach and preserving those to the gastric antrum. Next the posterior vagal is identified and those branches to the antrum are also preserved. The advantage of this procedure is that it denervates the mass of acid-secreting parietal cells but preserves the vagal innervation to the pylorus, thereby permitting near-normal gastric emptying, and obviates the need for a gastric drainage procedure.

b. Selective vagotomy (Fig. 2) – requires again the identification of the anterior vagal nerve. The hepatic branch is identified and preserved. The main right vagal trunk is severed below the origin of the hepatic branch, and branches arising to the left going to the fundus are divided. The posterior vagus nerve is next identified in the lesser omentum and the celiac branch is preserved. All neurovascular bundles between these branches and the lesser curvature are divided. Since the vagal innervation of the antrum is destroyed with this procedure, a pyloroplasty or a gastrojejunostomy must be performed to achieve adequate drainage.

c. Truncal vagotomy (Fig. 3) – requires mobilization of the abdominal esophagus in order to identify the anterior and posterior vagal nerves. After proper identification of these nerves, a 4-cm. segment of each nerve is resected. This procedure totally denervates the stomach from its parasympathetic vagal innervation, thereby necessitating a drainage procedure either by pyloroplasty or antrectomy. The continuity of the gastrointestinal tract may be achieved by the Billroth I gastroenterostomy (Plate 74, Fig. 4).

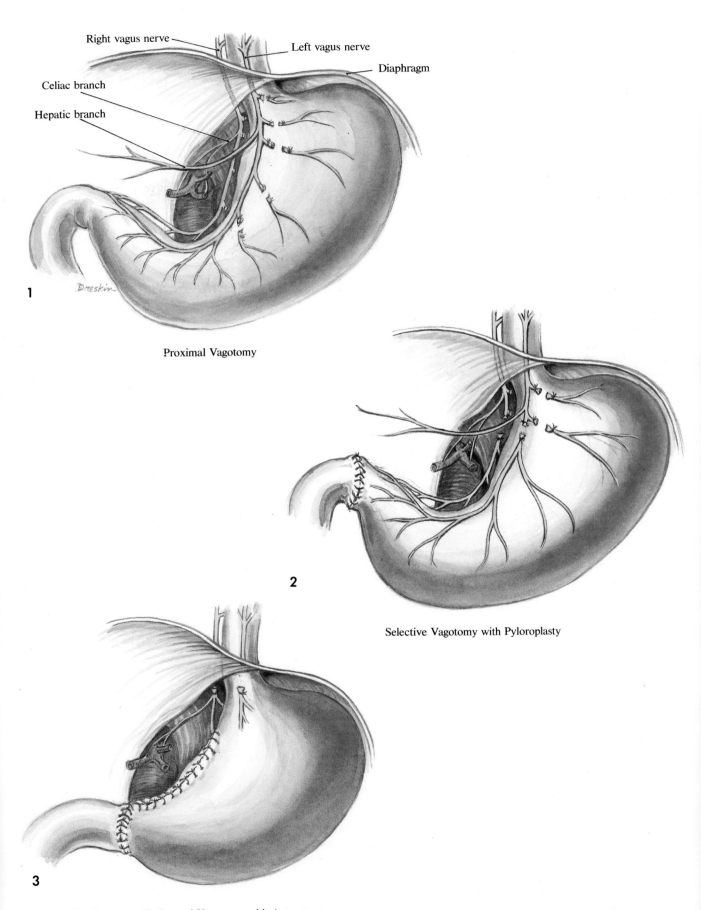

Right vagus nerve

Left vagus nerve

Diaphragm

Celiac branch

Hepatic branch

1

Proximal Vagotomy

2

Selective Vagotomy with Pyloroplasty

3

Subdiaphragmatic Truncal Vagotomy with Antrectomy

PANCREAS, DUODENUM, AND COMMON BILE DUCT:

These three structures are considered together because of their intimate embryologic relationships. They are located in relation to the primitive digestive tube near the junction of the foregut and midgut and will receive their vascular supply from both the celiac axis and superior mesenteric arteries (Fig. 1, page 149).

1. **Embryology**—the primitive foregut extends to the duodenojejunal junction and is suspended in its entire course by the dorsal mesentery. The primitive ventral mesentery, however, extends to about the midportion of the duodenum. It is in this location that the *hepatic diverticulum* extends forward as an entodermal outpouching from the foregut between the two layers of ventral mesentery (Fig. 1). The proximal portion of this diverticulum gives rise to the common bile duct. From this same hepatic diverticulum the *ventral pancreatic anlage* develops as a caudal outpouching. The *dorsal pancreatic anlage* arises from the dorsal wall of the duodenum and extends posteriorly between the two layers of dorsal mesentery (mesoduodenum) (Figs. 1 and 2). With the rotation of the foregut to the right in the longitudinal axis of the stomach (page 148) the ventral anlage pushes beneath the mesodermal covering of the duodenum and extends into the dorsal mesentery (Fig. 3) in juxtaposition with the dorsal anlage to form the definitive pancreas. As rotation of the foregut continues the mesoduodenum comes in apposition with the posterior parietal peritoneum and fuses. This fused layer is termed the *fascia of Treitz* (Fig. 4). In *the Kocher maneuver* for mobilization of the duodenum, the surgeon reconstructs the original mesoduodenum by dissection in this avascular fused peritoneal plane.

2. **Pancreatic Ducts**—after the fusion of the dorsal and ventral pancreatic anlage the ducts of these respective parts fuse. Although originally the smaller of the two ducts, that of the ventral anlage, becomes the *main pancreatic duct (Wirsung)* and the duct of the dorsal anlage, the *lesser pancreatic duct (Santorini).*

a. DUCT OF WIRSUNG—begins in the tail of the pancreas and extends to the right through the body and traverses the neck and head of the organ to end in the descending duodenum (Fig. 5).

b. DUCT OF SANTORINI—lies in the head of the pancreas and extends from the main duct and terminates in the duodenum about 2 cm. cranial to the orifice of the major duct (Fig. 5). In a small percentage of cases (7 per cent) this duct may persist as the major drainage of the pancreatic duct system.

3. **Relation of Common Bile Duct and Major Pancreatic Duct**—embryologically the major pancreatic duct arises as an outpouching from that portion of the hepatic diverticulum that gives rise to the common bile duct. It stands to reason, therefore, that in the majority of cases these two ducts will enter the duodenum in a common orifice. This common passage, *the ampulla of Vater,* opens into the *major duodenal papilla* about 8 to 10 cm. below the pylorus (Fig. 6A). A common finding, however, is the complete separation of the ductal

system by a septum extending into the ampulla (Fig. 6B) or less frequently, a septum extending to within only 1 cm. of the apex of the papilla (Fig. 6C). More detailed description of the ampulla of Vater is illustrated in Figure 1, page 173.

4. **Duodenum**—is, the widest part of the small intestine and extends from the pylorus to the duodenojejunal flexure. For convenience of description, it is divided into four parts:

a. SUPERIOR PORTION (duodenal bulb) (Fig. 7-1)—leads from the pylorus to the superior flexure.

b. DESCENDING PORTION (Fig. 7-2)—extends from the superior to the inferior flexure and receives the common bile and pancreatic ducts.

c. HORIZONTAL PORTION (Fig. 7-3)—passes from the inferior flexure and ascends slightly to become the:

d. ASCENDING PORTION (Fig. 7-4)—which terminates at the duodenojejunal junction.

5. **Pancreas**—as with the duodenum, arbitrary divisions are assigned to the various parts of this organ (Fig. 7):

a. HEAD—of the pancreas forms the enlarged right portion of the organ and lies in the concavity of the duodenum. The caudal and left portion of the head of the pancreas hooks around the posterior aspect of the superior mesenteric vessels and forms the *uncinate process.*

b. NECK—of the pancreas is located at the cranial and left aspect of the head and is grooved dorsally by superior mesenteric vessels.

c. BODY—of the pancreas extends from the neck on the right to the tail on the left extending transversely and cranialward. It is the largest part of this organ and presents an anterior, posterior, and inferior surface and three borders: inferior, anterior, and superior. The superior border is most important for practical purposes, for it is on this surface that the splenic artery lies. Pressure may be applied on the superior border to control hemorrhage.

d. TAIL—of the pancreas is almost invariably in contact laterally with the hilum of the spleen.

6. **Common Bile Duct**—begins in the hepatoduodenal ligament at the junction of the cystic and common hepatic ducts and terminates in the second portion of the duodenum. It may be divided into four parts (Fig. 7):

a. SUPRADUODENAL PORTION—lies in the hepatoduodenal ligament to the right of the hepatic artery and anterior to the portal vein.

b. RETRODUODENAL PORTION—descends behind the first portion of the duodenum.

c. INTRAPANCREATIC PORTION—begins at the upper margin of the head of the pancreas, then passes downward along the posterior surface which it grooves or tunnels, and terminates as it pierces the posteromedial wall of the midpart of the second portion of the duodenum.

d. INTRAMURAL PORTION—is the short segment which obliquely transverses the wall of the duodenum where it is joined by the main pancreatic duct to form the ampulla of Vater; the orifice of which is located on the major duodenal papilla.

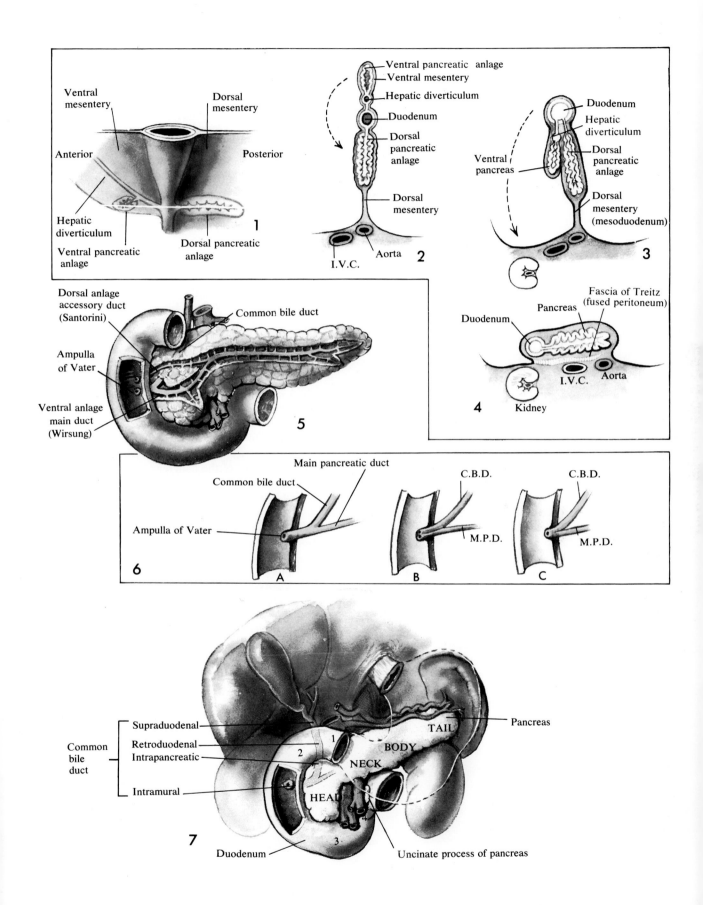

7. Arterial Supply (Figs. 1 to 3) — as previously mentioned, these structures with the exception of the common duct, will receive their arterial supply from both the celiac axis and the superior mesenteric arteries.

a. DUODENUM — is supplied primarily by two arterial arcades, anterior and posterior, the branches of which also supply the head of the pancreas and common bile duct. In the prevailing pattern, these arcades are formed by a branch of the common hepatic, the *gastroduodenal*, and the *inferior pancreaticoduodenal*, a branch of the superior mesenteric.

(1) *Gastroduodenal Artery* — arises from the common hepatic in the lesser omentum, descends behind the first portion of the duodenum where it gives rise to the *posterior superior pancreaticoduodenal artery (retroduodenal)* which enters into the formation of the posterior arcade. The gastroduodenal terminates at the lower margin of the duodenum by dividing into the right gastroepiploic and the *anterior superior pancreaticoduodenal* artery, the latter forming part of the anterior arcade.

(2) *Inferior Pancreaticoduodenal Artery* — is the first branch originating from the right side of the superior mesenteric. It divides into two branches, the *anterior and posterior inferior pancreaticoduodenal artery.*

(3) *Anterior Pancreaticoduodenal Arcade* — is formed by the anastomosis of the anterior superior and anterior inferior pancreaticoduodenal arteries. This arcade lies close to the pancreaticoduodenal sulcus and sends branches to the anterior wall of the second, third, and fourth portions of the duodenum as well as twigs to the head of the pancreas.

(4) *Posterior Pancreaticoduodenal Arcade* — lies on the posterior surface of the head of the pancreas and is composed of the posterior superior and posterior inferior pancreaticoduodenal arterial branches. From this arcade branches supply the posterior wall of the second, third, and fourth portions of the duodenum and to a lesser extent the head of the pancreas.

(5) *Supraduodenal Artery (Wilkie)* — is a small branch usually arising directly from the gastroduodenal and is the chief supply to the first portion of the duodenum. Small twigs from the right gastric, right gastroepiploic, and gastroduodenal trunk also supply this area.

(6) *First Jejunal Branch* — of the superior mesenteric artery sends branches to the distal part of the fourth portion of the duodenum and duodenojejunal junction.

b. PANCREAS — receives an arterial supply to the head of the organ from the anterior and posterior pancreaticoduodenal arcades previously described. The main contribution to the arterial supply of the remainder of the pancreas comes from the splenic artery branches which will be considered here.

(1) *Dorsal Pancreatic Artery* — usually arises from the splenic but not infrequently from the celiac, hepatic, or superior mesenteric. It descends behind the neck of the pancreas and divides into a right and left branch. The right branch is distributed to the head and uncinate process and anastomoses with the duodenal arterial arcades. The left branch is referred to as the inferior (transverse) pancreatic artery.

(2) *Inferior (transverse) Pancreatic Artery* — is actually the left branch of the dorsal pancreatic and extends to the left along the dorsal inferior surface of the body of the pancreas. In the tail of the pancreas it anastomoses with the caudal pancreatic artery.

(3) *Caudal Pancreatic Artery* — arises from the distal end of the splenic as a direct branch and joins the inferior pancreatic.

(4) *Pancreatica Magna* — is another large direct branch from the distal part of the splenic artery; it descends into the body and joins the inferior and caudal pancreatic branches.

(5) *Superior Pancreatic Rami* — are multiple small branches arising from the splenic as it courses along the superior border of the pancreas.

c. COMMON BILE DUCT (Fig. 2) — in its distal part is supplied mainly by descending branches of the *cystic* and may receive direct branches from the *hepatic propria*. The proximal portion is supplied by the *posterior superior pancreaticoduodenal (retroduodenal)* branch of the gastroduodenal. This artery has an important relationship with the common duct. After its origin from the gastroduodenal it crosses anterior to the duct, descends parallel to the duct on the right side, then passes posterior to it before joining the posterior inferior pancreaticoduodenal branch.

8. Venous Drainage (Fig. 4) — the drainage of this area has been inadequately studied although it is important in resections of these organs.

(Text continued on page 164.)

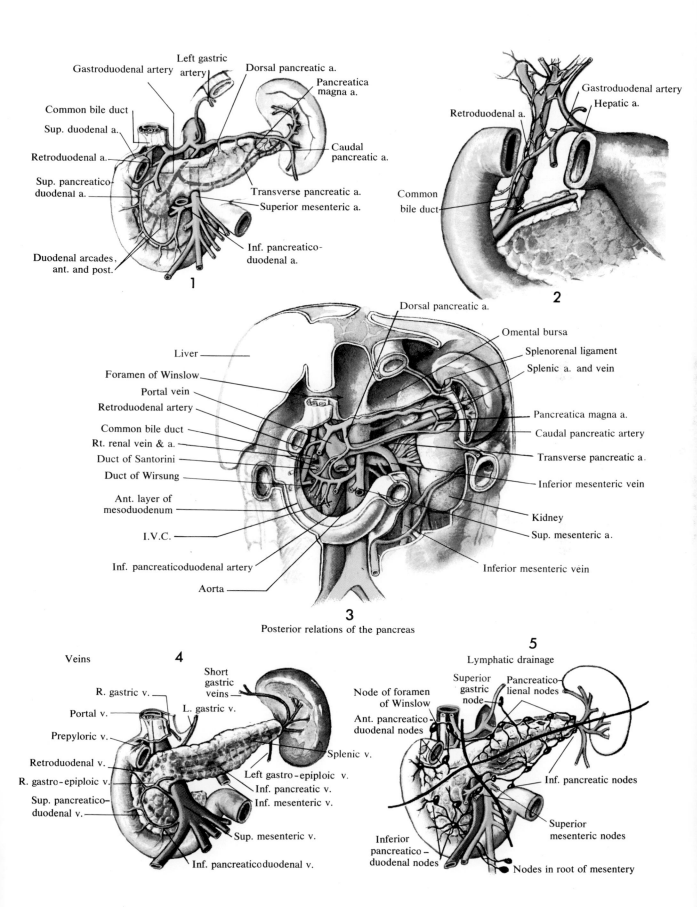

1

Gastroduodenal artery
Left gastric artery
Dorsal pancreatic a.
Pancreatica magna a.
Common bile duct
Sup. duodenal a.
Caudal pancreatic a.
Retroduodenal a.
Sup. pancreatico-duodenal a.
Transverse pancreatic a.
Superior mesenteric a.
Duodenal arcades, ant. and post.
Inf. pancreatico-duodenal a.

2

Gastroduodenal artery
Hepatic a.
Retroduodenal a.
Common bile duct

3

Dorsal pancreatic a.
Omental bursa
Splenorenal ligament
Splenic a. and vein
Liver
Foramen of Winslow
Portal vein
Retroduodenal artery
Common bile duct
Rt. renal vein & a.
Duct of Santorini
Duct of Wirsung
Ant. layer of mesoduodenum
I.V.C.
Inf. pancreaticoduodenal artery
Aorta
Pancreatica magna a.
Caudal pancreatic artery
Transverse pancreatic a.
Inferior mesenteric vein
Kidney
Sup. mesenteric a.
Inferior mesenteric vein

Posterior relations of the pancreas

4

Veins
Short gastric veins
R. gastric v.
Portal v.
L. gastric v.
Prepyloric v.
Retroduodenal v.
R. gastro-epiploic v.
Sup. pancreatico-duodenal v.
Splenic v.
Left gastro-epiploic v.
Inf. pancreatic v.
Inf. mesenteric v.
Sup. mesenteric v.
Inf. pancreaticoduodenal v.

5

Lymphatic drainage
Node of foramen of Winslow
Superior gastric node
Pancreatico-lienal nodes
Ant. pancreatico-duodenal nodes
Inf. pancreatic nodes
Inferior pancreatico-duodenal nodes
Superior mesenteric nodes
Nodes in root of mesentery

a. DUODENAL VEINS—closely follow the arteries and form anterior and posterior venous arcades. The *anterior and posterior inferior pancreaticoduodenal veins* both drain into the superior mesenteric. The *posterior superior pancreaticoduodenal vein* drains directly into the portal while its *anterior* counterpart empties into the right gastro-epiploic vein.

b. PANCREATIC VENOUS DRAINAGE—is by two main channels aside from the pancreaticoduodenal venous arcades previously described. The *splenic vein* receives numerous tributaries from the tail to the neck accompanying the arterial branches previously described: the dorsal and caudal pancreatic, pancreatic magna, and superior pancreatic. A second channel, the *inferior (transverse) vein* drains into the left side of the superior mesenteric.

9. **Lymphatic Drainage** (Fig. 5)—the lymph drainage of the pancreas is of main concern in this area because of the spread of cancer of the pancreas. No other organ in the abdomen has such a diffuse drainage, using both the supra- and infra-mesocolic compartments.

a. COLLECTING CHANNELS—emerge on the surface or along the border of the pancreas and are primarily directed in a superior and inferior direction. In addition, these collecting channels may be *arbitrarily* divided into right and left in line with the neck of the pancreas.

(1) *Left Superior Channels*—drain the upper part of the body and tail and end primarily in the *pancreaticolienal nodes* along the upper border of the pancreas. Direct channels may extend to the *superior gastric nodes* along the left gastric artery or directly into the *hepatic nodes*.

(2) *Left Inferior Channels*—drain the lower part of the body and tail and terminate in nodes along the inferior border (*inferior pancreatic nodes*) or into *superior mesenteric* and *left lumbar (paraortic) nodes*.

(3) *Right Superior Channels*—empty superiorly into the *subpyloric nodes* or directly into *hepatic nodes*. Some posterior channels pass to nodes on the posterior surface of the head of the pancreas (*posterior pancreaticoduodenal nodes*) thence to the *node of the foramen of Winslow* and *hepatic nodes*.

(4) *Right Inferior Channels*—from the anterior surface empty into *anterior pancreaticoduodenal* or directly into *nodes of the mesentery*. Posterior channels extend to *posterior pancreaticoduodenal nodes* or directly into the *superior mesenteric nodes* (Fig. 2, page 169).

PANCREAS: CLINICAL CONSIDERATIONS:

The pancreas is one of the most, if not the most, inaccessible of abdominal organs to the ordinary methods of physical examination. There is no method by which it can be delineated despite the advances in radiology and nuclear medicine. In spite of its physiological importance, clinical laboratory methods are still lacking in detection of any but the grossest abnormalities, with the exception of disturbances of the internal secretion of the islands of Langerhans. Symptoms produced by obstruction of the closely related common bile duct frequently are the first signs of disease of the pancreas.

1. **Pancreas Transplantation**—although the pancreas was the target of the earliest attempts at organ transplantation, success was not forthcoming. In recent years, however, with the successes achieved in renal transplants and the great strides made in vascular surgery and immunotherapy, new interest has ignited the field of surgical research.

As in other areas of organ transplantation a number of problems must be faced. Initially, pancreas transplants were reserved for those patients with *terminal* manifestations of diabetes mellitus. Many recipients were in need of or had had a renal transplant because of diabetic nephropathy. Best results are achieved, however, in patients who are nonuremic, non-kidney transplant recipients, i.e., those with *early* nephropathy, progressive retinopathy, and neuropathy.

The source of the donor pancreas may be a cadaveric specimen or a living donor who is tissue compatible. The graft may be a whole organ transplant with or without the duodenum or a segmental graft including the body and tail of the pancreas. Grafts may be stored in a hypothermic electrolyte solution, but the sooner the transplant is achieved, the greater the chance of survival in most cases.

The techniques involved in vascular and ductal reconstruction and drainage require maximal surgical skill, and they vary a great deal. The reader is referred to one of the latest textbooks of surgery for these variable alternatives. Whichever technique is chosen, rejection must be combated with one or a combination of the immunosuppressive drugs cyclosporine, azathioprine, and prednisone.

Although pancreatic transplants have not attained the success of renal transplants, they may in the future be an important factor in containing the progressive complications of diabetes mellitus.

(Text continued on page 166.)

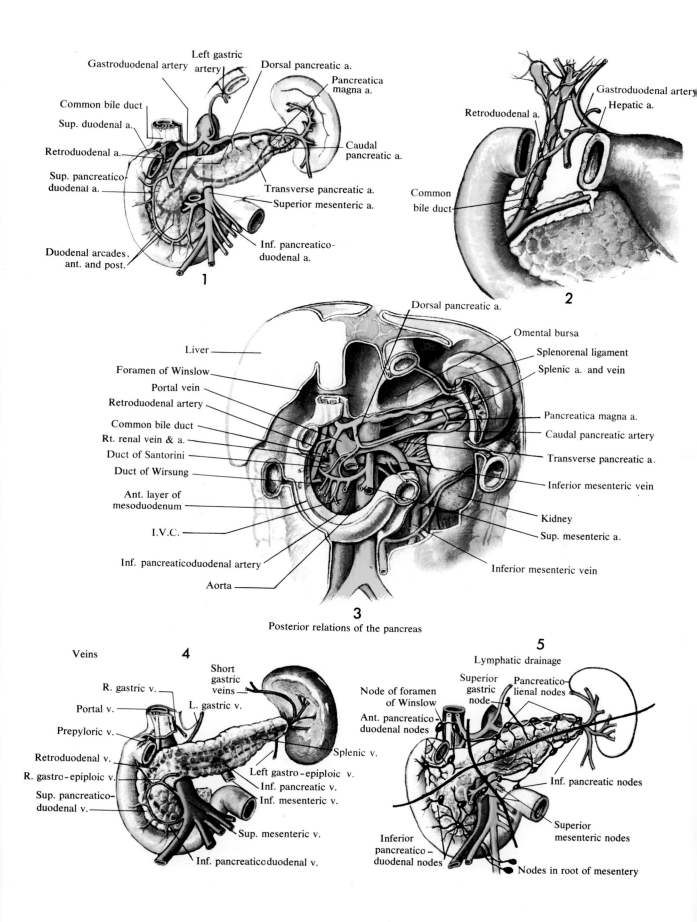

1

Left gastric artery
Gastroduodenal artery
Dorsal pancreatic a.
Pancreatica magna a.
Common bile duct
Sup. duodenal a.
Retroduodenal a.
Caudal pancreatic a.
Sup. pancreatico-duodenal a.
Transverse pancreatic a.
Superior mesenteric a.
Duodenal arcades, ant. and post.
Inf. pancreatico-duodenal a.

2

Gastroduodenal artery
Hepatic a.
Retroduodenal a.
Common bile duct

3

Dorsal pancreatic a.
Liver
Omental bursa
Foramen of Winslow
Splenorenal ligament
Portal vein
Splenic a. and vein
Retroduodenal artery
Common bile duct
Pancreatica magna a.
Rt. renal vein & a.
Caudal pancreatic artery
Duct of Santorini
Duct of Wirsung
Transverse pancreatic a.
Ant. layer of mesoduodenum
Inferior mesenteric vein
I.V.C.
Kidney
Sup. mesenteric a.
Inf. pancreaticoduodenal artery
Aorta
Inferior mesenteric vein

Posterior relations of the pancreas

4

Veins
Short gastric veins
R. gastric v.
L. gastric v.
Portal v.
Prepyloric v.
Splenic v.
Retroduodenal v.
R. gastro-epiploic v.
Left gastro-epiploic v.
Sup. pancreatico-duodenal v.
Inf. pancreatic v.
Inf. mesenteric v.
Sup. mesenteric v.
Inf. pancreaticoduodenal v.

5

Lymphatic drainage
Superior gastric node
Pancreatico-lienal nodes
Node of foramen of Winslow
Ant. pancreatico-duodenal nodes
Inf. pancreatic nodes
Inferior pancreatico-duodenal nodes
Superior mesenteric nodes
Nodes in root of mesentery

2. **Relational Anatomy**—the pancreas lies retroperitoneally in the epigastrium and left hypochondriac regions behind the posterior wall of the lesser peritoneal sac or omental bursa (Fig. 3, page 157). The important structures related to the posterior surface of the gland, including the inferior vena cava, aorta, superior mesenteric vessels, splenic and portal veins, and common bile duct, are shown in Figure 3, page 163. The splenic artery runs along the superior border of the pancreas, and the tail of the gland lies in contact with the hilum of the spleen. To the right the head of the pancreas is intimately related to the duodenum while in front the pancreas is separated from the stomach by the omental bursa. Any enlargement of the gland, either by tumor or cyst, will extend anteriorly due to the unyielding nature of the posterior abdominal wall. The layers of the transverse mesocolon attach to the anterior border of the gland. The anterior surface of the pancreas is therefore related to the lesser peritoneal cavity, whereas the inferior surface is related to the greater peritoneal cavity.

3. **Surgical Approaches**—access to the pancreas is usually accomplished by a transperitoneal route. Such an approach may be performed by entering the omental bursa through the gastrohepatic ligament, the gastrocolic ligament, or the transverse mesocolon (Fig. 8, page 149).

a. The gastrocolic ligament approach (Fig. 3)—is used in most surgical operations involving the pancreas, for it affords the best exposure of the entire gland. The stomach is retracted upward and the transverse colon downward. The incision through the gastrocolic ligament is made below the gastro-epiploic arterial arcade along the greater curvature of the stomach.

b. The gastrohepatic ligament approach—permits access to the superior surface of the pancreas but allows little room for surgical manipulation of the gland. Although this portion of the lesser omentum is usually avascular, an aberrant hepatic artery from the left gastric may be present.

c. The transverse mesocolon approach—likewise produces only limited exposure of the gland. The incision is made in the transverse mesocolon in the *avascular area of Riolan* located to the left of the midline between the middle colic artery on the right and the ascending branch of the left colic on the left side (Fig. 1, page 197).

4. **Congenital Anomalies**—several defects of pancreatic development produce clinical symptoms which necessitate surgical intervention.

a. Accessory pancreases—are not uncommon and develop as supernumerary primordia or displacement of parts of the original pancreatic anlage. They occur in relation to any derivative of the foregut or midgut as far distal as Meckel's diverticulum. They are most commonly found in the walls of the duodenum or stomach; rarely do they become so large as to produce intestinal obstruction and they may be discovered incidentally at operation. It should be kept in mind that these accessory pancreases may undergo the same pathological changes as may occur in the normally developed pancreas.

b. Annular pancreas—is unique in regard to congenital anomalies in that, although rare, in the majority of cases symptoms resulting from this deformity do not develop until later in life. In order to envision the development of this defect, the reader should refer to the embryology of the normal pancreas as described on page 160 and in particular of the ventral anlage of the pancreas. In the case of an annular pancreas, the ventral anlage divides into a right and left portion; the right rotating around the right side and the left around the left side of the duodenum. Both portions of the ventral anlage fuse with the dorsal anlage to form a ring of pancreatic tissue around the duodenum (Figs. 1 and 2). Duodenal obstruction is, of course, the major clinical finding. The surgical procedure of choice in cases which result in intestinal obstruction is to produce an anatomic bypass by means of a duodenojejunostomy. Direct attack upon the ring by dividing or resecting the pancreatic annulus frequently results in leakage of pancreatic juice which in turn produces further postoperative complications.

5. **Trauma**—because of its anatomic position, deep in the abdominal cavity and protected in part by the lower rib cage, the pancreas is only rarely involved in penetrating or nonpenetrating injuries to the abdominal wall. By far the most frequent cause of pancreatic trauma is operative injury particularly following gastric surgery. The surgeon should constantly alert his assistants during operative procedures involving supramesocolic organs of the possible injury retractors can cause to the pancreas.

6. **Pancreatic Cysts**—*true cysts* of the pancreas are rare and may be congenital or acquired. They may be retention cysts, hydatid and dermoid cysts, or cysts associated with adenoma or carcinoma of the gland. More frequent in occurrence is the presence of a so-called *pseudocyst*. This is a localized collection of fluid outside the substance of (but adjacent to) the pancreas. The fluid may be inflammatory exudate, pancreatic juices, or blood of the pancreas resulting from previous trauma or inflammation (pancreatitis) of the organ. The fluid lies in a retroperitoneal position and further enlargement proceeds in a forward direction producing a mass in the upper abdomen. The route of forward extension of these cysts vary; the most common varieties are illustrated in Figures 4 to 6.

7. **Sphincterotomy**—it has been suggested that pancreatitis may be due to regurgitation of bile into the pancreatic duct system as a result of either stricture or spasm of the ampulla of Vater. The anatomy of the ampulla is illustrated on page 173. In the relapsing form of pancreatitis it has been advocated that the muscular sphincter of the ampulla (*sphincter of Oddi*) be incised. The sphincterotomy may be performed by either of two anatomic approaches.

a. Endocholedochal sphincterotomy—requires a special instrument, the sphincterotome. An opening is made in the supraduodenal portion of the common bile duct and the instrument passed down the duct through the ampulla. Once in the lumen of the duodenum, the blade of the sphincterotome is released and

(Text continued on page 168.)

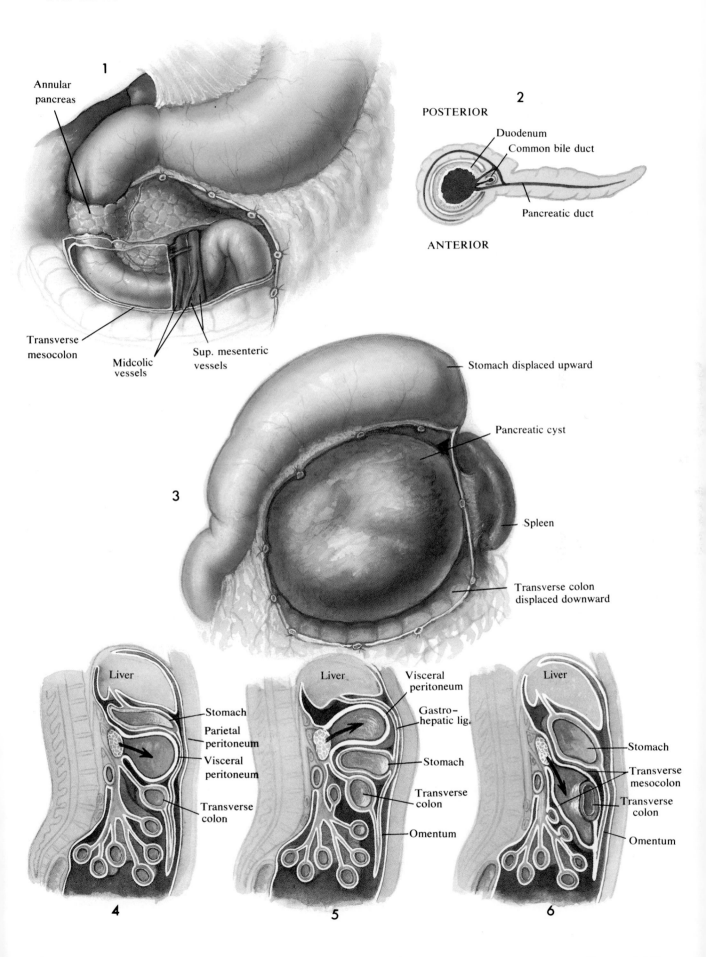

1

Annular
pancreas

Transverse
mesocolon

Midcolic
vessels

Sup. mesenteric
vessels

2

POSTERIOR

Duodenum

Common bile duct

Pancreatic duct

ANTERIOR

3

Stomach displaced upward

Pancreatic cyst

Spleen

Transverse colon
displaced downward

4

Liver

Stomach

Parietal
peritoneum

Visceral
peritoneum

Transverse
colon

5

Liver

Visceral
peritoneum

Gastro-
hepatic lig.

Stomach

Transverse
colon

Omentum

6

Liver

Stomach

Transverse
mesocolon

Transverse
colon

Omentum

hooked over the papilla. With the closure of the blade, the sphincter is cut.

b. TRANSDUODENAL SPHINCTEROTOMY—likewise requires an opening to be made in the supraduodenal portion of the common bile duct. Through this opening a probe is passed down the duct into the duodenum. The second portion of the duodenum is then opened and the ampulla with its sphincter is incised by direct vision over the end of the probe.

It must be remembered, however, that in only 75 per cent of people do the biliary and pancreatic ducts enter the duodenum as a common channel (page 160).

Endoscopic retrograde cannulation of the papilla of Vater (ERCP) has become a useful procedure for the diagnosis and treatment of biliary and pancreatic disease. By cannulating the papilla of Vater with a small tube introduced by way of the fiberoptic EGD scope and injecting contrast material, cholangiography and pancreatography can be performed.

Carcinoma of the papilla of Vater can be biopsied and stones in the common duct removed by electrosurgical papillotomy or sphincterotomy, performed by introducing a sphincterotome through the sheath of the fiberoptic scope.

Pancreatograms made by way of the papilla of Vater cannula outline the normal architecture of the pancreatic ducts and aid in the diagnosis of pancreatic cancer, chronic pancreatitis, annular pancreas, and disruption of the duct of Wirsung incidental to trauma. The alteration of the normal anatomy of the main pancreatic duct aids in determining the operability of pancreatic neoplasms.

8. **Anatomic Principles of Pancreaticoduodenal Resections**—the indications for partial resection of the pancreas can be found in any surgical textbook. In such a resection certain anatomic principles must be followed.

a. RESECTION OF THE HEAD AND NECK OF THE PANCREAS—also requires resection of the lower end of the common bile duct, the lower one-third of the stomach and the duodenum. An incision is made through the lesser omentum and, along the lesser curvature of the stomach and the superior border of the first portion of the duodenum (Fig. 1). The peritoneum to the right of the second portion of the duodenum is incised and the duodenum, along with the head of the pancreas, is reflected anteriorly and to the left (Fig. 2). This maneuver allows inspection of the posterior surface of the head and the removal of appropriate posterior pancreaticoduodenal lymph nodes for biopsy and the assessment of operability.

To completely mobilize the duodenum and the head and neck of the pancreas it is necessary to cut the gastrocolic ligament as shown in Figure 3. The stomach, duodenum, common bile duct, and neck of the pancreas are transected (Fig. 4). The pancreas is transected just to the left of the superior mesenteric vessels, and the venous tributaries from the posterior surface of the head and neck, which enter directly into the anterior and right lateral aspects of the portal vein (Fig. 4, page 163), are isolated and divided. This maneuver is tedious because the veins are small and thin-walled and if they are torn from the side of the major vein bleeding can be very brisk.

b. RECONSTRUCTION—of the biliary, gastrointestinal and pancreatic systems is necessary following the resection.

The biliary drainage may be re-established by a number of different procedures. The choice will depend upon the anatomic conditions encountered in the individual case. In the majority of instances the common bile duct is anastomosed to the jejunum *(choledochojejunostomy)* either end-to-end or end-to-side.

To re-establish pancreatic drainage the pancreatic stump is implanted into the jejunum *(pancreaticojejunostomy)* either by end-to-end or end-to-side anastomosis. This technique is advocated by the majority of surgeons. A few insist upon the identification and implantation of the major pancreatic duct into the jejunum.

The reconstruction of the gastrointestinal continuity will also vary depending upon the individual anatomic situation and the preference of the surgeon. But whatever technique is utilized, it will require a *gastrojejunostomy*. Whether or not a complimentary jejunojejunostomy need be performed will depend upon the overall anatomic arrangement.

9. **Anatomic Principles for Resection of the Body and Tail**—certain pathologic processes in the pancreas may require resection of only the body and tail of this organ. The blood supply of the body and tail of the pancreas comes chiefly from short branches of the splenic vessels (Fig. 1, page 163). It is virtually impossible to dissect and isolate individually these vessels if disease is present. The splenic vessels and spleen are, therefore, removed en bloc along with the pancreas.

a. RESECTION OF THE BODY AND TAIL—is initiated by incising the gastrocolic and gastrosplenic ligaments (Fig. 5), preserving the gastro-epiploic arterial arcade. The phrenicocolic ligament is severed in order to depress the splenic flexure of the large bowel from the operative area. The splenic artery is identified at the superior border of the pancreas and ligated well to the right of the spleen (Fig. 6). The peritoneal attachment to the lower border of the pancreas is incised, care being taken not to injure the superior mesenteric vessels and the middle colic artery. The tail of the pancreas is elevated with care so as not to injure the underlying left kidney and its hilar structures. Next the splenic vein is isolated along the superior border of the pancreas and ligated.

It is most important at this stage of dissection to identify the entrance of the inferior mesenteric vein, for the splenic vein *must* be ligated to the left of the entrance of the inferior mesenteric into the splenic vein (Fig. 6).

After resection of the neck of the pancreas, the body and tail along with the spleen are removed en bloc.

No reconstruction procedures are required following resection of the body and tail of the pancreas.

10. **Total Pancreatectomy**—should total pancreatectomy be indicated, a combination of the two above procedures are performed. The pancreas, of course, need not be transected. Again it must be emphasized that the splenic vein be ligated just to the left of the entrance of the inferior mesenteric tributary.

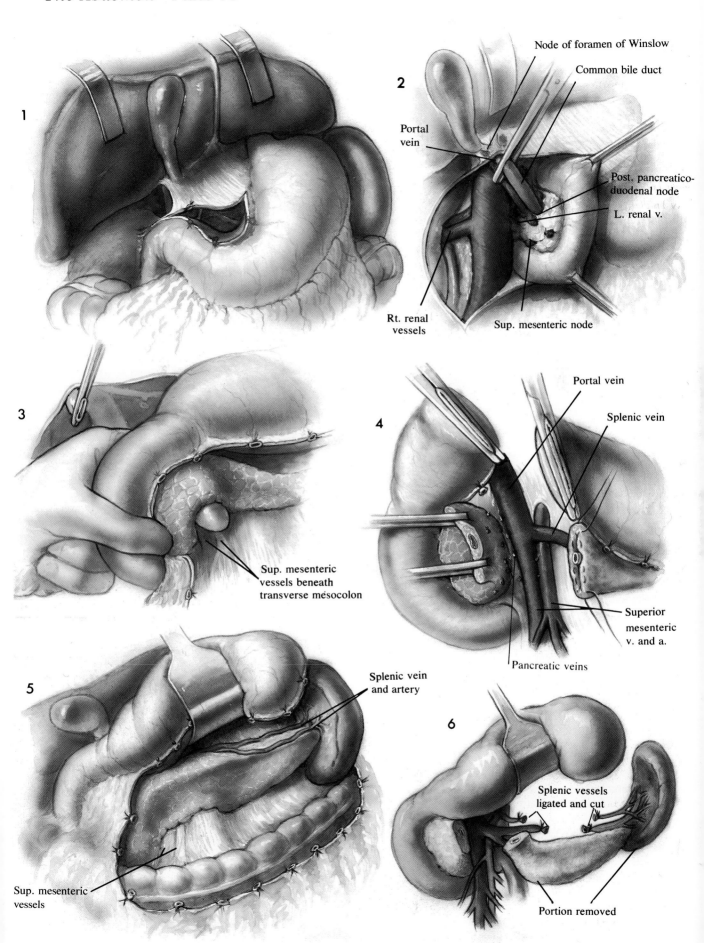

1

2

Node of foramen of Winslow

Common bile duct

Portal vein

Post. pancreatico-duodenal node

L. renal v.

Rt. renal vessels

Sup. mesenteric node

3

Sup. mesenteric vessels beneath transverse mesocolon

4

Portal vein

Splenic vein

Superior mesenteric v. and a.

Pancreatic veins

5

Splenic vein and artery

Sup. mesenteric vessels

6

Splenic vessels ligated and cut

Portion removed

SPLEEN:

The spleen is of concern to the surgeon when conditions indicate that it must be removed. Such conditions include trauma, tumors, and certain hematologic diseases resulting in splenic hyperactivity.

1. **Embryology**—the spleen develops within the double-layered dorsal mesogastrium as a condensation of mesenchymal cells and originally possesses two peritoneal ligaments: the *gastrosplenic* anteriorly and the *splenoaortic* posteriorly. With the rotation of the foregut, the latter becomes the *splenorenal (lienorenal) ligament.* (Figs. 2 and 3, page 149).

2. **Topography**—the spleen lies obliquely in the left hypochondrium under the cover of the ninth, tenth, and eleventh ribs. Because of this concealed position beneath the costal arch, the spleen is not normally palpable. The long axis of the organ runs parallel to the tenth rib (Fig. 1). The relationship of the costodiaphragmatic reflection of the parietal pleura is important. At the midaxillary line, this reflection occurs at the level of the tenth rib. This fact must be kept in mind during procedures such as *splenic needle biopsy* and the injection of radio-opaque media for *splenoportography* (Fig. 2).

3. **Ligaments**—the spleen is completely encased in double peritoneal coverings except in the hilar area where the peritoneal reflections to the neighboring organs are termed ligaments.

a. GASTROSPLENIC LIGAMENT (Figs. 3 and 4)—connects the left portion of the greater curvature of the stomach with the hilus of the spleen and is continuous with the greater omentum below. The short gastric vessels and the left gastro-epiploic vessels arise within this double layer of peritoneum and drain into the splenic vessels.

b. SPLENORENAL (LIENORENAL) LIGAMENT (Figs. 3 and 4)—is also a doubled layer of peritoneum extending between the hilus of the spleen and the ventral aspect of the left kidney. Within the layers of this ligament are located the splenic artery and vein.

c. PHRENICOCOLIC LIGAMENT (Fig. 3)—is a fold of peritoneum extending from the diaphragm at the level of the tenth and eleventh ribs to the left colic (splenic) flexure. Upon this ligament rests the inferior extremity of the spleen.

4. **Relations** (Figs. 3 and 4)—the shape of the spleen, like the liver is for the most part dependent upon the firmer related structures.

a. DIAPHRAGMATIC SURFACE—posterolaterally faces the concavity of the diaphragm.

b. GASTRIC SURFACE—consists of the ventral surface lying anterior to the hilus of the spleen and rests against the fundus and body of the stomach.

c. RENAL SURFACE—is that part of the ventral surface lying behind the hilus of the spleen and related to the anterior surface of the left kidney and adrenal gland.

d. COLIC SURFACE—is the base which is related to the splenic flexure of the colon and lies on the phrenocolic ligament.

e. ANTERIOR BORDER—forms a sharp convex line with notches which are of diagnostic importance in differentiating splenic enlargements from other abdominal enlargements.

5. **Arterial Supply** (Figs. 3 and 4)—in the majority of cases, the splenic artery arises from the celiac axis and extends along the upper border of the pancreas in a rather tortuous course and passes in front of the tail of the pancreas where it divides into terminal branches which are extremely variable. The pancreatic branches have been discussed on page 162). The splenic terminal branches are usually described as *superior* and *inferior terminal branches.*

a. SUPERIOR TERMINAL BRANCH—usually arises from the main trunk about 4 cm. from the hilus and after giving rise to the short gastric arteries enters the hilus.

b. INFERIOR TERMINAL BRANCH—artery gives rise to the left gastroepiploic artery before entering the hilus.

c. POLAR ARTERIES—are very common, both superior and inferior. The *superior polar artery* usually arises from the splenic trunk before its terminal division. An *inferior polar artery* is more common and usually arises from the left gastro-epiploic artery.

6. **Venous Drainage** (Fig. 4, page 163)—is conducted by several large veins that issue from the hilus of the spleen and unite after a short course to form the *splenic vein.* This large channel passes to the dorsal surface of the pancreas and extends from left to right. Behind the neck of the pancreas the splenic joins the *superior mesenteric* vein to form the *portal vein.* The *short gastric veins* draining the fundus of the stomach, the left *gastro-epiploic vein* and multiple *pancreatic* veins, also empty into the splenic vein. Another important tributary of the splenic vein is the *inferior mesenteric vein;* however, this vein may drain into the superior mesenteric or into the angle of union of the splenic and superior mesenteric.

7. **Lymphatic Drainage**—capillaries from the capsule and trabeculae form a subcapsular plexus from which lymph channels pass to the *splenic nodes (pancreaticolienal group)* along the splenic vessels. These nodes also receive channels from the stomach and pancreas.

8. **Splenectomy**—Two anatomic pathways are available to the surgeon in the approach to the splenic vessels. In one, the vessels are ligated before any attempt is made to mobilize the spleen. This approach is made through the gastrosplenic and gastrocolic ligaments, thus opening the omental bursa. The posterior parietal peritoneum is incised at the superior border of the pancreas about 2 inches from the hilus of the spleen, thus exposing the splenic vessels.

Another approach is possible if the spleen is free of adhesions and can be pulled forward through the abdominal wound; the left side of the splenorenal ligament may be exposed and the splenic vessels ligated at this location from the general peritoneal cavity. During a splenectomy, the surgeon must remember the intimate relationship of the tail of the pancreas to the hilus to prevent injury to this organ.

1

Midaxillary line

9th rib

10th rib

Point of puncture

2

Lung

Pleura

8th rib

Diaphragm

9th rib

10th rib

Spleen

11th rib

3

Esophagophrenic ligament

Esophagus

Left gastric artery

Omental bursa

Splenic artery

Hepatoduodenal lig.

Pancreas covered by posterior parietal peritoneum

Right gastro-epiploic a. and v.

Superior mesenteric artery and vein

Splenorenal ligament

Omental bursa

Gastrosplenic ligament

Short gastric arteries

Left gastro-epiploic artery

Gastrosplenic ligament

Transverse mesocolon

Phrenicocolic ligament

Transverse mesocolon

Posterior parietal peritoneum covering kidney

4

Right kidney

Diaphragm

Foramen of Winslow

Portal vein

Common bile duct

Hepatic arteries

Lesser omentum

I.V.C.

Aorta

Celiac artery

Pancreas

Left kidney

Splenorenal lig.

Spleen

Left gastro-epiploic a.

Gastrosplenic lig.

Parietal peritoneum

Omental bursa

Splenic artery

Stomach

GALLBLADDER, EXTRAHEPATIC DUCTS, AND HEPATIC PEDICLE:

The region of the hepatic pedicle is probably the most frequent site in the body for serious operative complications. This is due to the frequency of gallbladder surgery and the extreme variation in the anatomy of this area.

1. **Hepatic Ducts**—these ducts will be considered with the liver (see page 176).

2. **Gallbladder**—this organ develops as a secondary outpouching of the original hepatic diverticulum distal to the ventral anlage of the pancreas (Fig. 1, page 161). The proximal part of this secondary outpouching becomes the cystic duct.

a. PARTS—the gallbladder is a pear-shaped organ lying in a fossa on the visceral surface of the liver (Fig. 2). A portion usually extends beyond the lower border of the liver and is termed the *fundus* which is almost completely covered by peritoneum. The fundus may be folded upon itself which radiologists designate as the *phrygian cap*. Topographically, the fundus lies at the angle of the ninth costal cartilage and right lateral border of the rectus muscle. The parts include the *body* which continues into the tapering *neck* which opens into the cystic duct. On the ventral aspect of the bladder just proximal to the neck a dilatation may be present, *Hartmann's pouch* (Fig. 1A). Stones may lodge in this sac and if inflamed it may adhere to the cystic or even the common duct. It may also be used by the surgeon as a point of traction making for easier identification of the cystic duct.

b. BLOOD SUPPLY—the gallbladder is supplied by the *cystic artery* which is commonly a branch of the right hepatic. As it approaches the neck it divides into a *superficial* and *deep cystic* artery. The cystic artery usually lies in the *cystohepatic triangle (Calot)* which is bounded by the cystic and common hepatic ducts and the liver above (Fig. 2). The venous drainage of the gallbladder is usually by multiple channels which empty into the portal vein in the region of the porta hepatis.

c. LYMPHATIC DRAINAGE—lymphatic drainage of this organ is mainly into two constant nodes: one, the *node of the cystic angle*; the other, the node of the *foramen of Winslow* (Fig. 2).

3. **Cystic Duct**—this duct extends from the neck of the gallbladder to its union with the common hepatic duct (Fig. 1A). This union is predominately of the *angular* type in the hepatoduodenal ligament. However, a *parallel* type is not uncommon (20 per cent) and can be of particular significance when it is long and adheres to the common hepatic duct by connective tissue (Fig. 3A). A less common type (10 per cent) is the *spiral union* in which the cystic duct passes in front of or behind the common hepatic duct to enter from the left side (Fig. 3B). *Aberrant right hepatic ducts* (28 per cent) are of significance in regard to the cystic duct (Fig. 3C); indeed, the cystic duct may empty into one of these rather than the common hepatic duct. These ducts are usually erroneously referred to as *"accessory" right hepatic ducts*, but it has been shown that they are aberrant segments or subsegment ducts of the right lobe and

are the only drainage of that specific part of the liver (page 180). In the true definition of the word, therefore, "accessory" hepatic ducts do not exist. The cystic duct is guarded by the *spiral valve of Heister* (Fig. 1A).

4. **Common Bile Duct**—the anatomy of the common bile duct has already been discussed on pages 160 and 162. The sphincters of the common bile duct and pancreatic duct as well as their common sphincter (*sphincter of Oddi*) are illustrated in Figures 1B and C.

5. **Hepatic Pedicle** (Fig. 2)—The major components are:

a. HEPATODUODENAL LIGAMENT—is the lowermost portion of the lesser omentum which is derived from the ventral mesentery. It is a double layer of peritoneum surrounding the structures of the pedicle and forms the anterior boundary of the epiploic foramen.

b. EXTRAHEPATIC BILE DUCTS—have been discussed above and on pages 160 and 162. In the pedicle the common duct occupies a position anterior and to the right, while the cystic and common hepatic ducts along with the lower border of the liver form the important *cystohepatic triangle (Calot)*. It is in this triangle that one most frequently finds the cystic and right hepatic arteries as well as most aberrant segmental right hepatic ducts and arteries.

c. HEPATIC ARTERY—arises from the celiac axis as the common hepatic artery which courses between the layers of the original dorsal mesentery to the upper border of the first portion of the duodenum. Here it terminates by dividing into a descending branch, the *gastroduodenal*, and an ascending branch, the *hepatic propria*. The latter ascends in the hepatoduodenal ligament parallel and to the left of the common duct. The hepatic propria bifurcates into a right and left branch. The *right hepatic artery* usually passes behind the common hepatic duct (87 per cent) but may pass anterior to the duct (11 per cent). It terminates by dividing into an anterior and posterior segment artery (page 178). Rarely, the two segment arteries arise independently from the hepatic propria. Such cases are referred to as *double right hepatic arteries* (Fig. 4A). The *left hepatic artery* divides into medial and lateral segment arteries (page 178). In 25 per cent of people examined, these segment arteries may arise as separate trunks from the hepatic propria as *double left hepatic arteries* (Fig. 4B). "Accessory" hepatic arteries are frequently described in the literature which gives the surgeon the impression that such arteries are supplying a portion of the liver already supplied by the celiac hepatic. Such is not the case, for each artery entering the liver supplies a specific part of that organ without any gross anastomoses with other hepatic branches. The "accessory" hepatic arteries actually represent aberrant segment or subsegment arteries to the liver. The most frequent site of origin of *aberrant left hepatic arteries* is from the left gastric (23 per cent) and the *aberrant right hepatic* from the superior mesenteric (17 per cent) (Fig. 4C and D). The latter courses anterior and to the right of the portal vein in the hepatoduodenal ligament and its possible presence should be kept in mind during a portacaval shunt.

d. PORTAL VEIN—in the hepatic pedicle lies posterior in position behind the common duct and hepatic propria artery.

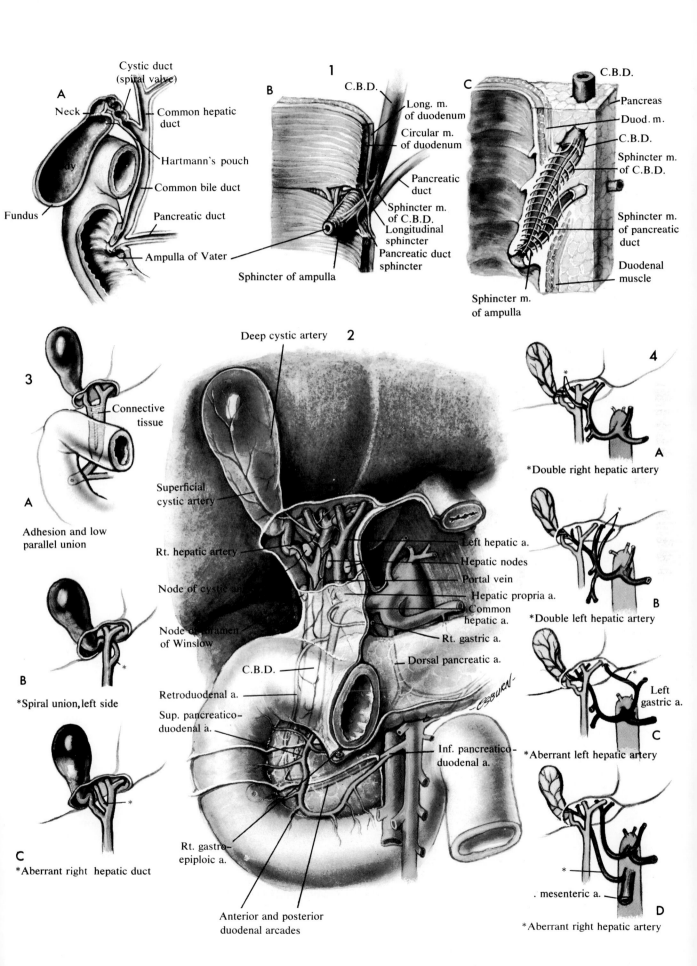

A

Cystic duct
(spiral valve)

Neck

Common hepatic
duct

Hartmann's pouch

Common bile duct

Pancreatic duct

Fundus

Ampulla of Vater

1

B

C.B.D.

Long. m.
of duodenum

Circular m.
of duodenum

Pancreatic
duct

Sphincter m.
of C.B.D.
Longitudinal
sphincter

Pancreatic duct
sphincter

Sphincter of ampulla

C

C.B.D.

Pancreas

Duod. m.

C.B.D.

Sphincter m.
of C.B.D.

Sphincter m.
of pancreatic
duct

Duodenal
muscle

Sphincter m.
of ampulla

3

Connective
tissue

A

Adhesion and low
parallel union

B

*Spiral union, left side

C

*Aberrant right hepatic duct

Deep cystic artery

2

Superficial
cystic artery

Rt. hepatic artery

Node of cystic

Node of foramen
of Winslow

C.B.D.

Retroduodenal a.

Sup. pancreatico-
duodenal a.

Rt. gastro-
epiploic a.

Anterior and posterior
duodenal arcades

Left hepatic a.

Hepatic nodes

Portal vein

Hepatic propria a.

Common
hepatic a.

Rt. gastric a.

Dorsal pancreatic a.

Inf. pancreatico-
duodenal a.

4

A

*Double right hepatic artery

B

*Double left hepatic artery

Left
gastric a.

C

*Aberrant left hepatic artery

. mesenteric a.

D

*Aberrant right hepatic artery

GALLBLADDER AND EXTRAHEPATIC BILE DUCTS: CLINICAL CONSIDERATIONS:

There is probably no other anatomic region in the human body that is so beset with variations of the "normal" pattern of arrangement than the hepatic pedicle. This normal arrangement is described on page 172. Because of the frequent need to operate on the gallbladder and extrahepatic biliary duct system, the surgeon should be fully cognizant of this prevailing pattern and aware that variations are extremely common. Some investigators claim that major variations of the ducts and arteries occur in about two-thirds of the bodies examined. *In order to avoid anatomic errors one should clearly identify all three biliary ducts, together with the cystic and hepatic arteries before dividing any of these structures.*

1. **Surgical Approach**—aside from the ignorance of variational anatomy of the hepatic pedicle, inadequate exposure of these deeply placed anatomic structures is the most frequent cause of surgical errors in this area. The choice of the surgical incision may vary with the planned procedure, the individual body build, and the preference of the operator. The most popular incisions include a right upper paramedian, a right upper transverse, or a right oblique subcostal.

2. **Congenital Anomalies**—congenital anomalies of the gallbladder such as agenesis, duplication, diverticula, and malposition produce no clinical symptoms and concern the surgeon only when the gallbladder is diseased. All developmental anomalies of the biliary duct system are of surgical significance.

   a. ATRESIA—may involve any or all of the biliary ducts. The gallbladder and extrahepatic ducts arise as entodermal tubular outpouchings (Fig. 1, page 161), which are at first patent, then become secondarily obliterated, and then are finally recanalized. Failure of recanalization of part or all of the ducts results in atresia. The most frequent patterns in order of occurrence are: (1) complete atresia of the gallbladder and all ducts, (2) atresia of the extrahepatic ducts only, (3) atresia of the hepatic ducts, and (4) atresia of the common bile duct. Such anomalies are incompatible with life; however, one-fifth of such cases may be surgically corrected.

   b. CYSTIC FORMATION (CHOLEDOCHAL CYST)—is a localized spherical enlargement of the whole or part of the common bile duct. This defect may arise during the stage of recanalization. Symptoms may not be present until the juvenile years. The anomaly is best treated by anastomosis of the biliary system to the intestinal tract.

   c. OTHER ANOMALIES OF THE EXTRAHEPATIC DUCTS—include doubling of the common bile duct, aberrant drainage of the hepatic, cystic, and common bile ducts, and the so-called "accessory" hepatic ducts. Some of these variations have already been discussed on page 172.

3. **Operative Procedures**—surgical operations upon the gallbladder and bile ducts are many and varied. They consist of simple incision, removal, by-pass, and reconstructive procedures.

   a. INCISION—of the gallbladder is used to create a temporary external biliary fistula by the insertion of a drainage tube into the cavity of the bladder and bringing it through the abdominal wall (*cholecystostomy*). An incision into the common duct (*choledochotomy*) is made to explore, dilate, and drain or to remove stones. It may be made in the supraduodenal or retroduodenal portions of the duct or directly through the duodenum (*transduodenal choledochoduodenostomy*).

   b. REMOVAL—of the gallbladder (*cholecystectomy*) may be performed either from the fundus downward or from the cystic duct upward. Following adequate surgery the individual may lead a normal life. If, however, a portion of the common bile duct is removed (as in a resection of the head of the pancreas) a by-pass or reconstructive procedure must be performed if life is to be maintained.

   c. BY-PASS PROCEDURE—may be accomplished after resection or obstruction of the common bile duct only if the gallbladder is intact. This is usually done by anastomosing the gallbladder to the intestines (*cholecystoenterostomy*) either into the duodenum or jejunum or, rarely, into the stomach (*cholecystogastrostomy*).

   d. RECONSTRUCTIVE—these procedures of the biliary tract system will vary depending upon the length and site of the obstruction. Both proximal and distal ends may be joined by direct end-to-end anastomosis, or the distal end of the duct may be joined preferably to the intestines (*choledochoenterostomy*) or to the stomach (*choledochogastrostomy*). Should only the common hepatic duct be patent, similar anatomic continuity can be re-established (*hepatoenterostomy* or *hepatogastrostomy*). Should there be insufficient length of the common hepatic duct direct anastomosis of the liver with the intestinal tract can be made either without (*hepatoenterostomy*) or with partial hepatectomy (*intrahepatic cholangiojejunostomy*).

4. **Extrahepatic Bile Duct Obstruction**—may be due to extramural, intramural, or intraluminal causes. Figures 1 to 8 illustrate some of these causes.

   Whatever the cause, obstruction anywhere from the ampulla to the junction of the right and left hepatic ducts will result in obstructive type jaundice (Fig. 6).

5. **Surgical Injury**—injury to the ductal system is far too frequent and often tragic. Awareness of the anatomic variations encountered in gallbladder surgery will help prevent many such accidents. Figure 7 illustrates one of the most common causes, i.e., excessive traction, particularly upon the fundus, resulting in injury to the common hepatic and common bile duct while clamping the cystic duct. Failure to recognize a long cystic duct of the parallel type is also common (Figs. 8 and 3A, page 173). A hurried blind clamping to control brisk hemorrhage, however, is the most common fault. Such a hemorrhage should be controlled by compression of the hepatoduodenal ligament between the thumb and index finger as shown in Figure 9 (Pringle's method).

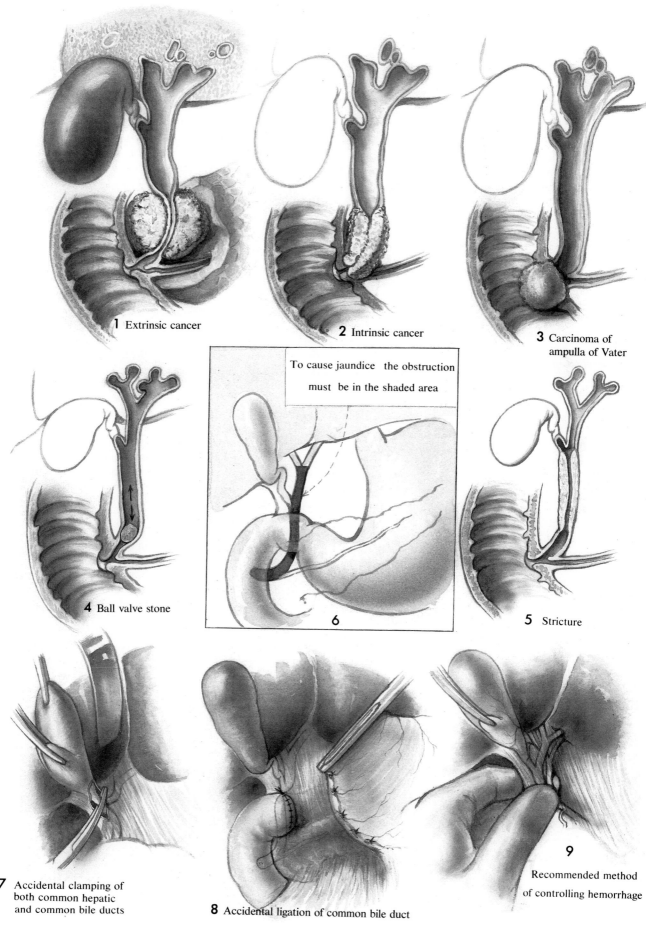

1 Extrinsic cancer

2 Intrinsic cancer

3 Carcinoma of ampulla of Vater

4 Ball valve stone

To cause jaundice the obstruction must be in the shaded area

6

5 Stricture

7 Accidental clamping of both common hepatic and common bile ducts

8 Accidental ligation of common bile duct

9 Recommended method of controlling hemorrhage

ANATOMY OF THE LIVER:

The liver arises as a ventral outpouching from the caudal portion of the foregut, extends into the ventral mesentery, and develops into the largest organ in the body. Newer diagnostic radiologic procedures, such as selective hepatic artery catheterization and portal venography and cholangiography, as well as the more frequent and radical surgical procedures now being performed require not only a knowledge of the extrahepatic but also the intrahepatic anatomy of this organ.

1. **Divisions of the Liver**—the true anatomic division of the liver into its right and left lobe is not in line with the attachment of the falciform ligament, but rather in line with the fossa of the gallbladder below and the inferior vena cava above as shown in cast specimens of the intrahepatic structures. This true anatomic division, termed the *main lobar fissure,* divides the liver into almost equal-sized right and left lobes. Each lobe is divided further in these cast specimens by fissures. The right lobe is divided by the *right segmental fissure* into an *anterior* and *posterior segment*, whereas the left lobe is divided by the *left segmental fissure* into a *medial* and *lateral segment* (Fig. 1*A, B,* and *C*). The term "quadrate lobe," in the older descriptions of the liver, is that portion lying on the visceral surface between the gallbladder fossa and the unbilical fossa. This area is actually a part of the medial segment (Fig. 1*C*). The *caudate lobe,* also seen on the visceral surface, lying between the fossa of the inferior vena cava and the fossa of the ligamentum venosum is a liver appendage which drains into both right and left hepatic duct systems.

2. **Ligamentous Attachments** (Fig. 2)—peritoneal reflections and remnants of the ventral mesentery form certain ligamentous attachments which aid in the fixation of the liver.

a. Coronary ligaments (anterior and posterior)—are formed by anterior and posterior reflections of peritoneum from the diaphragm upon the superior and posterior surface of the liver. The extraperitoneal area of the liver between these peritoneal reflections is referred to as the "bare area" (Fig. 2*A* and *B*). This bare area is roughly quadrangular in shape and at each of the four angles the layers of peritoneum join and are prolonged as ligaments.

b. Left triangular ligament—is a long, narrow prolongation of the coronary ligaments to the left. Patent bile ducts may occasionally (5 per cent) extend into this ligament.

c. Right triangular ligament—is similarly formed by the fusion of the coronary ligaments on the right side although it is much less conspicuous than the left triangular ligament.

d. Falciform ligament—extends between the liver and anterior abdominal wall as a remnant of the prehepatic portion of the ventral mesentery (Fig. 2, page 149) and is continuous with the anterior coronary ligaments. Its lower free border is termed the *ligamentum teres hepatis* and encloses the obliterated left umbilical vein.

e. Gastrohepatic ligament (lesser omentum)—represents the posthepatic portion of the ventral mesentery, the lower free border forming the hepatoduodenal ligament (Fig. 2, page 149), and is continuous with the posterior coronary ligament covering the obliterated fetal ductus venosus as the *ligamentum venosum.*

3. **Biliary Drainage of the Liver** (Fig. 3)—a segment duct emerges from each of the four major segments of the liver. The two segment ducts of each lobe join to form the right and left hepatic ducts which in turn unite to form the common hepatic duct.

a. Ducts of the right lobe—consist of *anterior* and *posterior segment ducts.* The segment ducts are formed by the union of the superior and inferior area (subsegment) ducts of each segment. The posterior duct is longer and somewhat superior in position. These ducts extend medially to the region of the porta hepatis where the two segment ducts join to form the *right hepatic duct.* Not infrequently (35 per cent) a long filamentous duct lies in the gallbladder bed and empties into either the anterior segment or right hepatic duct. This *subvesical duct* is superficial in position and is often attached to the undersurface of the gallbladder which places it in a very precarious position during cholecystectomies.

b. Ducts of the left lobe—taking exit from the two segments are termed the *lateral* and *medial segment ducts.* The lateral segment duct drains that portion of the liver described as the "left lobe" in the old terminology, and is formed by the union of the superior and inferior subsegment ducts. The medial segment duct joins the lateral segment duct in the porta hepatis and forms the *left hepatic duct.*

c. Ducts of the caudate lobe—are usually three in number: one draining the caudate process, one the right portion of the caudate lobe proper, and one the left portion. These ducts drain into both right and left hepatic duct systems. Communications between these two duct systems in the region of the caudate lobe could not be demonstrated.

d. Common hepatic duct—begins in the porta hepatis as a union of the right and left hepatic ducts and descends in the hepatoduodenal ligament for a variable distance where it is joined by the cystic duct coming in from the right side at a variable angle. The common hepatic duct averages about 4 cm. in length but varies considerably, depending upon the point of union with the cystic duct. Some of the variations have been discussed on page 172.

(Text continued on page 178.)

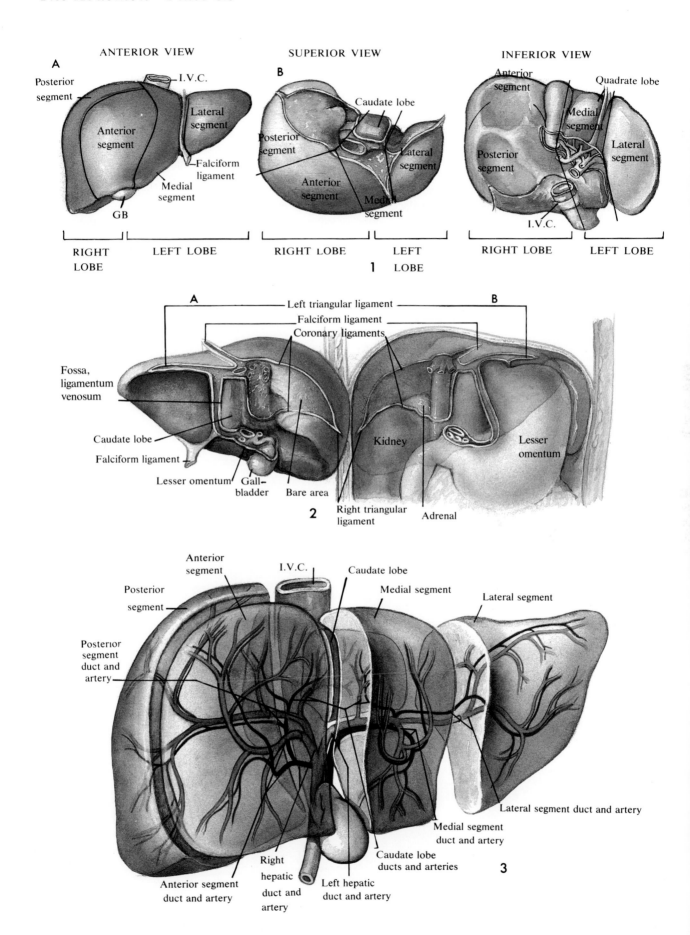

ANTERIOR VIEW

A

Posterior segment

I.V.C.

Anterior segment

Lateral segment

Falciform ligament

Medial segment

GB

RIGHT LOBE

LEFT LOBE

SUPERIOR VIEW

B

Caudate lobe

Posterior segment

Anterior segment

Lateral segment

Medial segment

RIGHT LOBE

LEFT LOBE

1

INFERIOR VIEW

Anterior segment

Quadrate lobe

Medial segment

Posterior segment

Lateral segment

I.V.C.

RIGHT LOBE

LEFT LOBE

A

Left triangular ligament

B

Falciform ligament

Coronary ligaments

Fossa, ligamentum venosum

Caudate lobe

Falciform ligament

Lesser omentum

Gall-bladder

Bare area

Right triangular ligament

Kidney

Adrenal

Lesser omentum

2

Anterior segment

I.V.C.

Caudate lobe

Posterior segment

Medial segment

Lateral segment

Posterior segment duct and artery

Anterior segment duct and artery

Right hepatic duct and artery

Left hepatic duct and artery

Caudate lobe ducts and arteries

Medial segment duct and artery

Lateral segment duct and artery

3

4. Arterial Supply to the Liver (Fig. 3)—the main arterial branch to the liver is via the *hepatica propria* branch of the common hepatic artery from the celiac.

a. HEPATICA PROPRIA—ascends in the hepato-duodenal ligament for a variable distance and divides into a right and left hepatic branch.

b. RIGHT HEPATIC—usually passes behind the common hepatic duct and after giving rise to the cystic artery as it transverses the hepatocystic triangle, terminates by dividing into an *anterior* and *posterior segment artery*. The anterior segment artery is more inferior in position and takes a serpentine course, looping downward toward the gallbladder fossa, which places this artery in a vulnerable position during operative procedures on the gallbladder. In its intrahepatic course the artery runs along the inferior border of the anterior segment duct and divides into a superior and an inferior area artery.

c. LEFT HEPATIC ARTERY—passes obliquely upward and to the left in the porta hepatis for a short distance and divides into two terminal branches: the *medial* and *lateral segment artery*. The medial segment artery in its *normal* anatomic position arises from the inferior surface of the left hepatic and descends into that portion of the liver formerly described as the quadrate lobe and divides into superior and inferior area branches. From extrahepatic dissections, this artery has been termed the ramus media, middle hepatic, or quadrate lobe artery.

d. CAUDATE LOBE ARTERIES—are usually two in number: one, arising from the right hepatic artery which supplies the caudate process and right portion of the caudate lobe proper; the other, from the left hepatic, supplies the left portion of the caudate lobe proper.

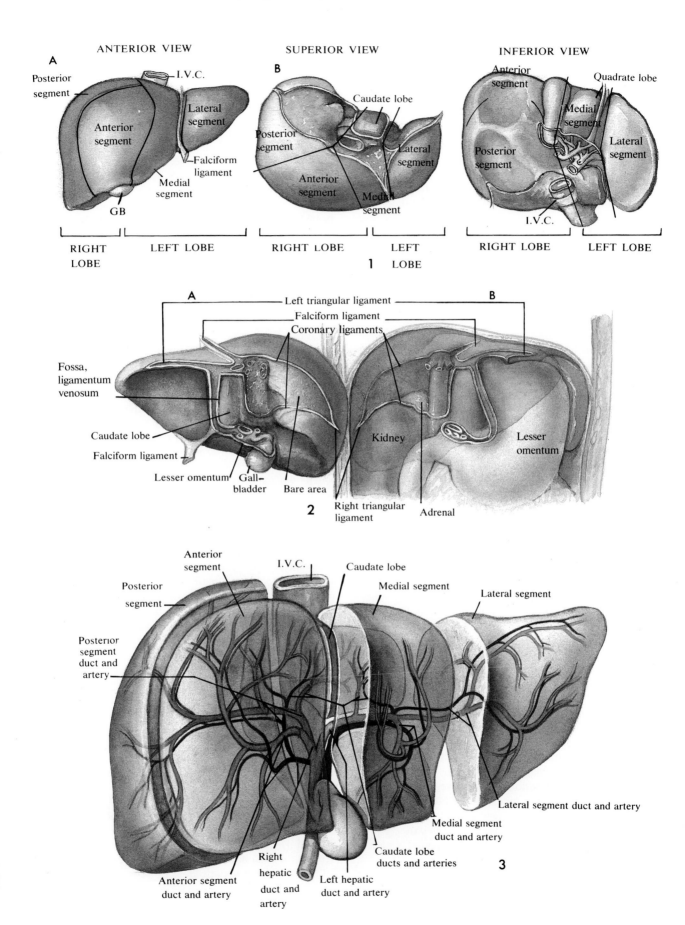

ANTERIOR VIEW

A

Posterior segment

I.V.C.

Anterior segment

Lateral segment

Falciform ligament

Medial segment

GB

RIGHT LOBE

LEFT LOBE

SUPERIOR VIEW

B

Caudate lobe

Posterior segment

Anterior segment

Lateral segment

Medial segment

RIGHT LOBE

LEFT LOBE

1

INFERIOR VIEW

Anterior segment

Quadrate lobe

Medial segment

Posterior segment

Lateral segment

I.V.C.

RIGHT LOBE

LEFT LOBE

Left triangular ligament

Falciform ligament

Coronary ligaments

A

B

Fossa, ligamentum venosum

Caudate lobe

Falciform ligament

Lesser omentum   Gall-bladder

Bare area

Right triangular ligament

Kidney

Adrenal

Lesser omentum

2

Anterior segment

I.V.C.

Caudate lobe

Medial segment

Lateral segment

Posterior segment

Posterior segment duct and artery

Anterior segment duct and artery

Right hepatic duct and artery

Left hepatic duct and artery

Caudate lobe ducts and arteries

Medial segment duct and artery

Lateral segment duct and artery

3

5. Portal Venous Supply (Fig. 1)—the portal vein ascends in the hepatoduodenal ligament posterior to the common bile duct and hepatic artery. As it reaches the porta hepatis it terminates in line with the main lobar fissure by dividing into a right and left portal vein.

a. RIGHT PORTAL VEIN—extends for a very short distance and divides into *anterior* and *posterior segment branches* which run their intrahepatic course accompanied by the segment branches of the right hepatic duct and artery. Like these structures they terminate as superior and inferior subsegment branches.

b. LEFT PORTAL VEIN—consists of two parts: a *pars transversus* which extends to the left in the porta hepatis and a *pars umbilicus* which descends into the umbilical fossa in line with the left segmental fissure. From the right side of the pars umbilicus the *medial segment veins* arise as multiple branches extending into the superior and inferior areas of the segment. The *lateral segment veins* take origin from the left side of the pars umbilicus as two separate branches: one to the superior, the other to the inferior subsegment.

c. CAUDATE LOBE VEINS—arise, like the duct and arteries, from both the right and left portal veins. The right vein supplies predominately the caudate process and right portion of the caudate lobe, while the left portal vein supplies the left portion of the caudate lobe.

6. Hepatic Venous Drainage (Fig. 1)—three major hepatic veins (the right, middle, and left) are formed in the liver and empty into the suprahepatic inferior vena cava. These major hepatic veins are *intersegmental* in position, each one lying in one of the aforementioned fissures of the liver (page 176). Because of this intersegmental position, the veins drain adjacent segments.

a. MIDDLE HEPATIC VEIN—lies in the main lobar fissure and drains the inferior areas of the medial and anterior segments.

b. RIGHT HEPATIC VEIN—is located in the right segmental fissure and receives tributaries from the entire posterior segment as well as the superior area of the anterior segment of the right lobe.

c. LEFT HEPATIC VEIN—which occupies the upper portion of the left segmental fissure drains the entire lateral segment and the superior area of the medial segment.

The middle and left hepatic veins usually (60 per cent) unite to form a single trunk before emptying into the inferior vena cava, while the right hepatic opens through a separate ostium. In addition to these main branches, one or two constant branches from the caudate lobe, as well as inconstant branches from the posterior segment of the right lobe, enter the inferior vena cava directly. The major hepatic veins may serve as landmarks for the interlobar or intersegmental planes during hepatic resection much as the pulmonary veins serve a similar purpose in segmental resection of the lung. Since no valves are present in the hepatic venous system, retrograde injection of radio-opaque material for roentgen visualization is possible.

7. Major Arterial and Ductal Variants—it is not our purpose to describe all possible variations of the arterial and ductal branches of the liver, for this invariably re-sults in nothing but confusion to the reader. We do wish, however, to correct certain erroneous concepts which have been handed down through generations of anatomists and surgeons.

a. **"Accessory" hepatic arteries**—are described in all surgical anatomy textbooks. The term "accessory" infers something that is additive and not in itself essential. The use of the term accessory hepatic artery gives the surgeon the impression that such an artery is supplying an area of the liver already supplied by the celiac hepatic. Such is not the case, for each artery entering the liver supplies a specific part of that organ without any gross anastomosis with other hepatic branches. These accessory hepatic arteries actually represent aberrant segment or subsegment arteries to the liver. Figure 2 represents a case in point. In this specimen, three hepatic arterial branches arise from the common hepatic. From an extrahepatic dissection they would have been designated as a right, middle, and left hepatic artery. In addition, an "accessory" right hepatic artery arises from the superior mesenteric and an "accessory" left hepatic from the left gastric artery. Injection of the specimen, however, reveals the following: right hepatic artery supplies only posterior segment, middle hepatic artery is the medial segment artery, left hepatic supplies the inferior area of lateral segment, the "accessory" left hepatic supplies the lateral superior area, and the "accessory" right hepatic is distributed to the anterior segment. *Accessory hepatic arteries, in the true definition of the term, do not exist.*

b. DOUBLE HEPATIC ARTERIES—is a term used when two major arterial branches enter the right lobe of the liver, but as previously described (page 172), these are actually separate origins of the segment arteries stemming from the hepatica propria. In these cases, a true right hepatic artery is not present (Fig. 4A, page 173). On the left side, a similar pattern is quite common (25 per cent), that is, the medial and lateral segment arteries originate separately from the hepatica propria. In these cases, however, rather than being referred to as double left hepatic arteries, the medial segment branch is termed the middle hepatic or quadrate lobe artery (Fig. 5).

c. "ACCESSORY" HEPATIC DUCT—carries with it the same connotation as does the term accessory hepatic artery. Like the arteries, however, each duct exiting from the liver drains a specific area of that organ. So-called accessory hepatic ducts are most frequently described as being present in the right lobe. In some 28 per cent of livers studied, two major ducts exited from the right lobe. The lower of the two would be described from extrahepatic dissection as an "accessory" duct. Injection studies revealed, however, that they actually were cases in which the anterior and posterior segment ducts did not join to form a right hepatic duct but entered the common hepatic duct separately (Figs. 3A and 4). Rarely (1 per cent) may a similar pattern of separate medial and lateral segment bile ducts draining into the common hepatic duct be seen. As on the right side, they are not "accessory" ducts but rather aberrant segment ducts.

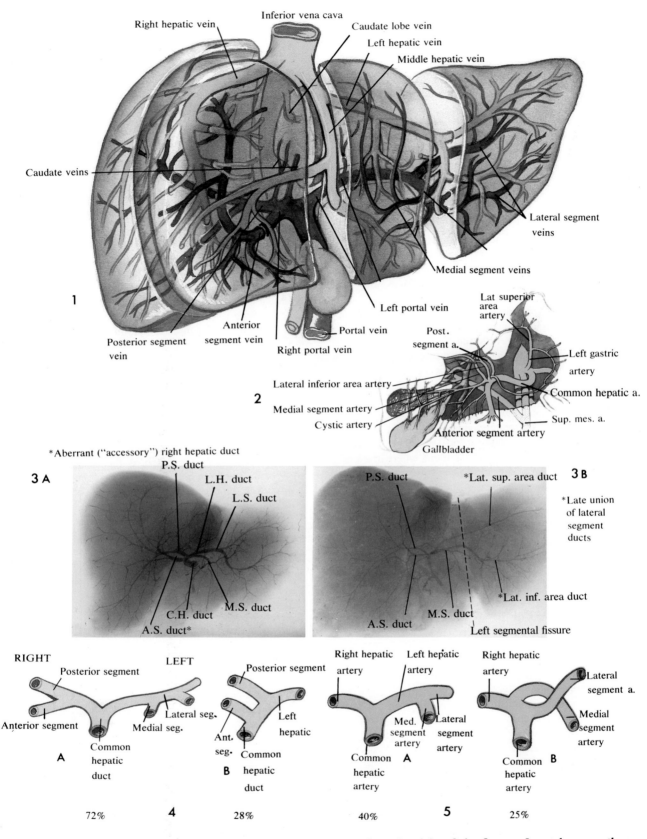

1

Right hepatic vein
Inferior vena cava
Caudate lobe vein
Left hepatic vein
Middle hepatic vein
Caudate veins
Lateral segment veins
Medial segment veins
Left portal vein
Portal vein
Right portal vein
Anterior segment vein
Posterior segment vein

2

Lat superior area artery
Post. segment a.
Left gastric artery
Lateral inferior area artery
Common hepatic a.
Medial segment artery
Sup. mes. a.
Cystic artery
Anterior segment artery
Gallbladder

3 A

*Aberrant ("accessory") right hepatic duct
P.S. duct
L.H. duct
L.S. duct
M.S. duct
C.H. duct
A.S. duct*

3 B

P.S. duct
*Lat. sup. area duct
*Late union of lateral segment ducts
*Lat. inf. area duct
A.S. duct
M.S. duct
Left segmental fissure

4

RIGHT   LEFT
Posterior segment
Anterior segment
Medial seg.
Lateral seg.
Common hepatic duct
A   72%

Posterior segment
Ant. seg.
Left hepatic
Common hepatic duct
B   28%

5

Right hepatic artery   Left hepatic artery
Med. segment artery   Lateral segment artery
Common hepatic artery
A   40%

Right hepatic artery
Lateral segment a.
Medial segment artery
Common hepatic artery
B   25%

d. LATE UNION OF LATERAL SEGMENT DUCTS—is the most frequent variation of the biliary drainage of the left lobe. In these cases, the superior and inferior area ducts do not join in line with the left segmental fissure but well to the right of the fissure. In such cases, the medial segment duct usually drains into the inferior duct of the lateral segment (Fig. 3B).

THE LIVER: CLINICAL CONSIDERATIONS:

The liver, because of its great size and vascularity, has caused surgeons to hesitate to operate upon it. With the newer concepts of the intrahepatic anatomy as discussed on pages 176, 178 and 180 such fear is being somewhat allayed. Still, the majority of the operative procedures are performed in the immediate region of the liver for extrahepatic pathology or upon extrahepatic structures to alleviate interhepatic pathology.

1. **Surgical Approach** — incisions to expose the liver may range from a simple incision through the anterior abdominal wall in order to drain a suprahepatic anterior abscess to a thoracoabdominal incision for a major hepatic resection. Incisions may be extraperitoneal, transperitoneal, extrapleural, transpleural, or combinations of these approaches.

2. **Surgery of Hepatic Cirrhosis** — for the patient with portal cirrhosis, surgery is not curative but only a palliative procedure performed to allieviate the complications of ascites and esophageal varices. Surgery, therefore, is performed primarily to promote collateral circulation from the portal to the caval venous system thereby reducing the increased portal pressure produced by the diseased liver. Although the intrahepatic distribution of the portal vein has been described on page 180, a knowledge of its extrahepatic anatomy is necessary in order to understand the rationale of such operative attempts.

a. THE EXTRAHEPATIC PORTAL VEIN — begins behind the neck of the pancreas as a union of the splenic vein and the superior mesenteric vein (Fig. 1). It ascends in the hepatoduodenal ligament where the common bile duct lies anterior and to the right, and the hepatic propria artery anterior and to the right (Fig. 2, page 173). At the porta hepatis it divides into a right and left branch, each of which pursues an intrahepatic course (Fig. 1, page 181). Within the liver the portal vein terminates in the sinusoids from which the central veins of the hepatic venous system take origin.

The portal vein receives blood from the foregut, midgut, and hindgut derivatives of the abdominal portion of the digestive tract. The direct tributaries from these parts consist of the splenic, superior mesenteric (at times, 25 per cent, the inferior mesenteric), the left gastric (coronary), the right gastric (pyloric), the retroduodenal, and cystic veins.

b. COLLATERAL CHANNELS — between the portal and systemic venous systems are extremely important in portal hypertension. Such channels may on one hand produce natural shunts which aid in diverting the partially obstructed portal blood back to the heart. On the other hand, certain of these channels may become markedly dilated (varices) resulting in rupture, hemorrhage, and often death. Such retrograde flow exists in the portal system because of the absence of valves.

Several important collateral sites are normally present. The most obvious, of course, is the *portal-hepatic* anastomosis within the liver (Fig. 1*A*). Pathologic interference with this shunt, regardless of the etiologic factor, is by far the most common cause of portal hypertension. A second important collateral is the *portal-azygos* anastomosis in the lower esophagus (Fig. 1*B*).

This consists of a communication between the esophageal branches of the left gastric (coronary) branch of the portal vein and the azygos system of veins within the thorax. Rupture of these *esophageal varices* is a common cause of death in cirrhosis. A third important site is the *portal-hemorrhoidal* anastomosis between the superior hemorrhoidal branch of the inferior mesenteric and the hemorrhoidal plexus of the hypogastric veins (Fig. 1*C*). Dilatation of this anastomotic site results in the production of *piles* or *hemorrhoids*. A *portal-retroperitoneal* venous anastomotic plexus may become prominent with increased portal pressure. This plexus consists of retroperitoneal branches of the colic veins and lumbar veins (Fig. 1*D*), pancreaticoduodenal veins with the renal veins (Fig. 1*E*), and the subcapsular veins of the liver with phrenic veins. Such communicating venous channels are collectively termed the *veins of Retzius*. A final site of collateral circulation is the *portal-umbilical* anastomosis. This consists of a venous communication located in the ligamentum teres hepatis between the portal vein branches above and the paraumbilical veins (Sappey) on the superficial abdominal wall. Varices of these vessels produce the *caput medusae* which is seen more frequently in textbooks than in patients with cirrhosis.

It must be kept in mind that portal hypertension with resultant development of varices may result from causes other than intrahepatic obstruction (Fig. 2*A*). Suprahepatic obstruction of the hepatic veins (*Budd-Chiari Syndrome*) or congestive heart failure may result in an increased pressure in the entire portal system. Extrahepatic obstruction of the main portal trunk (Fig. 2*B*) or a major tributary such as the splenic (Fig. 2*C*) may occur, due to either congenital or acquired factors. In any case, the formation of esophageal varices is most significant clinically.

c. SURGICAL PROCEDURES — are performed in cirrhotic patients in order to (1) control bleeding of esophageal varices and (2) decompress the portal venous system, thus helping to relieve both bleeding and ascites.

A diagnosis of bleeding esophageal varices requires immediate emergency intervention because of the very high mortality rate associated with such bleeding. Nonsurgical emergency procedures include *esophageal balloon tamponade, gastroesophageal hypothermia, endoscopic sclerotherapy,* and *intravenous injection of posterior pituitary extract.* Unfortunately, such procedures still result in a poor rate of survival. Direct operative methods are advocated, such as transesophageal ligation of the varices, resection of the varices-bearing area by *esophagogastrectomy* followed by a reconstructive procedure, or an *emergency portacaval shunt.*

Whatever emergency intervention is performed, consideration must be given to produce portal decompression by reducing portal flow or to achieve surgically created portal-systemic shunts which relieve not only the bleeding but also the ascites. This may be accomplished by an *anastomosis* between the portal vein and the inferior vena cava either by a side-to-side or an end-to-side technique (portacaval shunt, Fig. 3).

The procedure of choice at present is the anastomosis of the splenic vein into the renal vein (distal splenorenal shunt) as shown in Figure 4.

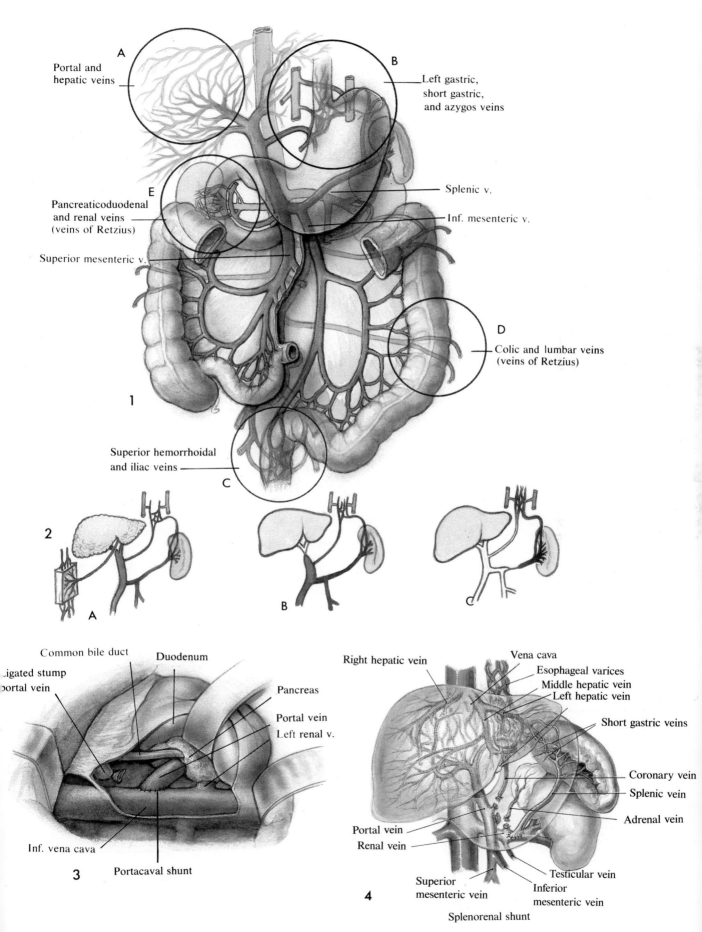

Portal and
hepatic veins

A

B

Left gastric,
short gastric,
and azygos veins

Splenic v.

E

Pancreaticoduodenal
and renal veins
(veins of Retzius)

Inf. mesenteric v.

Superior mesenteric v.

D

Colic and lumbar veins
(veins of Retzius)

1

Superior hemorrhoidal
and iliac veins

C

2

A

B

C

Common bile duct

Duodenum

Ligated stump
portal vein

Pancreas

Portal vein
Left renal v.

Inf. vena cava

3

Portacaval shunt

Right hepatic vein

Vena cava

Esophageal varices

Middle hepatic vein
Left hepatic vein

Short gastric veins

Coronary vein

Splenic vein

Adrenal vein

Portal vein

Renal vein

Testicular vein

Superior
mesenteric vein

Inferior
mesenteric vein

4

Splenorenal shunt

3. **Abscesses** — abscesses located within the liver or in the adjacent peritoneal cavity require surgical drainage.

a. INTRAHEPATIC ABSCESSES — may be due to a variety of factors, chiefly pyogenic organisms or histolytic amoeba. Such organisms spread to the liver via the bile ducts, hepatic artery, or portal vein. Direct extension of contiguous abscesses into the liver may occur when Glisson's capsule is eroded. A tear in the capsule secondary to trauma may also permit bacterial continuation and abscess formation. Intrahepatic abscesses may be multiple or single. In both types appropriate bacteriocidal or amebicidal drugs should be administered. Only the solitary abscess lends itself to surgical drainage as discussed below.

b. EXTRAHEPATIC ABSCESS — is a collection of pus in any of the several potential spaces formed in relation to the peritoneal attachments of the liver. This area includes the entire supramesocolic region of the peritoneal cavity and is termed the *subphrenic* or *subdiaphragmatic space*. This space is limited by the diaphragm above, by the posterior abdominal wall behind, and by the ventrolateral abdominal wall and diaphragm in front. Below, the space extends to the transverse colon and mesocolon but is in continuity with the inframesocolic compartment via the *paracolic gutters*.

The liver and its peritoneal attachments divide the subphrenic space into a *suprahepatic space* and an *infrahepatic space*. The suprahepatic space is further divided by the falciform ligament into a right and left space (Fig. 1). The *right suprahepatic space* lies between the inferior surface of the diaphragm and the anterosuperior surface of the right lobe and medial segment of the liver. Above the liver, the space is bounded behind by the right anterior coronary and right triangular ligaments. Below, the space is in continuity with the general peritoneal cavity. The *left suprahepatic space* is separated from its right counterpart by the falciform ligament. It is located between the diaphragm and abdominal wall in front and the lateral segment of the liver behind. The left anterior coronary and left triangular ligaments bound the space above and behind the liver.

On the right side, below the liver, is the *right infrahepatic space*, also known as the *hepatorenal pouch of Morison* (Fig. 2). The space is bounded by the diaphragm and posterior abdominal wall behind and the right lobe of the liver in front. It is limited superiorly by the right posterior coronary and right triangular ligaments. Medially, the hepatoduodenal ligament limits the pouch. Here it communicates with the omental bursa through the epiploic foramen. Below, the space is continuous with the general peritoneal cavity.

The left infrahepatic space is further divided into an anterior and posterior space. This division is due to the presence of the gastrohepatic ligament, stomach, and gastrocolic ligament. Lying anterior to these structures is the *left anterior infrahepatic space*, also referred to as the *perigastric space* (Fig. 1). The *left posterior infrahepatic space* is actually the lesser peritoneal cavity or omental bursa (Fig. 3, page 157).

Subphrenic abscesses occur far more frequently on the right side. The frequency of ruptured appendices, duodenal ulcers, and gallbladders accounts for this fact. Figures 1 and 2 illustrate the sources of infection and the routes of spread to the subphrenic spaces. An extraperitoneal abscess located in the "bare area" of the liver may result from a ruptured right perinephric or an intrahepatic abscess. On the left side, the abdominal esophagus or kidney may be a source of an extraperitoneal abscess.

c. SURGICAL TREATMENT — once a diagnosis is made and the abscess accurately located, drainage should be established. An extraperitoneal-extrapleural approach is used.

A *posterior extraserous* drainage is usually indicated for abscesses located in the right infrahepatic, the upper part of the right suprahepatic, or the extraperitoneal spaces. A similar approach may be utilized on either the right or left side. The skin incision is made parallel to the twelfth rib, and the rib completely removed subperiosteally. The deep transverse incision is made at the level of the spinous process of the first lumbar vertebra (Fig. 3A and B). The abscess is opened through the retroperitoneal space (Fig. 3C). A common mistake is to make the deep incision parallel to the periosteal bed of the twelfth rib. Such an incision will most likely open the pleural cavity (Fig. 1, page 147). A similar approach may be used to drain an intrahepatic abscess which presents posteriorly.

In order to drain anteriorly placed intrahepatic or right suprahepatic space abscesses, as well as those in the left suprahepatic or left anterior infrahepatic space, an *anterior extraserous approach* may be used. A short subcostal abdominal incision divides the layers of the ventral abdominal wall down to but not including the peritoneum. By blunt dissection the peritoneum is stripped from the diaphragm until the abscess is reached (Fig. 4A and B).

At times it is impossible to drain adequately a subphrenic abscess by the extraserous approaches. In such cases, a *transabdominal, transperitoneal,* or, rarely, a *transthoracic (transpleural* or *extrapleural)* approach may be indicated.

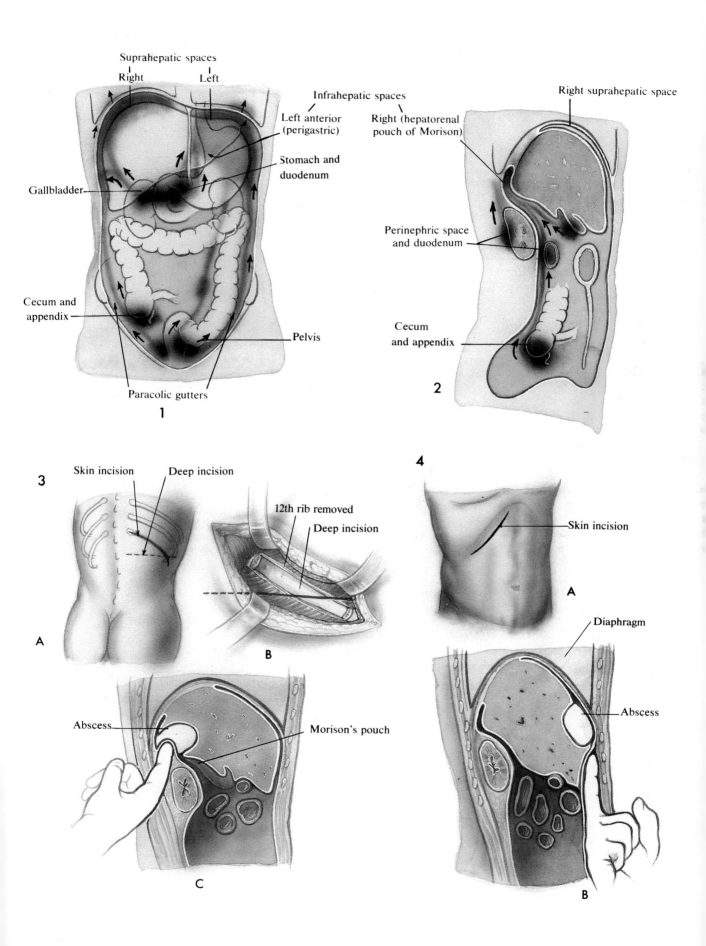

Suprahepatic spaces
Right
Left

Infrahepatic spaces
Left anterior (perigastric)
Right (hepatorenal pouch of Morison)

Stomach and duodenum

Gallbladder

Cecum and appendix

Pelvis

Paracolic gutters

1

Right suprahepatic space

Perinephric space and duodenum

Cecum and appendix

2

3

Skin incision   Deep incision

A

12th rib removed
Deep incision

B

Abscess   Morison's pouch

C

4

Skin incision

A

Diaphragm

Abscess

B

4. **Liver Resections** — were performed as early as 1716. In 1888 Langenbeck performed the first partial hepatectomy, and in 1890 Keen was the first American surgeon to do a partial hepatic resection. In subsequent years, little advancement was made in the surgical technique of such resections and the mortality was prohibitive. The techniques were extremely crude, consisting of the use of Paquelin's cautery, the employment of large strangulating through-and-through mattress sutures, and mass ligation of vessels and ducts to that part of the liver which was to be resected. Such procedures were frowned upon if applied to other organs of the body. In the early 1950s, the intrahepatic distribution of vascular and biliary channels was first clarified and their segmental distribution described. This advance in the knowledge of gross intrahepatic anatomy resulted in the development of much more refined techniques for segmental resection of the organ utilizing an individual ligation technique. The intrahepatic anatomy is described on pages 176 through 181.

The most common indication for hepatic resection is primary liver cancer or solitary metastatic lesions. Benign tumors, cysts, abscesses, and trauma have also been treated by liver resection. The resection may be a total lobectomy, segmentectomy, trisegmentectomy, or subsegmental resection (wedge resection).

a. FUNDAMENTAL SURGICAL CONSIDERATIONS OF HEPATIC RESECTION — include adequate exposure, which may be best achieved by a right thoracicoabdominal approach; however, for a lateral segmentectomy or a subsegmental (wedge) resection, an upper midline abdominal incision may be sufficient. Exploration of the abdomen is done to determine operability of the lesion and whether metastasis has occurred. Adequate mobilization of that part of the liver must be achieved. This will require the division of the peritoneal attachments, again depending upon the part of the organ to be resected. These attachments include the ligamentum teres, the coronary ligaments (anterior and posterior), the right and left triangular ligaments, the falciform ligament, and the gastrohepatic ligament (pages 176 to 177). In transecting the left triangular ligament, one must be aware that in 5 per cent of cases a patent bile duct may be present in this location.

Most important are the identification and isolation of the biliary and vascular structures in the hepatic pedicle and awareness of the variational patterns in this area (Fig. 1). Equally important is knowledge of the anatomy of the hepatic veins, because the main branches — right, middle, and left — lie in the intersegmental planes.

The identification of interlobar and intersegmental planes is more difficult because, unlike the lung, the liver has no lobar or segmental fissures. The main lobar fissure which divides the liver into the true right and left lobes has no demarcation on the anterior surface of the organ. On the posterior surface, it is in line with the gallbladder fossa below and the fossa for the inferior vena cava above. This fissure on the anterior surface begins about 3 to 4 cm. to the left of the line between the gallbladder and caval fossae and angulates through the hepatic parenchyma at proximally 75 degrees to the right. The left segmental fissure is marked on the anterior surface by the attachment of the falciform ligament and enters through the liver at approximately a 45-degree angle to the right. The right segmental fissure takes about a 30-degree angle through the right lobe, dividing it into anterior and posterior segments. The major trunks of the right, middle, and left hepatic veins lie in the interlobar and intersegmental

planes (Fig. 1, page 181). The right hepatic vein drains into the right side of the vena cava and the middle and left hepatic veins drain as a single or common trunk into the left side of the inferior vena cava.

b. RIGHT HEPATIC LOBECTOMY (Fig. 2) — is approached by a right thoracicoabdominal incision through the eighth intercostal space. The diaphragm is incised to the inferior vena cava in order to obtain adequate exposure of the vessel. The falciform ligament, the ligamentum teres, the right triangular, and the anterior and posterior coronary ligament are severed (Fig. 2, page 177), which allows displacement of the right lobe anteriorly and upward, thus exposing the structures in the porta hepatis.

The cystic duct is ligated, and a "subvesical duct" must be carefully sought (35 per cent) and, if present, ligated. Individual ligation of the cystic artery, followed by ligation of the right hepatic duct and right hepatic artery (keeping in mind the many variations that may be present, particularly an "afferent" right hepatic artery) and the right portal vein, is next performed.

After ligation of the right hepatic artery, a blanching over the anterior surface takes place which delineates the main lobar fissure and is a guide to the proper plane of dissection. With the electrocoagulating cautery or with the YAG laser, an incision is made through Glisson's capsule, and dissection can be performed by the finger fracture technique or by utilizing the ultrasonic dissector and YAG laser. By moving the electrosonic dissector horizontally over the liver surface, the liver parenchyma is fragmented without injury to the vessels and ducts, thus allowing control by conventional means. The surgeon and operating personnel must wear protective glasses if the YAG laser is used.

Most important in the transection of the liver parenchyma is to keep in mind the angle of the main lobar fissure (75-degree angle from the anterior surface directed toward the right) and the identification of the middle hepatic vein which lies in the depth of the fissure. The dissection is carried along the plane of demarcation proceeding along the right edge of the lobar fissure and vein toward the diaphragm. By general traction of the liver anteriorly and medially, the short veins draining into the inferior vena cava are ligated. The right hepatic vein is doubly ligated and transfixed at its entrance to the vena cava.

c. LEFT LATERAL SEGMENTECTOMY (Fig. 3) — may be adequately approached through an upper midline abdominal incision. Such an incision may be extended to a left thoracicoabdominal approach should more exposure be required. The peritoneal attachments are incised. These include the left triangular ligament (in 5 per cent of cases a patent bile duct may be present), the coronary ligaments, the ligamentum teres, and the falciform ligament. With such mobilization of the lateral segment, the porta hepatis can be readily exposed.

The lateral segment artery and bile duct are identified and ligated. Here again variational patterns must be kept in mind (Fig. 3B, page 181). Of particular importance in this procedure is the dissection of the left portal vein. The vein has two segments: a pars transversa, which lies in the porta hepatis, and a pars umbilicus, which descends into the umbilical fossa. The lateral segment branches, superior and inferior, arise from the left border of the pars umbilicus. Dissection must extend 1 to 2 cm. along the left side of the vein to ligate these vessels and preserve the medial segment veins.

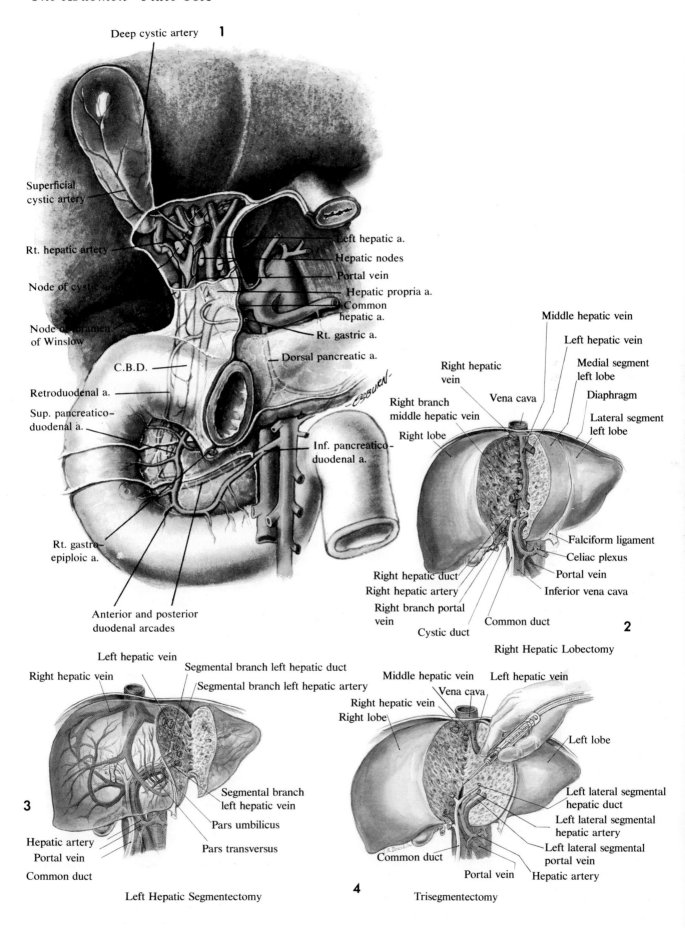

1

Deep cystic artery

Superficial cystic artery

Rt. hepatic artery

Node of cystic n.

Node of foramen of Winslow

C.B.D.

Retroduodenal a.

Sup. pancreatico-duodenal a.

Rt. gastro-epiploic a.

Anterior and posterior duodenal arcades

Left hepatic a.

Hepatic nodes

Portal vein

Hepatic propria a.

Common hepatic a.

Rt. gastric a.

Dorsal pancreatic a.

Inf. pancreatico-duodenal a.

2

Middle hepatic vein

Left hepatic vein

Medial segment left lobe

Diaphragm

Lateral segment left lobe

Right hepatic vein

Vena cava

Right branch middle hepatic vein

Right lobe

Falciform ligament

Celiac plexus

Portal vein

Inferior vena cava

Right hepatic duct

Right hepatic artery

Right branch portal vein

Cystic duct

Common duct

Right Hepatic Lobectomy

3

Left hepatic vein

Right hepatic vein

Segmental branch left hepatic duct

Segmental branch left hepatic artery

Segmental branch left hepatic vein

Pars umbilicus

Pars transversus

Hepatic artery

Portal vein

Common duct

Left Hepatic Segmentectomy

4

Middle hepatic vein

Left hepatic vein

Right hepatic vein

Right lobe

Vena cava

Left lobe

Left lateral segmental hepatic duct

Left lateral segmental hepatic artery

Left lateral segmental portal vein

Hepatic artery

Common duct

Portal vein

Trisegmentectomy

Incision through Glisson's capsule is made 1 to 2 cm. to the left of the attachment of the falciform ligament, and the line of resection is aligned with the left side of the vena cava, leaving 1 cm. of liver tissue protecting the middle hepatic vein. Dissection through the parenchyma is made at a 45-degree angle toward the right to expose the left hepatic vein. Care must be taken to identify the hepatic venous branches draining the superior subsegment of the medial segment and ligation performed just to the left of its entrance into the left hepatic vein (Fig. 1, page 181). An alternative method of performing left lateral lobe segmentectomy is with the use of hepatic occlusive and hepatic resection clamps.

d. TRISEGMENTECTOMY (Fig. 4) — is also referred to as extended right lobectomy. It consists of the removal of the entire right lobe and the medial segment of the left lobe. The parenchymal dissection may proceed in a fashion similar to that described for lateral segmentectomy. Beginning 1 to 2 cm. to the right of the falciform ligament, the origin of the vessels and ducts to the medial segment are encountered as the hilar dissection is extended from the inferior surface of the liver medial to the umbilical fissure. However, in this procedure, the lateral segment vessels and ducts are preserved, as is the left hepatic vein. The right and middle hepatic veins are both ligated as they enter the inferior vena cava near the diaphragm.

e. OTHER LIVER RESECTIONS — have been performed, including left lobectomy, medial segmentectomy, and anterior or posterior right segmentectomy. Another type of resection performed is known as subsegmental or wedge resection. Such a resection is, as the name suggests, a simple wedge removal of a portion of the liver with no anatomic basis, so that the bleeding and biliary seepage must be controlled by suture techniques.

5. **Liver Transplantation** — first introduced in 1963 by Thomas Starzl, has progressively become more refined, resulting in higher survival rates. Liver transplants are being done with increasing frequency, as are transplants of other visceral organs such as kidneys, heart, lungs, and pancreas. The liver is the largest visceral organ in the body and certainly the most complex in its multitude of functions. Its transplantation is a difficult procedure and has been beset with many problems.

In kidney transplantation, if early signs of rejection are identified, renal dialysis can sustain the organ until the complication is overcome. There is no such support system for the liver because of its multifunctional activities. The time interval between obtaining the donor organ and the transplant into the recipient also differs in the two procedures. The kidney may be preserved for much longer periods (optimally, less than 24 hours); however, time is extremely critical for the donor liver.

Another major problem in the early years of liver transplantation was the rejection phenomenon. With conventional immunosuppressive drugs (usually azathioprine and steroids) results were disappointing — about 33 per cent 1-year and 20 per cent 5-year survivals. However, in 1980 a new drug, cyclosporine plus prednisone, was introduced. In a very short time, survival improved to 70 per cent at 1 year and 63 per cent at 5 years.

a. SELECTION OF THE RECIPIENT — the operation is indicated for patients with liver failure, usually due to biliary atresia, postnecrotic cirrhosis, inborn error of metabolism, primary biliary cirrhosis, or sclerosing cholangitis. Inoperable hepatic tumors were an initial indication, but because of the very high incidence and rapidity of recurrence, this indication has fallen in disfavor.

b. SELECTION OF THE DONOR — is critical because the donor liver must be removed immediately after the death pronouncement and total body hypothermia instituted to prevent liver autolysis. The donor must, of course, have normal liver function studies. Blood type compatibility is also required.

c. PREPARATION OF THE DONOR ORGAN — is accomplished by making a right thoracicoabdominal incision into the corpse while it is undergoing hypothermic extracorporeal circulation. The diaphragmatic peritoneal attachments to the liver are incised and the organ retracted to the left, exposing the upper abdominal inferior vena cava. This vessel is exposed from the diaphragm to the level of the renal veins. The posterior tributaries, including the right adrenal vein, are ligated and divided. The porta hepatis is next exposed and its contents (i.e., the common bile duct, hepatic artery, and portal vein) exposed. Variant patterns of the artery and duct must be kept in mind. The lesser omentum is severed up to the diaphragm and an incision made in the fundus of the gallbladder; all bile is aspirated to prevent autolysis.

Removal of the donor liver, at the appropriate time, is achieved by transecting the inferior vena cava just above the renal veins and just below the diaphragm. Structures in the porta hepatis are next ligated, leaving lengthy segments of the vascular structures and bile ducts. Once removed, the liver must be perfused with a chilled Ringer's solution.

d. PREPARATION OF THE RECIPIENT — like the donor, the recipient is approached through a right thoracicoabdominal incision to ensure adequate exposure. The peritoneal attachments to the liver are incised and the common bile duct, portal vein, and hepatic artery are exposed along with the inferior vena cava from the diaphragm to just above the level of the renal veins. This segment of the cava is transected as well as the biliary and vascular structures in the porta hepatis. Before devascularization of the liver, attention must be directed to stabilization of the body's hemodynamics. This may be accomplished either by a femoral vein — internal jugular by-pass or by rapid perfusion of blood into the superior vena cava via the internal jugular vein. The diseased liver is removed and the donor liver ready for implantation (Fig. 1).

e. IMPLANTATION OF THE DONOR LIVER (Fig. 2) — is begun by careful anastomosis of the upper end of the vena cava, followed by the lower end of the cava. Clamps are removed and the caval circulation re-established. Next, the portal vein anastomosis is performed, clamps removed, and the portal circulation re-established. Then the hepatic artery continuity between donor and recipient is completed, followed by reconstruction of the common bile duct. A T-tube is placed in the duct for a temporary period. Should the donor common bile duct be inadequate or inaccessible, a cholecystoduodenostomy or a cholecystojejunostomy may be performed to achieve adequate biliary drainage.

f. RETRANSPLANTATION — may be necessary because of technical complications, rejection, or graft failure in some 20 per cent of patients receiving liver transplants.

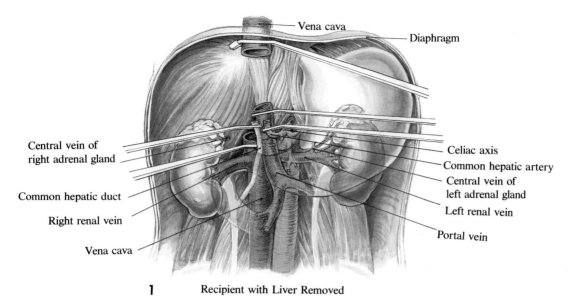

Vena cava

Diaphragm

Central vein of
right adrenal gland

Celiac axis

Common hepatic artery

Central vein of
left adrenal gland

Common hepatic duct

Left renal vein

Right renal vein

Portal vein

Vena cava

1 Recipient with Liver Removed

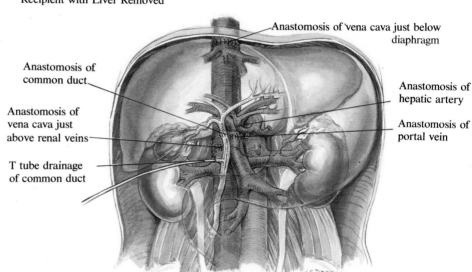

Anastomosis of vena cava just below
diaphragm

Anastomosis of
common duct

Anastomosis of
hepatic artery

Anastomosis of
vena cava just
above renal veins

Anastomosis of
portal vein

T tube drainage
of common duct

2 Completed Liver Transplant

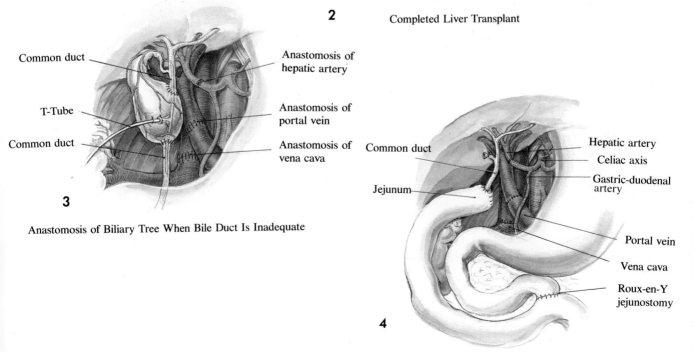

Common duct

Anastomosis of
hepatic artery

T-Tube

Anastomosis of
portal vein

Common duct

Anastomosis of
vena cava

Common duct

Hepatic artery

Celiac axis

Jejunum

Gastric-duodenal
artery

Portal vein

Vena cava

Roux-en-Y
jejunostomy

3

Anastomosis of Biliary Tree When Bile Duct Is Inadequate

4

Alternate Biliary Drainage - Choledochojejunostomy

ANATOMY OF SMALL INTESTINE:

The small intestine extends from the pylorus to the cecum and consists of the duodenum, jejunum, and ileum. The duodenum has already been considered (pages 160 and 162). The portion of the bowel, which extends from the duodenojejunal junction to the cecum, averages 22 feet in length.

1. **Peritoneal Attachments** — the small bowel, except for the duodenum, retains most of its original dorsal mesentery but is thrown from its original midline attachment by fixation of the mesentery of the duodenum and ascending colon.

a. ROOT OF THE MESENTERY — of the small bowel extends in an oblique manner from the left side of the second lumbar vertebra to the right sacroiliac joint, a distance of approximately 6 inches. At its point of attachment to the posterior wall, it crosses the third portion of the duodenum, aorta, inferior vena cava, psoas muscle, right ureter, and right internal spermatic (ovarian) vessels (Fig. 1). The root of the mesentery may fail to fuse over the entire length of the posterior parietal peritoneum, in which case a defect between the mesentery and posterior peritoneum may be the site of an internal hernia, the *mesentericoparietal hernia of Waldeyer*. Within the two layers of the mesentery run the neurovascular structures and lymphatic supplying the small bowel.

b. DUODENOJEJUNAL JUNCTION (Fig. 1) — may also be the site of an internal hernia because of the presence of certain peritoneal folds and fossae. When the jejunum is pulled to the right, a *superior* and *inferior duodenojejunal fold* extending to the posterior abdominal wall may be observed. Beneath the free edge of the folds are the *superior* and the *inferior duodenojejunal fossa*. At times the two folds may be in continuity laterally with a fold of peritoneum which encloses the inferior mesenteric vein, in which case a *paraduodenal fossa (Landzert)* may also be formed. In this same area, a retroperitoneal fibromuscular band may extend from the duodenojejunal junction to the right crus of the diaphragm and aids in the fixation of the duodenum. This structure is termed the *ligament of Treitz* or *suspensory muscle of the duodenum* (Fig. 2).

2. **Differentiation Between Jejunum and Ileum** — although there is no sharp morphological demarcation between the jejunum (upper two-fifths) and ileum (lower three-fifths) there are certain anatomic characteristics which enable the surgeon to differentiate the jejunum from the ileum at the operating table.

(a) The jejunum has a thicker wall due to the fact that the circular folds (plicae circulares) are larger in the proximal end of the small bowel.

(b) The jejunum is of greater diameter because the small bowel tapers in size from proximal to distal ends.

(c) The jejunal mesentery contains less fat than that of the ileum, so that the arterial arcades are easier to visualize.

(d) The jejunal arterial arcades are simple or double with long vasa recti, whereas the arterial branches in the ileal region form four to five arcades and have, therefore, short vasa recti (Fig. 3).

3. **Bowel Wall** (Fig. 5) — the wall of the small bowel consists of four layers:

a. SEROSAL LAYER — is the visceral peritoneum encasing the bowel; it is continuous with the mesentery.

b. MUSCULAR LAYER — is made up of two well defined layers of smooth muscle; an outer longitudinal and an inner circular. Between the two layers is located a plexus of nerve fibers and parasympathetic ganglia known as the *plexus of Auerbach*.

c. SUBMUCOSAL LAYER — is the strongest part of the bowel wall and is most important in suture anastomosis. In this layer, a second parasympathetic plexus is present *(Meissner's plexus)*.

d. MUCOSAL LAYER — consists of a lining epithelium, a lamina propria with its glands, and a limiting membrane. the *muscularis mucosae*. The most characteristic feature of this layer is the presence of numerous *villi*, circular folds *(plicae circulares)*, and lymphoid aggregations known as *Peyer's patches*. The latter are located mainly in the distal ileum along the antimesenteric border.

4. **Blood Supply** — The superior mesenteric artery alone supplies blood to the jejunum and ileum.

a. SUPERIOR MESENTERIC ARTERY — arises as an unpaired artery from the abdominal aorta at the level of the first lumbar vertebra. It lies behind the neck of the pancreas, then passes over the uncinate process and anterior to the third part of the duodenum (Fig. 7, page 161) and enters the root of the mesentery. The branches to the small bowel are the *inferior pancreaticoduodenal artery* (page 162) and the jejunal-ileal arteries. The *jejunal* and *ileal* arteries consist of ten to sixteen branches arising from the left side of the superior mesenteric trunk (Fig. 3). They extend into the mesentery where adjacent arteries unite to form loops or arcades. These *arcades* are single or double in the ileal region, but become more complex in the jejunal area where tertiary or even quaternary loops are formed. From the peripheral arcades, *vasa recti* arise and pass to the mesenteric border of the bowel without anastomosing with one another. The vasa recti alternately pass to one side or the other or split at the mesenteric border and form a *subserosal plexus*. Deep branches extend through the muscular wall sending short muscular branches and lateral anastomotic channels between adjacent segments of the small bowel. Deep branches extending further into the bowel wall form a *submucosal plexus* (Figs. 4 and 5). The terminal portion of the ileum is supplied not by direct intestinal branches but by the *ileal branch of the ileocolic artery* which anastomoses with the terminal intestinal branch of the superior mesenteric.

5. **Venous Drainage** — the venous drainage of the duodenum is discussed on page 164. The remainder of the small bowel is drained by the direct tributaries which correspond to the branches of the superior mesenteric artery and which form the *superior mesenteric vein*. It joins the splenic vein to form the portal vein.

6. **Lymphatic Drainage** — collecting channels exit from the small bowel at its mesenteric border and terminate in either of three groups of *mesenteric nodes* — a

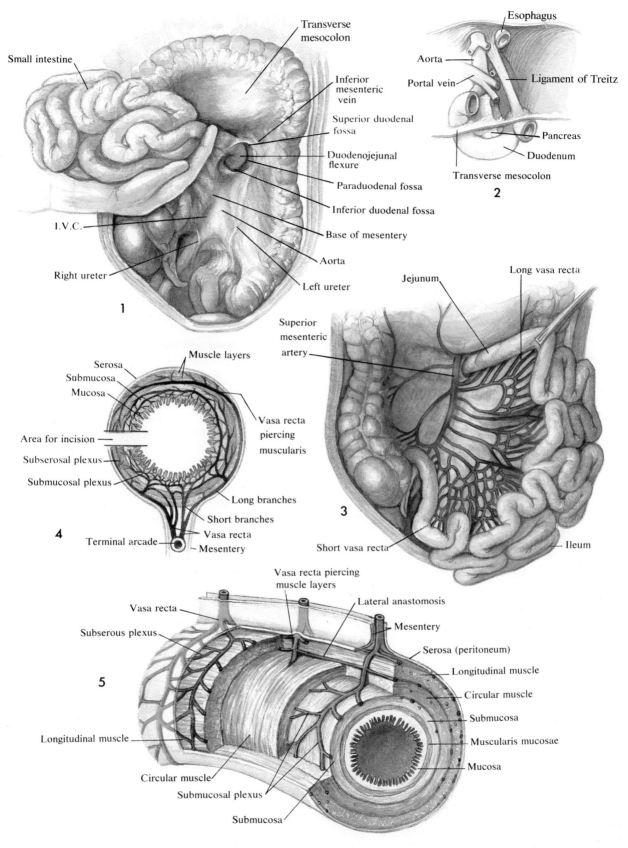

Small intestine

Transverse mesocolon

Esophagus

Aorta

Portal vein

Ligament of Treitz

Inferior mesenteric vein

Superior duodenal fossa

Duodenojejunal flexure

Paraduodenal fossa

Inferior duodenal fossa

Base of mesentery

Aorta

Left ureter

Pancreas

Duodenum

Transverse mesocolon

2

I.V.C.

Right ureter

1

Jejunum

Long vasa recta

Superior mesenteric artery

Muscle layers

Serosa

Submucosa

Mucosa

Vasa recta piercing muscularis

Area for incision

Subserosal plexus

Submucosal plexus

Long branches

Short branches

Vasa recta

Mesentery

Terminal arcade

4

Short vasa recta

Ileum

3

Vasa recta piercing muscle layers

Lateral anastomosis

Vasa recta

Mesentery

Subserous plexus

Serosa (peritoneum)

Longitudinal muscle

Circular muscle

Submucosa

Muscularis mucosae

Mucosa

5

Longitudinal muscle

Circular muscle

Submucosal plexus

Submucosa

peripheral group located near the mesenteric border, a *middle group* within the mesentery, and a *central group* (actually *preaortic — superior mesenteric nodes*).

This nodal group draining the small bowel are the most numerous in the body, consisting of from one to two hundred nodes in all.

SMALL INTESTINE: CLINICAL CONSIDERATIONS:

The jejunoileal portion of the alimentary tract is intimately involved in the rotational process of the embryonic bowel and, therefore, presents significant embryological malformations. Malignant tumors of the small intestine are uncommon, but nonetheless resection of portions of the small bowel is frequently indicated.

1. **Enterostomy**—in this procedure an artificial fistula is created between a loop of the small intestine and the skin of the abdominal wall. A *jejunostomy* is created to provide nutrition to a patient when such a fistula cannot be made through the stomach. An *ileostomy*, on the other hand, is performed as a temporary or permanent procedure to relieve a large bowel obstruction.

2. **Enterectomy**—resection of a portion of the small bowel may be indicated in instances of inflammatory lesions, tumors, or gangrene. Such a resection requires not only the removal of a part of the bowel but a portion of the mesentery as well. Figure 1 illustrates the fundamental anatomic principle in performing such a procedure in order to preserve the blood supply to the remaining bowel.

3. **Ileal Conduit (Bricker's Pouch)**—a short loop of ileum may be used as a substitute urinary bladder. Should a resection of the urinary bladder be indicated, the ureters may be anastomosed into the proximal end of an ileal loop and the distal end of the bowel exteriorized to the abdominal wall. In contrast to resection of the bowel it is imperative in such procedures that the blood supply to the resected ileal loop be preserved (Fig. 2).

4. **Small Bowel Anastomosis**—Most surgeons prefer two layers of suture as shown in Figure 8. The inner layer approximates the mucosal surfaces and the outer layer includes the seromuscular layer by an everting technique. Lembert's principle of serosa-to-serosa apposition for bowel closure has been greatly emphasized in surgical textbooks. However, of greater significance is Halsted's plea that the outer seromuscular suture *must* include the submucosal layer—the strongest anatomic layer of the bowel wall.

5. **Congenital Anomalies**—developmental defects of the small bowel result chiefly as malrotations of the midgut, defective luminal developments, or persistence of the yolk stalk.

a. ANOMALIES OF THE MIDGUT ROTATION—which include the jejunum and ileum are often asymptomatic. Frequently, however, an improper rotation will produce intestinal obstruction. The normal mechanism of rotation has been discussed on page 150 and some of the major anomalies on page 152.

b. ANOMALIES OF LUMINAL DEVELOPMENT—of the small bowel may result in atresia, stenosis, or duplication of the bowel lumen. At about the sixth week of embryonic life there is a rapid proliferation of the epithelial lining extending from the esophagus to the rectum. This epithelial proliferation results in temporary luminal obliteration of varying degrees in different parts of the alimentary tract. Following this stage, vacuoles appear in this solid epithelial cord and eventually coalesce. This stage of vacuolorization and coalescence results again in normal luminal patency.

Failure of complete coalescence of these vacuoles, i.e., a persistent *transverse* septum between adjacent vacuoles, may result in complete obliteration of the lumen resulting in an *atresia* of the bowel.

A *stenosis* or narrowing of the alimentary tract results from the same defective process that produces an atresia. However, in such cases the septum is partially perforated.

Duplication (enteric or enterogenous cysts) of a portion of the bowel lumen may also result due to the persistence of a *longitudinal* septum between vacuoles. As shown in Figure 3, duplications may occur in any part of the alimentary tract. They may, but usually do not, communicate with the intestinal lumen (in which case they may be termed *enteric diverticula*).

It is important to differentiate between these duplications and *mesenteric cysts*. These cysts are most commonly found in relation to the jejunum and ileum between the leaves of the mesentery, usually near the mesenteric border of the bowel. They are considered to be lymphatic cysts. Their walls are thin in contrast to the thick walled duplication. Their linings are smooth whereas the lining of a duplication contains intestinal mucosa. The fluid content is serous or chylous while that of a duplication is mucoid. The blood supply to the related segment of bowel passes anterior to the mesenteric cyst. The duplication of small bowel has the same blood supply as its adjacent bowel. A cleavage plane exists between the cyst and adjacent bowel whereas the wall of the duplication is usually contiguous with the bowel wall. A mesenteric cyst can therefore be excised without injury to the bowel or its blood supply. Removal of an intestinal diverticulum, on the other hand, requires removal of the adjacent segment of bowel and restoration of intestinal continuity.

c. PERSISTENCE OF THE YOLK SAC (VITELLINE, OMPHALOMESENTERIC DUCT)—is one of the commonest of the anomalies of the intestinal tract and is known as *Meckel's diverticulum*. The stalk is an entodermal outpouching through the umbilical cord communicating with the yolk sac. As development proceeds this stalk is usually obliterated, but in some 2 per cent of persons partial persistence of the structure is evident. It may persist as a blind pouch of varying size with no parietal attachment (Fig. 5), as a diverticulum with a fibrous band attachment to the umbilicus, or as a complete fistulous communication between the intestine and abdominal wall at the umbilicus (*umbilicointestinal fistula*) (Fig. 6). Occasionally, only cystic remnants of the stalk may remain. It is said to communicate with any part of the last 5 feet of ileum, and is twice as common in men than women.

The diverticulum may become inflamed giving rise to symptoms mimicking appendicitis. Of more significance, however, is the unexplained fact that the mucosa may be gastric, pancreatic, duodenal, colonic, as well as ileal. Ulceration (Fig. 7) and hemorrhage may therefore be the significant pathologic findings.

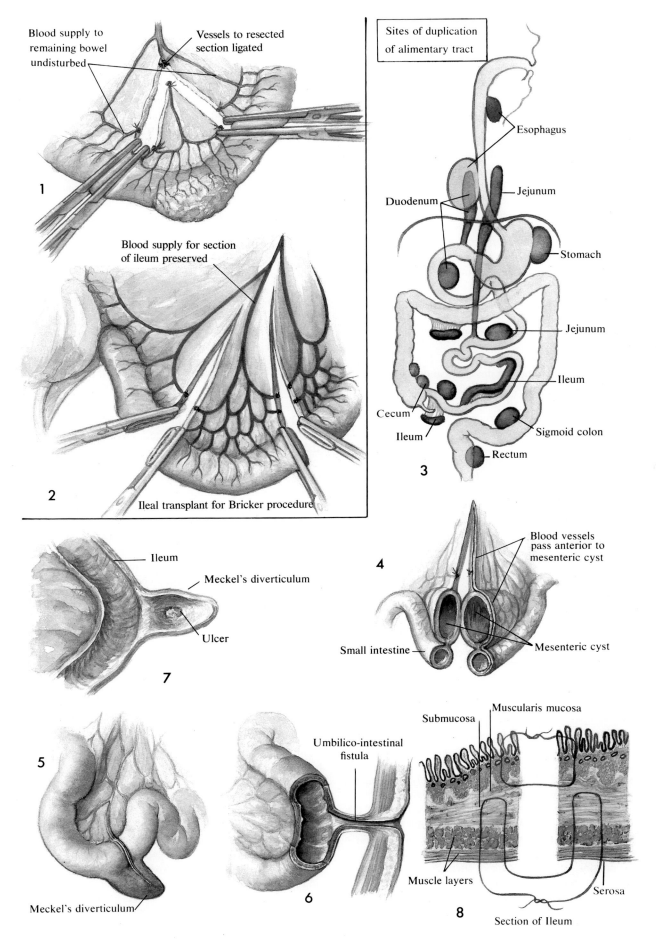

1

Blood supply to remaining bowel undisturbed

Vessels to resected section ligated

Blood supply for section of ileum preserved

2

Ileal transplant for Bricker procedure

Sites of duplication of alimentary tract

3

Esophagus

Jejunum

Duodenum

Stomach

Jejunum

Ileum

Cecum

Ileum

Sigmoid colon

Rectum

4

Blood vessels pass anterior to mesenteric cyst

Small intestine

Mesenteric cyst

7

Ileum

Meckel's diverticulum

Ulcer

5

Meckel's diverticulum

6

Umbilico-intestinal fistula

8

Submucosa

Muscularis mucosa

Muscle layers

Serosa

Section of Ileum

The Abdomen

ANATOMY OF LARGE INTESTINE:

The large intestine extends from the ileocecal junction to the anus. Its parts consist of the cecum and appendix, the colon (ascending, transverse, descending, and sigmoid), the rectum, and anal canal. The latter two parts are located in the pelvis and described on page 224.

1. **Peritoneal Attachments** – on page 150 we have described the rotation of the gut and the fixation of the dorsal mesentery related to the parts of the large bowel. Only the mesentery of the transverse colon (*transverse mesocolon*) and sigmoid colon (*mesosigmoid*) persist in the adult. During rotation the mesentery of the ascending and descending colon are thrown against the posterior parietal peritoneum to which they fuse as the *fascia of Toldt* (Fig. 5). Peritoneal folds and associated fossae are found particularly in the ileocecal region. They are:

a. SUPERIOR ILEOCECAL FOLD – produced by the passage of the anterior cecal branch of the ileocolic artery which extends anterior to the junction of cecum and ileum (Fig. 2).

b. SUPERIOR ILEOCECAL FOSSA – lies deep to the above fold with its opening directed caudalward (Fig. 2).

c. INFERIOR ILEOCECAL FOLD – extends from the antimesenteric border of the lower ileum to the mesoappendix. It is usually devoid of blood vessels and is, therefore, termed *"the bloodless fold of Treves"* (Fig. 2).

d. INFERIOR ILEOCECAL FOSSA – is fairly constant with its opening directed caudally (Fig. 2).

e. MESOAPPENDIX – is a triangular peritoneal fold extending from the mesentery of the ileum. In its free margin runs the appendicular artery, an indirect branch of the ileocolic (Fig. 2).

f. RETROCECAL FOSSA – results from failure of fixation of the mesentery of the cecum to the posterior peritoneum. The appendix is most commonly located in this retrocecal position (Fig. 6).

g. INTERSIGMOID FOSSA (Fig. 3, page 197) – is a small depression in the mesosigmoid over the bifurcation of the left iliac vessels. In the fossa, one may see the peritoneal reflection over the left ureter.

In addition to the folds, certain inconstant *peritoneal bands* related to the large bowel may be observed. These colic bands are of significance in that they may provide a fixed attachment of bowel about which a volvulus may form or which may result in constriction or acute angulation of the bowel.

h. JACKSON'S PARACOLIC MEMBRANE (Fig. 4) – is a vascular band extending from the posterior abdominal wall to the anterior surface of the ascending colon or cecum. It may be distinguished from peritoneal adhesions by the parallel pattern of its blood vessels.

i. INTERCOLIC MEMBRANES – are located at the hepatic and splenic flexures between the transverse colon and the ascending and descending colons on their respective sides. They are believed to be extensions of the greater omentum across the hepatic or splenic flexures.

j. CYSTOCOLIC MEMBRANE – passes from the gallbladder to the hepatic flexure or may in fact extend as far as the liver as the *hepatocystocolic ligament*. These bands are thought to be a persistence of parts of primitive ventral mesentery.

2. **Gross Characteristics** (Fig. 1) – several anatomic features of the large bowel distinguish it from other parts of the digestive tract; they are:

a. TAENIAE COLIC – result from the realignment of the longitudinal muscle of the small bowel into three longitudinal bands. All three bands begin at the base of the appendix and terminate at the rectum where they spread out again as a complete longitudinal layer. They are termed the *taenia mesocolica, taenia omentalis,* and *taenia libera.* The latter is important to the surgeon since it lies on the anterior surface of the cecum and may be used as a guide to the base of the appendix (Figs. 2, 3 and 5).

b. HAUSTRA – or sacculations of the large bowel are produced by the large intestine (5 feet) adapting in length to the three shorter taeniae (4 feet).

c. APPENDICES EPIPLOICAE – are fat-containing peritoneal pouches related to all parts of the colon except the cecum, appendix, and rectum. They are closely related to the taeniae and are most numerous in the sigmoid colon.

3. **Cecum and Appendix** – these parts constitute the first portion of the large bowel and are situated below the entrance of the ileum. The appendix extends from the caudal end of the cecum.

a. ILEOCECAL VALVE (Fig. 1) – is located in the dorsal-medial wall of the large bowel. It consists of a *superior* and *inferior lip (labrum)* between which is a transverse slit about 1.2 cm. in length. The lips join at each end of the slit to form a *frenulum*, each of which partially surrounds the intestine demarcating the cecum from the ascending colon.

b. CECUM PROPER – usually lies in the false pelvis on the iliopsoas muscle but, depending upon the peritoneal fixation, may be located anywhere from a subhepatic position to the true pelvis. These abnormal positions are of practical significance when its appendage, the appendix, becomes diseased. Since it is the thinnest walled part of the large bowel, distal obstruction of the colon may result in rupture of the uninvolved cecum. In its most common form, the development of that part of the cecum lateral to the taenia libera (anterior) is excessive so that the appendix arises close to the ileocecal junction. Rarely does the fetal conical-shaped cecum persist; the appendix arises therefore, from the apex of the cone. Other variations in form may be found but, in any case, the taenia libera leads the surgeon to the base of the appendix.

c. APPENDIX (VERMIFORM PROCESS) – is a blind tube which varies extremely in both length and position. Major variations in position are illustrated in Figure 5 and are dependent upon the variations of the fixation of the cecum, for the relationship of the base of the appendix to the cecum is constant. Its peritoneal relation has been discussed above.

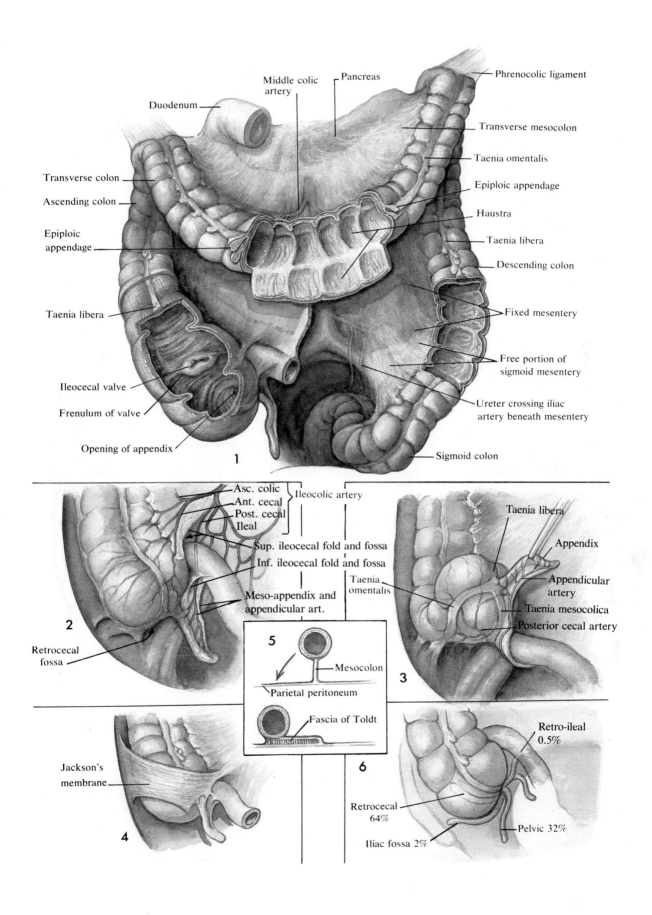

1

Duodenum

Middle colic artery

Pancreas

Phrenocolic ligament

Transverse mesocolon

Taenia omentalis

Epiploic appendage

Haustra

Taenia libera

Descending colon

Transverse colon

Ascending colon

Epiploic appendage

Taenia libera

Ileocecal valve

Frenulum of valve

Opening of appendix

Fixed mesentery

Free portion of sigmoid mesentery

Ureter crossing iliac artery beneath mesentery

Sigmoid colon

2

Asc. colic
Ant. cecal
Post. cecal
Ileal

Ileocolic artery

Sup. ileocecal fold and fossa

Inf. ileocecal fold and fossa

Meso-appendix and appendicular art.

Retrocecal fossa

3

Taenia libera

Appendix

Appendicular artery

Taenia mesocolica

Posterior cecal artery

Taenia omentalis

5

Mesocolon

Parietal peritoneum

Fascia of Toldt

4

Jackson's membrane

6

Retro-ileal 0.5%

Retrocecal 64%

Pelvic 32%

Iliac fossa 2%

4. **Blood Supply** (Fig. 1)—that portion of the large bowel derived from the midgut is supplied by the superior mesenteric artery and that portion derived from the hindgut, by the inferior mesenteric artery.

a. SUPERIOR MESENTERIC ARTERY—arises from the aorta at the level of the first lumbar vertebra. Its jejunal and ileal branches arising from the left side of the main trunk have been described on page 190. The large bowel branches arise from the right side of the artery as it descends through the root of the mesentery. The *middle colic artery* arises at the lower border of the pancreas and *descends* into the transverse mesocolon where it divides into a branch which passes to the left to anastomose with the ascending branch of the left colic and into one or two branches which curve to the right to join the ascending branch of the right colic. The *right colic artery* passes to the right and divides into an ascending branch which anastomoses with the middle colic and a descending branch which anastomoses with the colic branch of the ileocolic artery. Although usually a direct branch of the superior mesenteric, it may arise as a common trunk with the middle colic or with the ileocolic. The *ileocolic artery* is the chief supply of the cecum and appendix. This artery arises as the lowest branch from the right side of the superior mesenteric and descends toward the cecum. It terminates by dividing into a *colic* branch which ascends to anastomose with the right colic, and an *ileal* branch which joins the terminal intestinal branch of the superior mesenteric. Near the division, the ileocolic gives rise to the *anterior* and *posterior cecal arteries*. From the latter, the *appendicular artery* takes origin (Fig. 2, page 195).

b. INFERIOR MESENTERIC ARTERY—arises from the aorta at the level of the third lumbar vertebra as an impaired anterior visceral branch. It passed downward and to the left behind the peritoneum and gives rise to the following branches: the *left colic artery* runs in a transverse direction and near the mesocolic margin of the bowel divides into an ascending branch which anastomoses with the middle colic and a descending branch which joins the upper sigmoid artery. Usually two to three *sigmoid arteries* run downward and to the left in the sigmoid mesocolon. Each artery divides into an ascending and descending branch which anastomose with each other and with the left colic above and the superior hemorrhoidal below. The *superior hemorrhoidal artery* is a continuation of the inferior mesenteric trunk and is described on page 226.

c. MARGINAL ARTERY OF DRUMMOND—is made up of a number of anastomotic arcades paralleling the mesenteric border of the colon and formed by the arterial vessels supplying the large bowel. It consists therefore of the connecting vessels between ileocolic, right colic, and middle colic branches of the superior mesenteric artery with the left colic, sigmoid, and superior hemorrhoidal interconnecting channels from the inferior mesenteric artery. From this anastomotic arcade arise the vasa recta to the colon. The marginal artery may serve as a collateral pathway when a major vessel supplying the colon is ligated. The adequacy of this collateral channel in its entirety is questionable. In particular, the anastomosis between the middle colic and left colic arteries and that between the lowest sigmoid and superior hemorrhoidal in some people may be inadequate. For the surgeon, it is probably safest to assume that the marginal artery, although anatomically a true collateral pathway, is not so physiologically efficient as to support that portion of the large bowel supplied by a major vessel which has been ligated. This fact is taken into consideration, along with the lymphatic drainage of the involved portion of bowel (page 198), when resections of the large bowel are planned. Between the middle colic artery and the ascending branch of the left colic in the transverse mesocolon is an area devoid of blood vessels and termed the *avascular area of Riolan*. In a posterior gastroenterostomy the intestinal loop is passed through this area.

d. INTRAMURAL BLOOD SUPPLY—is by *vasa recta* arising from the marginal artery and is illustrated in Figure 2.

5. **Venous Drainage**—the veins draining the large bowel closely follow the arteries and are similarly named. The ileocolic, right, and middle colic, are tributaries of the *superior mesenteric vein*. The middle colic often joins the right gastroepiploic vein to form the *gastrocolic trunk* before emptying into the superior mesenteric. Behind the neck of the pancreas, the superior mesenteric joins the splenic to form the portal vein. The superior hemorrhoidal, sigmoid veins, and left colic drain into the *inferior mesenteric* which usually empties into the splenic vein (Fig. 1, page 183).

6. **Mobilization of the Colon**—since both the transverse and sigmoid colon retain their primitive mesenteries, it is only the ascending and descending colon and rectum which require mobilization prior to resection. Mobilization of the rectum is illustrated on page 231. The basic principle in mobilization of either the ascending or descending colon is to reconstruct the original dorsal mesentery. It should be recalled that during rotation of the gut, the ascending and descending colon are thrown upon the posterior abdominal peritoneum and become fused with that layer (page 150). These fused peritoneal layers form an avascular fascial layer known as *Toldt's fascia* (Fig. 5, page 195).

a. ASCENDING COLON—must be first freed from the posterior parietal wall by incising the lateral peritoneal reflection in the *right paracolic gutter*. Since the blood vessels approach the colon from the medial side, such an incision is safe. The colon is retracted to the left and the fused peritoneal fascial plane (Toldt's) is identified. By blunt dissection through this cleavage plane the ascending colon and its mesentery are separated from the underlying retroperitoneal structures shown in Figure 4.

b. DESCENDING COLON—is mobilized much as is the ascending colon. The incision is made in the *left paracolic gutter* and the bowel is reflected to the right. It is again important to identify the fused peritoneal structures. If dissection proceeds on a plane deep to Toldt's fascia, the ureter and internal spermatic (ovarian) vessels may be reflected with the mesentery of the bowel and damaged during resection (Fig. 5).

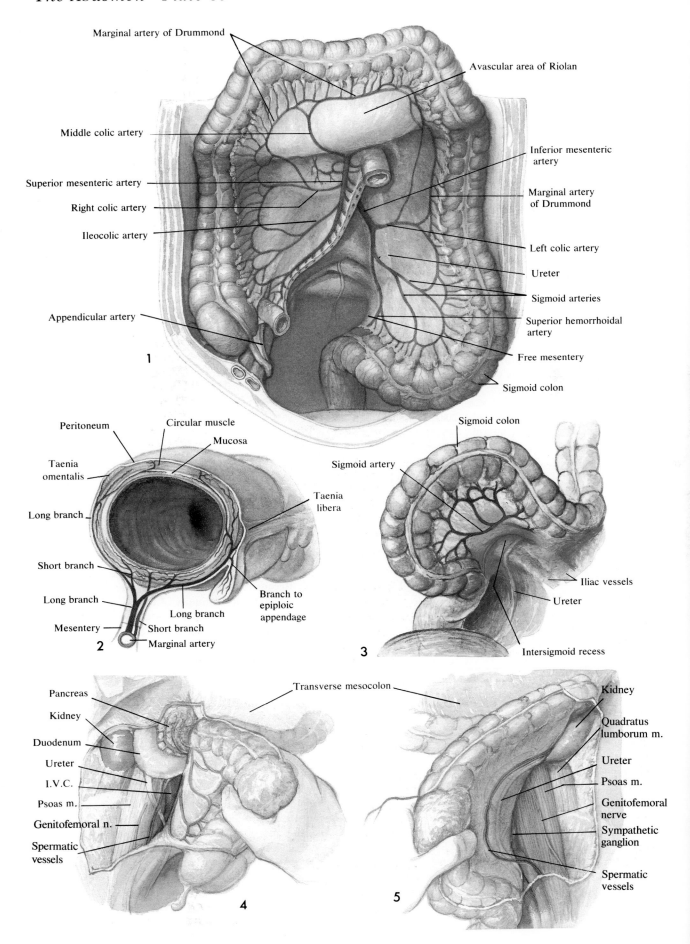

Marginal artery of Drummond

Avascular area of Riolan

Middle colic artery

Inferior mesenteric artery

Superior mesenteric artery

Marginal artery of Drummond

Right colic artery

Left colic artery

Ileocolic artery

Ureter

Sigmoid arteries

Superior hemorrhoidal artery

Appendicular artery

Free mesentery

Sigmoid colon

1

Peritoneum

Circular muscle

Mucosa

Sigmoid colon

Sigmoid artery

Taenia omentalis

Long branch

Taenia libera

Short branch

Long branch

Mesentery

Long branch

Short branch

Branch to epiploic appendage

Marginal artery

Iliac vessels

Ureter

2

3

Intersigmoid recess

Pancreas

Transverse mesocolon

Kidney

Kidney

Quadratus lumborum m.

Duodenum

Ureter

Ureter

I.V.C.

Psoas m.

Psoas m.

Genitofemoral n.

Genitofemoral nerve

Spermatic vessels

Sympathetic ganglion

Spermatic vessels

4

5

7. Lymphatics of the Large Bowel—treatment of malignant lesions of the large bowel requires the removal not only of the primary tumor but the regional lymph nodes as well.

a. CAPILLARY LYMPHATIC PLEXUSES—are located in the mucosal, submucosal, muscular, and subserosal layers of the bowel wall.

b. COLLECTING CHANNELS—arise from these capillary plexuses of the large bowel and drain into various nodal groups. They include the epicolic, paracolic, intermediate, and principle nodes. Lymphatic channels may traverse all four of these nodal groups or enter any of the groups directly without traversing the others.

c. REGIONAL NODES (Fig. 1)—related to the large bowel are arranged in four nodal groups:

(1) *Epicolic Nodes*—are subserous in position in the epiploic appendices and most numerous in the sigmoid colon.

(2) *Paracolic Nodes*—lie along the mesenteric border of the large bowel but are less numerous in relation to the descending colon.

(3) *Intermediate Nodes*—are located along the major arterial branches supplying the large bowel., i.e., ileocolic, right colic, middle colic, left colic, and sigmoid arteries.

(4) *Principal Nodes*—are actually preaortic nodes of the retroperitoneal group (page 208). They are related to the superior and inferior mesenteric arteries.

d. TERMINAL COLLECTING CHANNELS—from the superior mesenteric nodes and upper inferior mesenteric nodes join those of the celiac nodes to form the *intestinal trunk*. Collecting trunks from the lower inferior mesenteric nodes enter the left lateral aortic (lumbar) chain directly.

8. Resection of the Large Bowel—if resection of a portion of the large bowel is performed for a benign or malignant lesion, *it is most imperative that an adequate blood supply be preserved to the remaining segments.* In benign conditions the blood supply to the remaining segments is the major anatomic consideration. If resection of the large bowel is performed for removal of a malignant lesion, the regional lymphatic drainage of that segment of bowel which is to be removed must be considered as well.

a. CECUM (Fig. 2)—a malignant lesion of the cecum requires the removal of the lymphatic channels and nodes draining this area, but the blood supply of the remaining colon must be preserved. To accomplish this the terminal ileum ascending colon and first portion of the transverse colon are resected. The terminal ileal branches, the ileocolic, and right colic arteries are ligated at their origin from the superior mesenteric artery and these vessels along with the mesentery and aforementioned bowel segments are removed in toto.

b. ASCENDING COLON AND HEPATIC FLEXURE (Figs. 3 and 4)—resection of malignant lesions involving any part of the ascending colon or hepatic flexure requires a procedure similar to that described above except that two-thirds of the transverse colon is resected.

This requires the ligation of the middle colic branch of the superior mesenteric in addition to the right colic, ileocolic, and terminal ileal branches.

c. TRANSVERSE COLON (Fig. 5)—the lymphatics of the transverse colon are numerous and capillary channels may end directly in the intermediate nodes of the middle colic artery. Resection of a malignant lesion of transverse colon should include the transverse mesocolon with ligation of the middle colic at its origin from the superior mesenteric artery in order to remove the regional nodes.

d, SPLENIC FLEXURE (Fig. 6)—lesions in this area require resection of the distal one-third of the transverse colon and upper portion of the descending colon. Ligation of the left colic branch with preservation of the remaining inferior and superior mesenteric artery is required.

e. DESCENDING COLON (Fig. 7)—carcinoma of the descending colon requires resection not only of the specific part involved but of the distal third of the transverse colon as well. Ligation of the left colic artery at its origin from the inferior mesenteric and the upper sigmoidal arteries is required in order to remove adequate mesentery with lymphatic nodes and capillaries.

f. SIGMOID COLON (Fig. 8)—this area of bowel is heavily endowed with lymphatic channels. In resection of this segment of bowel the inferior mesenteric artery is ligated just below the origin of the left colic artery. This segment of bowel with its mesentery is totally removed.

g. COLECTOMY—a total colectomy requires removal of the terminal ileum, ascending, transverse, descending, and sigmoid colon, as well as the rectum and anal canal. A permanent ileostomy is constructed. In a *subtotal colectomy* the rectum and anus are preserved and bowel continuity restored by anastomosing the ileum to the rectum. A colectomy is usually indicated in diffuse benign diseases of the large bowel.

9. Reconstruction Procedures—several methods are used to reestablish continuity of the bowel.

a. PRIMARY END-TO-END ANASTOMOSIS—may be used following resection of short segments of bowel or resection of the transverse, descending, or sigmoid colon.

b. ILEOCOLOSTOMY—is required following a right hemicolectomy or subtotal colectomy.

c. COLOSTOMY—establishes an opening between the colon and the skin of the abdominal wall. The more *mobile* portions of the large bowel are usually used, i.e., *cecostomy, transverse colostomy,* and *sigmoidostomy.* Colostomies may be constructed so as to form a temporary fecal fistula or a permanent artificial anus.

d. INTERNAL BY-PASS PROCEDURES—may serve the same purpose as a colostomy. A by-pass may be established by a side-to-side anastomosis of the bowel proximal and distal to the site of the lesion. More frequently the bowel may be transected proximal to the lesion and continuity reestablished by anastomosing the proximal loop of bowel to a segment of bowel distal to the lesion.

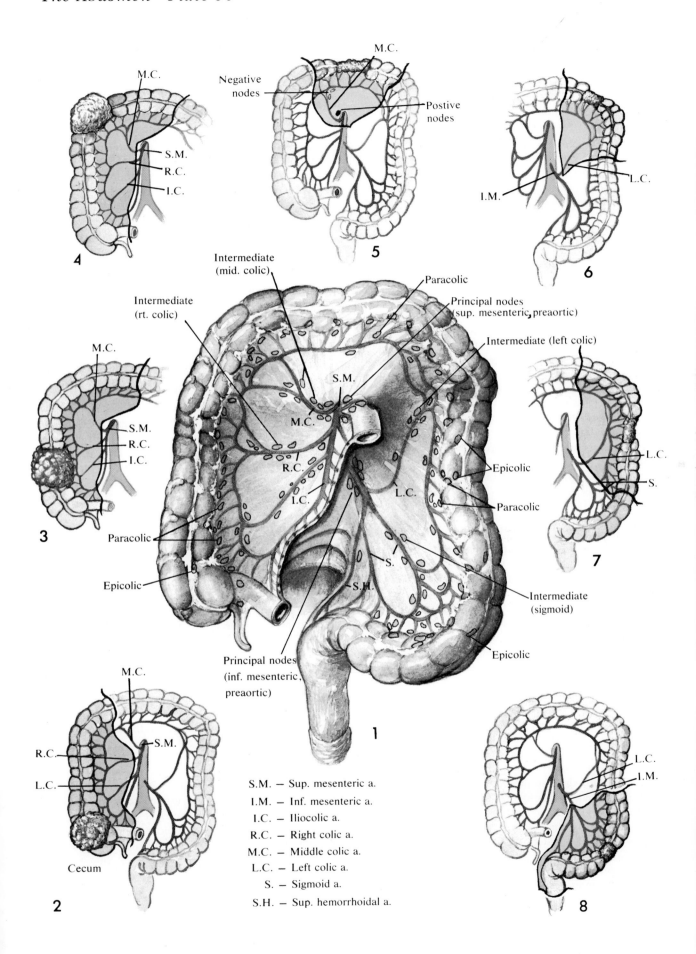

M.C.

Negative nodes

M.C.

Postive nodes

5

I.M.

L.C.

6

M.C.

4

S.M.
R.C.
I.C.

Intermediate (mid. colic)

Paracolic

Intermediate (rt. colic)

Principal nodes (sup. mesenteric, preaortic)

Intermediate (left colic)

M.C.

S.M.
R.C.
I.C.

S.M.

M.C.

3

R.C.

I.C.

L.C.

Epicolic

Paracolic

L.C.

S.

Paracolic

Epicolic

S.

7

Intermediate (sigmoid)

S.H.

Epicolic

Principal nodes (inf. mesenteric, preaortic)

1

M.C.

S.M.

R.C.

L.C.

Cecum

2

L.C.

I.M.

8

S.M. — Sup. mesenteric a.

I.M. — Inf. mesenteric a.

I.C. — Iliocolic a.

R.C. — Right colic a.

M.C. — Middle colic a.

L.C. — Left colic a.

S. — Sigmoid a.

S.H. — Sup. hemorrhoidal a.

RETROPERITONEAL VISCERA:

The true embryonic retroperitoneal viscera consists of the adrenal glands, kidneys, ureters, and gonads. Since the gonads migrate downward they are considered in the discussions of the testicle and ovary.

1. **Adrenal (Suprarenal) Glands**—these organs are part of the endocrine (ductless) glands of the body. Each adrenal gland consists of a cortex derived from the mesoderm and a medulla derived from ectodermal tissue. These two parts differ histologically as well as physiologically.

The *posterior surface* of both adrenals is firmly attached to the diaphragm. The *base* rests upon the upper pole of the kidneys. The base of the left adrenal extends inferiorly over the anteromedial surface to the renal hilus (Fig. 1). The upper half of the anterior surface of the left adrenal is covered by posterior parietal peritoneum and is related to the lesser peritoneal cavity. The lower half of this surface is covered by the splenic vessels and the pancreas (Fig. 1). On the right side the anterior surface of the gland is related in its upper part to the bare area of the liver (Fig. 1). Medially the upper part of the gland may extend behind the inferior vena cava (Fig. 3). The remainder of the right adrenal is covered by the parietal peritoneum related to the general peritoneal cavity.

2. **Kidneys**—each organ lies between the endo-abdominal fascia behind and the posterior parietal peritoneum in front surrounded by areolar and fascial coverings.

a. RENAL (GEROTA'S) FASCIA (Figs. 2 and 3)—is also referred to as *perirenal fascia* or the *false capsule* of the kidney. It is a condensation of the extraperitoneal fatty tissue layer of the abdominal wall. This fascial layer extends over the anterior and posterior surfaces of the kidneys. Medially it becomes adherent to the adventitial coverings of the renal vessels, aorta, and inferior vena cava. Above, the anterior and posterior layers fuse at the upper pole of the kidney but also extend upward to form a special compartment for the adrenal gland. Some investigators claim the anterior and posterior layers of renal fascia do not fuse below, while others state that a fusion does occur and that the fascia extends inferiorly as a *periureteral sheath*. Proof that this fascial fusion does not occur is offered clinically by the fact that air injected into the extraperitoneal fatty tissue in the presacral area can outline the kidneys in radiologic examination (*retroperitoneal air insufflation*) and by the clinical condition referred to as *nephroptosis*.

b. PARARENAL (RETRORENAL) FAT CAPSULE—is in continuity with the extraperitoneal fatty layer of the anterolateral and posterior abdominal wall. This fat depot lies between the renal fascia and endoabdominal fascia posteriorly and the renal fascia and posterior parietal peritoneum anteriorly. It is most marked on the posterolateral abdominal wall and varies in thickness from a few millimeters in asthenic patients to a layer of enormous proportions in obese patients.

c. RENAL CAPSULE—is the true fibrous capsule of the kidney. It is attached to the overlying renal fascia by multiple fibrous trabeculae.

d. PERIRENAL FAT CAPSULE—is located between the renal fascia externally and the renal capsule internally. This fatty capsule, part of the extraperitoneal fatty tissue, occupies an area termed the *perinephric space*.

e. PERITONEAL RELATIONS (Fig. 1)—of the anterior surface of the kidneys in the embryo to the posterior parietal layer of peritoneum is illustrated in Figure 2, page 149. With the rotation of the gut, this simple relationship changes due to fixation of the original dorsal mesentery to the posterior parietal peritoneum. The upper three-fourths of the anterior surface of the right kidney remains covered by the original posterior parietal peritoneum and is directly related to the *hepatorenal pouch (Morison)* (Fig. 2, page 185). The descending portion of the duodenum becomes fixed to the original peritoneal covering of the medial border of the right kidney by fusion of the embryonic dorsal mesentery to the posterior parietal peritoneum (Fig. 4, page 161). The dorsal mesentery of the upper portion of the ascending colon becomes fused with the posterior peritoneum covering the lower pole of the right kidney during rotation of the gut (Fig. 5, page 195).

As a result of the rotation of the foregut the embryonic mesogastrium fuses with the original peritoneal covering of the upper anterior surface of the left kidney. This upper portion of the kidney is therefore related to the omental bursa (Fig. 3, page 157). The midportion of the left kidney loses direct peritoneal relationship due to the growth of the tail of the pancreas. The lower pole of the kidney retains its original posterior parietal peritoneal covering and is related to the upper portion of the left paracolic gutter.

3. **Ureters**—fibromuscular tubes are divided into abdominal, pelvic, and intravesical parts. The latter two parts will be described in the discussion of the pelvic viscera.

a. ABDOMINAL URETER (Fig. 1)—extends from the renal pelvis to the pelvic brim and its lumen is narrowest at these two points. At the kidney pelvis it lies posterior to the renal artery and vein. It courses downward and medialward over the psoas muscle and genitofemoral nerve, crosses the bifurcation of the common iliac artery anterior to the sacroiliac joint, and enters the pelvis. The anatomic relationship with the genitofemoral nerve may explain the testicular pain sometimes associated with the passage of an ureteral stone.

Anteriorly the ureter is closely related to the posterior parietal peritoneum—a relationship extremely important in the mobilization of the ascending and descending colon (page 196). The right ureter is covered anteriorly by the descending duodenum, the internal spermatic (ovarian), the right colic and ileocolic vessels, and the root of the mesentery. On the left side, the internal spermatic (ovarian), left colic, and sigmoid vessels cross this portion of the ureter.

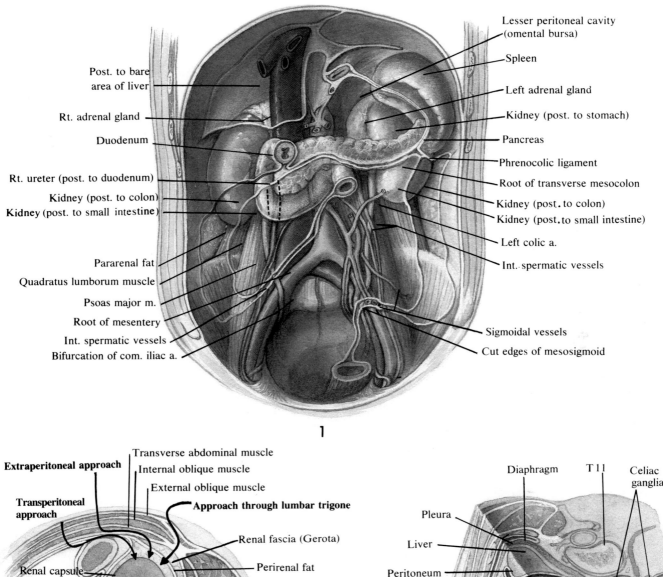

Lesser peritoneal cavity (omental bursa)

Spleen

Left adrenal gland

Kidney (post. to stomach)

Pancreas

Phrenocolic ligament

Root of transverse mesocolon

Kidney (post. to colon)

Kidney (post. to small intestine)

Left colic a.

Int. spermatic vessels

Sigmoidal vessels

Cut edges of mesosigmoid

Post. to bare area of liver

Rt. adrenal gland

Duodenum

Rt. ureter (post. to duodenum)

Kidney (post. to colon)

Kidney (post. to small intestine)

Pararenal fat

Quadratus lumborum muscle

Psoas major m.

Root of mesentery

Int. spermatic vessels

Bifurcation of com. iliac a.

1

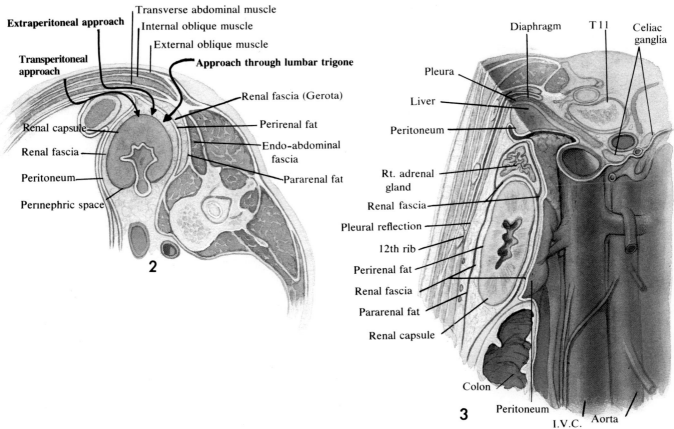

Transverse abdominal muscle

Internal oblique muscle

External oblique muscle

Extraperitoneal approach

Transperitoneal approach

Approach through lumbar trigone

Renal fascia (Gerota)

Perirenal fat

Endo-abdominal fascia

Pararenal fat

Renal capsule

Renal fascia

Peritoneum

Perinephric space

2

Diaphragm   T 11   Celiac ganglia

Pleura

Liver

Peritoneum

Rt. adrenal gland

Renal fascia

Pleural reflection

12th rib

Perirenal fat

Renal fascia

Pararenal fat

Renal capsule

Colon

Peritoneum

I.V.C.   Aorta

3

4. **Arterial Supply** (Fig. 1)—the blood vessels supplying the adrenals, ureters, kidneys, and gonads arise chiefly from the three paired visceral branches of the abdominal aorta; the middle suprarenal, renal, and internal spermatic (ovarian) arteries.

a. ADRENAL GLAND—of each side is classically described as being supplied by three arteries: a *superior suprarenal* artery from the inferior phrenic branch of the aorta, a *middle suprarenal* directly from the aorta, and an *inferior suprarenal* arising from the renal artery. Actually each of these arteries may give rise to multiple branches which enter the periphery of the organ. In fact, the major branches themselves may arise as multiple branches from their parent vessels. Relatively speaking, the adrenal gland is probably the most vascular organ in the body.

b. KIDNEY—the *renal arteries* arise from the lateral surfaces of the aorta usually at the level of the upper border of L_2. Variations in origin frequently occur to the extent that they may arise at a full vertebral level above or below the normal point of origin. Supernumerary arteries supplying the kidney are not infrequent, being as high as 35 per cent in some series. The single right renal artery passes behind the inferior vena cava. Both the right and left renal arteries lie between the renal vein in front and the renal pelvis at the hilus of the kidney. In its course toward the hilus each renal artery gives off the inferior suprarenal artery and a ureteric branch. At the hilus the artery divides into anterior and posterior branches in relation to the renal pelvis. Both branches, according to recent investigation, are segmental branches. Like the segmental arteries of the lung and liver there is little if any anastomosis between these segmental branches. Aberrant polar arteries may be present as discussed on page 204.

c. URETER—the arterial supply to the ureter is both multiple and variable. The abdominal part of the ureter receives arterial branches from the renal artery above, from the internal spermatic (ovarian) artery in the intermediate area, and from the common iliac artery below. Each of these ureteric branches gives rise to ascending and descending anastomotic channels. The pelvic portion of the ureter receives branches from the uterine, inferior vesical, and middle hemorrhoidal arteries.

5. **Venous Drainage**—the veins of all true retroperitoneal viscera drain into the inferior caval system.

a. ADRENALS—unlike the multiplicity of the adrenal arteries, the major adrenal vein on each side is singular. The *central vein* of each adrenal exits from the gland at a slit-like area termed the *adrenal hilus.* On the left side the hilus is located at the lower part of the medial border, whereas on the right gland it is located on the anteromedial surface. The *central vein of the right adrenal* exits from the hilus and takes a short and almost transverse course to empty into the inferior vena cava. Because of its short course, this vein may be easily torn

during manipulation of the right adrenal gland. The *central vein of the left adrenal,* on the other hand, extends inferiorly over the anterior surface of the adrenal and after joining the left inferior phrenic vein terminates in the left renal vein.

b. RENAL VEINS—exit from the renal parenchyma at the renal hilus anterior to the renal artery. The renal vein is longer and slightly higher on the left side as compared to the right vein, but both enter the inferior vena cava at nearly a right angle. The renal veins, although less frequently than the arteries, may be multiple, particularly on the right side. The left renal vein receives the left suprarenal and left inferior phrenic vein either separately or as a single tributary, the left spermatic (ovarian) vein, and the left upper ureteric vein. The right renal vein because of its very short course receives only the ureteric vein.

c. URETERIC VEINS—specific information regarding the venous drainage is lacking. Most anatomic textbooks simply state that the veins tend to follow the arterial supply. One can only surmise, therefore, that ureteric veins are tributaries of the renal, internal spermatic (ovarian), common iliac, and hypogastric veins.

6. **Lymphatic Drainage**—of these retroperitoneal organs is usually described, if considered at all, in most surgical textbooks as emptying into "regional nodes" (see page 208).

a. ADRENAL—lymphatic capillaries of the cortex follow the superior and middle suprarenal arterial branches while the medullary capillaries follow the central veins. The collecting channels from these capillary networks drain into the para-aortic nodes at the level of the superior mesenteric artery on the left side and into laterovenous or retrovenous nodes related to the inferior vena cava at the same body level on the right. The medullary collecting channels terminate in preaortic or para-aortic nodes just below the renal vessels. Of most particular importance is the fact that collecting channels from both glands may directly communicate with the posterior mediastinal nodes of the thorax. The clinical significance of this anatomic continuity becomes apparent when one reflects upon the high incidence of metastatic carcinoma of the adrenal from primary lung cancer and the similar relationship between adrenal insufficiency and tuberculosis.

b. KIDNEYS—capsular and parenchymal lymphatic networks form collecting channels that drain from the right kidney to prevenous, laterovenous, and retrovenous nodes of the right lumbar chain extending from the renal pedicle to the level of the aortic bifurcation. From the left kidney collecting channels terminate in the left para-aortic chain in the region of the renal pedicle.

c. URETER—lymphatic drainage of the ureter is of least importance in regard to the retroperitoneal viscera. Suffice it to say that the upper segment collecting channels join the renal lymphatics or empty directly into the

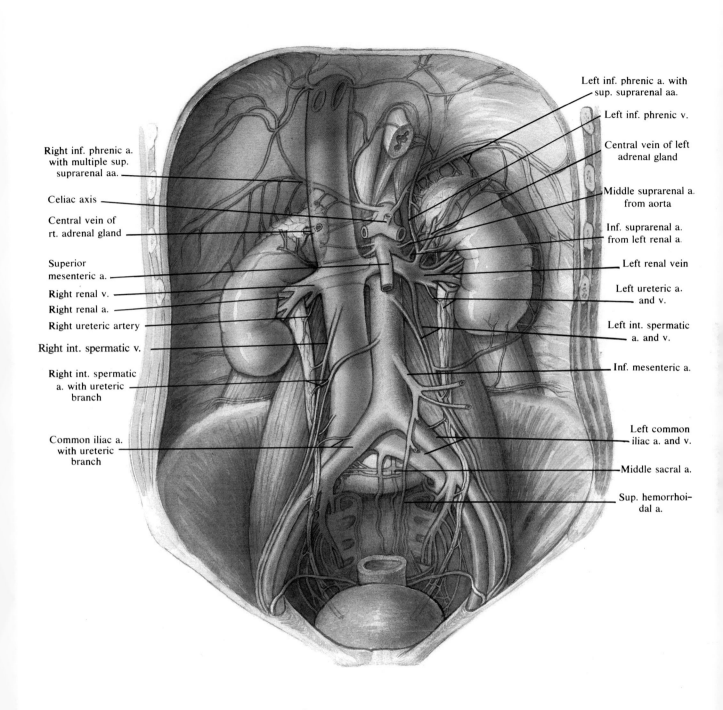

Right inf. phrenic a. with multiple sup. suprarenal aa.

Celiac axis

Central vein of rt. adrenal gland

Superior mesenteric a.

Right renal v.

Right renal a.

Right ureteric artery

Right int. spermatic v.

Right int. spermatic a. with ureteric branch

Common iliac a. with ureteric branch

Left inf. phrenic a. with sup. suprarenal aa.

Left inf. phrenic v.

Central vein of left adrenal gland

Middle suprarenal a. from aorta

Inf. suprarenal a. from left renal a.

Left renal vein

Left ureteric a. and v.

Left int. spermatic a. and v.

Inf. mesenteric a.

Left common iliac a. and v.

Middle sacral a.

Sup. hemorrhoidal a.

right and left lumbar nodes. The lymphatic channels draining the middle segment, which extends from the internal spermatic vessels to the pelvic brim, empty into the para-aortic nodes adjacent to the inferior mesenteric artery or into a common iliac node.

7. **Nerve Supply**—the nerve supply of these retroperitoneal viscera will not be considered here. Such information may be obtained by consulting any of the textbooks on neuroanatomy or the autonomic nervous system.

CLINICAL CONSIDERATIONS: KIDNEYS, URETERS, AND ADRENALS:

These retroperitoneal abdominal organs may be exposed by a variety of surgical incisions. Such incisions may be made from a lumbar extraperitoneal approach, a posterolateral extraperitoneal approach, or an anterior transperitoneal approach (Fig. 2, page 201).

1. **Congenital Anomalies**—anomalies are frequent in relation to the kidney and ureters. Some of these anomalies require early surgical intervention; all such anomalies are important in the preoperative evaluation prior to any surgical procedure upon the upper urinary tract.

a. STRUCTURAL ANOMALIES—include *hypoplasia,* a failure of the kidney to fully develop, or a *hyperplasia,* a uniform enlargement of one kidney because of the absence or hypoplasia of the opposite kidney. A *polycystic* kidney, which probably results from a failure of the collecting tubules arising from the ureters to connect completely with the secreting (uriniferous) tubules of the kidneys, is of serious clinical import. One of the most frequent anomalies is the *horseshoe kidney.* During the ascent of the primordial embryonic kidney of each side, portions of these bilateral structures may fuse, usually at the lower pole, to form a commissure between the two formed kidneys. This commissure may be composed of true renal or fibrous tissue. These fused kidneys are usually at a lower level than normal. Very rarely a *congenital stricture of the ureter* may occur resulting in an enlargement of the ureters proximal to the narrowing *(megalo-ureter).*

b. POSITIONAL ANOMALIES—are termed *ectopic kidneys.* The primordial kidneys develop in the pelvic region and ascend to their normal lumbar position during development. Disturbance in this normal developmental procedure may result in an adult kidney being located anywhere between the pelvic cavity and its normal lumbar position. In addition, the ascent of one kidney may deviate across the midline so that both kidneys develop on the same side of the body. Such an ectopic kidney may be mistaken for a tumor. The ureteric orifice may be ectopic in position, particularly in the female. In most instances it usually opens below the normal vesical opening.

c. NUMERICAL ANOMALIES—vary from *agenesis* or congenital absence, an extremely important clinical entity, to the extremely rare *supranumerary kidneys.* The most frequent anomaly of the ureter is that of the *double ureter.* This condition may be complete duplication or incomplete duplication *(forked ureter).* They are usually of no clinical significance except that the complete type may be of concern during gynecological procedures since they are three times more frequent in the female.

d. VASCULAR ANOMALIES—are a common cause of congenital hydronephrosis. Some 35 to 40 per cent of obstructions at the ureteropelvic junction is due to an aberrant renal artery (Fig. 1). These polar arteries are not "accessory" vessels, but are normal segmental arteries that arise from an aberrant site as an early branch of the renal artery or directly from the aorta.

2. **Trauma**—because of the deep retroperitoneal position of the kidney, ureters, and adrenals, anterior abdominal wall injuries rarely involve these organs. In posterior abdominal wall contusions or penetrating wounds they are more vulnerable and possible injury to these structures should always be considered in the evaluation of such injuries.

The most vulnerable of these retroperitoneal organs to trauma is the ureter. Operative injury is the primary case. This is particularly true in intra-abdominal operative procedures. Emphasis has already been placed upon this fact on page 196. The possible surgical injury to the ureter in pelvic procedures is illustrated on page 239.

Damage to the blood supply may also cause damage to the ureters as a result of ischemic necrosis. The blood supply of the ureters has already been discussed on page 202. Variation in the blood supply is considerable. The supply to the lower abdominal portion of the ureter is particularly sparse and isolation of the ureters for a length of more than 2.5 cm. may cause ureteral necrosis.

3. **Surgical Anatomy of the Kidney**—the relation of the anatomy of the kidney to the abdominal cavity has been discussed on pages 200 and 202. The topographic anatomy and the practical application of renal percutaneous biopsy are discussed on page 146. Surgical procedures upon the kidney may vary from a total removal of the organ *(total nephrectomy),* partial removal *(partial nephrectomy),* an incision into the renal parenchyma with *(nephrostomy)* or without *(nephrotomy)* drainage.

If an incision into the renal parenchyma is necessary it is best performed through *Brödel's line* (Fig. 2). This line is described as being located slightly behind the convex border of the kidney. It is a relatively avascular zone where the anterior and posterior vessels meet. Nephrotomy through this line is far from bloodless, but such an incision is less likely to produce an ischemia necrosis of the adjacent renal parenchyma.

Renal transplantation is discussed on page 214.

4. **Surgical Anatomy of the Adrenal Glands**—the adrenal glands may be approached by both the posterolateral extraperitoneal and anterior transperitoneal approach. The latter approach is particularly preferred for the removal of a *pheochromocytoma.* This anterior approach has several advantages: the lateral localization of the tumor may not be apparent preoperatively, the tumor may be bilateral (10 per cent), or the tumor may be ectopic in position. The most common abdominal ectopic locations of such tumors are along the sympathetic trunks or the preaortic plexuses. The anterior transabdominal approach allows careful search of these areas (Fig. 4). Adrenal tumors may at times be recognized radiographically by the displacement of the upper pole of the kidney (Fig. 3).

The adrenal veins are the object of special attention by the surgeon. On the right gland, the vein is short and passes from the medial aspect of the gland into the inferior vena cava (Fig. 5). It cannot be exposed until the gland is mobilized. The left central adrenal vein, however, lies in an anterior position and is 2 to 3 cm. long (Fig. 6).

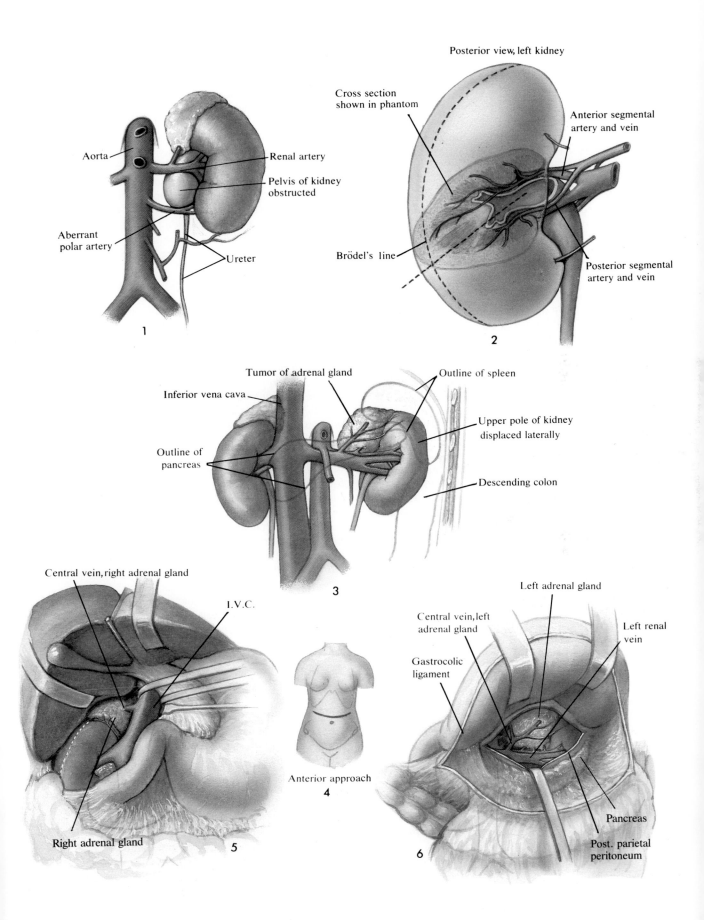

Aorta

Renal artery

Pelvis of kidney obstructed

Aberrant polar artery

Ureter

1

Posterior view, left kidney

Cross section shown in phantom

Anterior segmental artery and vein

Brödel's line

Posterior segmental artery and vein

2

Tumor of adrenal gland

Outline of spleen

Inferior vena cava

Upper pole of kidney displaced laterally

Outline of pancreas

Descending colon

3

Central vein, right adrenal gland

I.V.C.

Left adrenal gland

Central vein, left adrenal gland

Left renal vein

Gastrocolic ligament

Anterior approach

4

Right adrenal gland

5

Pancreas

Post. parietal peritoneum

6

RETROPERITONEAL ANATOMY:

All retroperitoneal anatomic structures lie in the extraperitoneal fatty tissue between the posterior peritoneum in front and the endo-abdominal fascia behind. In addition to the retroperitoneal viscera, which has been discussed on page 200, the inferior vena cava and its tributaries, the abdominal aorta and its branches, the lumbar plexus and its rami, and the sympathetic trunk are located in this same anatomic plane.

1. **Inferior Vena Cava** (Fig. 1) – the inferior vena cava in the adult begins at the union of the right and left common iliac veins between the right common iliac artery anteriorly and the fifth lumbar vertebra posteriorly. The vein ascends to the right of the midline paralleling the aorta. Above the renal tributaries it is separated from the aorta by the right medial crus of the diaphragm. In its suprarenal portion, the inferior vena cava first forms the posterior boundary of the epiploic foramen, then is related to the liver lying in the fossa of the inferior vena cava. It traverses the diaphragm through the caval orifice and enters the right atrium.

The inferior vena cava receives *parietal* tributaries draining the lower extremities, pelvis, and posterolateral abdominal wall. *Visceral* tributaries drain the retroperitoneal viscera as well as the liver.

a. PARIETAL TRIBUTARIES – consist of the common iliac, lumbar, and inferior phrenic veins. The *common iliac veins* are formed by the union of the external and internal iliac veins on either side. The *lumbar veins* drain the posterolateral abdominal wall and have direct posterior connections with the vertebral venous plexus. There is usually a communicating channel, the *ascending lumbar vein*, between the four or five lumbar veins on each side. The *inferior phrenic veins* follow the corresponding arteries. The vein on the right side is a direct tributary of the inferior vena cava. The left inferior phrenic vein usually empties into the left suprarenal vein but occasionally empties into the renal vein or inferior vena cava.

b. VISCERAL TRIBUTARIES – consist of the *renal, adrenal,* and *ureteric veins,* which have been discussed on page 202. The *gonadal veins* in the male are the *internal spermatic veins* and in the female, the *ovarian veins.* These gonadal veins on the right side enter the inferior vena cava directly, whereas, on the left side they empty into the left renal vein. The *hepatic veins* are the largest visceral tributaries of the inferior vena cava. Usually right, left, and middle hepatic veins are described, but in the majority of cases the middle and left branches empty as a common trunk. Veins from the caudate lobe and the right lobe of the liver may drain independently into the cava.

2. **Abdominal Aorta** (Fig. 2) – like the inferior vena cava, aortic branches may be divided into parietal and visceral branches.

a. PARIETAL BRANCHES – are distributed to the abdominal wall. The *inferior phrenic arteries* are the first branches of the abdominal aorta but frequently arise from the celiac axis. The *lumbar arteries* are usually arranged as four paired branches related to the upper four lumbar vertebrae. They send off branches which supply the skin and muscles of the back, and anteriorly anastomose with arterial branches of the anterolateral abdominal wall.

b. VISCERAL BRANCHES – consist of three paired and three unpaired branches. The unpaired branches supply the gastrointestinal tract and its accessory organs. The paired branches supply the true retroperitoneal viscera, i.e., the kidneys, adrenals, and gonads.

(1) *Celiac Artery (axis)* – is the largest branch of the abdominal aorta. It arises from the anterior surface of the aorta at the level of the upper border of L_1. Prevailingly, three arteries arise from this trunk: the left gastric, splenic, and the common hepatic.

(2) *Superior Mesenteric* – arises at the lower border of L_1. Its branches and areas of distribution are described on page 190.

(3) *Inferior Mesenteric* – takes origin from the anterior surface of the aorta at the level of L_3. The anatomy of this vessel is discussed on page 196.

(4) *Middle Suprarenal Arteries* – are paired vessels arising from the aorta just above the first lumbar arteries (page 200).

(5) *Renal Arteries* – are also described on page 200.

(6) *Gonadal Arteries* – in the male are the paired *internal spermatic* and in the female the *ovarian arteries.*

c. TERMINAL BRANCHES – include the *common iliac arteries* and the *middle sacral* which are discussed in the anatomy of the pelvis.

3. **Lumbar Plexus** (Fig. 3) – this nerve plexus is formed by the anterior primary divisions of the upper four lumbar nerves plus a branch from T_{12}. Branches from this plexus have an intimate relationship with the psoas major muscle. They lie in the substance of the muscle and exit from its medial border (*obturator nerve*), its anterior surface (*genitofemoral nerve*), or its lateral border. The branches innervate the ventrolateral abdominal wall, the scrotum (labia), the thigh, and the gluteal region.

a. ILIOHYPOGASTRIC NERVE (T_{12}–L_1) – extends to the anterior abdominal wall between the internal oblique and transversus abdominis muscles (Fig. 1, page 137) and supplies the skin over the symphysis pubis.

b. ILIOINGUINAL NERVE (L_1) – passes forward in the same muscular interval as the iliohypogastric. It extends into the inguinal region and exits through the superficial inguinal ring to supply the skin of the thigh and scrotum (labia).

c. GENITOFEMORAL NERVE (L_1 and L_2) – pierces the psoas, enters the spermatic cord at the abdominal inguinal ring, and supplies a motor branch to the cremaster muscle (*external spermatic nerve*) and a sensory branch to the inner thigh (*lumboinguinal nerve*).

d. LATERAL FEMORAL CUTANEOUS NERVE (posterior secondary L_2 and L_3) – crosses the iliac muscles and passes into the thigh deep to the inguinal ligament just medial to the anterior superior iliac spine.

e. FEMORAL NERVE (posterior secondary L_2, L_3, and L_4) – emerges from the lateral border of the psoas, supplies branches to the iliac muscles, and enters the thigh deep to the inguinal ligament.

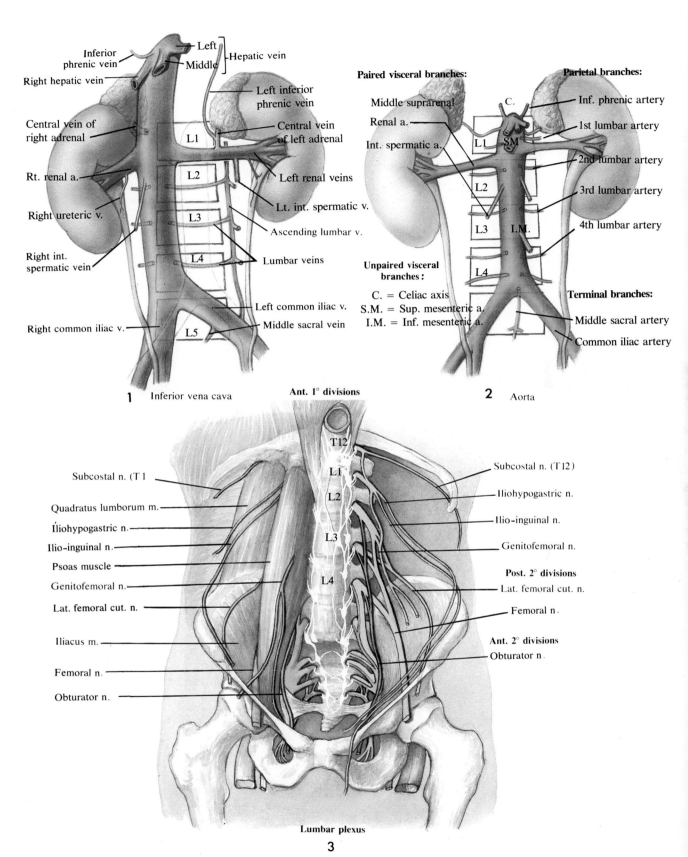

1 Inferior vena cava

Inferior phrenic vein
Right hepatic vein
Central vein of right adrenal
Rt. renal a.
Right ureteric v.
Right int. spermatic vein
Right common iliac v.

Left | Hepatic vein
Middle |
Left inferior phrenic vein
Central vein of left adrenal
Left renal veins
Lt. int. spermatic v.
Ascending lumbar v.
Lumbar veins
Left common iliac v.
Middle sacral vein

L1, L2, L3, L4, L5

2 Aorta

Paired visceral branches:
Middle suprarenal
Renal a.
Int. spermatic a.

Unpaired visceral branches:
C. = Celiac axis
S.M. = Sup. mesenteric a.
I.M. = Inf. mesenteric a.

Parietal branches:
Inf. phrenic artery
1st lumbar artery
2nd lumbar artery
3rd lumbar artery
4th lumbar artery

Terminal branches:
Middle sacral artery
Common iliac artery

C., SM, I.M.

3 Lumbar plexus

Ant. 1° divisions
T12, L1, L2, L3, L4

Subcostal n. (T1)
Quadratus lumborum m.
Iliohypogastric n.
Ilio-inguinal n.
Psoas muscle
Genitofemoral n.
Lat. femoral cut. n.
Iliacus m.
Femoral n.
Obturator n.

Subcostal n. (T12)
Iliohypogastric n.
Ilio-inguinal n.
Genitofemoral n.
Post. 2° divisions
Lat. femoral cut. n.
Femoral n.
Ant. 2° divisions
Obturator n.

f. Obturator nerve (anterior secondary L₂, L₃, and L₄)—is the only branch of the plexus which emerges from the medial border of the psoas major. It proceeds forward into the pelvis in the extraperitoneal fatty tissue and exits from the pelvis through the obturator foramen.

4. **Sympathetic Trunk**—located in this same anatomic plane; will be considered on page 210.

Page 207

RETROPERITONEAL LYMPHATICS:

Refinements in the radiologic diagnostic methods of lymphangiography have emphasized to the surgeon the importance of the retroperitoneal lymph nodes. Many operative procedures for the removal of cancer of the gastrointestinal tract and particularly the genital organs are extended to include a retroperitoneal lymph node dissection. A knowledge of these nodes is therefore of increasing significance to the surgeon.

1. **Retroperitoneal Lymph Nodes** (Figs. 1 and 2):

a. PREAORTIC NODES—are nodal aggregations located on the anterior surface of the abdominal aorta around the three unpaired visceral branches.

(1) *Inferior Mesenteric Nodes*—receive lymphatic channels draining the descending colon, sigmoid colon, and rectum. Usually two nodes are present.

(2) *Superior Mesenteric Nodes*—usually number two, and receive vessels from the small bowel, cecum, transverse colon, and pancreas as well as channels from the inferior mesenteric nodes.

(3) *Celiac Nodes*—are one to three in number and receive channels from the superior gastric, hepatic, pancreaticolineal, and superior mesenteric nodes.

b. LEFT LUMBAR (PARA-AORTIC) CHAIN (Fig. 1)—is made of five to ten nodes which extend along the left side of the abdominal aorta. They are in direct continuity with the common iliac nodes below and drain into the thoracic duct above.

c. RETROAORTIC NODES—are variable in number and are not true regional nodes. They receive channels from either the preaortic or left lumbar (para-aortic) nodes.

d. RIGHT LUMBAR CHAIN OF NODES—is more complex because of the interposition of the inferior vena cava around which the nodes are distributed. Some are in front, some behind, some to the right, and some to the left of this vessel.

(1) *Interaorticovenous Nodes*—may be found between the inferior vena cava and aorta at any level from the aortic bifurcation to the left renal vein.

(2) *Prevenous Nodes*—may also be found at any level but two are fairly constant. An inferior node is located at the level of the aortic bifurcation and a superior node immediately below the level of the termination of the right renal vein.

(3) *Laterovenous Nodes*—are aligned with the right side of the inferior vena cava. They vary in number but one node has a constant position inferior to the angle formed by the entrance of the right renal vein into the inferior vena cava. This node is of particular importance in the spread of cancer from the right testicle.

(4) *Retrovenous Nodes*—lie on the psoas muscle and the right medial crus of the diaphragm.

2. **Lymphatic Drainage of the Adrenal Gland**—the lymphatic drainage of the adrenal gland per se is not as important as its lymphatic connections with other viscera. The lymphatic capillaries of the cortex follow the arterial supply while those of the medulla follow the veins. In either case, the first echelon nodes receiving adrenal lymphatics are the lumbar (para-aortic) nodes extending from the level of the celiac axis to the renal pedicle. The adrenal gland has important direct lymphatic connections, however, with the posterior mediastinal nodes. Such connections are significant in the incidence of adrenal involvement in tuberculosis and in metastatic lung cancer.

3. **Lymphatic Drainage of the Kidney**—lymphatic collecting channels from the left kidney terminate in the left lumbar (para-aortic) nodes at the level of the left renal vein. On the right side collecting channels terminate in right lumbar nodes anywhere within the level of the renal pedicle or in retrovenous nodes at this same level.

4. **Lymphatic Drainage of the Testicle**—from four to eight collecting channels ascend in the spermatic cord. On the right side they terminate in the laterovenous nodes, particularly in the node located in the angle between the right renal and inferior vena cava. Other channels from the right testis empty into the precaval nodes, especially those at the level of the aortic bifurcation. From the left testis lymph channels enter the left lumbar (para-aortic) nodes; however, some may terminate in the preaortic (inferior mesenteric) nodes. It has been claimed that some lymphatic channels of the testicle follow the vas deferens into the pelvis and end in the external iliac nodes.

5. **Lymphatic Drainage of the Ovaries**—the rich plexus of lymphatic capillaries of the ovaries gives rise to collecting channels which on the right side drain into the laterovenous and prevenous nodes anywhere from the level of the aortic bifurcation to the renal pedicle. On the left side, lymph channels terminate in the left lumbar (para-aortic) and preaortic nodes below the level of the renal pelvis. A connecting channel may also extend laterally through the broad ligament and terminate in a node of the external iliac chain.

6. **Thoracic Duct**—this main collecting channel of body lymph begins in the abdomen. It is formed by the union of the right and left lumbar trunks and the intestinal trunk. Efferent lymph vessels from the interaorticovenous, prevenous, laterovenous, and retrovenous nodes coalesce to form the *right lumbar trunk*. The left lumbar (para-aortic) and retroaortic efferent channels form a *left lumbar trunk*. The efferent vessels of the preaortic nodes join to form an *intestinal trunk*. This latter trunk usually drains into the left lumbar trunk. The site of this union is variable—occurring anywhere from the eleventh thoracic vertebral level to the second lumbar. If the union occurs low, however, a dilated portion of the ductal system results—the *cisterna chyli*. This union of the right and left lumbar trunks plus the intestinal trunk forms the *thoracic duct* (Fig. 3), which ascends into the thoracic cavity through the aortic orifice of the diaphragm. Its intrathoracic course is described on pages 96 and 98.

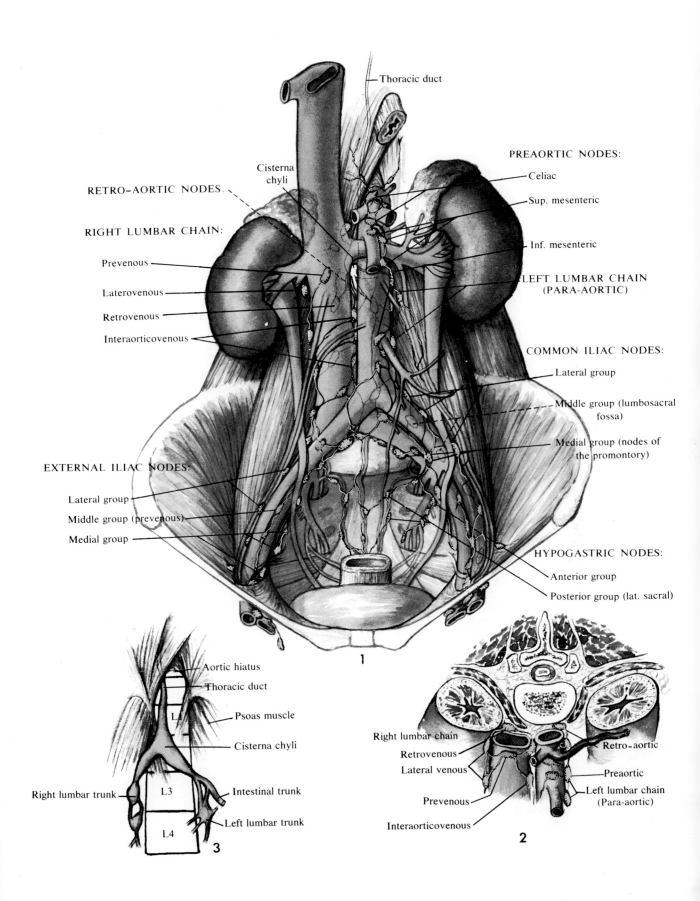

Thoracic duct

PREAORTIC NODES:

Celiac

Sup. mesenteric

Inf. mesenteric

LEFT LUMBAR CHAIN
(PARA-AORTIC)

Cisterna
chyli

RETRO-AORTIC NODES.

RIGHT LUMBAR CHAIN:

Prevenous

Laterovenous

Retrovenous

Interaorticovenous

COMMON ILIAC NODES:

Lateral group

Middle group (lumbosacral
fossa)

Medial group (nodes of
the promontory)

EXTERNAL ILIAC NODES:

Lateral group

Middle group (prevenous)

Medial group

HYPOGASTRIC NODES:

Anterior group

Posterior group (lat. sacral)

1

Aortic hiatus

Thoracic duct

Psoas muscle

Cisterna chyli

Intestinal trunk

Left lumbar trunk

Right lumbar trunk

L3

L4

3

Right lumbar chain

Retrovenous

Lateral venous

Prevenous

Interaorticovenous

Retro-aortic

Preaortic

Left lumbar chain
(Para-aortic)

2

RETROPERITONEAL VISCERAL NERVES:

All nerve fibers concerned with nerve impulses *to* and *from* the glands and the smooth and cardiac muscles of the body are collectively termed the *visceral nervous system*. The glands which this system supplies include those of the skin, the head, and the visceral structures of the body. In addition to cardiac muscles, these nerves innervate the muscles of the respiratory, alimentary, and urogenital tracts as well as the smooth muscles in the blood vessels, skin, and eyes.

1. **Visceral Afferent (Sensory) Fibers** — these fibers arise from receptors in the mucous membranes and the walls of visceral organs from all parts of the body. Nerve impulses from these receptors do not give rise to conscious sensations except for the *special visceral afferents* of taste and smell. However, they do play a part in visceral reflex arcs and particularly in producing referred pain, i.e., a conscious reception of visceral pain.

2. **Visceral Efferent (Motor) Fibers** — all nerve cells and nerve fibers by means of which motor impulses pass to tissues other than the multinucleated striated muscles constitute the *autonomic nervous system*. The autonomic nerve fibers are divided into two groups: the *parasympathetic* and *sympathetic*. Each group consists of a preganglionic and a postganglionic nerve fiber. The cell body of the preganglionic fiber is located in a nucleus within the central nervous system while that of the postganglionic fiber is located in an autonomic ganglion.

The two portions of the autonomic system differ in several ways. They differ in the source of preganglionic fibers from the central nervous system. The parasympathetic nuclei are associated with the oculomotor, facial, glossopharyngeal, and vagus nerves as well as the second, third, and fourth sacral nerves. These fibers are referred to as the *craniosacral outflow*. The sympathetic preganglionic fibers arise from the thoracic and lumbar segments of the spinal cord — the *thoracolumbar outflow*.

The parasympathetic and sympathetic nerves also differ in that the postganglionic parasympathetic fibers arise in *terminal autonomic ganglia* while the sympathetic postganglionic fibers arise from *vertebral* or *prevertebral ganglia*.

a. TERMINAL GANGLIA — consist of the ciliary, otic, submaxillary, cardiac, pulmonary, and enteric (Auerbach's and Meissner's) plexuses. Terminal ganglia of the sacral parasympathetic outflow are located within the walls of the pelvic viscera.

b. VERTEBRAL GANGLIA — of the thoracolumbar sympathetic outflow are located in relation to the cervical (pages 14 and 22), thoracic (page 98), and lumbar and sacral vertebrae.

The ganglia of the lumbar chain, usually four in number, are located on each side of the vertebral column and continue into the pelvis as the sacral chain (Fig. 1). The lumbar chain lies along the medial edge of the psoas major muscle. The left lumbar chain is slightly overlapped by the aorta and the right chain by the inferior vena cava (Fig. 2). The surgeon must retract these vessels medially in order to expose these sympathetic chains (Fig. 3). They are usually seen in the groove between the psoas major muscle laterally and the vertebral bodies medially. However, they may be obscured by fat or lymphatic tissue. The lumbar sympathetic chains are also intimately related to the lumbar vessels. The vessels usually lie posterior to the chain, but one or more vessels may pass anterior to the nerve trunk or in fact may split around the trunk (Fig. 3).

The lumbar ganglia vary in number, size, and position which makes total denervation difficult.

c. PREVERTEBRAL GANGLIA — which also contain postganglionic sympathetic nuclei are two in number in the retroperitoneal abdominal area: the celiac and hypogastric ganglia or plexuses. The *celiac ganglion* surrounds the celiac axis and from this plexus several subordinate plexuses arise. They consist of the paired phrenic, adrenal, renal, and spermatic (ovarian) plexuses, and the unpaired hepatic, splenic, gastric, superior, and inferior mesenteric plexuses. These are collectively termed the *aortic plexus*. A second major ganglion is the hypogastric plexus which will be discussed on page 220.

Aside from these anatomic differences, the two parts of the autonomic nervous system also differ pharmacologically in their reaction to certain drugs and physiologically in their function.

3. **Surgical Considerations** — the principle indication for lumbar sympathectomy is for relief of vasospastic diseases of the lower extremities. There are other less frequent indications such as severe hyperhidrosis, causalgia, and other painful post-traumatic disorders. Interruption of the visceral nerve impulses to the lower extremities may be accomplished by a temporary pharmacological block of these fibers (see Lumbar Sympathetic Block, page 270), or by surgical removal of certain of the lumbar ganglia and division of their rami communicantes.

a. SURGICAL ACCESS — to the lumbar chain is usually accomplished through a lateral *extraperitoneal approach*. The muscles of the abdominal wall are split and the peritoneum is swept medially and forward to expose the anterior margin of the psoas major muscle. The sympathetic trunk on the left side lies on the anterolateral margin of the vertebral bodies in a sulcus between the medial border of the psoas muscle and the aorta. On the right side, the trunk lies in the sulcus between the psoas and the inferior vena cava. If visual identification is difficult, palpation may guide the surgeon to the chain.

A *transperitoneal approach* for lumbar sympathectomy is a common supplementary procedure in operations involving the aorta and iliac arteries for obliterative disease.

b. EXTENT OF RESECTION — is still a controversial issue. Fortunately total denervation is not necessary for clinical success either in the management of vascular disease or hyperhidrosis. Removal of the second and third lumbar ganglia is important. Removing the first ganglion will increase the probabilities of complete denervation but in young men it should be preserved lest the power of ejaculation be lost. Removal of the fourth ganglion adds little to the operation and has the disadvantage of adding to the technical difficulties.

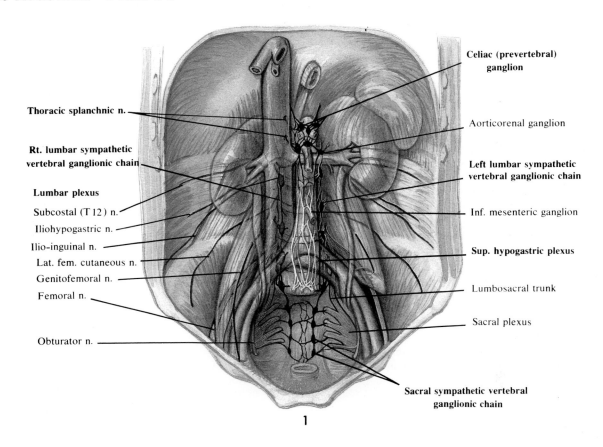

Celiac (prevertebral) ganglion

Aorticorenal ganglion

Left lumbar sympathetic vertebral ganglionic chain

Inf. mesenteric ganglion

Sup. hypogastric plexus

Lumbosacral trunk

Sacral plexus

Thoracic splanchnic n.

Rt. lumbar sympathetic vertebral ganglionic chain

Lumbar plexus

Subcostal (T 12) n.

Iliohypogastric n.

Ilio-inguinal n.

Lat. fem. cutaneous n.

Genitofemoral n.

Femoral n.

Obturator n.

Sacral sympathetic vertebral ganglionic chain

1

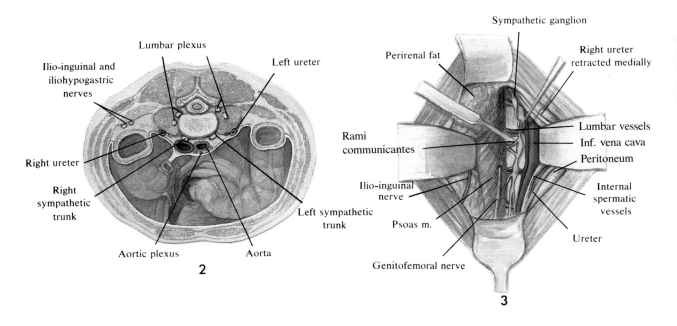

Ilio-inguinal and iliohypogastric nerves

Lumbar plexus

Left ureter

Right ureter

Right sympathetic trunk

Aortic plexus

Left sympathetic trunk

Aorta

2

Sympathetic ganglion

Perirenal fat

Right ureter retracted medially

Lumbar vessels

Inf. vena cava

Peritoneum

Rami communicantes

Ilio-inguinal nerve

Psoas m.

Internal spermatic vessels

Ureter

Genitofemoral nerve

3

c. SURGICAL ERRORS—during lumbar sympathectomy are frequent. *Identification* of the chain is a particularly troublesome technical problem Its location has been described above but it can be missed by the surgeon who can mistakenly remove in its stead such structures as the genitofemoral nerve, the lumbar lymphatics, the psoas minor tendon, or even a segment of the ureter. A second technical problem may be *bleeding* from the lumbar tributaries of the inferior vena cava. Finally the intimate relationship of the right lumbar chain to the inferior vena cava and the left chain to the aorta exposes both these vessels to possible injury during the course of operation. Because of the thinness of the wall of the cava it is the more vulnerable of the two vessels to injury. Special care and gentleness in retraction of the vena cava is mandatory in preventing *laceration* of its wall.

CLINICAL CONSIDERATIONS: AORTA AND INFERIOR VENA CAVA:

Operative procedures upon these retroperitoneal vascular structures are quite commonplace today. Particularly important is the resection and surgical replacement of a part of the abdominal aorta by prosthetic grafts in the treatment of aortic aneurysms. Ligation or plication of the abdominal inferior vena cava is advocated by many surgeons to prevent pulmonary emboli following thrombosis of veins of the pelvis or lower extremities.

1. **Aorta**—the aorta is approximately 4 inches in length and extends from the aortic hiatus of the diaphragm opposite the twelfth thoracic vertebra to its bifurcation at the level of the fourth lumbar vertebra. Topographically, this bifurcation terminates on the plane extending transversely across the abdomen on a level with the highest points of the iliac crests (supracristal line) slightly to the left of midline.

Of the branches of the aorta the following are of major clinical significance:

The *celiac (axis) artery* arises immediately below the aortic opening of the diaphragm opposite the twelfth thoracic vertebra.

The *superior mesenteric artery* arises approximately $1/2$ inch below the origin of the celiac artery opposite the lower border of the first lumbar vertebra.

The *inferior mesenteric artery* takes origin from the aorta at the level of the third lumbar vertebra about $1\frac{1}{2}$ inches above the aortic bifurcation.

The paired *renal arteries* prevailingly arise from the lateral surface of the aorta approximately $1/2$ inch below the origin of the superior mesenteric artery at the level of the upper border of the second lumbar vertebra.

a. RELATIONAL ANATOMY—of the abdominal aorta is most important in surgical procedures upon this structure and other retroperitoneal structures.

The third (horizontal) and fourth (ascending) parts of the duodenum lie in intimate relationship to the anterior surface of the aorta about the level of the renal arteries. The duodenum, therefore, lies at the level of the upper portion of most abdominal aortic aneurysms. This portion of the bowel must be carefully mobilized and retracted in order to place an occluding clamp across the aorta above the aneurysm but below the renal arteries (Fig. 1). Aneurysms have ruptured into the duodenum at this anatomic site. Also a number of cases have been reported in which a faulty suture line at the upper end of an aortic prosthesis has led to the development of an aorticoduodenal fistula.

Another important structure related to the abdominal aorta is the root of the mesentery of the small bowel. The mesentery is related to the posterior abdominal wall. It extends from the left side of the second lumbar vertebra obliquely downward and to the right to the level of the right sacroiliac joint. The mesentery which contains the superior mesenteric vessels supplying the small bowel must be displaced when the aorta is surgically exposed (Fig. 1).

An obvious structure which is related to the aorta and must be considered is the inferior vena cava. All along its course this vein is in intimate contact with the right wall of the aorta. During removal of the abdominal aortic aneurysms special care and attention must be made to avoid injury to the inferior vena cava (Fig. 1). In addition, because of the intimate relationship of these two anatomic structures penetrating wounds of the abdomen may simultaneously damage both the aorta and inferior vena cava and lead to the development of an arteriovenous fistula.

Another noteworthy relationship is that of the abdominal aorta to the left lumbar sympathetic chain. This chain lies just posterior and to the left of the aorta. In order to expose the chain for resection, the aorta must be retracted to the right.

Finally, the posterior relationship of the aorta to the vertebral column should be recalled (Fig. 2). This intimate relation explains the erosion of the spine which may occur with an aortic aneurysm or with injuries to the aorta or its terminal branches in operations for intervertebral disc disease (see below).

2. **Inferior Vena Cava**—the topography of the inferior vena cava parallels that of the abdominal aorta. It commences at the level of L_5, ascends to the right of the aorta, and pierces the diaphragm at the level of T_8.

a. RELATIONAL ANATOMY—of the inferior vena cava to the aorta and the importance of this relationship in the resection of abdominal aortic aneurysms have already been described above. Further emphasis should be placed upon the relationship of the left renal tributary during this same procedure. The left renal vein crosses the aorta at the level of the second lumbar vertebra and is intimately related to the upper end of an abdominal aortic aneurysm (Fig. 1).

As shown in Figure 2, page 211, the right lumbar sympathetic chain lies behind the inferior vena cava. The inferior vena cava must be retracted to the left in order to gain adequate exposure of this chain.

Posteriorly, the inferior vena cava and its main tributaries, the common iliac veins, lie in close relationship with the vertebral bodies and intervertebral discs (Fig. 2).

Surgical exposure of the inferior vena cava is usually performed for ligation or plication of the vessel in order to prevent pulmonary emboli following thrombosis of the veins of the pelvis or lower extremity. Such an exposure may be made either by a transperitoneal or extraperitoneal approach from the right side of the abdominal wall. The latter approach is the procedure of choice.

3. **Vascular Injuries in Disc Surgery**—these injuries are not commonly reported yet do pose a threat in operative procedures for a herniated nucleus pulposus. The intimate relationship of the aorta, the inferior vena cava, and the common iliac vessels to the anterior aspect of the vertebral column accounts for these vascular injuries. As already pointed out, the aorta terminates anterior to the body of L_4 or on the disc below, 2 cm. to the left of the midline. The inferior vena cava begins at the level of L_5 to the right of the midline. The common iliac vessels (the veins in a plane posterior to the arteries) lie close to the fifth intervertebral disc.

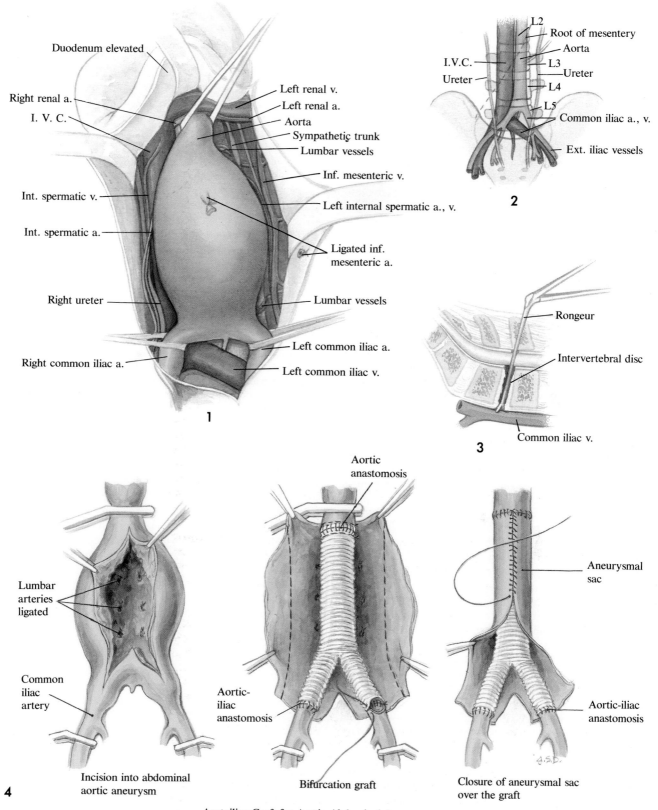

1

Duodenum elevated

Right renal a.

I. V. C.

Left renal v.

Left renal a.

Aorta

Sympathetic trunk

Lumbar vessels

Inf. mesenteric v.

Int. spermatic v.

Int. spermatic a.

Left internal spermatic a., v.

Ligated inf. mesenteric a.

Right ureter

Lumbar vessels

Right common iliac a.

Left common iliac a.

Left common iliac v.

2

L2

Root of mesentery

Aorta

I.V.C.

L3

Ureter

Ureter

L4

L5

Common iliac a., v.

Ext. iliac vessels

3

Rongeur

Intervertebral disc

Common iliac v.

4

Lumbar arteries ligated

Common iliac artery

Incision into abdominal aortic aneurysm

Aortic anastomosis

Aortic-iliac anastomosis

Bifurcation graft

Aneurysmal sac

Aortic-iliac anastomosis

Closure of aneurysmal sac over the graft

Aortoiliac Graft for Aortic Abdominal Aneurysm

Injury is produced by the rongeur being unintentionally pushed through the interval of the fourth or fifth lumbar disc (Fig. 3). The common iliac vessels are most frequently injuried and venous injuries are more common than arterial injuries. Certain anatomic factors may account for this finding: the veins have thinner walls, lie closer to the vertebral column and are more fixed in position. Venous injuries are more likely to remain clinically unrecognized.

RENAL TRANSPLANTATION:

Since the first renal transplant was reported by Murray in 1954, successful transplantation has been made possible by the careful criteria and selection of the donor and recipient. The surgical technique, development of peritoneal dialysis and hemodialysis, and advances in immunosuppressive agents (azathioprine, cyclosphosphamide, cyclosporine, corticosteroids, and antilymphocytic antibodies), and assessment and preparation of patients by determining ABO blood groups and histocompatibility have greatly enhanced survival rates and decreased the rejection of renal allografts. Transplantation between HLA-compatible siblings is successful in over 90 per cent of cases.

The most common indication for renal transplantation is chronic renal failure secondary to glomerulonephritis, pyelonephritis, polycystic kidneys, malignant hypertension, metabolic disease (e.g., diabetes mellitus), amyloidosis, renal calculi, malignant tumors, and so forth. The recipient must be selectively assessed by history, physical examination, voiding cystourethrography, cystourethric studies, cystoscopy, cardiopulmonary work-up, and renal angiography. The donor is selected on the basis of healthy kidneys, lack of systemic disease, normal bilateral renal function, histocompatibility, and emotional stability. If a cadaver kidney is used, it must be free of disease and removed quickly from the deceased donor as soon as brainstem death or circulatory arrest has been established. The kidney is cooled by perfusion with heparinized electrolyte solution and is stored under hypothermic conditions.

After the donor kidney is available, the patient is taken to surgery. An incision is made from the anterior superior spine to the pubic symphysis, the iliac fossa is exposed retroperitoneally, and the kidney is placed in the iliac fossa. The left donor kidney is implanted on the right side and the right is placed in the left iliac fossa. The common, internal, and external iliac arteries are dissected free and the lymphatics ligated. The common, internal, and external iliac veins are dissected. The donor right renal artery is anastomosed to the recipient right hypogastric artery. The donor right renal vein is anastomosed to the recipient right hypogastric vein. However, the donor right renal artery may be anastomosed to the right common iliac and the donor right renal vein to the recipient right common iliac vein.

The donor ureter is anastomosed to the recipient bladder (ureteroneocystostomy). The anterior wall of the bladder is opened lateral to the midline and the ureter inserted submucosally in a tunnel created by the lateral wall of the bladder. An alternative method is to make an incision into the mucosa in the anterolateral or superior wall and anastomose the ureter to the mucosal opening.

DIALYSIS:

Dialysis is indicated when the kidney fails to remove toxic substances from the blood and does not maintain fluid, electrolyte, and acid-base balance. The type of dialysis may be peritoneal or hemodialysis. Indications are acute renal failure due to retention of urea, creatinine, and uric acid; hyperkalemia; excessive extracellular fluid; and metabolic acidosis. Patients with uremia, oliguria, increasing acidosis, and congestive heart failure or acute drug intoxication may benefit from dialysis. Dialysis may be used in patients with chronic renal failure until renal transplantation can be performed. Peritoneal dialysis requires placing a sterile plastic catheter under local anesthesia through the abdominal wall into the pelvic gutter at a site in the midline one-third the distance from the umbilicus to the pubic symphysis. The peritoneum is irrigated with sterile dialysate hypertonic solution composed of glucose, sodium, potassium, chloride, calcium, and magnesium.

Hemodialysis is accomplished by using the kidney machine which has a membrane unit. The tubing system conveys blood from the patient to the membrane unit, where blood and dialysate from the dialysate supply system come into contact with the opposite surface of the cellophane membrane and dialysis occurs. Access to the circulation for hemodialysis is established through arteriovenous shunts. These shunts may be external or internal, beginning with vessels at the wrist, i.e., anastomosing the cephalic vein and radial artery side to side or end to end. Internal arteriovenous fistulas are more commonly preferred and are established in the distal forearm by side-to-side anastomosis between the radial artery and an adjacent vein. Another site is in the lower antecubital fossa, anastomosing the lower brachial artery to an adjacent vein.

A segment of long saphenous vein or Gore-Tex graft can be anastomosed end to side from the distal brachial artery to the cephalic vein below the elbow.

If the upper extremity vessels are thrombosed and exhausted, lower extremity vessels may be used for dialysis. Through a mid-thigh incision, the long saphenous vein is anastomosed to the proximal superficial femoral artery. Above the ankle, the long saphenous may be anastomosed to the posterior tibial artery. Patients with fistulas may require several hours of dialysis two to three times a week in preparation for renal transplantation.

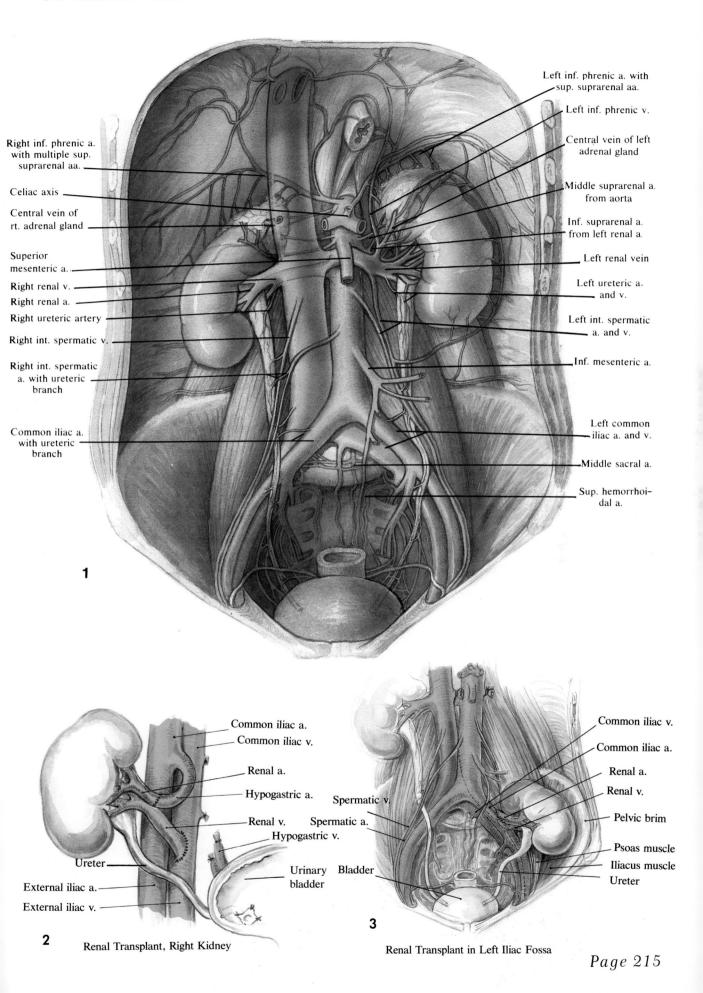

Right inf. phrenic a.
with multiple sup.
suprarenal aa.

Celiac axis

Central vein of
rt. adrenal gland

Superior
mesenteric a.

Right renal v.

Right renal a.

Right ureteric artery

Right int. spermatic v.

Right int. spermatic
a. with ureteric
branch

Common iliac a.
with ureteric
branch

Left inf. phrenic a. with
sup. suprarenal aa.

Left inf. phrenic v.

Central vein of left
adrenal gland

Middle suprarenal a.
from aorta

Inf. suprarenal a.
from left renal a.

Left renal vein

Left ureteric a.
and v.

Left int. spermatic
a. and v.

Inf. mesenteric a.

Left common
iliac a. and v.

Middle sacral a.

Sup. hemorrhoi-
dal a.

1

Common iliac a.
Common iliac v.

Renal a.

Hypogastric a.

Renal v.
Hypogastric v.

Urinary
bladder

Ureter

External iliac a.

External iliac v.

2 Renal Transplant, Right Kidney

Spermatic v.

Spermatic a.

Bladder

Common iliac v.

Common iliac a.

Renal a.

Renal v.

Pelvic brim

Psoas muscle

Iliacus muscle

Ureter

3 Renal Transplant in Left Iliac Fossa

The Pelvis

GENERAL CONSIDERATIONS:

The basic construction of the pelvis (L: basin) is similar in both the male and female except for the alterations produced by the genital organs. It may be divided into a false pelvis and a true pelvis. The former is that portion above the pelvic brim and can best be considered as part of the abdominal cavity since it contains abdominal viscera. The true pelvis is formed by bony and ligamentous walls but is open above and below. Muscle covers its lateral sides and a muscular diaphragm incompletely closes the outlet. These muscles are covered by a fascial layer, the endopelvic fascia, which also reflects upon the pelvic viscera. An extraperitoneal layer of fatty tissue contains the vascular and neural structures supplying the pelvic viscera. The peritoneum covers the pelvis from within.

1. **Bony and Ligamentous Parts** (Fig. 1)—the pelvis is bounded behind by the sacrum and coccyx and in front and laterally by the innominate bone. The *pelvic inlet* is formed by the pectineal lines of the pubic bones, the arcuate line of the ilium, and the promontory of the sacrum. The *pelvic outlet* anteriorly is formed by the pubic arch made up of the inferior rami of the pubis and ischium. Laterally the bony boundary is the ischial tuberosity and posteriorly the tip of the coccyx. The large notch between these latter two bony points is bridged by two ligaments, the sacrotuberous and the sacrospinal (Fig. 2). The *sacrotuberous ligament* arises from the posterior superior iliac spine and the lateral border of the sacrum and coccyx and inserts on the ischial tuberosity. The *sacrospinous ligament* arises from the pelvic side of the lateral border of the sacrum and coccyx and inserts on the ischial spine. These ligaments convert the notch into the *greater sciatic foramen* which is the major exit of structures from the pelvis and the *lesser sciatic foramen*. Only one structure leaves the pelvis via the lesser foramen, the obturator internus muscle.

2. **Lateral Muscular Wall** (Figs. 2 and 3)—on each side of the pelvis, buffering the lateral bony walls, are two muscles both lateral rotators and abductors of the thigh, and both innervated by the sacral plexus (page 260).

a. PIRIFORMIS—arises from the ventral surfaces of the second to the fourth sacral vertebra, exits from the pelvis through the greater sciatic foramen, and inserts on the greater trochanter of the femur.

b. OBTURATOR INTERNUS—has an extensive origin from the pelvic surfaces of the pubis ramus surrounding the obturator foramen, the obturator membrane, and the pelvic surface of the ischium between the ischial spine and foramen. It is fan-shaped and converges to exit through the lesser sciatic foramen to insert on the medial side of the greater trochanter of the femur.

3. **Pelvic Diaphragm** (Fig. 4)—a muscular sling consisting of two muscles on either side, the coccygeus and levator ani, forms an incomplete closure of the pelvic outlet. The muscular interval between the anterior-most fibers of the levator ani is termed the *urogenital hiatus* and is reinforced by the urogenital diaphragm (see Perineum, page 238). Both muscles are innervated by branches from the anterior primary division of the second and third sacral nerves. Their primary function is to support the pelvic floor.

a. COCCYGEUS—has an apical origin from the ischial spine and fans out to insert into the lateral margin of the lower sacral and coccygeal vertebrae.

b. LEVATOR ANI—is a complex and variable muscle. For instructive purposes it is divided into three parts: The *iliococcygeus* extends from the ischial spine to the superior ramus of the pubis near the obturator canal arising mainly from the arcus tendineus (see Endopelvic Fascia). It inserts into the coccyx and a median raphe just anterior to the coccyx, the *anococcygeal raphe*. The *pubococcygeus* arises from the os pubis from the symphysis to the origin of the iliococcygeus. Its lateral fibers insert into the anococcygeal raphe whereas the medial fibers attach to the pelvic viscera, particularly the rectum. The third portion, the *puborectalis*, takes origin from the pubis below the origin of the pubococcygeus and forms a thick band on each side of the vagina and rectum. Although some fibers insert in the anococcygeal raphe, the majority unite with fibers of the opposite side forming a sling behind the rectum. Many consider this muscle as part of the external sphincter mechanism.

4. **Pelvic Viscera**—the viscera in the pelvic cavity are identical in position in both male and female except that the genital organs of the male have a common outlet with the urinary system, whereas the female has a separate genital outlet. Their pelvic relationships, however, are similar with the urinary tract anterior in position and the digestive tract posterior with the genital tract interposed between the other two.

5. **Endopelvic Fascia**—is a continuation of the endoabdominal fascia. That portion covering the iliacus and psoas muscle in the false pelvis is referred to as the *iliopsoas fascia* (Fig. 3). In the true pelvis three parts to this fascial plane are distinguished.

a. PARIETAL LAYER (Fig. 5)—covers the muscles lining the lateral pelvic wall, the piriformis and internal obturator. It is continuous above with the iliopsoas and transversalis fascia and attaches below to the bony and ligamentous boundaries of the pelvic outlet. All *somatic* motor nerves except for the obturator nerve lie deep to this fascial plane within the pelvis. A thickening of this fascia extending from the pelvic surface of the pubis to the ischial spine is termed the *arcus tendineus*. It is from this fascial thickening that the iliococcygeal portion of the levator ani arises.

b. DIAPHRAGMATIC PORTION (Fig. 6)—covers

(Text continued on page 218.)

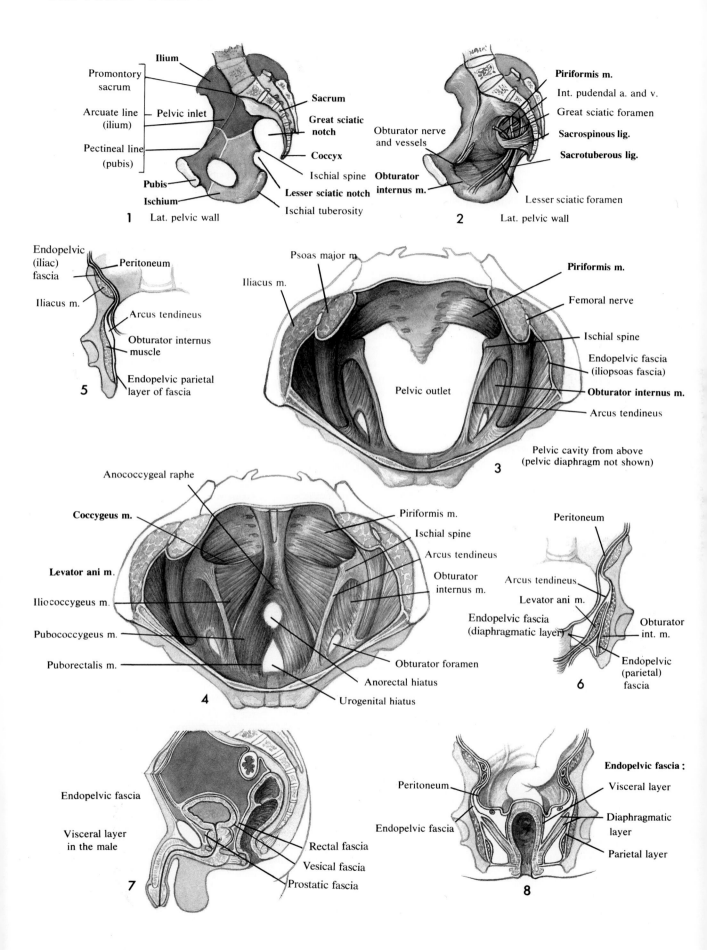

1 Lat. pelvic wall

- Promontory sacrum
- Arcuate line (ilium)
- Pectineal line (pubis)
- Pubis
- Ischium
- **Ilium**
- Pelvic inlet
- **Sacrum**
- **Great sciatic notch**
- **Coccyx**
- Ischial spine
- **Lesser sciatic notch**
- Ischial tuberosity

2 Lat. pelvic wall

- **Piriformis m.**
- Int. pudendal a. and v.
- Great sciatic foramen
- **Sacrospinous lig.**
- **Sacrotuberous lig.**
- Obturator nerve and vessels
- **Obturator internus m.**
- Lesser sciatic foramen

5

- Endopelvic (iliac) fascia
- Peritoneum
- Iliacus m.
- Arcus tendineus
- Obturator internus muscle
- Endopelvic parietal layer of fascia

3 Pelvic cavity from above (pelvic diaphragm not shown)

- Psoas major m.
- Iliacus m.
- **Piriformis m.**
- Femoral nerve
- Ischial spine
- Endopelvic fascia (iliopsoas fascia)
- **Obturator internus m.**
- Arcus tendineus
- Pelvic outlet

4

- Anococcygeal raphe
- **Coccygeus m.**
- **Levator ani m.**
- Iliococcygeus m.
- Pubococcygeus m.
- Puborectalis m.
- Piriformis m.
- Ischial spine
- Arcus tendineus
- Obturator internus m.
- Obturator foramen
- Anorectal hiatus
- Urogenital hiatus

6

- Peritoneum
- Arcus tendineus
- Levator ani m.
- Endopelvic fascia (diaphragmatic layer)
- Obturator int. m.
- Endopelvic (parietal) fascia

7

- Endopelvic fascia
- Visceral layer in the male
- Rectal fascia
- Vesical fascia
- Prostatic fascia

8

- Peritoneum
- Endopelvic fascia
- Endopelvic fascia:
  - Visceral layer
  - Diaphragmatic layer
  - Parietal layer

the two muscles on each side of the pelvis which make up the pelvic diaphragm, the coccygeus, and levator ani. This is a double fascial layer ensheathing the diaphragm. The inferior layer of diaphragmatic fascia forms the superior layer of the urogenital diaphragm (page 252).

c. VISCERAL PORTION (Figs. 7 and 8, page 217) – is that part of the endopelvic fascia continuous with the superior layer of diaphragmatic fascia which reflects upward upon the pelvic viscera. It extends upon the pelvic organs for a variable distance blending with their outer fibrous coats. Various terms are used to describe parts of this portion of the endopelvic fascia in accordance with the viscera to which it is related, e.g., rectal, prostatic, vesical, and vaginal.

6. **"Ligaments" of the Pelvis** – the pelvic viscera receive support by thickenings of endopelvic fascia and by thickenings of extraperitoneal fatty tissue reinforced by extensions of the endopelvic fascia upon the neurovascular structures supplying the pelvic organs. The former are related to the anterior and posterior pelvic walls, while the latter extend from the lateral walls and are related to the urinary, genital, and digestive tracts.

a. PUBOPROSTATIC (VESICAL) LIGAMENTS – consist of medial and lateral ligaments of either side of the pelvis. The *medial puboprostatic ligaments* are paired thickenings of endopelvic fascia extending from the posterior surface of the pubis to the prostate in the male (*pubovesical* in the female). The *lateral puboprostatic ligaments* extend from the superior diaphragmatic layer of endopelvic fascia to the prostate (or bladder in the female).

b. FASCIA OF WALDEYER – in both male and female is a thickening of endopelvic fascia which extends from the anterior surface of the second, third, and fourth sacral segment to the posterior wall of the rectum (Fig. 4, page 225).

c. LATERAL TRUE LIGAMENTS OF THE BLADDER – extend from the lateral pelvic wall to the lateral wall of the urinary bladder. Each is formed by a thickening of endopelvic fascia and extraperitoneal tissue surrounding the neurovascular bundle supplying the bladder. In the male it also includes the vas deferens.

d. LATERAL RECTAL STALKS – consist of fascial thickenings over the middle hemorrhoidal vessels and hemorrhoidal autonomic plexus which pass from the posterolateral pelvic wall to the sides of the rectum.

e. LATERAL CERVICAL (CARDINAL, MACKENRODT'S) LIGAMENT – is a thickening of endopelvic and perivascular tissue extending from the lateral pelvic wall to the cervix of the uterus and the upper part of the vagina. It is located at the base of the broad ligament of the uterus and is regarded as the main ligamentous support of this organ. The uterine artery runs along the upper portion of this ligament and the ureter pierces the ligament near its uterine attachment.

7. **Extraperitoneal Fatty Tissue** – between the overlying pelvic peritoneum and the parietal and superior layers of diaphragmatic endopelvic fascia is a layer of adipose tissue in which the internal iliac (hypogastric) vessels and autonomic nerve fibers supplying the pelvic viscera are located. Only one somatic motor nerve, the obturator, is located in this anatomic plane in the pelvis.

a. INTERNAL ILIAC (HYPOGASTRIC) ARTERY (Fig. 1) – is the most superficial structure on the lateral pelvic wall. It arises from the common iliac at the level of the lumbosacral joint and descends into the true pelvis where it branches at the upper border of the piriformis into an anterior and posterior division. From these divisions parietal and visceral branches arise:

	POSTERIOR	ANTERIOR
Parietal	Iliolumbar	Obturator
	Lateral sacral	Internal pudendal
	Superior gluteal	Inferior gluteal
Visceral		Umbilical (superior vesical)
		Inferior vesical
		Middle hemorrhoidal

N.B. In the female, the *uterine* is a direct anterior visceral branch from the internal iliac, whereas its homologue in the male, the *deferential* artery, usually arises as a branch of the inferior vesical.

Since the visceral branches remain in the pelvis they will be discussed in connection with the viscera they supply. Of the parietal branches, the *superior* and *inferior gluteal* and *internal pudendal* arteries take immediate leave from the pelvis via the greater sciatic foramen. The *obturator artery* proceeds forward through the extraperitoneal tissue and exits from the pelvis to the thigh through the obturator foramen. The *lateral sacral* remains in the true pelvis descending on the sacrum medial to the anterior foramina. It sends off spinal branches through the foramina and several small rectal branches. The *iliolumbar* passes laterally deep to the common iliac vessels and is distributed to the false pelvis.

In addition to the branches of the hypogastric artery, the pelvis is supplied by the *middle sacral* and *superior hemorrhoidal arteries* (page 226).

b. INTERNAL ILIAC (HYPOGASTRIC) VEIN – is formed in part by tributaries draining the pelvic viscera. These visceral veins form interconnecting plexuses draining the rectum (*hemorrhoidal*), genital organs (*prostatic* and *uterovaginal*), and bladder (*vesical*). From these plexuses veins corresponding to the visceral branches of the artery join tributaries accompanying parietal arterial branches to form the internal iliac vein which in turn joins the external iliac vein at the sacroiliac articulations to form the common iliac vein. Tributaries from the perineum unaccompanied by arterial branches drain into the hypogastric system: the *dorsal vein of the penis* in the male, and *veins of the clitoris* in the female.

(*Text continued on page 220.*)

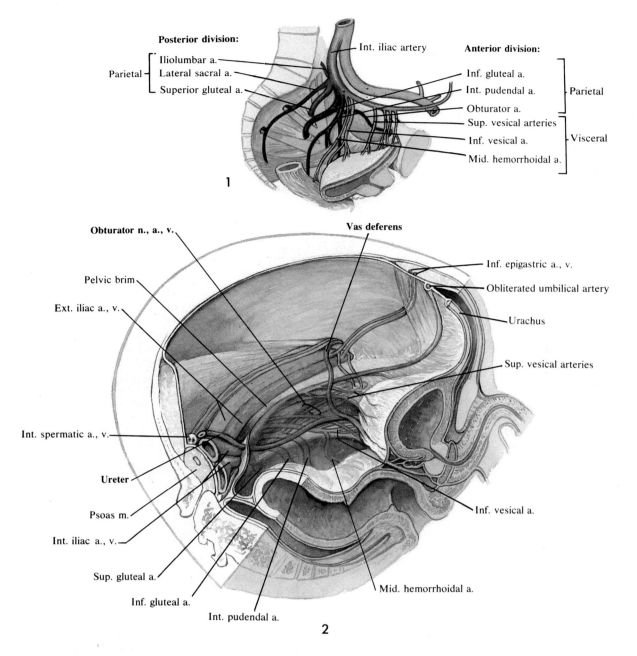

Posterior division:

Parietal
- Iliolumbar a.
- Lateral sacral a.
- Superior gluteal a.

Int. iliac artery

Anterior division:
- Inf. gluteal a.
- Int. pudendal a. — Parietal
- Obturator a.
- Sup. vesical arteries
- Inf. vesical a. — Visceral
- Mid. hemorrhoidal a.

1

Obturator n., a., v.

Vas deferens

Pelvic brim

Inf. epigastric a., v.

Obliterated umbilical artery

Ext. iliac a., v.

Urachus

Sup. vesical arteries

Int. spermatic a., v.

Ureter

Psoas m.

Inf. vesical a.

Int. iliac a., v.

Sup. gluteal a.

Mid. hemorrhoidal a.

Inf. gluteal a.

Int. pudendal a.

2

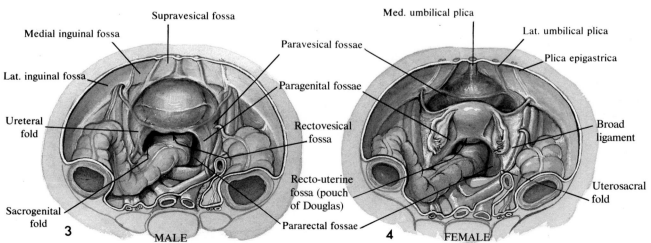

Supravesical fossa

Med. umbilical plica

Medial inguinal fossa

Lat. umbilical plica

Paravesical fossae

Plica epigastrica

Lat. inguinal fossa

Paragenital fossae

Ureteral fold

Rectovesical fossa

Broad ligament

Recto-uterine fossa (pouch of Douglas)

Uterosacral fold

Sacrogenital fold

3

MALE

Pararectal fossae

4

FEMALE

The *middle sacral vein*, a tributary of the left common iliac, and the *superior hemorrhoidal vein* which empties into the inferior mesenteric vein also aid in the venous drainage of the pelvis.

c. PELVIC NERVES (Fig. 5, page 225) — consist of branches of the sacral plexus and the abdominal sympathetics. A single branch of the lumbar plexus, the *obturator nerve*, traverses the pelvis through the extraperitoneal fatty tissue plane, but all other somatic motor branches of the sacral plexus lie deep to the endopelvic fascia and exit from the pelvis via the greater sciatic foramen. They will be discussed on page 274. The *parasympathetic branches of* S_2, S_3, and S_4 (*pelvic splanchnics* and *nervi erigentes*) extend from the sacral plexus and join the pelvic visceral plexus. The *sympathetic nerves* enter the pelvis as branches from the *superior hypogastric plexus* located at the bifurcation of the aorta. Fibers then descend as a cord-like structure, the *presacral nerve*, over the promontory of the sacrum and diverge to form the *inferior hypogastric (pelvic) plexuses* on the sides of the rectum where they are joined by pelvic parasympathetic fibers. From the pelvic plexuses, fibers extend along branches of the hypogastric artery to form secondary plexuses — *middle hemorrhoidal, prostatic (uterovaginal),* and *vesical.* Sympathetic fibers also enter the pelvis by following the superior hemorrhoidal artery. This *superior hemorrhoidal plexus* supplies the upper rectum and joins the middle hemorrhoidal plexus.

d. STRUCTURES ON LATERAL PELVIC WALL (Fig. 2) — extending parallel along the pelvic brim, from superior to inferior in direction, are anatomic structures important in surgical orientation. They are the internal spermatic vessels, the psoas muscle, external iliac vessels, the pelvic brim, and within the pelvic cavity the obturator nerve, artery, and vein. Crossing these structures from the abdominal side is the ureter, and crossing them below is the vas deferens.

8. **Pelvic Peritoneum** — the parietal layer of peritoneum of the abdominal cavity extends into the pelvis and forms the roof of this body cavity. As it reflects over the pelvic visceral structures it is thrown into folds and corresponding peritoneal fossae. Several of these folds and fossae are related to the anterior abdominal wall and are described on page 136. The remainder of the folds and fossae are related to the urinary, genital, and digestive tracts (Figs. 3 and 4).

a. URINARY TRACT REFLECTIONS — consist of parietal peritoneal reflections from the anterior abdominal wall to the superior surface of the bladder (*anterior false ligament of the bladder*), from the lateral pelvic wall to the bladder (*lateral false ligaments of the bladder*), and from the posterior surface of the bladder into the genital organs (the *posterior false ligaments of the bladder*). The most lateral true peritoneal fold, prominent in the male, is the *ureteral fold* over the ureter. In the female, its counterpart is the *broad ligament.* Ventral to these folds, on either side of the pelvis, are located the *paravesical fossae.*

b. GENITAL TRACT REFLECTIONS — are most prominent in the female as the *uterosacral (rectouterine, Douglas's)* fold extending from the uterus to the sacrum. This fold is less distinct in the male and is termed the *sacrogenital fold.* Between the broad ligament and uterosacral fold in the female is the *paragenital fossa.* In the male this fossa is less prominent and lies between the ureteric and sacrogenital folds.

c. DIGESTIVE TRACT REFLECTIONS — provide little support to the rectum. The mesocolon of the sigmoid terminates at the level of S_3 where the rectum begins. The peritoneum is related to the anterior and lateral walls of the upper one-third of the rectum and to the anterior wall of the middle third. The lower third, however, has no peritoneal relationship. In the female, between the uterosacral folds and lateral wall of the rectum, is the *pararectal fossa.* It communicates with the fossa of the opposite side by the *rectouterine fossa (pouch of Douglas).* In the male the pararectal fossa is located between the sacrogenital fold and rectum and communicates with its fellow of the opposite side through the less distinct *rectovesical fossa.*

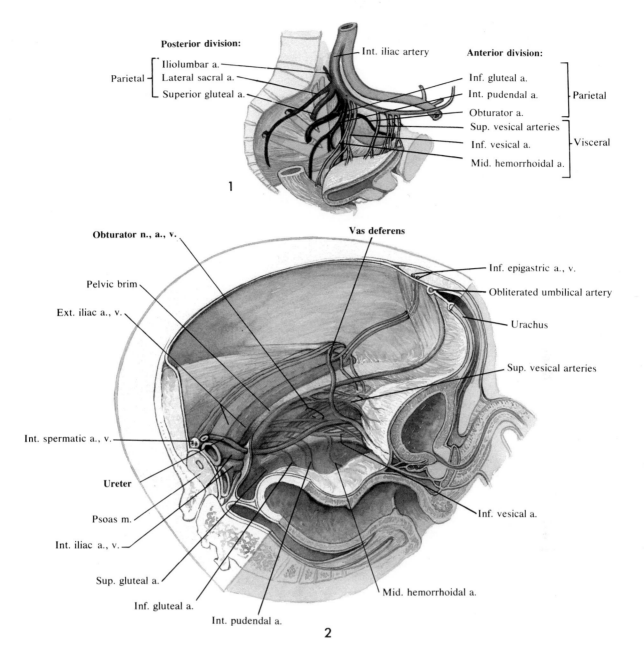

Posterior division:
Parietal
Iliolumbar a.
Lateral sacral a.
Superior gluteal a.

Int. iliac artery

Anterior division:
Inf. gluteal a.
Int. pudendal a.
Obturator a.
Parietal
Sup. vesical arteries
Inf. vesical a.
Mid. hemorrhoidal a.
Visceral

1

Obturator n., a., v.

Vas deferens

Inf. epigastric a., v.

Obliterated umbilical artery

Pelvic brim

Ext. iliac a., v.

Urachus

Sup. vesical arteries

Int. spermatic a., v.

Ureter

Psoas m.

Int. iliac a., v.

Inf. vesical a.

Sup. gluteal a.

Inf. gluteal a.

Int. pudendal a.

Mid. hemorrhoidal a.

2

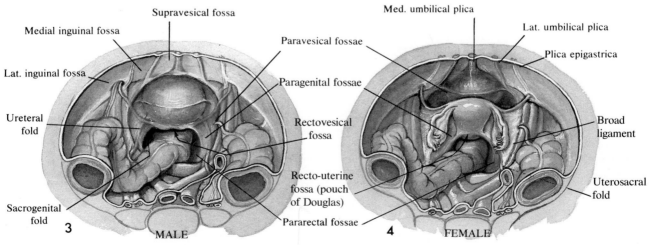

Supravesical fossa

Medial inguinal fossa

Med. umbilical plica

Lat. umbilical plica

Lat. inguinal fossa

Paravesical fossae

Plica epigastrica

Paragenital fossae

Ureteral fold

Rectovesical fossa

Broad ligament

Recto-uterine fossa (pouch of Douglas)

Uterosacral fold

Sacrogenital fold

3   MALE

Pararectal fossae

4   FEMALE

CLINICAL CONSIDERATIONS:

A knowledge of the relational anatomy of the pelvic walls and the visceral components are of the utmost importance to the physician in the diagnosis of intra-pelvic and intra-abdominal pathology. The orifices of the digestive tract and, in the female, of the genital tract permit an excellent opportunity for a sweeping examination of the pelvic cavity by simple digital examination.

1. **Digital Rectal Examination** (Fig. 1)—passage of the gloved finger through the anal sphincter in both sexes permits examination of the lumen of the anal canal and rectum for a distance of about 7 to 7.5 cm. Fecal impactions and foreign bodies may be detected. Within the wall of the rectum, tumors, strictures, and granulomas may be palpated. The retrorectal area including the coccyx and lower portion of the sacrum may be palpated posteriorly. Anteriorly in the male the bulbourethral (Cowper's) gland, the prostate gland, and seminal vessels can be contacted by the examining finger. In the female, the posterior vaginal wall, the cervix, and uterine body can be examined, particularly if anterior abdominal pressure is applied. Assessment of dilatation of the cervical os during parturition may be determined, as might be any enlargement, displacement, or tumor formation of the corpus uteri.

With lateral rotation of the finger in both sexes, one may survey the ischiorectal fossa and lateral pelvic walls in order to detect any abscess formation or pelvic wall tumors. This is an especially important manuever in examining the female, for the fallopian tubes and ovaries may be contacted by the examining finger.

Superiorly in the male the condition of the recto-vesical space and, in the female, the rectouterine fossa or pouch of Douglas may be determined. Because of the dependent location of these cul-de-sacs in both the erect and supine positions of the body, a number of secondary changes may occur in these fossae. It is a favorite site for purulent collections secondary to perforation of abdominal viscera (such as the appendix), sigmoid diverticula, or duodenal or gastric ulcers. Such abscesses in these fossae may drain through the rectum. Impalement injuries of the rectum may penetrate into the peritoneal cavity. Gastric cancer may spread over the peritoneal surface and form metastatic deposits in these fossae. A palpable metastatic deposit here is referred to as a "rectal shelf."

2. **Vaginal Examination**—in the female a more thorough examination can be made of the pelvic cavity because of the access to the genital orifice. Direct palpation of the walls of the vaginal cavity can be made to determine the presence of any abnormal growths or the strength or lack of strength of the vaginal or uterine supports (cystocele, rectocele, or degree of uterine prolapse). The cervix uteri may be examined for lacerations, inflammation, tumor formation, etc. The uterus may be more readily surveyed for malposition, enlargements, and tumors. Anteriorly, the urethra and bladder are readily accessible to the examining finger. Lateral palpation permits assessment of the adnexa, including the tubes, ovary, and lateral pelvic walls.

Superior examination of the rectouterine fossa, in addition to revealing the secondary lesions that occur in the male, may, in the female, reveal a variety of others. These include changes secondary to disease of the female genital tract—ovarian tumors, endometrial implants, blood from ruptured ovarian cysts, or tubal pregnancies, to name only a few.

In addition to the palpable detection, direct visual examination of the vaginal vault can be made by the insertion of a speculum. Abscesses in the rectouterine fossa may be drained by incising the vaginal wall at the posterior fornix (Fig. 2). Through this same route, but with the patient in a knee-chest prone position, *culdoscopy* (the passage of a scope into the cul-de-sac) may be performed. The procedure has proven useful in the diagnosis of a number of pelvic diseases.

3. **Internal Pelvic Hernias** (Fig. 3)—internal herniation of the gastrointestinal tract may occur in the region of the pelvic cavity just as it may occur in the abdominal cavity. Such hernias are usually the result of a developmental muscular defect in either the lateral wall or pelvic diaphragm. They rarely occur and are rarely considered by the surgeon in the assessment of pelvic pain.

a. Obturator hernia—occurs through the obturator canal. The pelvic peritoneal sac of the hernia usually presents itself in the canal medial to the obturator vessels and nerve. Pressure on the nerve may produce pain along the inner aspect of the thigh from the groin to the knee (*Howship-Romberg sign*). The herniated sac is usually small and lies beneath the pectineus muscle; therefore, little if any external deformity is present. Internal rotation of the abducted thigh will usually intensify the pain.

b. Sciatic hernias—present in the buttocks beneath the gluteus maximus muscle. Such hernias may occur through the greater sciatic foramen above the piriformis muscles (suprapiriformis) or below the muscle (infrapiriformis).

c. Ischiorectal hernia—is a protrusion of peritoneal sac through the *hiatus of Schwalbe*. In most cases the levator ani muscle arises from the pubis anteriorly, from the ischial spine posteriorly, and from the arcus tendineus of the obturator fascia between these bony points. Occasionally, however, the arcus tendineus separates from the obturator internus muscle, and the levator fibers are suspended from this tendenous sling. Between the arcus tendineus and the obturator internus is an opening through which a peritoneal sac and loop of bowel may extend through the pelvic wall into the ischiorectal fossa.

d. Perineal hernias—are protrusions through weakened portions of the levator ani usually between its ileococcygeal and pubococcygeal portions.

4. **Pelvic Fractures** (Fig. 4)—the real danger of fractures of the pelvis is due not to the damage done to the pelvic bones but to injury of the pelvic contents which so frequently complicate these fractures. Injury to the urinary bladder, urethra, rectum, vagina, and pelvic blood vessels and nerves are the chief com-

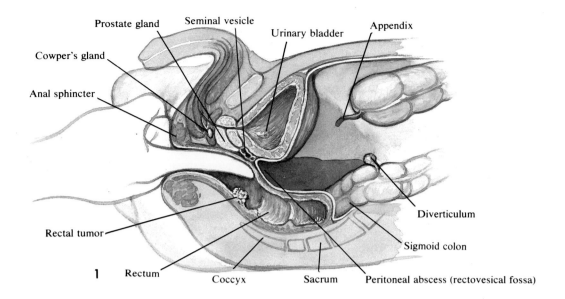

1

Cowper's gland · Prostate gland · Seminal vesicle · Urinary bladder · Appendix

Anal sphincter

Rectal tumor · Rectum · Coccyx · Sacrum · Diverticulum · Sigmoid colon · Peritoneal abscess (rectovesical fossa)

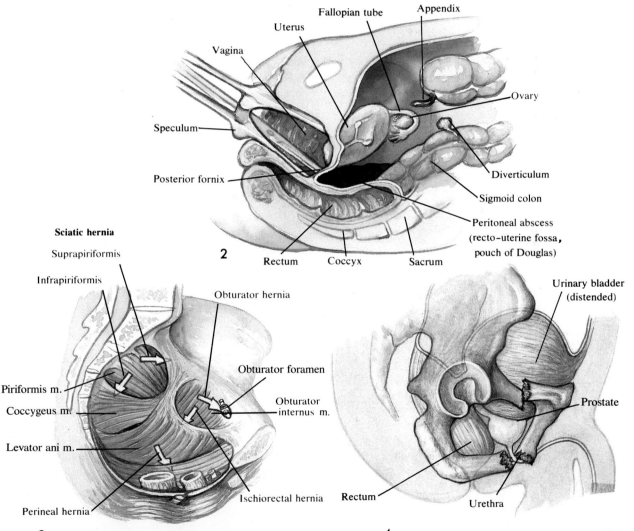

2

Vagina · Uterus · Fallopian tube · Appendix

Speculum · Ovary

Posterior fornix · Diverticulum · Sigmoid colon

Rectum · Coccyx · Sacrum · Peritoneal abscess (recto-uterine fossa, pouch of Douglas)

Sciatic hernia

Suprapiriformis

Infrapiriformis

Obturator hernia

Obturator foramen

Piriformis m.

Obturator internus m.

Coccygeus m.

Levator ani m.

Perineal hernia

Ischiorectal hernia

3   ROUTES OF INTERNAL HERNIA

Urinary bladder (distended)

Prostate

Rectum

Urethra

4   PELVIC FRACTURES

plications of such injuries. By far the most vulnerable structure is the urinary bladder, particularly when this organ is distended. Rupture of the bladder always results in extravasation of urine. This extravasation may be intraperitoneal or extraperitoneal. Immediate surgical intervention is imperative. Crushing injury to the pelvis must be carefully scrutinized for possible injury to any of the underlying pelvic viscera.

ANATOMY OF RECTUM AND ANAL CANAL:

The terminal part of the digestive tract extends from the third sacral segment to the anus and is divided into two parts: the *rectum* and *anal canal*. The rectum extends to the level of the pelvic diaphragm and the anal canal continues caudally to the anus.

1. **Rectum** — the external layer of the rectal wall is comprised of peritoneum above and rectal fascia below. The muscular coat differs from other parts of the large bowel, for in addition to the inner circular layer, there is a *complete* longitudinal muscular layer resulting from the coalescence of the taenia coli. The submucosal and mucosal layers make up the remainder of the rectal wall.

The rectum in man is curved in both anterior-posterior and lateral directions and measures 10 to 12 cm. in length. The anterior-posterior curvatures are an upper *sacral flexure* which is concave forward and a lower *perineal flexure* which curves dorsally and caudally and joins the anal canal (Figs. 1, 2, and 4). The lateral curvatures are due to the presence of three transverse folds of mucosa, submucosa, and circular muscular fibers, the *rectal valves of Houston*. The upper and lower valves are on the left, and the middle valve on the right wall (Fig. 3). The lower third of the rectum, which lies below the pelvic peritoneum, is dilated and termed the *ampulla*.

a. RECTAL SUPPORTS — aside from the pelvic diaphragm, there are chiefly two rectal supports: the *fascia of Waldeyer* (Fig. 4), a thickening of endopelvic fascia extending from the anterior surface of the third and fourth sacral segment to the posterior rectal wall, and the *lateral rectal stalks* which are bilateral fascial thickenings over the middle hemorrhoidal vessels and the pelvic splanchnics passing from the posterolateral pelvic wall to the lateral walls of the rectum. The peritoneal reflections add little support.

b. RELATIONS — of the rectum have already been discussed on page 222 under Digital Rectal Examination. Figures 1 and 2 illustrate the direct anterior and posterior relationships in the male and female. Figure 3 illustrates the lateral relationship to the pelvic diaphragm and *supralevator space*.

2. **Anal Canal** — this terminal portion of the digestive tract extends from the anorectal line to the anus and measures approximately 3.5 cm. in length. The muscular walls of the anal canal derived from the longitudinal and circular coats of the rectum become modified into internal and external sphincters of the anus. The anal canal is related dorsally to the anococcygeal ligament and laterally to the levator ani whose puborectalis fibers aid in the sphincter control of the anus. Anteriorly in the male is the dorsal margin of the urogenital diaphragm, and in the female the well defined *perineal body*.

a. PECTINATE (DENTATE) LINE — is the outstanding gross structure on proctoscopic examination and is located about 2 cm. above the anus. Below the pectinate line the anal canal is lined with squamous epithelium and above by stratified columnar. For this reason it is also referred to as the *mucocutaneous line*. The blood supply above the line is via the superior hemorrhoidal vessels whereas below, the anal canal is supplied by the inferior hemorrhoidals (Fig. 1, page 227). This line also marks the site of portocaval anastomosis; the internal hemorrhoids are located above the pectinate line and external hemorrhoids below (Fig. 3, page 227). The lymphatics above the line drain into pelvic and lumbar nodes while those below empty into the inguinal nodes (Fig. 1, page 231). The nerve supply to the area of anal canal above the pectinate line is via sympathetic fibers, whereas the area below is supplied by the inferior hemorrhoidal (somatic) nerves.

Extending upward from the pectinate line are a varying number of longitudinal mucosal vascular folds, the *rectal columns (Morgagni)*. The thickened bases of the rectal columns are the *anal papillae*. Joining the bases of adjacent columns on a level with the pectinate line are folds of mucous membrane termed the *anal valves*; these valves are remnants of the cloacal membrane (page 228). The fossae formed between adjacent columns and valves are referred to as *rectal crypts (sinuses)* frequently the seat of proctocologic pathology (Fig. 3).

b. ANORECTAL LINE — is located about 1.5 cm. proximal to the pectinate line and probably represents the true embryologic division between rectum and anal canal for it is here that mucosal epithelium of the rectum changes from its typical simple columnar to stratified columnar type. This line is seen microscopically rather than grossly.

c. INTERSPHINCTERIC (HILTON'S WHITE LINE) LINE — marks the interval between the internal and external sphincters of the anus. This "line" is a *palpable* landmark and is approximately 1.5 cm. above the anal orifice.

d. PECTEN — is that portion of the anal canal located between the pectinate line above and the intersphincteric line below. It is covered with stratified squamous epithelium beneath which is a heavy deposit of connective tissue. This latter tissue is derived from that portion of the longitudinal muscle of the rectum that forms the anal intermuscular septum between the external and internal sphincters and attaches to the skin of the anal canal.

e. ANOCUTANEOUS LINE (ANAL VERGE) — is the line of junction of the perianal skin, which contains hair follicles, with the squamous epithelium of the lower anal canal which is hair-free.

f. ANUS (L-RING) — is a muscular ring surrounding the distal orifice of the digestive tract comprised chiefly of an internal and external sphincter. The *internal sphincter* is formed by a thickening of the circular involuntary muscle of the gut. The *external sphincter* is more complex, being composed of a deep, a superficial, and a subcutaneous portion. The *subcutaneous* division has no bony attachments and encircles the anal orifice. The *superficial* division lies deeper and attaches to the coccyx behind and to the perineal body anteriorly. The *deep* division has no bony attachments and forms a muscular ring blending with the puborectalis fibers of

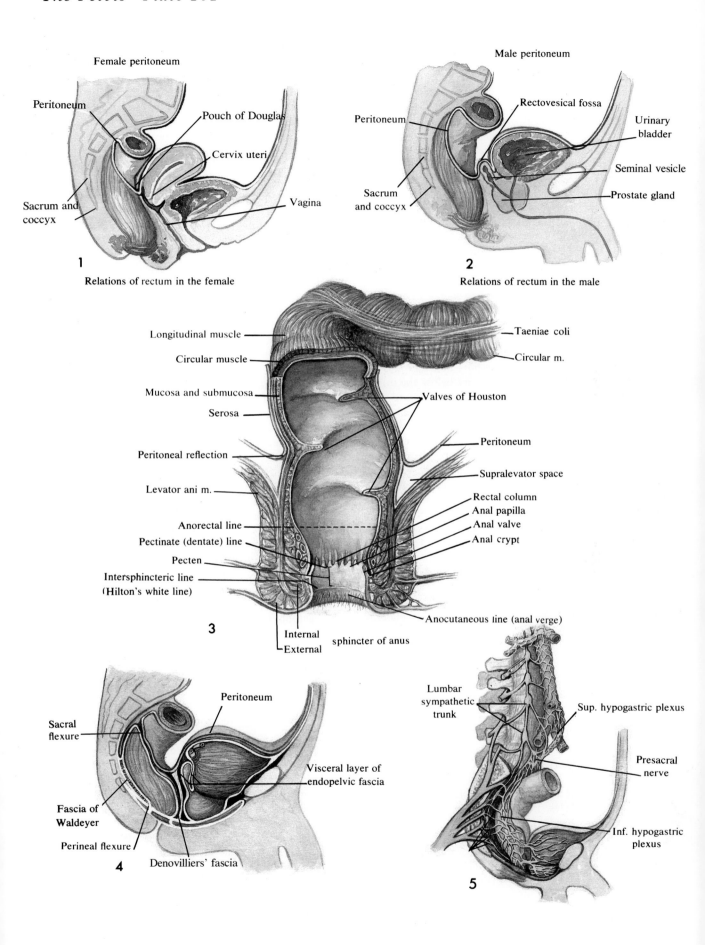

Female peritoneum

Peritoneum

Pouch of Douglas

Cervix uteri

Sacrum and coccyx

Vagina

1

Relations of rectum in the female

Male peritoneum

Peritoneum

Rectovesical fossa

Urinary bladder

Seminal vesicle

Prostate gland

Sacrum and coccyx

2

Relations of rectum in the male

Longitudinal muscle

Circular muscle

Mucosa and submucosa

Serosa

Peritoneal reflection

Levator ani m.

Anorectal line

Pectinate (dentate) line

Pecten

Intersphincteric line (Hilton's white line)

Taeniae coli

Circular m.

Valves of Houston

Peritoneum

Supralevator space

Rectal column

Anal papilla

Anal valve

Anal crypt

Anocutaneous line (anal verge)

Internal

External

sphincter of anus

3

Sacral flexure

Peritoneum

Fascia of Waldeyer

Perineal flexure

Denovilliers' fascia

Visceral layer of endopelvic fascia

4

Lumbar sympathetic trunk

Sup. hypogastric plexus

Presacral nerve

Inf. hypogastric plexus

5

the levator ani and with fibers of the internal sphincter. These muscles forming the external sphincter are innervated by the inferior hemorrhoidal branch of the pudendal nerve.

4. **Arterial Supply** (Figs. 1 and 2)—the rectum and anal canal receive their arterial blood supply from six vessels: two paired and two unpaired vessels. The unpaired rectal vessels are direct (*middle sacral artery*) and indirect (*superior hemorrhoidal artery*) branches from the abdominal aorta. The paired anal canal vessels are direct (*middle hemorrhoidal artery*) and indirect (*inferior hemorrhoidal artery*) branches arising from the internal iliac (hypogastric) arteries.

a. MIDDLE SACRAL ARTERY—arises as a terminal branch from the posterior wall of the abdominal aorta just above the bifurcation and descends into the pelvis over the anterior surface of the sacrum extending to the coccyx. In addition to the lowest lumbar branches and the lateral sacral branches, the middle sacral sends small arterial twigs to the posterior wall of the rectum.

b. SUPERIOR HEMORRHOIDAL (RECTAL) ARTERY— is a continuation of the inferior mesenteric branch of the abdominal aorta into the pelvis. Where this artery begins is controversial. Some authors consider this to be at the point in the abdominal cavity below the origin of the lowest sigmoid branch, while others state that the superior hemorrhoidal begins after the inferior mesenteric trunk crosses the pelvic brim. The main trunk descends in the sigmoid mesentery and at the rectosigmoid junction (S_3) divides into right and left branches which extend inferiorly along the lateral rectal walls and anastomose with branches of the middle and inferior hemorrhoidal arteries near the anorectal junction. If the superior hemorrhoidal artery is considered as beginning at the pelvic brim, an important branch (sometimes two) arises about 1 to 2 cm. below the brim. This vessel takes origin just above the bifurcation of the superior hemorrhoidal and is termed the *rectosigmoid* or *sigmoid ima*. It anastomoses with the lowest sigmoid above and parallels the superior hemorrhoidal trunk in its descent on the posterior bowel wall. It supplies the anterolateral surfaces of the upper fifth of the rectum, overlapping in part the upper distribution of the superior hemorrhoidal. However, adequate anastomosis between this latter vessel and the rectosigmoid artery could be demonstrated in only one-half of the largest series of bodies studied. It is therefore important that if the rectosigmoid junction is to be preserved during resection, the superior hemorrhoidal should be ligated above the origin of the rectosigmoid artery.

c. MIDDLE HEMORRHOIDAL (RECTAL) ARTERIES— take origin from within the pelvis usually as direct branches from the anterior division of the internal iliac (hypogastric) arteries. Frequently, however, they arise from the internal pudendal. The middle hemorrhoidals extend from the posterolateral pelvic wall to the sides of the lower rectum and contribute to the formation of the lateral rectal stalks (page 218). These vessels anastomose freely with the superior hemorrhoidal arteries above and the inferior hemorrhoidals below.

d. INFERIOR HEMORRHOIDAL (RECTAL) ARTERIES—

arise from the internal pudendal branches of the internal iliacs. The internal pudendal takes immediate exit from the pelvis through the greater sciatic foramen and enters the gluteal region. At this point, it winds around the ischial spine and via the lesser sciatic foramen gains access to the perineum on the lateral wall of the ischiorectal (ischioanal) fossa, where it lies in a duplication of obturator fascia (*pudendal* or *Alcock's canal*). It is here that the internal pudendal gives rise to the inferior hemorrhoidal artery which extends medially across the ischiorectal fossa and supplies the perianal skin, external sphincter musculature, anal canal, and lower rectum. It anastomoses above with the middle and superior hemorrhoidal arteries in the rectal wall. This vessel is apparently more significant in the vascular supply of the rectum than most anatomic descriptions would indicate since it can be shown at operation that vascularity of a relatively large distal rectal stump may be preserved despite ligation of both middle hemorrhoids and the superior hemorrhoidal arteries.

5. **Venous Drainage** (Fig. 3)—within the walls of the rectum and anal canal are located three venous plexuses which give rise to six major venous tributaries corresponding in name to the arterial trunks described above. Of clinical significance is the fact that from these plexuses blood is returned to two different venous systems which intercommunicate: the portal and caval. This anorectal area is therefore important as a site of portocaval anastomosis (page 182).

a. EXTERNAL (INFERIOR) HEMORRHOIDAL PLEXUS— is located in the submucosal area of the anal canal below the pectinate line and in the subcutaneous tissue of the perianal area. This plexus connects above with the internal hemorrhoidal plexus and below with tributaries from the *inferior hemorrhoidal (rectal) vein* which in turn empties into the internal pudendal tributary of the internal iliac vein. Dilatation of these vessels within this plexus are termed *external hemorrhoids (piles)*.

b. INTERNAL (SUPERIOR) HEMORRHOIDAL PLEXUS— is located in the submucosal layer of the upper anal canal and rectum. The greatest aggregation of venules of this plexus is located in the rectal columns above the pectinate line. Tributaries from the internal plexus ascend in the submucosa for approximately 10 cm. above the pectinate line and pierce the muscular coat on either side of the rectal wall where they coalesce to form the *superior hemorrhoidal (rectal) vein* on the posterior wall of the rectum. The latter continues upward into the abdominal cavity as the inferior mesenteric tributary of the portal system of veins. Vessels from this internal plexus communicate below with the external plexus and laterally with the perimuscular rectal plexus. Since the superior hemorrhoidal veins are devoid of valves, any increase in portal venous pressure such as that seen in cirrhosis of the liver may produce dilatation of the internal plexus or *internal hemorrhoids*. It has also been demonstrated that the superior hemorrhoidal veins in the female may have direct connection with the uterine veins which again because of lack of valvular obstruction may well be a more important site of portocaval anastomosis than the other rectal veins.

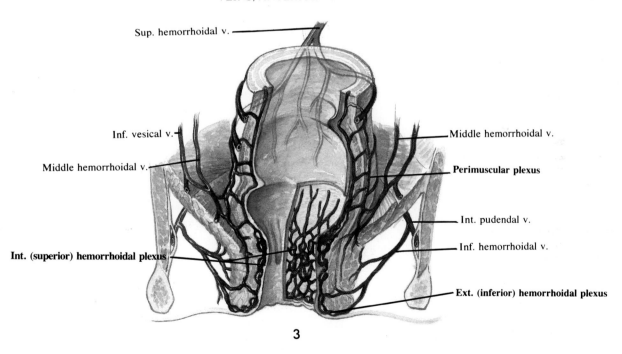

ARTERIES, ANTERIOR VIEW

Inferior mesenteric a.

Aorta

Sigmoid arteries

Common carotid a.

Middle sacral a.

Sup. hemorrhoidal a.

Rectosigmoid a.

Ext. iliac a.

Int. iliac a.

Internal iliac a.

Middle hemorrhoidal a.

Int. pudendal a.

Inferior hemorrhoidal a.

1

ARTERIES, POSTERIOR VIEW

Inferior mesenteric

Middle sacral a.

Rectosigmoid a.

Sigmoid arteries

Sup. hemorrhoidal a.

Mid. hemorrhoidal a.

Inf. hemorrhoidal a.

2

VEINS, ANTERIOR VIEW

Sup. hemorrhoidal v.

Inf. vesical v.

Middle hemorrhoidal v.

Middle hemorrhoidal v.

Perimuscular plexus

Int. pudendal v.

Inf. hemorrhoidal v.

Int. (superior) hemorrhoidal plexus

Ext. (inferior) hemorrhoidal plexus

3

c. PERIMUSCULAR HEMORRHOIDAL (RECTAL) PLEXUS—receives its tributaries primarily from the muscular wall of the rectum. Although the plexus communicates with the superior hemorrohoidal veins above, the principle drainage of this plexus is into the paired *middle hemorrhoidal veins* which in turn empty into the internal iliac (hypogastric) veins, a part of the caval system. Some vessels of the perimuscular plexus drain into the *middle* sacral vein which normally terminates in the left common iliac vein.

6. **Lymphatic Drainage**—the lymphatic drainage of the rectum and anal canal is discussed on page 230.

DEVELOPMENTAL DEFECTS OF THE RECTUM AND ANAL CANAL:

Congenital anorectal malformations occur infrequently and are more common in male infants. These defects are due to an abnormality of development during the sixth to eighth week of embryonic life.

1. **Normal Development** (Figs. 1 and 2)—almost as soon as the hindgut is established in the embryo, a ventral diverticulum, the *allantois,* arises from the hindgut and extends into the yolk stalk. That portion of the hindgut caudal to the allantois enlarges and forms a blind entodermal sac, the *cloaca* (L.: a sewer). This term is most appropriate, for in vertebrates other than placental mammals, this chamber persists, and all fecal, urinary, and reproductive products are expelled through it to the exterior. An ectodermal depression, the *proctodeum,* comes in contact with the cloaca. The area of union is termed the *cloacal membrane* and consists of an inner layer of entoderm and an outer layer of ectoderm.

At its cephalic end the cloaca gives off the allantois and laterally receives the mesonephric ducts from which arise metanephric ducts. The *mesonephric ducts* give rise to the vas deferens in the male, while the *metanephric ducts* become the ureters in both sexes. The ventral portion of the primitive cloaca undergoes further change. The proximal part of the allantois and the ventral cephalic portion of the cloaca become greatly dilated to form the *urinary bladder.* The distal portion of the allantois becomes the *urachus* which in the adult obliterates to form the median umbilical ligament. The posterior portion of the cloaca receives the hindgut.

At the angle between the hindgut and allantois a wedge of mesoderm, the *urorectal septum,* descends toward the cloacal membrane and divides the primitive cloaca into a posterior rectum and an anterior urinary bladder and *urogenital sinus.* The urogenital sinus is further divided into pelvic and phallic parts. In the male, the pelvic portion forms the prostatic and membranous urethra whereas the phallic portion becomes the cavernous urethra. In the female, the pelvic portion remains as the permanent urethra and the phallic portion forms the vestibule of the female external genitalia. When the separation of the cloaca is complete (seventh-week), the cloacal membrane ruptures resulting in separate openings for the anal canal behind and the urogenital ostium in front. In the female, the Müllerian ductal system which forms the uterovaginal canal develops in conjunction with the posterior wall of the urogenital sinus. Any abnormal connection existing between the rectum and urogenital sinus in the female must therefore involve the vaginal wall.

2. **Congenital Anorectal Malformations**—three phases in the development of the anorectal canal are significant in the development of anomalies in this region. They are the formation of the proctodeum, the rupture of the cloacal (anal) membrane, and the division of the primitive cloaca by the urorectal septum.

a. ANOMALIES OF THE PROCTODEUM—are rare. There may be a complete *absence of the anus* due to failure of the proctodeum to invaginate. An *aberrant anus* may develop due to invagination of the proctodeum at an abnormal location.

b. ANOMALIES OF THE CLOACAL (ANAL) MEMBRANE RUPTURE—are the most frequent malformations of the anorectal canal. Clinically several varieties are described which are collectively referred to as an *imperforate anus.* They are frequently (70 per cent) associated with anomalies of the urorectal septum with resultant fistula formation.

Type I—*congenital anorectal stenosis* is the result of incomplete disintegration of the anal (cloacal) membrane.

Type II (Fig. 3)—*true imperforate anus* is the result of complete persistence of the anal membrane and is the least common of these malformations of the anorectal canal. If not associated with a fistula, complete intestinal obstruction results.

Type III (Fig. 4)—*imperforate anus with rectal atresia* results from a combination of persistence of the anal membrane and partial failure of recanalization of the rectum. During the embryonic period of development, the lumen of the rectum becomes occluded by proliferation of epithelial cells and is normally recanalized. In this malformation such recanalization is incomplete, resulting in a blind rectal pouch located well above the imperforate anus. This is by far the most common anomaly (87 per cent) and is associated with fistula formation in some 80 per cent of the patients.

Type IV (Fig. 5)—*perforate anus with rectal atresia* is not an anomaly associated with the malformation of the anal membrane although it is classified as such in most surgical texts. Actually this anomaly represents an atresia of the rectum due to failure of recanalization, but there is normal development of the anal canal. It is rarely if ever associated with a fistula.

c. ANOMALIES OF THE RECTAL SEPTUM—frequently (70 per cent) occur in association with the anomalies of anorectal membrane rupture or imperforate anus.

(1) *Persistent Cloaca* (Fig. 6)—is an extremely rare anomaly resulting from failure of complete development of the urorectal septum. In such an anomaly the urinary, genital, and digestive tracts have a common external orifice.

(2) *Rectovaginal Fistula* (Fig. 7)—is the most common of this type of anomaly.

(3) *Rectoperineal Fistula* (Fig. 8)—occurs equally in males and females and has its opening in front of the anal dimple.

(4) *Rectovesical Fistula* (Fig. 9)—occurs almost invariably in the male.

(5) *Rectourethral Fistula* (Fig. 10)—is confined to male infants. Fistulas associated with the rectum almost never enter the urinary system in the female because of the interposition of the Müllerian ductal system between the urogenital sinus and rectum during the partitioning of the primitive cloaca. The Müllerian ducts persist in the female as the uterovaginal canal. In the male, however, the Müllerian ducts degenerate so that the rectum and urinary systems are in direct relationship.

It should be kept in mind that although the symp-

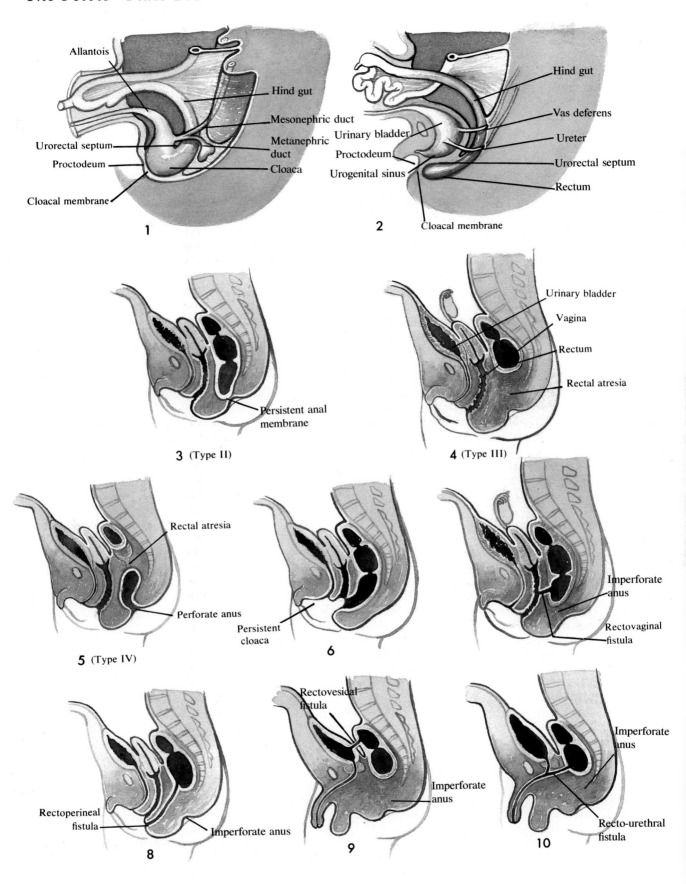

1

Allantois · Hind gut · Mesonephric duct · Metanephric duct · Urorectal septum · Proctodeum · Cloaca · Cloacal membrane

2

Hind gut · Vas deferens · Ureter · Urinary bladder · Urorectal septum · Proctodeum · Rectum · Urogenital sinus · Cloacal membrane

3 (Type II) — Persistent anal membrane

4 (Type III) — Urinary bladder · Vagina · Rectum · Rectal atresia

5 (Type IV) — Rectal atresia · Perforate anus

6 — Persistent cloaca

7 — Imperforate anus · Rectovaginal fistula

8 — Rectoperineal fistula · Imperforate anus

9 — Rectovesical fistula · Imperforate anus

10 — Imperforate anus · Recto-urethral fistula

toms of anorectal malformations may be obvious in these newborn infants, in almost 50 per cent of patients associated congenital anomalies may be present, the most common being congenital heart disease. To correct one deformity and overlook the other may prove disastrous.

THE RECTUM AND ANAL CANAL: CLINICAL CONSIDERATIONS:

Many pathologic conditions confront the surgeon in this part of the alimentary tract. Some of the benign disorders of the rectum and anal canal are considered on page 266. Of particular significance to the surgeon is the problem of anorectal cancer which comprises almost half of all cancers involving the large intestine.

1. **Lymphatic Drainage** (Fig. 1)—the lymphatic drainage of the rectum and anal canal, so important in the dissemination of cancer from this part of the digestive tract, spreads through lymph channels to three different sets of regional nodes. A diffuse *intramural lymphatic capillary plexus* is present in the submucous and subserous layers of the anorectal wall. Some of these channels terminate in intercalated *pararectal nodes* while the majority terminate in other first echelon nodes. The *extramural collecting channels* may be divided into superior, middle, and inferior groups.

a. SUPERIOR COLLECTING CHANNELS—are most important. They drain primarily that portion of the rectum above the middle rectal valve. These lymph vessels follow the superior hemorrhoidal artery and terminate in the *preaortic (inferior mesenteric)* and *paraortic nodes* of the left lumbar chain. Of particular significance is the node located at the third sacral vertebral level at the bifurcation of the superior hemorrhoidal artery. This node is termed the *principal node of the rectum* since it receives most of the superior collecting channels.

b. MIDDLE COLLECTING CHANNELS—drain mainly the area between the middle rectal valve and the pectinate line. They follow the middle hemorrhoidal vessels to the *hypogastric (internal iliac) nodes* which lie in the fat and fascia lying in relation to the upper surface of the levator ani muscles and lateral pelvic walls. Some of the channels from the posterior wall pass directly to the *lateral sacral nodes* thence to the *common iliac nodes* overlying the promontory of the sacrum.

c. INFERIOR COLLECTION CHANNELS—extend exclusively from the anal canal and follow the inferior hemorrhoidal vessels across the ischiorectal fossa and terminate in the *inguinal nodes*. The area of the anal canal between the pectinate line above and the intersphincteric line below is often referred to as the transitional zone. Lesions in this area may metastasize above and follow the middle collecting channels or below and follow the inferior collecting channels.

Inguinal node metastasis may occur even in rectal cancer. But this is rare and occurs only in advanced lesions in which the superior lymphatic channels are blocked and a retrograde metastasis to nodes below the primary lesion results.

2. **Excision of the Rectum**—whether the decision of the surgeon, based on pathologic and anatomic factors, has been to sacrifice or preserve the anal sphincter in an operation undertaken for cancer of the rectum, the extent of the intra-abdominal dissection is the same. The operation with the greatest prospect for cure includes the removal en bloc of all or part of the sigmoid and rectum with their mesenteric attachments containing the regional lymph nodes. In accomplishing this goal completely and cleanly, the surgeon must at the same time avoid injury to the ureters, the iliac vessels, aorta, and inferior vena cava. It is also most important to preserve the blood supply to the proximal segment if it is to be exteriorized as a permanent colostomy. These points are simple in principle, but, particularly in the obese, may be difficult in execution.

a. MOBILIZATION OF THE RECTUM—is accomplished by first incising the peritoneum along the base of the mesosigmoid on the left side (Fig. 2). This incision is extended inferiorly across the brim of the pelvis along the sides of the rectum to the rectovesical fossa in the male or the rectovaginal fossa in the female. As dissection is extended into the retroperitoneal space the left ureter and testicular (ovarian) vessels are exposed and protected.

The peritoneum forming the base of the right leaf of the mesosigmoid is incised and carried downward parallel with the incision made on the left side (Fig. 3). The two lateral incisions are connected in front of the rectum in the rectovesical or rectovaginal fossa. The right ureter must be identified and protected.

The inferior mesenteric vessels must next be ligated and divided. The site of this ligation will depend upon the level of transection of the proximal bowel and the level of the palpable lymph nodes. The ligation site of choice is just below the origin of the left colic artery (Fig. 3). Ligation at this level assures the proximal bowel segment of an adequate blood supply.

Following the ligation of the inferior mesenteric artery, the rectum is freed from its posterior attachment in the presacral space by blunt dissection as far as the tip of the coccyx. Sharp dissection is required to separate the rectum anteriorly from the bladder, seminal vesicle, and prostate in the male, and the uterus and upper vagina in the female. Laterally, dissection must extend to the superior surface of the levator ani muscles and the *lateral rectal stalks* containing the middle hemorrhoidal vessels must be ligated and divided.

b. PERINEAL RESECTION—of the rectum and anal canal is required in those cases in which a sphincter-saving procedure is deemed inadvisable. After mobilization of the rectum by the abdominal route as described above, and the establishment of a sigmoid or transverse colostomy, the rectum and anal canal can only be removed in their entirety by this perineal approach.

After closure of the anus by a purse string suture, an elliptical incision is made around the anus. The inferior hemorrhoidal vessels are ligated and divided on each side in the ischiorectal fossa (Fig. 4). Posteriorly the anococcygeal ligament is divided from its coccygeal attachment (Fig. 5). The levator ani muscles are then divided on either side (Fig. 6) and the dissection carried anteriorly to separate the rectum from the posterior surface of the prostate (or vaginal wall) and the posterior edge of the urogenital diaphragm by dividing the perineal body.

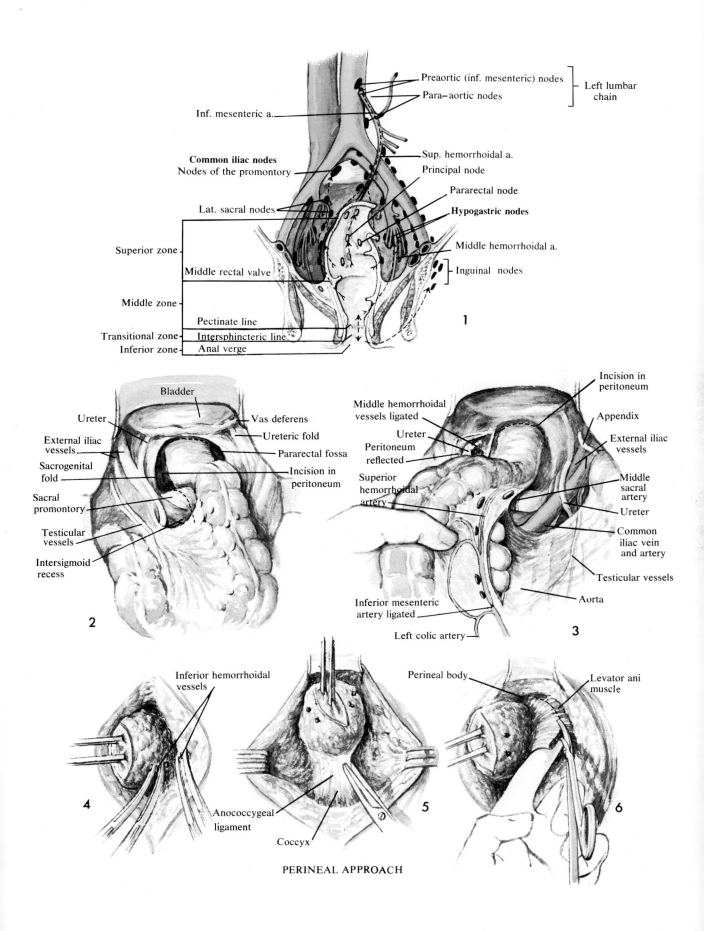

1

Preaortic (inf. mesenteric) nodes
Para–aortic nodes
} Left lumbar chain

Inf. mesenteric a.

Sup. hemorrhoidal a.
Principal node
Pararectal node
Hypogastric nodes
Middle hemorrhoidal a.
} Inguinal nodes

Common iliac nodes
Nodes of the promontory

Lat. sacral nodes

Superior zone
Middle rectal valve
Middle zone
Pectinate line
Transitional zone — Intersphincteric line
Inferior zone — Anal verge

2

Bladder
Ureter
External iliac vessels
Sacrogenital fold
Sacral promontory
Testicular vessels
Intersigmoid recess

Vas deferens
Ureteric fold
Pararectal fossa
Incision in peritoneum

3

Incision in peritoneum
Appendix
External iliac vessels
Middle sacral artery
Ureter
Common iliac vein and artery
Testicular vessels
Aorta

Middle hemorrhoidal vessels ligated
Ureter
Peritoneum reflected
Superior hemorrhoidal artery
Inferior mesenteric artery ligated
Left colic artery

4

Inferior hemorrhoidal vessels

Anococcygeal ligament
Coccyx

5

6

Perineal body
Levator ani muscle

PERINEAL APPROACH

PELVIC URINARY ORGANS:

Basically there is little difference between the pelvic portions of the urinary tract of the male and female. The differences that are prevalent arise as a result of the variation in the development of the respective genital organs. In the pelvis of each gender, one finds the pelvic ureter, the urinary bladder, and the urethra.

1. **Ureter**—the abdominal portion of this structure has already been described on page 200. Its pelvic portion begins at the pelvic brim (Fig. 4). It is related posteriorly to the sacroiliac joint, and descends on the lateral pelvic wall anterior to the internal iliac vessels inclining slightly laterally and dorsally in the extraperitoneal fatty tissue in conformity with the curvature of the lateral pelvic wall. At the level of the ischial spine it turns anteriorly and medially to enter the bladder.

Its anterior relations differ in the two sexes. In the male, the ureter is crossed by the vas deferens (water passes under the bridge) and passes under the free edge of the seminal vesicle. In the female, the ureter passes under the uterine artery in the base of the broad ligament 8 to 10 mm. lateral to the cervix of the uterus before entering the bladder (Figs. 1 and 2, page 251).

The intravesical portion of the ureter extends for approximately 2 cm. in an anteromedial and inferior direction through the bladder wall. They are about 5 cm. apart on entering the bladder on either side, but their *ureteral orifices* are only 2.5 cm. apart in the empty bladder.

The blood supply to the pelvic portion of the ureter is by ureteric branches from the common iliac and inferior vesical arteries (Fig. 1, page 203).

2. **Urinary Bladder**—for descriptive purposes, the empty bladder may be described as having a superior, posterior, and two inferior lateral surfaces. When distended the bladder becomes spherical in shape and ascends to an intra-abdominal position—a fact every surgeon must be aware of. Because of the small size of the pelvis in children under three years of age, the bladder is, in fact, intra-abdominal although extraperitoneal in position.

a. PERITONEAL RELATIONS—of the bladder in the male and female are illustrated in Figures 1 and 2. In both sexes, the reflections from the anterior abdominal wall to the superior surface of the bladder and from the lateral pelvic walls to the superior surface are respectively known as the *anterior* and *lateral false ligaments of the bladder*. In the female, the posterior reflection of peritoneum from the superior surface is upon the uterus forming the *vesicouterine fossa* (Fig. 1). In the male, a similar reflection upon the rectum forms the *vesicorectal fossa* (Fig. 2).

b. FIXATION OF THE BLADDER—is attained by certain thickenings of the endopelvic fascia, the *true ligaments of the bladder*. Anteriorly in the female these ligaments extend between the bladder and pubis as the *medial* and *lateral pubovesical ligaments* (Fig. 1). In the male they extend between the intervening prostate gland and pubis as the *medial and lateral puboprostatic ligaments* on either side (Fig. 2). Thickenings of the endopelvic fascia and extraperitoneal fatty tissue surrounding the neurovascular bundle from the lateral pelvic wall to the bladder constitute the *lateral true ligaments of the bladder*. From the apex of the bladder extending to the umbilicus the obliterated urachus forms the *medial umbilical ligament* which also aids in fixation of the bladder.

c. RELATIONAL ANATOMY—of the bladder is similar anteriorly and inferior laterally in both sexes. Anteriorly the symphysis pubis is separated from the bladder by the *prevesical space of Retzius* which contains the prevesical plexus of veins in the extraperitoneal fatty tissue (Figs. 1 and 2). The inferior lateral surfaces lie in relation to the levator ani and obturator internus muscles. In the extraperitoneal fatty tissue of these surfaces the superior vesical arteries lie anterior in position while the vas deferens enters posteriorly (Fig. 4).

The superior surface of the bladder in both sexes is covered by peritoneum with coils of small bowel and sigmoid colon overlying it. In the female, the body of the uterus in its normal antiverted antiflexed position overlaps the posterior superior aspect (Fig. 1).

The main difference in relational anatomy concerns the posterior surface of the bladder, the difference being due to the genital organs. In the female, the vagina and supravaginal portion of the uterine cervix are directly related (Fig. 1). In the male, the rectum and seminal vesicles are in immediate posterior relationship (Fig. 2).

Inferiorly, the apex, or vesical neck, also differs in its relationship in the two sexes. In the female it lies in intimate contact with the urogenital diaphragm (Fig. 1). In the male, however, the prostate gland intervenes between the vesical neck and the urogenital diaphragm (Fig. 2).

d. BLOOD SUPPLY OF THE URINARY BLADDER—is carried exclusively by branches of the hypogastric (internal iliac) artery (Fig. 4). The embryonic umbilical arteries provide the chief supply by their unobliterated proximal parts which usually give rise to two or three *superior vesical arteries*. The *inferior vesical arteries* are either direct or, more commonly, indirect branches from the hypogastric. They supply most of the inferior lateral wall of the bladder as well as the prostate in the male. A third set of arteries, the *deferential arteries*, supplies most of the posterior surface of the bladder. They are variable in origin and have as their homologue in the female, the uterine arteries.

The veins do not follow the arteries but form a plexus which, in the male, is termed the prostatic plexus and in the female, the vesicle plexus. These vessels ultimately terminate as tributaries of the hypogastric vein.

(Text continued on page 234.)

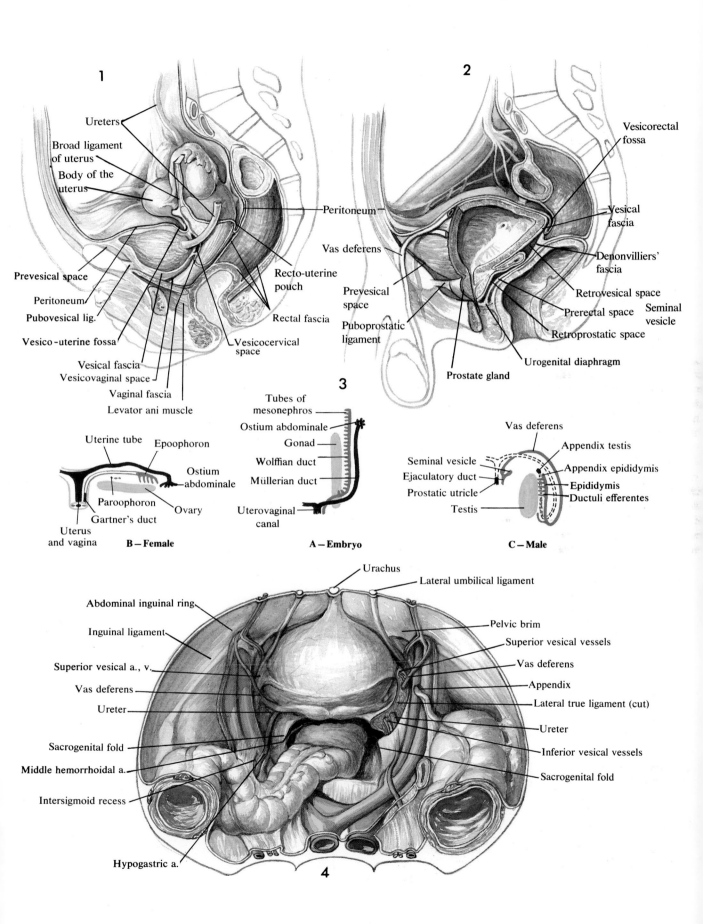

1

Ureters

Broad ligament
of uterus

Body of the
uterus

Prevesical space

Peritoneum

Pubovesical lig.

Vesico-uterine fossa

Vesical fascia

Vesicovaginal space

Vaginal fascia

Levator ani muscle

Peritoneum

Recto-uterine
pouch

Rectal fascia

Vesicocervical
space

2

Vesicorectal
fossa

Vesical
fascia

Denonvilliers'
fascia

Retrovesical space

Prerectal space   Seminal
vesicle

Retroprostatic space

Urogenital diaphragm

Prostate gland

Vas deferens

Prevesical
space

Puboprostatic
ligament

3

Uterine tube   Epoophoron

Ostium
abdominale

Paroophoron   Ovary

Gartner's duct

Uterus
and vagina   **B—Female**

Tubes of
mesonephros

Ostium abdominale

Gonad

Wolffian duct

Müllerian duct

Uterovaginal
canal

A—Embryo

Vas deferens

Appendix testis

Appendix epididymis

Seminal vesicle

Ejaculatory duct

Prostatic utricle

Testis

Epididymis

Ductuli efferentes

C—Male

4

Urachus   Lateral umbilical ligament

Abdominal inguinal ring

Inguinal ligament

Superior vesical a., v.

Vas deferens

Ureter

Sacrogenital fold

Middle hemorrhoidal a.

Intersigmoid recess

Hypogastric a.

Pelvic brim

Superior vesical vessels

Vas deferens

Appendix

Lateral true ligament (cut)

Ureter

Inferior vesical vessels

Sacrogenital fold

e. LYMPHATICS OF THE BLADDER—are described on page 238.

f. NERVE SUPPLY OF THE BLADDER—is derived from the hypogastric sympathetic plexus and the pelvic splanchnics (nervi erigentes) and has been discussed on page 220. But aside from this known anatomic fact there is much discrepancy in the literature as to the innervation of the bladder and the physiologic reactions in micturition and pain conduction. It is far beyond the scope of this book to enter into the controversy.

3. **Urethra**—the urethra in the female simply serves as a conduit for the excretion of the urinary bladder contents. Since the bladder neck lies directly upon the urogenital diaphragm, the female urethra does not lie within the pelvic cavity. The male urethra, however, serves not only the purpose of the passage of urinary secretions but also conducts the discharges from the male germinal organs. It must traverse the prostate gland before taking exit from the pelvis. It does, therefore, have clinical significance in consideration of intrapelvic pathology. Because of this intimate anatomic relationship with the prostate gland, the pelvic or prostatic portion of this structure will be considered on page 236.

PELVIC GENITAL ORGANS: EMBRYOLOGY:

In the embryo, an indifferent stage of sex development is present, consisting of the gonads and a double set of sexual duct systems which terminate in the urogenital sinus (Fig. 3A).

1. **Gonads**—in both sexes, the gonads arise from a germinal ridge of mesoderm in the posterior wall of the abdomen. This gonadal tissue, in the male, gives rise to the testes which descends through the abdominal wall into the scrotum. This descent of the testes is described on page 138. In the female, the *ovaries* develop from the same germinal ridge and, like the testes, descend from their original position on the posterior abdominal wall. This descent in the female is more limited; the ovaries descend into the pelvis.

2. **Wolffian (mesonephric) Duct**—this, the male sexual duct, develops just lateral to the gonads (Fig. 3A). Tubules from this duct communicate with the developing testes and are restricted as the *efferent ductules of the testes*. That part of the Wolffian duct into which they enter constitutes the *epididymis*. The most caudal part of the tube above the epididymis remains as the *appendix of the epididymis*. Some of the caudal mesonephric tubules are rudimentary and persist as the *paradidymis*. Caudal to the epididymis, the Wolffian duct receives a thick smooth muscle layer and becomes the

vas deferens. Just before the vasa enter the urogenital sinus, an evagination of the duct occurs to form the *seminal vesicles*. The terminal part of the Wolffian duct between the seminal vesicles and urethra constitutes the *ejaculatory duct* (Fig. 3C).

In the female, the Wolffian duct degenerates for the most part. The most cranial portion of the duct and tubules persists in the female as the *epoophoron* and *paroophoron*, and the most distal part as the *duct of Gartner* (Fig. 3B).

3. **Müllerian Duct** (Fig. 3A)—this female sexual tube disappears in the male except for its most cranial and caudal tip. The former persists as the *appendix of the testes*, and the latter as the *prostatic utricle* (Fig 3C). In the female, the tube forms the uterine tube, uterus, and upper vagina (Fig. 3B).

Homologues of the Major Genital Organs

MALE	FEMALE
Testis	Ovary
Appendix testis	Ostium abdominale of the uterine tube
No homologue	Uterine tube
No homologue	Uterus
No homologue	Vagina (upper)
Prostatic utricle	Vagina (lower)
Gubernaculum testis	Round and ovarian ligaments
Appendix epididymidis	Epoophoron-distal longitudinal duct
Ductuli efferentes	Epoophoron-transverse ducts
Paradidymis (tubuli)	Paroophoron
Paradidymis (collecting duct)	No homologue
Ductus epididymidis (proximal)	Epoophoron-proximal longitudinal duct
Ductus epididymidis (distal)	No homologue
Ductus deferens (proximal)	No homologue
Ductus deferens (distal)	Duct of Gartner
Seminal vesicle	No homologue
Urethra (above prostatic utricle)	Urethra
Urethra (below prostatic utricle)	Vestible
Colliculus seminalis	Hymen
Scrotum	Labia majora
Processus vaginalis testis	Canal of Nuck
Penis	Clitoris
Urethral surface of penis	Labia minora
Prostate	Urethral glands
Bulbo urethral glands (Cowper)	Major vestibular gland (Bartholin)
Urethral glands (Littré)	Minor vestibular glands
Corpus cavernosum urethrae	Bulbi vestibuli
Corpus cavernosum penis	Corpus cavernosum clitoridis

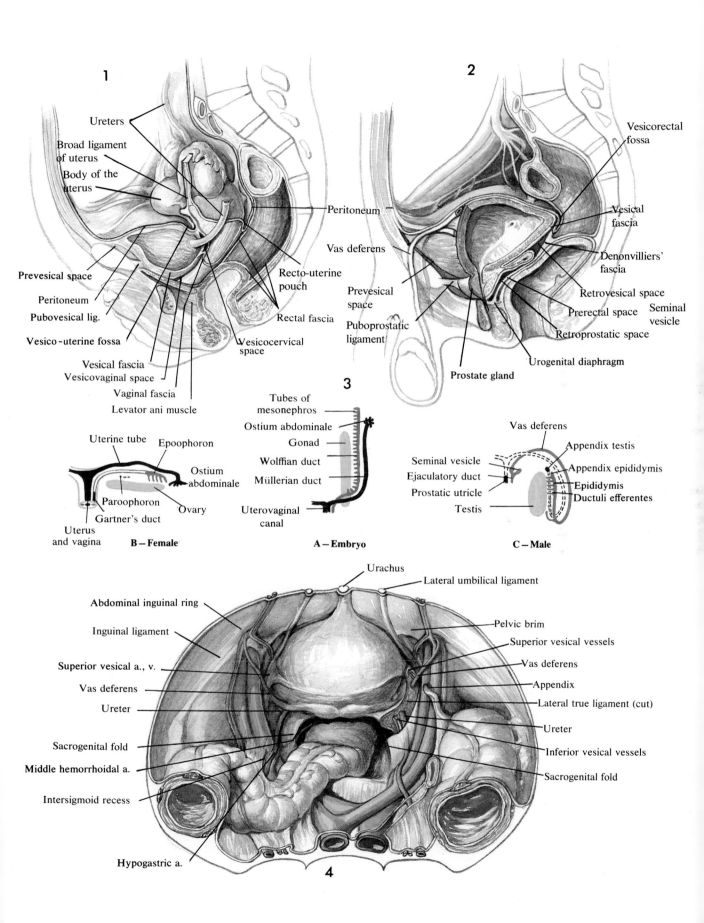

1

Ureters

Broad ligament
of uterus

Body of the
uterus

Prevesical space

Peritoneum

Pubovesical lig.

Vesico-uterine fossa

Vesical fascia

Vesicovaginal space

Vaginal fascia

Levator ani muscle

Peritoneum

Recto-uterine
pouch

Rectal fascia

Vesicocervical
space

2

Vesicorectal
fossa

Vesical
fascia

Denonvilliers'
fascia

Retrovesical space

Prerectal space

Retroprostatic space

Urogenital diaphragm

Vas deferens

Prevesical
space

Puboprostatic
ligament

Prostate gland

Seminal
vesicle

3

Tubes of
mesonephros

Ostium abdominale

Gonad

Wolffian duct

Müllerian duct

Uterovaginal
canal

A — Embryo

Uterine tube

Epoophoron

Ostium
abdominale

Ovary

Paroophoron

Gartner's duct

Uterus
and vagina

B — Female

Vas deferens

Appendix testis

Appendix epididymis

Epididymis

Ductuli efferentes

Seminal vesicle

Ejaculatory duct

Prostatic utricle

Testis

C — Male

Urachus

Lateral umbilical ligament

Abdominal inguinal ring

Inguinal ligament

Superior vesical a., v.

Vas deferens

Ureter

Sacrogenital fold

Middle hemorrhoidal a.

Intersigmoid recess

Hypogastric a.

Pelvic brim

Superior vesical vessels

Vas deferens

Appendix

Lateral true ligament (cut)

Ureter

Inferior vesical vessels

Sacrogenital fold

4

PELVIC GENITAL ORGANS: MALE:

The vas deferens, seminal vesicles, and ejaculatory ducts develop from the Wolffian ducts (Fig. 3, page 235). The prostate gland arises as multiple evaginations from the urethra. The prostatic urethra is a derivative of the urogenital sinus (page 228). The testicle and epididymis, the extrapelvic portions of the male genital organs, are shown on page 139, and the penis on page 256.

1. **Vas (Ductus) Deferens** — this duct which conveys the spermatozoa from the testes begins at the tail of the epididymis, ascends through the spermatic cord and inguinal canal to enter the abdominal cavity (Fig. 5, page 139). Upon entering the abdominal inguinal ring it passes medially into the pelvis overlying the structures of the pelvic brim (Fig. 4, page 235). It passes just beneath the peritoneum to the posterior wall of the bladder, lying medial to the seminal vesicle where it becomes dilated as the *ampulla* (Fig. 3).

2. **Seminal Vesicles** — these are bilateral, coiled, sacculated tubes about 5 cm. in length. They rest upon the posterior surface of the bladder lying parallel and lateral to the vas deferens (Fig. 3). Anteriorly, the capsule of the vesicle is firmly affixed to the posterior wall of the bladder. Posteriorly, its upper portion is covered by peritoneum of the rectovesical fossa, while the remainder of the posterior surface is separated from the rectum by a thick double layer of fascia *(Denonvilliers' fascia)*.

3. **Ejaculatory Ducts** — each duct is formed by the union of the vas deferens and the duct of the seminal vesicles (Fig. 3). The ducts pierce the prostate gland and empty into the prostatic urethra on the *colliculus seminalis* just lateral to and below the opening of the *prostatic utricle* (Fig. 4).

4. **Prostate Gland** — the prostate is a pyramidal-shaped, fibromuscular and glandular organ which secretes an alkaline fluid which aids in the motility of the sperm cells. The gland arises from multiple outgrowths of the urethral epithelium into the surrounding connective tissue. The prostatic urethra and the two ejaculatory ducts pierce the gland (Fig. 1).

The base of the prostate is in intimate relationship with the neck of the bladder. The urethra pierces this surface of the prostate near its anterior border. The apex of the prostate rests upon the urogenital diaphragm. Anteriorly, the prostate is separated from the symphysis pubis by the extraperitoneal *prevesical (retropubic) space of Retzius*. In this space, the prostatic venous plexus and puboprostatic ligaments are found. Posteriorly, the prostate is related to the rectum and may be palpated by digital rectal examination. Laterally, the prostate lies upon the levator ani muscles (Fig. 3).

Four lobes of the prostate are usually described: two lateral lobes, a posterior lobe, and a middle lobe. The *lateral lobes* make up the major portion of the gland. These lobes are a frequent site of benign adenomas. The *posterior lobe* is considered by many as a part of the lateral lobes. It arises as urethral outpouchings below the entrance of the ejaculatory ducts and grows posterior and superior in direction (Fig. 1). This part of the gland is readily palpable by digital examination and is a frequent site of cancer of the prostate. A *middle lobe* lies between the urethra and ejaculatory ducts and is intimately related to the vesical neck. Because of this anatomic relationship even small adenomas in this lobe may obstruct the vesical outlet. An *anterior lobe* is described by some investigators. However, the anterior evaginations from the urethra no longer retain their glandular components in the adult, and the lobe is considered only as an isthmus between the two lateral lobes anterior to the urethra.

The prostate possesses a *true capsule*, a thin fibromuscular sheath that surrounds the gland. The *false capsule* is part of the visceral layer of endopelvic fascia (page 216). An important posterior fascial relationship is a fascial plane separating the prostate from the rectum — the *fascia of Denonvilliers* (Fig. 2, page 235).

5. **Prostatic Urethra** (Fig. 4) — this portion of the male urethra extends from the neck of the bladder to the urogenital diaphragm. It traverses the prostate for about 2.5 cm. of its length and extends 0.5 cm. beyond the apex of the gland before piercing the diaphragm. On its dorsal surface a large fold, the *urethral crest*, extends throughout its length, on the middle of which is an eminence, the *colliculus seminalis (verumontanum)*. On the colliculus is the opening of the *prostatic utricle*, homologous to the lower portion of the vagina, and the *orifices of the ejaculatory ducts*. On either side of the colliculus are numerous openings of the ducts of the prostatic glands.

6. **Blood Supply of the Pelvic Genital Organs** (Figs. 2 to 4) — the *inferior vesical artery* is the major arterial supply to these organs. This artery is usually a direct visceral branch of the anterior division of the internal iliac (hypogastric artery). The inferior vesical gives rise to a *deferential artery*, homologous to the uterine artery in the female. This vessel divides into an ascending branch which follows the vas into the spermatic cord and a descending branch which supplies the ampulla of the vas and seminal vesicles. The inferior vesical artery divides into *capsular branches,* which supply the major portion of the gland, and *urethral branches* which supply the deep periurethral parts of the prostate (Fig. 4).

The venous and lymphatic drainage of these organs is described on page 240.

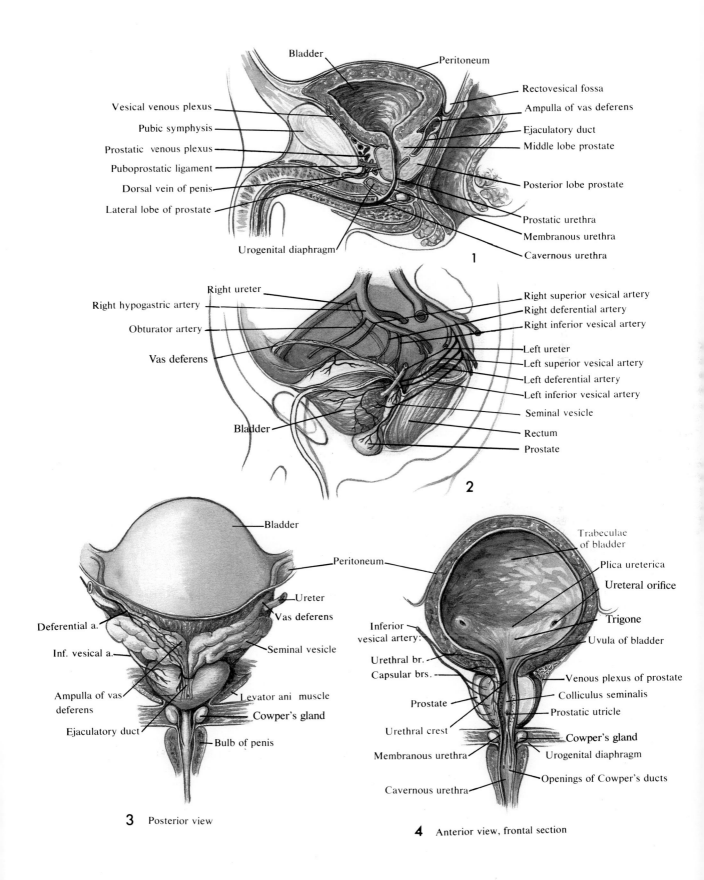

Bladder

Peritoneum

Rectovesical fossa

Ampulla of vas deferens

Ejaculatory duct

Middle lobe prostate

Posterior lobe prostate

Vesical venous plexus

Pubic symphysis

Prostatic venous plexus

Puboprostatic ligament

Dorsal vein of penis

Lateral lobe of prostate

Prostatic urethra

Membranous urethra

Cavernous urethra

Urogenital diaphragm

1

Right ureter

Right hypogastric artery

Obturator artery

Vas deferens

Bladder

Right superior vesical artery

Right deferential artery

Right inferior vesical artery

Left ureter

Left superior vesical artery

Left deferential artery

Left inferior vesical artery

Seminal vesicle

Rectum

Prostate

2

Bladder

Peritoneum

Ureter

Vas deferens

Seminal vesicle

Deferential a.

Inf. vesical a.

Ampulla of vas deferens

Ejaculatory duct

Levator ani muscle

Cowper's gland

Bulb of penis

3 Posterior view

Trabeculae of bladder

Plica ureterica

Ureteral orifice

Trigone

Uvula of bladder

Inferior vesical artery

Urethral br.

Capsular brs.

Prostate

Urethral crest

Membranous urethra

Cavernous urethra

Venous plexus of prostate

Colliculus seminalis

Prostatic utricle

Cowper's gland

Urogenital diaphragm

Openings of Cowper's ducts

4 Anterior view, frontal section

PELVIC URINARY ORGANS: CLINICAL CONSIDERATIONS:

Traumatic injury to the pelvic urinary organs is one of the most common pathologic conditions confronting the general surgeon in this anatomic area. This is especially true in regard to the pelvic ureters. The presence of urinary calculi, bladder tumors, prostatic tumors requiring an intravesical approach, and congenital disorders are also indications for surgical intervention.

1. **Pelvic Ureters** — aside from the common bile duct, the pelvic ureters are the most abused ductal structures in the body as a result of surgery performed on related organs. They are rarely injured in penetrating wounds of the abdomen or pelvis but are frequently injured during lower abdominal and especially pelvic operations. Injuries to the ureters must be immediately repaired to prevent extravasation of urine into the peritoneal cavity which is inevitably followed by peritonitis. Unfortunately, many instances occur in pelvic surgery where the injury may not be apparent during the operative procedure.

a. OPERATIVE TRAUMA — may occur as a result of many factors. Figures 1 and 2 illustrate a few of these causes. Because of the close relationship of the ureter with the ovarian vessels it may be accidentally ligated in the stump of the infundibulopelvic ligament. It may be crushed by the clamp applied to the parametrial tissue, or accidentally ligated as the tie is placed upon the uterine artery and cardinal ligaments. During a supravaginal hysterectomy, the ureter may be partially severed by the needle during closure of the lateral cuff of the vaginal vault. Although these illustrations show the possibilities of ureteral injury in gynecologic procedures, the chance of injury is present in any pelvic operation.

Careful anatomic exposure and identification of the ureter in all abdominal and pelvic operative maneuvers is the procedure of choice in order to prevent injury to this structure.

b. URETERAL REPAIR OR TRANSPLANT — is necessary should injury occur. Reconstruction of anatomic continuity by direct end-to-end anastomosis *(ureterouterostomy)* is the procedure of choice. If this is not possible, implantation of the proximal end of the ureter into the urinary bladder should be performed.

In many instances where a large segment of the ureter must be sacrificed or the bladder removed, other means of diverting the urinary stream to the exterior must be utilized. These include the transplantation of the ureter to the skin of the abdominal wall, an *external ureterostomy;* the transplantation of the ureter to the sigmoid colon, an *ureterosigmoidostomy;* or the *construction of an ileal conduit.* In the latter, an isolated segment of ileum is exteriorized onto the abdominal wall and the ureters transplanted into this loop of bowel (page 192).

2. **Urinary Bladder** — operations upon the urinary bladder are performed for temporary drainage of the urinary tract because of urethral obstruction or for removal of stones *(cystostomy). Partial cystectomy* is indicated for chronic ulcers, diverticuli, fistulae, benign tumors, or localized cancer. *Total cystectomy* is indicated in selected cases of cancer of the bladder or other pelvic viscera or in exstrophy of the bladder.

a. OPERATIVE APPROACH — to the bladder depends upon the pathology. An *intravesical approach* may be used to treat small benign tumors or stones by cystoscopic means. In the major portion of bladder disorders, an *extraperitoneal cystostomy* or *cystectomy* is required.

b. LYMPHATIC DRAINAGE — of the bladder is important in the treatment of cancer of this organ. Three bilateral collecting lymph channels exit from the capillary plexus of the bladder (Fig. 3).

(1) *Anterior Collecting Trunk* — drains the anterior portion of the lateral surface of the bladder and terminates in the node of the medial group of the external iliac nodes situated near the femoral ring *(retrofemoral node).*

(2) *Superior Collecting Trunk* — receives channels from the anterior portion of the superior surface and posterior part of the inferior lateral surface. This trunk terminates in the *middle node of the medial chain* of external iliac nodes.

(3) *Posterior Collecting Trunk* — of the bladder drains the remainder of the superior and posterior surfaces of the bladder. These channels may extend directly to the *superior node* of the medial group of the external iliac chain, follow the deferential or uterine artery to the *hypogastric nodes* or the lateral sacral artery to the *lateral sacral nodes,* or pass directly to the *nodes of promontory* of the common iliac group.

c. VESICOVISCERAL FISTULAE — are rather rare but anatomically important pathologic entities. The developmental fistula has been discussed on page 228. Trauma, infection, or neoplastic disease may cause such fistulae. In the female, fistulae between the bladder and vagina *(vesicovaginal fistulae)* are most common, whereas those between the bladder and uterus are rare *(vesicouterine fistulae)* (Fig. 4). In the male, for reasons discussed on page 228, fistulae usually occur between the bladder and rectum *(vesicorectal fistulae).*

d. STRESS INCONTINENCE — is the most common type of involuntary loss of urinary control in the female. It is usually the result of obstetrical trauma to the supporting elements of the bladder neck and urethra. Of particular importance in support of these structures are the *pubovesical* and *vesicouterine* ligaments (Fig. 5; Fig. 4, page 243). Injury to these ligaments results in a downward and backward displacement of the urethra. The urethral walls relax and the internal bladder sphincter opens. The upper portion of the urethra becomes an extension of the bladder and voluntary control is impeded. Any increase in intra-abdominal pressure, such as heavy lifting, sneezing, coughing, or laughing will result in the loss of urine. Stress incontinence should be distinguished from a *cystocele* (page 264). In the latter, the obstetrical trauma involves supportive structures at the base of the bladder, rather than anteriorly at the vesical neck.

Many different operative procedures are utilized to correct a stress incontinence, but all are designed to restore the normal anatomic relation of the bladder neck to the urethra.

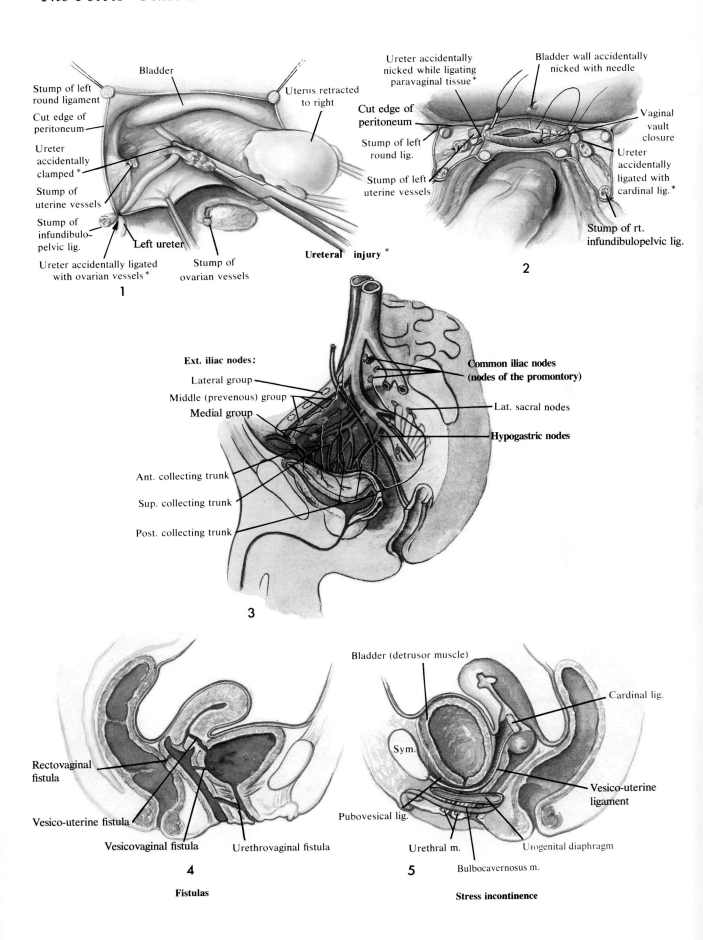

Stump of left
round ligament

Cut edge of
peritoneum

Ureter
accidentally
clamped *

Stump of
uterine vessels

Stump of
infundibulo-
pelvic lig.

Ureter accidentally ligated
with ovarian vessels *

Bladder

Uterus retracted
to right

Left ureter

Stump of
ovarian vessels

1

Ureteral injury *

Ureter accidentally
nicked while ligating
paravaginal tissue *

Bladder wall accidentally
nicked with needle

Cut edge of
peritoneum

Stump of left
round lig.

Stump of left
uterine vessels

Vaginal
vault
closure

Ureter
accidentally
ligated with
cardinal lig. *

Stump of rt.
infundibulopelvic lig.

2

Ext. iliac nodes:

Lateral group

Middle (prevenous) group

Medial group

Ant. collecting trunk

Sup. collecting trunk

Post. collecting trunk

Common iliac nodes
(nodes of the promontory)

Lat. sacral nodes

Hypogastric nodes

3

Rectovaginal
fistula

Vesico-uterine fistula

Vesicovaginal fistula

Urethrovaginal fistula

4

Fistulas

Bladder (detrusor muscle)

Sym.

Pubovesical lig.

Urethral m.

Bulbocavernosus m.

Cardinal lig.

Vesico-uterine
ligament

Urogenital diaphragm

5

Stress incontinence

PELVIC MALE GENITAL ORGANS: CLINICAL CONSIDERATIONS:

Of the pelvic genital organs in the male, the prostate gland is most important to the surgeon. Infection with abscess formation, benign hypertrophy, or malignant tumors are the most common indications for surgical intervention. The prostatic urethra may also be of surgical significance.

1. **Rupture of the Prostatic Urethra** — as described on page 236, this portion of the male urethra extends from the neck of the bladder to the urogenital diaphragm. Although most of its length (2.5 cm.) traverses the prostate gland, a portion, usually about 0.5 cm., extends beyond the apex of the gland before piercing the diaphragm. Rupture of the prostatic urethra is usually associated with a fracture of the pelvis. Such an injury results in hematoma formation, extravasation of urine, and subsequent infection. An immediate cystostomy is indicated to divert the urinary flow and prevent further leakage. The extravasated urine collects in the extraperitoneal fatty tissue layer of the pelvis (Fig. 1). It is usually limited posteriorly by Denonvilliers' fascia unless this facial layer is torn as well, and is limited inferiorly by the urogenital diaphragm. Its path of least resistance is therefore anteriorly into the space of Retzius.

2. **Surgical Approach to the Prostate** — to gain access to the prostate gland for either partial or complete resection, any of four anatomical routes may be used (Fig. 2). The selection of the approach will vary with the operator and the specific indications for which the procedure is performed.

a. SUPRAPUBIC APPROACH (Fig. 2) — may be performed for either partial (intracapsular) or complete (extracapsular) removal of the gland. The approach is made through the abdominal wall and the urinary bladder is opened. Since the prostate gland lies outside the bladder wall, the gland must be removed by blind digital enucleation. In the case of an extracapsular enucleation, the danger of hemorrhage from rupture of the prostaticovesical venous plexus is ever present. Should hemorrhage occur, it is difficult to control.

b. RETROPUBIC APPROACH (Fig. 2) — also utilizes an abdominal wall incision, but in this technique the urinary bladder is not entered. Instead, the space of Retzius is enlarged and the prostate directly approached in its extravesical position.

c. PERINEAL APPROACH (Fig. 2) — is a procedure that is definitely indicated when carcinoma of the gland has invaded the capsule. The surgical approach is made through the skin of the perineum anterior to the anus (Fig. 4, page 263). The central tendon of the perineum is divided and the rectum retracted posteriorly and the corpus cavernosum penis anteriorly. The fascial interval between the two layers of Denonvilliers' fascia is then entered to expose the prostate gland which can be removed under direct vision.

d. TRANSURETHRAL APPROACH (Fig. 2) — is utilized to relieve obstruction at the vesical neck, primarily for benign enlargements of the gland, particularly the middle lobe, or as a palliative procedure in obstruction from malignant disease of the gland. Electrocautery is used to resect the obstructive tissues.

3. **Lymphatic Drainage of the Prostate** (Fig. 3) — four major collecting trunks arise from the lymphatic capillaries of the prostate gland.

a. EXTERNAL ILIAC PEDICLE — extends from the superior and upper part of the posterior surface and terminates in the medial and middle (prevenous) nodes of the external iliac chain.

b. HYPOGASTRIC PEDICLE — is represented by collecting channels from the posterior and lateral surfaces of the gland which follow the inferior vesical artery to the hypogastric nodes.

c. POSTERIOR PEDICLE — is composed of lymph channels from the posterior surface of the prostate which terminate either in the lateral sacral nodes or pass directly to the nodes of the promontory (common iliac nodes).

d. INFERIOR PEDICLE — arises from a single collecting trunk from the apex of the gland, passes through the perineum, and follows the internal pudendal artery back into the pelvis to terminate in a hypogastric node.

4. **Lymphatic Drainage of the Seminal Vesicles and Vas Deferens** — numerous collecting channels issue from the vas deferens. These channels accompany the deferential artery and empty into the lateral and middle (prevenous) nodes of the external iliac chain and into the hypogastric nodes.

Lymphatic channels draining the seminal vesicles likewise drain into the external iliac chain (prevenous) and hypogastric nodes.

5. **Venous Drainage of the Male Pelvic Genital Organs** (Fig. 4) — the venous drainage of the vas deferens is via the *deferential vein*. This vein is a tributary of the *seminal venous plexus* which receives the venous tributaries of the seminal vesicle.

The veins of the prostate gland form a rich plexus, the *prostatic (pudendal) plexus,* located between the true and false capsules of the gland. Anteriorly, this plexus receives the dorsal vein of the penis, superiorly it receives the vesicle veins, and posteriorly the tributaries of the seminal venous plexus. Posteriorly, the prostatic plexus also communicates with the hemorrhoidal plexus. The prostatic plexus drains laterally through the lateral true ligaments of the bladder with the hypogastric (internal iliac vein).

An important communication exists between the prostatic plexus of veins and the vertebral venous plexus. These veins are valveless and may explain the frequency of vertebral metastasis in prostatic carcinoma.

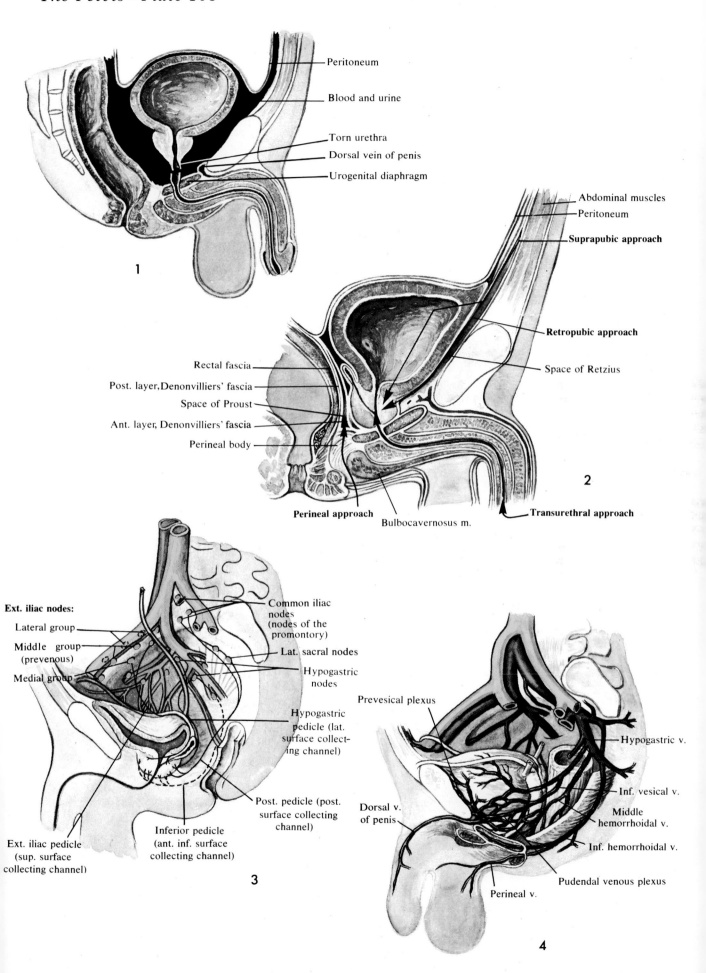

1

- Peritoneum
- Blood and urine
- Torn urethra
- Dorsal vein of penis
- Urogenital diaphragm

Abdominal muscles
Peritoneum
Suprapubic approach

Retropubic approach

Space of Retzius

Rectal fascia
Post. layer, Denonvilliers' fascia
Space of Proust
Ant. layer, Denonvilliers' fascia
Perineal body

Perineal approach

Bulbocavernosus m.

Transurethral approach

2

Ext. iliac nodes:

Lateral group

Middle group
(prevenous)

Medial group

Common iliac
nodes
(nodes of the
promontory)

Lat. sacral nodes

Hypogastric
nodes

Hypogastric
pedicle (lat.
surface collect-
ing channel)

Post. pedicle (post.
surface collecting
channel)

Inferior pedicle
(ant. inf. surface
collecting channel)

Ext. iliac pedicle
(sup. surface
collecting channel)

3

Prevesical plexus

Hypogastric v.

Inf. vesical v.

Middle
hemorrhoidal v.

Inf. hemorrhoidal v.

Dorsal v.
of penis

Pudendal venous plexus

Perineal v.

4

PELVIC FEMALE GENITAL ORGANS:

The pelvic female genital organs are derivatives of the gonadal tissue and Müllerian ducts, although some remnants of the Wolffian duct system remain (page 234). These female organs are the ovaries, uterine tubes, uterus, and vagina.

1. **Peritoneal Relations** (Figs. 1 to 3)—from the anterior abdominal wall the parietal peritoneum in the midline passes over the superior surface of the bladder onto the anterior surface of the uterus as the *vesicouterine reflection*. The peritoneum then passes over the fundus of the uterus onto the posterior surface and extends inferiorly covering the upper part of the vagina before reflecting upon the rectum. This reflection forms the *rectouterine pouch of Douglas*.

Of particular importance is the fold of peritoneum related to the pelvic genital organs, the *broad ligament*. This structure is actually a bilateral mesentery formed by a double layer of peritoneum related to the ovary, the uterine tubes, and the uterus. It is roughly triangular in shape extending from the lateral wall of the uterus to the lateral pelvic wall. Its free upper border in part encases the uterine tube and is directed anteriorly. Medially, the two layers envelop the uterus and are continuous with the layers of the opposite side. Inferiorly and laterally the two layers, anterior and posterior, extend over the floor of the true pelvis. The anterior surface is directed inferiorly as well as anteriorly and the posterior surface, superiorly and posteriorly. The outer fifth of the upper free border contains the ovarian vessels and is termed the *infundibulopelvic (suspensory) ligament of the ovary*. The ovary projects from the posterior surface of the broad ligament suspended by a small peritoneal fold termed the *mesovarium*. The portion of the ligament above this is termed the *mesosalpinx* and is related to the uterine tube. That portion of the broad ligament below the mesovarium is referred to as the *mesometrium*.

2. **Support of the Pelvic Genital Organs** (Figs. 2 to 4)—the support of the uterus is dependent upon two elements: the musculature of the pelvic diaphragm and the intrinsic ligaments of the uterus. The musculature of the pelvic diaphragm has been described on page 216.

a. OVARIAN LIGAMENTS—are fibromuscular cords extending from the inferior pole of the ovary to the uterus. They are encased in the medial portion of the mesovarium of the broad ligament and are homologous to the upper part of the gubernaculum testis.

b. ROUND LIGAMENTS—are fibromuscular cords extending from the anterior surface of the uterus to the abdominal inguinal ring. They are the homologues of the lower portion of the gubernaculum testis. They extend through the inguinal canal to attach to connective tissue of the labium majorus. These ligaments aid in sustaining the uterus in its normal anteverted position.

c. LATERAL CERVICAL (MACKENRODT'S, CARDINAL) LIGAMENTS—are bilateral thickenings of endopelvic fascia and perivascular tissue extending from the lateral pelvic wall to the cervix of the uterus and upper portion of the vagina. They are located at the base of the broad ligament of the uterus. The uterine artery runs along the upper portion of this ligament and the ureter pierces the ligament near its uterine attachment. These ligaments are the main supportive elements for the pelvic genital organs.

d. UTEROSACRAL LIGAMENTS—are bilateral condensations of endopelvic fascia. Anteriorly, the ligaments attach to the sides of the cervix and upper vagina. They extend posteriorly around the rectum on either side of the pelvis to attach to the anterior surface of the bodies of the second to the fourth sacral vertebra. The medial border of the ligament is distinct and forms the wall of the pararectal and rectouterine fossa (page 220). These ligaments aid in maintaining the uterus in an anteverted position, but add little to the actual support of the organ.

3. **Ovaries** (Fig. 3 to 5)—these bilateral organs in the nullipara lie in relation to the peritoneum covering the lateral pelvic wall in an area described as the *ovarian fossa*. This depression is bounded by the external iliac vessels above, the obturator vessels below, the broad ligament anteriorly, and the ureter posteriorly. This position will vary considerably in the multiparous woman. The ovaries may, in fact, be found in any part of the posterior portion of the pelvic cavity.

The ovary is suspended from the posterior layer by a mesentery, the *mesovarium*. Extending from the upper pole to the lateral pelvic wall is the *infundibulopelvic (suspensory) ligament* containing perivascular connective tissue surrounding the ovarian vessels. From the lower pole a fibromuscular cord, the *ovarian ligament* (described above), extends to the lateral uterine wall.

Two surfaces and two borders are also described. The *lateral surface* lies in relation to the ovarian fossa, whereas the *medial surface* is related to the fimbriated end of the uterine tube and loops of small bowel. This medial surface in the middle-aged woman appears puckered and scarred because of markings of developing and ruptured Graafian follicles. The *posterior border* lies free while the *anterior border* is related to the mesovarium.

4. **Uterine (fallopian) Tubes** (Fig. 5)—these structures are encased in the inner four-fifths of the upper free border of the broad ligament. The adjacent portion of the ligament is termed the *mesosalpinx*.

The uterine tube has two openings. The *abdominal ostium* opens into the general peritoneal cavity of the pelvis. The *uterine ostium* opens directly into the uterine cavity.

Four parts of the tube are described. From lateral to medial, they are: (1) the *infundibulum*, a bugle-shaped extremity with a fimbriated mouth that overlies the ovary, to which one long fimbria actually adheres, the *fimbria ovarica*; (2) the *ampulla*, which is wide, thin-walled, and somewhat tortuous and the largest portion of the tube; (3) the *isthmus*, a narrow, straight, thin-walled portion of the tube immediately adjacent to the uterus; and (4) the *intramural* portion whose lumen narrows to approximately 1 mm. or less as it pierces the uterine wall. The tube serves as a conduit for passage of the ova from the ovary to the uterus.

The blood supply of the ovaries and tubes is described on page 246 and their lymphatic drainage on page 208.

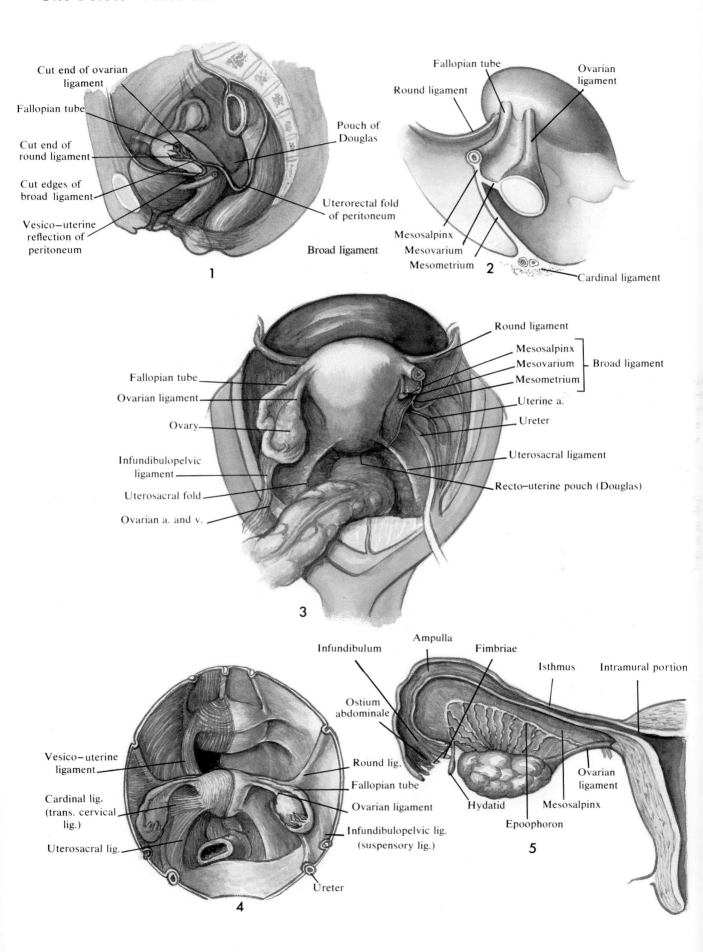

1

Cut end of ovarian ligament

Fallopian tube

Cut end of round ligament

Cut edges of broad ligament

Vesico—uterine reflection of peritoneum

Pouch of Douglas

Uterorectal fold of peritoneum

Broad ligament

2

Fallopian tube

Round ligament

Ovarian ligament

Mesosalpinx

Mesovarium

Mesometrium

Cardinal ligament

3

Fallopian tube

Ovarian ligament

Ovary

Infundibulopelvic ligament

Uterosacral fold

Ovarian a. and v.

Round ligament

Mesosalpinx

Mesovarium

Mesometrium

Broad ligament

Uterine a.

Ureter

Uterosacral ligament

Recto—uterine pouch (Douglas)

4

Vesico—uterine ligament

Cardinal lig. (trans. cervical lig.)

Uterosacral lig.

Round lig.

Fallopian tube

Ovarian ligament

Infundibulopelvic lig. (suspensory lig.)

Ureter

5

Infundibulum

Ampulla

Fimbriae

Isthmus

Intramural portion

Ostium abdominale

Round lig.

Fallopian tube

Ovarian ligament

Hydatid

Mesosalpinx

Epoophoron

Ovarian ligament

5. **Uterus**—this unpaired, pear-shaped muscular organ measures approximately 7 to 8 cm. in length. Its peritoneal relationships and the description of its supportive ligaments have been described on page 242. The uterus consists of three layers: an inner mucosal layer, the *endometrium*; a thick muscular layer, the *myometrium*; and the serosal coat, the *perimetrium*. The serosal layer over most of the uterus is firmly adherent to the underlying muscular coat; however, over the posterior surface of the cervix and the lower portion of the anterior surface of the body loose connective tissue separates the two layers. This tissue extends upward along the sides of the uterus in the broad ligament and is termed the *parametrium* (metra, Gr., uterus).

The uterus is made up of the fundus, body, and cervix (Fig. 5). The *fundus* is that part of the organ lying above the entrance of the uterine tubes. These tubes enter at the superolateral angle (the *cornu*). The *body* (*corpus uteri*), along its lateral margin, is devoid of peritoneum and related to the aforementioned tissue between the layers of the broad ligament, the parametrium. The ovarian ligaments posteriorly and the round ligaments anteriorly attach to the lateral walls just below the cornua. A flat anterior (vesical) surface and a convex posterior (intestinal) surface may be described. The body narrows to an area termed the *isthmus* which continues into the *cervix*. The cervix is 1.5 cm. in length and its lower portion protrudes into the vagina; a *supravaginal* and an *infravaginal* portion of the cervix may therefore be defined. The latter portion presents an opening of the uterine cavity, the *external os*, bounded by an *anterior* and a *posterior labium*. In the nonpregnant woman, the cervix has the firm consistency similar to the nose, whereas the cervix in a pregnant woman has the soft consistency of the lips (*Goodell's sign*).

The *uterine cavity* as viewed on coronal section is triangular in shape. At the base on each side is the uterine ostia of the uterine tubes. The cavity narrows and at the level of the isthmus communicates via the *internal os* with the cervical canal which, in turn, opens into the vagina by the *external os*. In the nulliparous woman the external os is circular but after childbirth it becomes a transverse slit.

The position of the uterus can be extremely variable for it is not a fixed organ (Figs. 1 to 3). The degree of distention of the bladder and rectum may vary its position, as may development defects, adhesions, endometriosis, inflammation, or pelvic tumors. It is stated that normally the uterus is bent forward (*anteflexed*) in line with the horizontal axis at the level of the internal os. But it is also bent forward in line with its vertical axis (*anteverted*), so that the uterus lies in an almost horizontal plane. A uterus may be *retroverted* or *retroflexed* or have a combination of both. Such positions

may be symptomless; however, should the supportive elements (pelvic floor musculature or uterine ligaments, particularly the lateral cardinal ligaments) be weakened, the uterus may prolapse to various degrees into the vaginal vault.

The relational anatomy of the uterus is illustrated in Figures 4 and 5.

a. ANTERIORLY—the body is related to the vesicovesical pouch of peritoneum and lies either on the superior surface of the bladder or on coils of intestines. The supravaginal cervix is related directly to the bladder. The infravaginal cervix abuts upon the anterior fornix of the vagina.

b. POSTERIORLY—lies the rectouterine pouch of Douglas.

c. LATERALLY—the broad ligament and its contents are related. Of particular significance is the close proximity of the ureter to the supravaginal cervix.

6. **Vagina**—the vagina is a flattened but dilatable musculomembraneous canal extending from the cervix of the uterus above to the vestibule below. It pierces the pelvic floor and therefore has an upper pelvic portion which is derived from the Müllerian ducts and a lower perineal portion derived from the urogenital sinus. It is directed downward and forward. With the uterus in a normal anteverted, anteflexed position, the cervix enters the anterior wall of the vagina at almost a right angle (Fig. 4). For this reason the anterior vaginal wall (7.5 cm.) is shorter than the posterior wall (9 cm.).

The walls of the vagina are in contact except where the cervix uteri projects into the vaginal cavity. A space then exists between the infravaginal portion of the cervix and the vaginal walls. This space is termed the *fornix of the vagina* and for descriptive purposes an anterior, posterior, and two lateral fornices are distinguished.

The support of the vagina is an extremely important clinical consideration, yet much controversy exists in regard to the supportive elements. As mentioned on page 242, both the lateral cervical ligaments and the uterosacral ligaments insert in part into the upper vaginal walls and lend support to this organ. Where the vagina pierces the pelvic floor, some fibers of the levator ani insert into the wall. In addition, the vagina is firmly affixed to the perineal body posteriorly and the urethra anteriorly which aid in its support. The existence of other fascial supports have been emphasized by surgeons but questioned by anatomists. One such structure is the *pubocervical (vesicovaginal) ligament* (Fig. 5, page 239), another is the *rectovaginal septum*. Although surgeons emphasize the importance of these structures in the causation of cystocele and rectocele, most surgical anatomy texts make no reference to their existence.

(*Text continued on page 246.*)

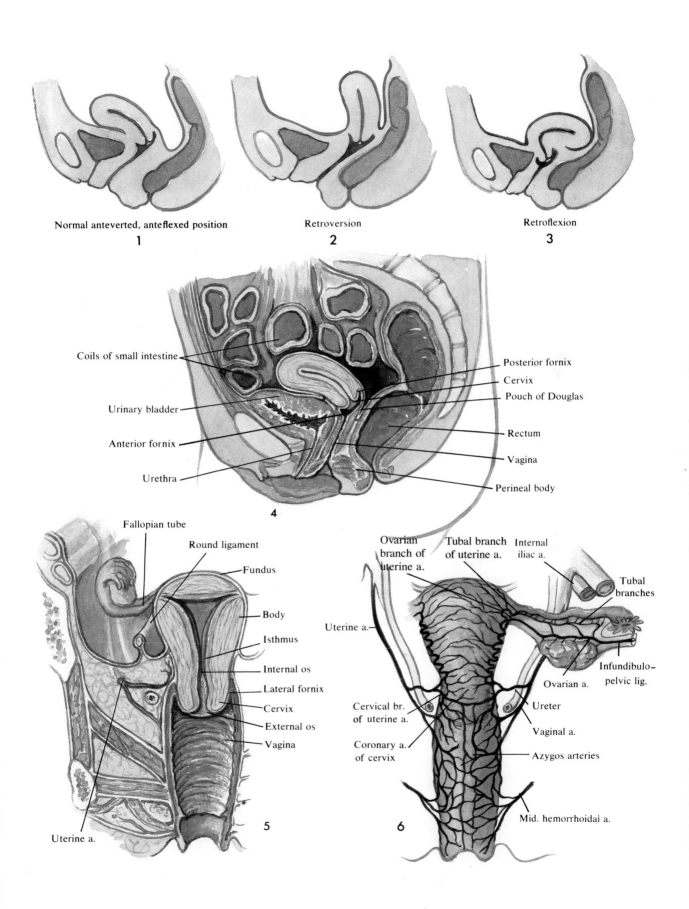

Normal anteverted, anteflexed position
1

Retroversion
2

Retroflexion
3

Coils of small intestine

Urinary bladder

Anterior fornix

Urethra

Posterior fornix

Cervix

Pouch of Douglas

Rectum

Vagina

Perineal body

4

Fallopian tube

Round ligament

Fundus

Body

Isthmus

Internal os

Lateral fornix

Cervix

External os

Vagina

Uterine a.

5

Ovarian branch of uterine a.

Tubal branch of uterine a.

Internal iliac a.

Tubal branches

Uterine a.

Infundibulo-pelvic lig.

Cervical br. of uterine a.

Ovarian a.

Ureter

Coronary a. of cervix

Vaginal a.

Azygos arteries

Mid. hemorrhoidai a.

6

The relational anatomy of the vagina is shown on the accompanying Figures 4 and 5. Structures related are:

a. ANTERIORLY—the base of the bladder and the urethra;

b. POSTERIORLY—the rectouterine pouch of Douglas (upper fourth), the rectum (middle half), and perineal body (lower fourth);

c. LATERALLY—levator ani and pelvic fascia, the bulb of the vestibule, the uterine artery, and the ureter.

7. **Blood Supply of the Female Pelvic Genital Organs** (Fig. 6)—the pelvic portion of the female genital organs is supplied by two bilateral arteries, the ovarian and the uterine.

a. OVARIAN ARTERIES—arise as direct branches from the abdominal aorta about 1.5 to 2 cm. below the renal arteries. In their descent through the abdominal cavity they pass over the ureter supplying a *ureteric branch*. The ovarian arteries then enter the pelvis and cross the common iliac vessels to enter the infundibulo-pelvic ligament. The arteries then enter the mesovarium where they anastomose with the ovarian branch of the uterine artery (both supply branches to the ovary) and send off several *tubal branches* to the infundibulum and ampulla of the uterine tube.

b. UTERINE ARTERIES—are branches of the anterior division of the internal iliac (hypogastric) artery. It descends in the pelvis and extends medially lying on the upper surface of the lateral cervical ligament and passes over the ureter. The main trunk ascends along the lateral uterine wall in the parametrium. During the ascent, it gives rise to anterior and posterior branches to the body of the uterus and at the upper portion terminates by dividing into a tubal and ovarian branch. The *tubal branch* extends laterally in the mesosalpinx supplying the tube and anastomosing with the tubal branches of the ovarian artery. The *ovarian branch* extends into the mesovarium supplying the ovary and anastomosing with the main ovarian artery.

At the level of the isthmus the uterine artery gives rise to the *cervical branch* which divides into anterior and posterior rami which in turn anastomose with similar branches of the opposite side to form the *coronary artery of the cervix.*

Just before the uterine artery passes over the ureter, it gives rise to the *vaginal artery*. This artery corresponds to the inferior vesicle artery of the male. It passes beneath the ureter and is distributed to the vaginal wall by anterior and posterior branches. Rami from the vaginal and cervical branches form a midline arterial anastomosis on both the anterior and posterior walls of the vagina. These anastomotic channels are referred to as the *azygos arteries of the vagina*. The lower portion of the vagina is supplied by the middle hemorrhoidal artery, also a branch of the internal iliac artery.

8. **Venous Drainage of the Female Genital Pelvic Organs**—the general arrangement of the veins of the pelvis has already been described on page 218. The veins of the pelvis form plexuses related to the urinary, genital, and digestive organs; these venous plexuses communicate freely with one another.

The veins draining the uterus and vagina form the *uterovaginal venous plexus*. This plexus has connections anteriorly with the vesical plexus and posteriorly with the hemorrhoidal plexus. The lower portion of the uterovaginal plexus drains through the internal pudendal vein to the internal iliac (hypogastric) vein. The upper portion of the plexus drains laterally via the *uterine veins*, which also are tributaries of the internal iliac veins.

The veins draining the uterine tube extend medially to join the uterovaginal plexus and laterally to empty into the *ovarian pampiniform plexus*. From the ovarian plexus, a single *ovarian vein* is eventually formed which accompanies the ovarian artery. The ovarian vein on the right side empties directly into the inferior vena cava, whereas the left ovarian vein is a tributary of the left renal vein.

9. **Lymphatic Drainage of the Female Genital Pelvic Organs**—the lymphatic drainage of the ovary has been previously discussed on page 208. The principal lymph channels and nodes of the uterine tubes are identical to those of the ovaries. The lymphatic drainage of the uterus is described on page 250. From the lymphatic plexus of the vagina the collecting channels give rise to several pedicles:

a. SUPERIOR PEDICLE—drains the upper vagina and follows the uterine artery to terminate in the external iliac chain of nodes.

b. MIDDLE PEDICLE—consists of several collecting channels following the vaginal artery. This pedicle drains into the hypogastric nodes.

c. INFERIOR PEDICLE—extends posteriorly and terminates in either the lateral sacral nodes or the nodes of the promontory.

That portion of the lower vagina derived from the urogenital sinus drains into the superior-medial group of superficial inguinal nodes.

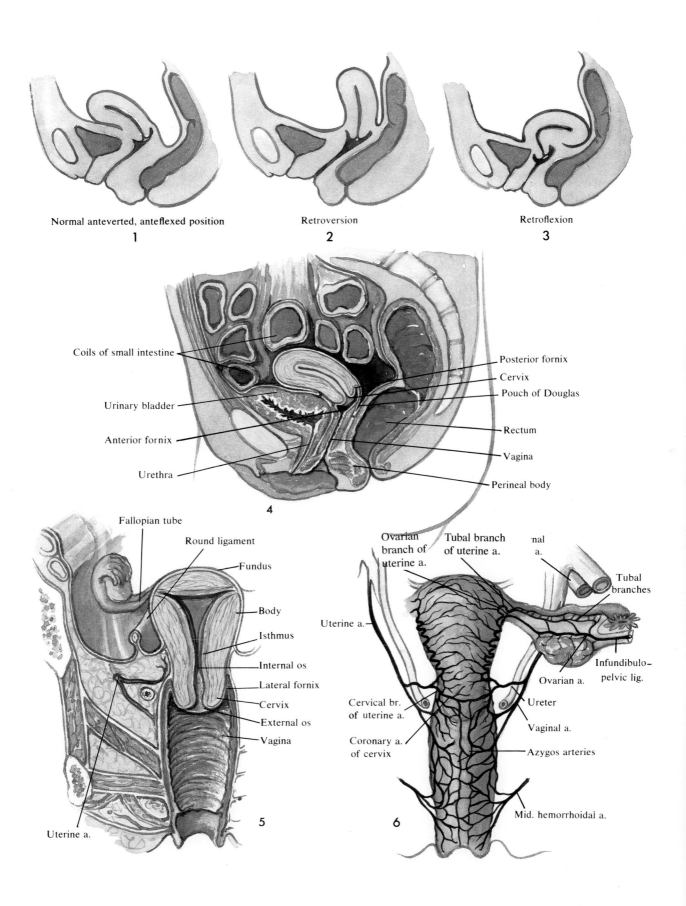

Normal anteverted, anteflexed position
1

Retroversion
2

Retroflexion
3

Coils of small intestine

Urinary bladder

Anterior fornix

Urethra

Posterior fornix

Cervix

Pouch of Douglas

Rectum

Vagina

Perineal body

4

Fallopian tube

Round ligament

Fundus

Body

Isthmus

Internal os

Lateral fornix

Cervix

External os

Vagina

Uterine a.

5

Ovarian branch of uterine a.

Tubal branch of uterine a.

...nal a.

Tubal branches

Uterine a.

Cervical br. of uterine a.

Coronary a. of cervix

Ovarian a.

Ureter

Vaginal a.

Azygos arteries

Mid. hemorrhoidal a.

Infundibulo-pelvic lig.

6

PELVIC FEMALE GENITAL ORGANS: CLINICAL CONSIDERATIONS:

Surgical procedures upon the female pelvic genital organs make up a great proportion of the total operative procedures performed by general surgeons. This is one of the reasons that the female pelvis has been referred to as "the surgeon's playground." Many procedures are used in the diagnosis of pathology of the female pelvic genital organs. The most fundamental and simplest procedures are the vaginal and rectal examinations. These procedures are described on page 222.

1. **Ovary**—the chief indication for surgical removal of part or all of the ovary (*oophorectomy*) is the presence of benign or malignant tumors or cysts. The three anatomic structures commonly involved with ovarian cysts or tumors are the ureters, bladder, and intestines. These structures must be carefully identified and protected. This may be a difficult chore particularly in those cases of long-standing inflammatory disease where extensive adhesions may greatly distort the regional anatomy.

a. OVARIAN CYSTS—are of many varieties. In the benign types, of which the *follicular cyst*, due to persistence of the Graafian follicle, is most common, resection of the cyst and retention of as much ovarian tissue as possible is the procedure of choice (Fig. 1). This is particularly important in women of childbearing age.

b. PARAOVARIAN CYSTS—are cystic enlargements of the vestigial remnants of the Wolffian duct system in the female (page 234 and Fig. 3, page 235). These cysts lie in the broad ligament and may be enucleated by blunt dissection (Fig. 1). They may possess a vascular pedicle which must be carefully clamped, for bleeding deep in the broad ligament is extremely difficult to control. The position of the ureter must be kept in mind during removal of these paraovarian cysts.

2. **Uterine Tubes**—surgical removal of the uterine tubes (*salpingectomy*) is most frequently indicated in those diseases involving the ovaries or the uterus requiring removal of all these organs.

Removal of the tube alone, in its entirety or in part, is indicated in patients with a chronic inflammation of the tube or an ectopic tubal pregnancy or in sterilization procedures.

3. **Vagina**—although operative procedures upon the vagina are frequent, they are usually performed via the perineal approach. These considerations are discussed on page 264. Such operations are primarily plastic procedures used to correct abnormal relaxation of the anterior and posterior vaginal walls when childbirth results in a prolapse of the bladder (*cystocele*) or rectum (*rectocele*) into the vaginal vault. Congenital deformaties of the vagina are discussed below in conjunction with such deformities of the uterus.

a. POSTERIOR COLPOTOMY—is a procedure in which an incision is made through the posterior fornix of the vagina into the uterorectal pouch of the peritoneal cavity. Intraperitoneal pelvic abscesses may be drained by such an anatomic approach.

Through this same approach, an endoscopic instrument may be introduced (*culdoscopy*) which has proven valuable in the diagnosis of intrapelvic disease (Fig. 2, page 223).

b. VAGINAL FISTULAE—may be associated with any of adjacent hollow viscera. These viscera include the digestive tract (rectum, sigmoid, or small bowel) or the urinary tract (ureter, bladder, or urethra). Such fistulae may be caused by trauma (mainly childbirth or operative), infection, or carcinomatous invasion. Figure 2 illustrates a *rectovaginal fistula* resulting from contiguous extension of a carcinoma of the posterior lip of the cervix. In Figure 3, a fistula between the vagina and sigmoid colon (*sigmoidovaginal fistula*) in a patient who has undergone a hysterectomy is illustrated. Urinary tract fistulae are illustrated in Figure 4, both a *vesicovaginal* and an *ureterovaginal fistula*. The operative causative factors are shown in Figure 5. In the process of closure of the vaginal vault in a supravaginal hysterectomy, the ureter or the bladder may be accidentally entered in the repair.

4. **Congenital Defects of Uterus and Upper Vagina**—these structures are derived from the Müllerian ducts (page 234). The lower ends of each duct fuse to form the uterus and upper vagina. The fused portions retain a midsaggital septum which later disappears. The absorption of this septum begins at the region of the vestibule below and proceeds upward to the fundus. Anomalies of these organs result from failure of complete fusion of the Müllerian ducts, persistence or incomplete absorption of the partitioning septum, or a combination of these two factors.

a. DUPLEX UTERUS AND VAGINA (Fig. 6*A*)—results as a failure of fusion of the Müllerian tubes.

b. UTERUS SEPTUS DUPLEX WITH DOUBLE VAGINA (Fig. 6*B*)—occurs after normal fusion of the Müllerian tubes but with complete persistence of the septum.

c. UTERUS SEPTUS DUPLEX (Fig. 6*C*)—is a result of an incomplete absorption of the septum. A single vagina is present but the uterus is completely partitioned.

d. UTERUS BICORNIS UNICOLLIS (BICORNUATE) (Fig. 6*D*)—is due to incomplete fusion of the fundic portion of the uterus with persistence of the fundic portion of the septum.

e. UTERUS SUBSEPTUS UNICOLLIS (Fig. 6*E*)—exhibits a normal fundus but with a partially partitioned uterine cavity.

These are but a few of many varieties of congenital malformations of the uterus and vagina. Very rarely there may be an arrest in the development of the paranephric or Müllerian duct resulting in *absence of the uterus or vagina*.

Of particular clinical significance is the atresia or stenosis of the lower portion of the uterovaginal canal. Like many ductule systems in the embryo, a stage of epithelial proliferation occludes the Müllerian ducts. This is later followed by recanalization. Failure of recanalization may result in *atresia* or *stenosis*. This occurs most frequently in the region of the vagina and results in a collection of menses in that cavity proximal to the obstruction (*hematocolpos*).

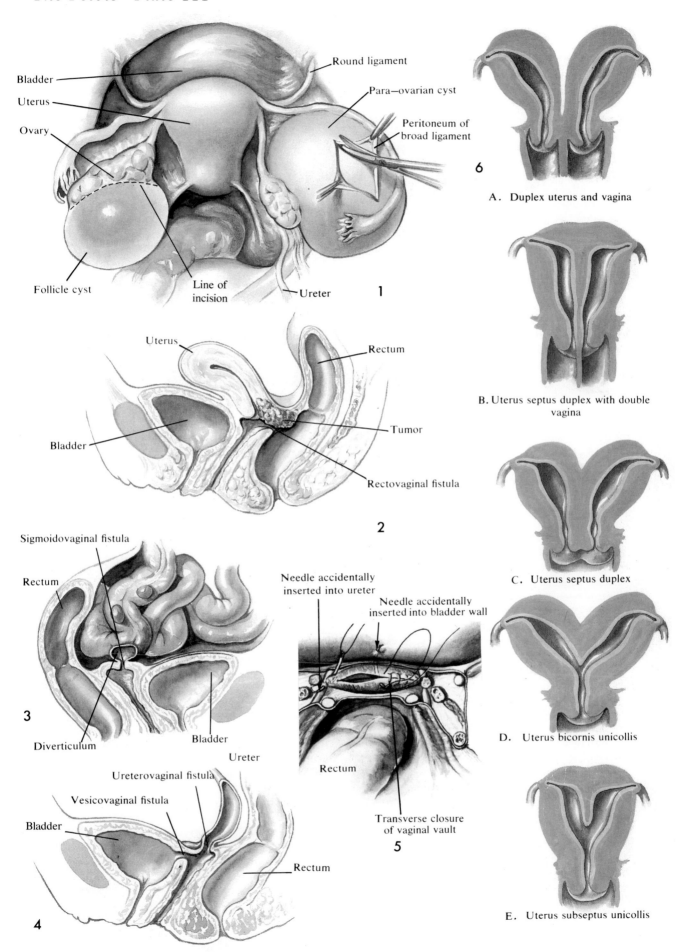

Bladder

Uterus

Ovary

Round ligament

Para—ovarian cyst

Peritoneum of broad ligament

Follicle cyst

Line of incision

Ureter

1

6

A. Duplex uterus and vagina

Uterus

Rectum

Bladder

Tumor

Rectovaginal fistula

2

B. Uterus septus duplex with double vagina

Sigmoidovaginal fistula

Rectum

Needle accidentally inserted into ureter

Needle accidentally inserted into bladder wall

C. Uterus septus duplex

3

Diverticulum

Bladder

Ureter

Rectum

Ureterovaginal fistula

Vesicovaginal fistula

Bladder

Transverse closure of vaginal vault

5

Rectum

D. Uterus bicornis unicollis

4

E. Uterus subseptus unicollis

5. **Uterus**—numerous surgical operations are performed upon this organ, ranging from simple cervical procedures to complete removal of the uterus. The organ may be approached by either a vaginal or an abdominal route.

The endometrial tissue may be scraped for diagnostic purposes or the endometrial cavity evacuated in order to remove retained fetal membranes. In this procedure (*curettage*) the curet is introduced through a previously dilated external os. Great care must be taken to prevent perforation of the uterine wall, and the procedure is contraindicated in cases of acute infection of the uterus or tubes.

The cervix is a frequent site of chronic infection, erosion, lacerations, benign hypertrophy, and cancer. Several operations are designed to treat these conditions. The most common gynecologic procedure indicated in most cases of cervicitis or erosion, is *cauterization of the cervix*. The deeply scarred, lacerated, noninfected cervix may be repaired by a plastic procedure, a *trachelorrhaphy*, in which the cervical canal is reconstructed. A third procedure used is *amputation of the cervix* which is usually indicated in rigid, scarred, and hypertrophied, chronically infected cervices. The cervix is amputated above its diseased portion in such a manner that the mucous membrane covering the lips of the cervix may be sutured to the mucosa of the cervical canal in order to cover the defect.

Surgical incisions into the walls of the body of the uterus are performed to remove benign myomata in women of childbearing years, a procedure termed *myomectomy*. Such tumors may be removed by either a vaginal or an abdominal approach. A second surgical procedure which requires a surgical incision through the uterine wall is a *cesarian section* which allows removal of a child from the uterus through an incision in the abdominal wall.

In many instances, displacements of the uterus may require surgical intervention. Retrodisplacements, either retroflexion or retroversion (page 244), or prolapse of the uterus may be an indication. In *prolapse* there is an abnormal protrusion of the uterus into the vaginal cavity. When partial, the prolapse is termed *descensus uteri* and when complete, a *procidentia*. The surgical correction of these displacements is essentially achieved by various plication procedures upon the major supporting ligaments of the uterus.

6. **Hysterectomy**—this term refers to the surgical removal of the uterus, either partial or complete. A *partial hysterectomy* is also referred to as a *subtotal* or *supravaginal hysterectomy*. Total removal of the uterus is termed a *panhysterectomy* and may be performed by a vaginal approach (*vaginal panhysterectomy*), or an abdominal approach (*abdominal panhysterectomy*). A *radical panhysterectomy* refers to the procedure in which not only the uterus, but the tubes, ovaries, and regional lymphatics are removed.

Figure 1 illustrates what the surgeon views on his approach through the abdominal wall with the peritoneum intact on the left and the anatomic structures he must visualize on the right.

The *round ligaments* are first divided and ligated about 1 inch from the uterus. Next, the *vesicouterine peritoneal reflection* is incised and dissection proceeds downward to the vaginal fornix. The *infundibulopelvic ligaments* are ligated and divided. Within these ligaments are the ovarian vessels. An incision is made in the *uterorectal reflection* of peritoneum close to the cervical wall, and the *uterosacral ligaments* are ligated and divided.

Next the *broad ligaments* are clamped, divided, and securely tied by transfixing sutures since the uterine artery is included. Special care must be taken during this phase to be assured that the ureter is not included in the clamp or ligature (Fig. 2).

The *vaginal vault* is incised anteriorly and posteriorly to remove the uterus and its adnexa. The anterior and posterior walls of the vagina are then approximated by interrupted sutures. Figure 3 illustrates the anatomic situation at this stage of the operation.

To complete the operation, the stumps of the round, infundibulopelvic, and uterosacral ligaments are firmly affixed to the lateral margins of the vaginal cuff and the peritoneal edges approximated.

7. **Lymphatic Drainage**—lymphatic drainage of the uterus is complex and extremely important because of the incidence of cancer involving this organ. From the diffuse mucosal, muscular, and serous capillary plexuses, important collecting channels arise. These channels originate from the region of the fundus, body, and cervix (Fig. 4).

a. COLLECTING CHANNELS FROM THE FUNDUS AND BODY—form three lymphatic pedicles:

(1) *Anterior Pedicle*—extends from the fundus and follows the round ligament through the inguinal canal to the superior-medial group of superficial inguinal nodes (Fig. 2, page 305).

(2) *Principal (Uteroovarian) Pedicle*—arises from collecting channels of the fundus and upper portion of the body of the uterus and anastomoses with the collecting channels of the tubes and ovaries to terminate in first echelon nodes of the lumbar chain.

(3) *Transverse Pedicle*—extends from channels below the cornu and drains into the uppermost node of the external iliac chain at the bifurcation of the common iliac artery.

b. COLLECTING CHANNELS FROM THE CERVIX—also form three lymph pedicles:

(1) *Anterior Pedicle*—extends from the cervix and terminates in first echelon nodes of the medial and middle external iliac chain.

(2) *Hypogastric Pedicle*—drains into the hypogastric (internal iliac) node at the origin of the uterine artery.

(3) *Posterior Pedicle*—consists of several collecting channels which terminate in either the lateral sacral nodes or nodes of the promontory (common iliac group).

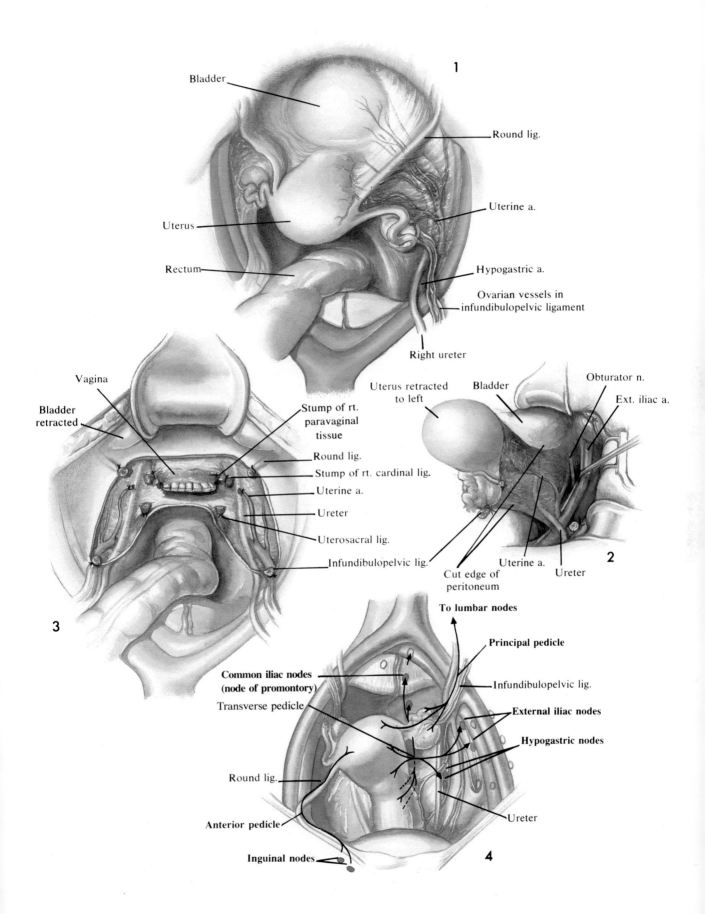

1

Bladder

Round lig.

Uterine a.

Uterus

Hypogastric a.

Rectum

Ovarian vessels in
infundibulopelvic ligament

Right ureter

Vagina

Uterus retracted
to left

Bladder

Obturator n.

Ext. iliac a.

Bladder
retracted

Stump of rt.
paravaginal
tissue

Round lig.

Stump of rt. cardinal lig.

Uterine a.

Ureter

Uterosacral lig.

Infundibulopelvic lig.

Cut edge of
peritoneum

Uterine a.

Ureter

2

3

To lumbar nodes

Principal pedicle

**Common iliac nodes
(node of promontory)**

Infundibulopelvic lig.

Transverse pedicle

External iliac nodes

Hypogastric nodes

Round lig.

Ureter

Anterior pedicle

Inguinal nodes

4

The Perineum

GENERAL CONSIDERATIONS:

The perineum in the normal (erect) anatomic position is actually a narrow area between the musculature of the thigh and gluteal region. With the thighs in an abducted position, however, the perineum becomes a wide diamond-shaped area bounded by the gluteal region behind, the thighs laterally, and the eminence over the symphysis pubis anteriorly. In the perineum are found the orifices of the urinary, genital, and digestive tracts and the external genitalia of both sexes. For descriptive purposes, the perineum may be divided into an anterior urogenital triangle and a posterior anal triangle.

1. **Bony and Ligamentous Boundaries**—the perineum is an area between the thighs marking the inferior end of the torso of the body. Its bony and ligamentous boundaries form the pelvic outlet and consist of the symphysis pubis in front, the tip of the coccyx behind, and laterally, from front to rear, the combined ischiopubis rami, ischial tuberosities, and the sacrotuberous and sacrospinal ligaments. An imaginary line drawn between the ischial tuberosities divides the perineum in the urogenital triangle anteriorly and the anal triangle posteriorly (Fig. 1).

2. **Muscular Diaphragm of the Pelvic Outlet**—the pelvic outlet, bounded by the bony and ligamentous structures described above, must be closed in order to support the pelvic viscera. Such a closure is accomplished for the most part by the muscular pelvic diaphragm. This muscular layer does not accomplish full closure of the pelvic outlet anteriorly. The defect referred to as the *urogenital hiatus* requires the formation of a second muscular diaphragm (Fig. 4, page 217). The latter lies below the pelvic diaphragm and is known as the urogenital diaphragm.

a. PELVIC DIAPHRAGM—consists of two muscles; the coccygeus and levator ani. These muscles have already been described on page 216.

b. UROGENITAL DIAPHRAGM—is also made up of two muscles; the sphincter of the membranous urethra and the deep transverse perineal muscle. Both muscles lie on the same plane in the deep perineal pouch and are closely united. They are less well developed in the female. The more anterior of the two muscles, the *sphincter urethra*, arises from the inferior ramus of the pubis of each side. The fibers extend toward the midline and pass in front and behind the urethra in both sexes. The more posterior fibers in the female insert into the vagina and perineal body. The *deep transverse perinei* arise from the inner aspect of the ramus of the

ischium and insert into a median raphe, the perineal body.

3. **Fascia of the Perineum:**
a. ENDOPELVIC FASCIA—described on page 216, extends into the perineum. That part of the *parietal layer* of endopelvic fascia which covers the obturator internus attaches to the margins of the pelvic outlet and forms the lateral boundaries of the perineal area. In the region of the anal triangle, there is a duplication of this fascial layer, *pudendal (Alcock's) canal* in which run the internal pudendal vessels and nerves (Fig. 2). The double-layered diaphragmatic portion of endopelvic fascia crosses the pelvic diaphragm, the inferior layer of which bounds the perineum above.

b. DEEP PERINEAL FASCIA—is a double-layered fascial encasement of the muscles of the urogenital diaphragm. It is described as having a deep (superior) and a superficial (inferior) layer which fuse both anteriorly and posteriorly forming the deep perineal pouch (Fig. 3). The fusion of these layers anteriorly forms the *transverse perineal (pelvic) ligament*. Between this ligament and the *arcuate ligament* of the symphysis pubis is a gap through which passes the dorsal vein of the penis. (clitoris) (Fig. 7, page 257). The *superficial (inferior) layer* of deep perineal fascia is a well developed structure composed of strong bands of fibrous tissue extending transversely between the ischiopubic rami. It is also referred to as the *perineal membrane*. The *deep (superior) layer* also extends between the ischiopubic rami and is much less distinct than the superficial fascial layer. Anteriorly it also fuses with the fascia of the pelvic diaphragm.

c. SUPERFICIAL PERINEAL FASCIA (COLLES' FASCIA)—is a perineal extension of the fused Scarpa's and Camper's fasciae of the ventrolateral abdominal wall (page 132). This fused fascial layer passes into the penis as penile fascia, into the scrotum as dartos fascia, and continues in the urogenital triangle of the perineum as Colles' fascia. This fascia attaches laterally to the ischiopubic rami and ischial tuberosity and posteriorly fuses with the two fascial layers of the urogenital diaphragm (Fig. 3).

4. **Anal Triangle**—the boundaries of this triangle are illustrated in Figure 1. The most conspicuous anatomic structure in this region is the anal orifice.

a. SKIN—of the anal triangle is thick but thins out around the anal orifice. In this immediate perianal area the skin is thin, pigmented in appearance, and contains hair follicles and sweat glands. The *anal orifice (anus)* is normally closed by its sphincters, and the surround-

(Text continued on page 254.)

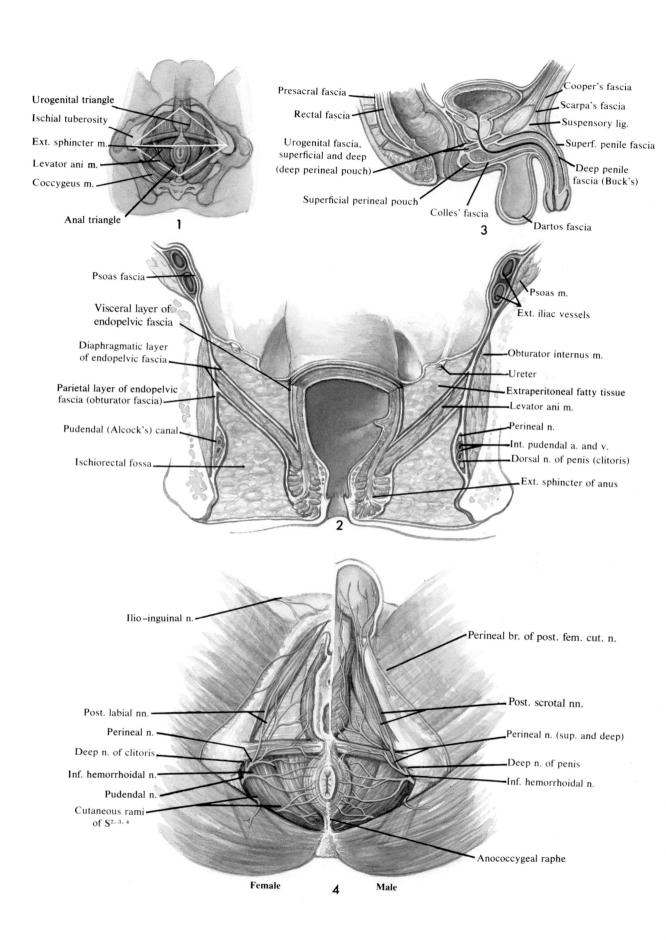

Urogenital triangle
Ischial tuberosity
Ext. sphincter m.
Levator ani m.
Coccygeus m.

Anal triangle

1

Presacral fascia
Rectal fascia
Urogenital fascia, superficial and deep (deep perineal pouch)
Superficial perineal pouch

Cooper's fascia
Scarpa's fascia
Suspensory lig.
Superf. penile fascia
Deep penile fascia (Buck's)

Colles' fascia
Dartos fascia

3

Psoas fascia
Visceral layer of endopelvic fascia
Diaphragmatic layer of endopelvic fascia
Parietal layer of endopelvic fascia (obturator fascia)
Pudendal (Alcock's) canal
Ischiorectal fossa

Psoas m.
Ext. iliac vessels
Obturator internus m.
Ureter
Extraperitoneal fatty tissue
Levator ani m.
Perineal n.
Int. pudendal a. and v.
Dorsal n. of penis (clitoris)
Ext. sphincter of anus

2

Ilio-inguinal n.

Post. labial nn.
Perineal n.
Deep n. of clitoris
Inf. hemorrhoidal n.
Pudendal n.
Cutaneous rami of $S^{2, 3, 4}$

Perineal br. of post. fem. cut. n.

Post. scrotal nn.

Perineal n. (sup. and deep)

Deep n. of penis
Inf. hemorrhoidal n.

Anococcygeal raphe

Female **4** **Male**

ing skin is puckered and wrinkled in appearance because of the action of the surrounding *corrugator cutis ani* muscle which is a continuation of the longitudinal muscle coat of the rectum into the skin. Anterior to the anus is the perineal body and posterior, the anococcygeal raphe.

b. SUPERFICIAL FASCIA—of the anal triangle is ladened with fat, filling a fascial-lined wedge-shaped space, the *ischiorectal fossae*, on either side of the anus (Fig. 3). Each fossa is bounded by obturator fascia laterally, the diaphragmatic portion of the endopelvic fascia covering the inferior surface of the pelvic diaphragm medially. The apex is formed at the junction of the medial and lateral wall and the base by the skin of the perineum. A short *anterior recess* extends towards the body of the pubis between the pelvic and urogenital diaphragms. A *posterior recess* is also seen extending between the pelvic diaphragm above and the gluteus maximus and sacrotuberous ligament below.

A reduplication of the obturator fascia *(Alcock's canal)* in the lateral wall of the ischiorectal fossa contains the internal pudendal branch of the internal iliac artery and its accompanying vein. Also with the canal is the *pudendal nerve* (S_2, S_3, and S_4), which terminates here by dividing into three branches: the inferior hemorrhoidal nerve, the perineal nerve, and the dorsal nerve of the penis (clitoris). In the region of the ischiorectal fossa, the *inferior hemorrhoidal* branches of the internal pudendal vessels and the inferior hemorrhoidal nerve pierce the medial wall of Alcock's canal and pass forward and medially to supply the external sphincter of the anus and adjacent skin (Fig. 4).

5. **Superficial Nerves of the Perineum** (Fig. 4)—as described above, the internal hemorrhoidal nerve (a branch of the pudendal) is the main nerve supply, both motor and sensory, to the region of the ischiorectal fossa. A second branch of the pudendal, the *perineal nerve*, divides within the canal into a superficial and deep branch. While in the ischiorectal fossa the *deep branch* sends twigs which pierce Alcock's canal and innervate the anterior-most fibers of the external sphincter and levator ani muscles, its main branch continues through the superficial pouch of the urogenital diaphragm (see page 258). The *superficial branch* also enters the superficial pouch and branches into medial and lateral posterior scrotal (labial) nerves which pierce the pouch almost immediately to be distributed in the subcutaneous tissue. The *perineal branch of the posterior femoral cutaneous nerve (nerve of Soemmering)* also enters into the cutaneous innervation of the perineum. This nerve supplies the skin of the anterior lateral part of the perineum and continues forward to the skin of the posterior lateral surfaces of the scrotum (labia majora). The skin of the anterior-most portion of the perineum is supplied by the anterior scrotal (labial) branches of the ilioinguinal nerve (L_1) and by twigs of the genital branches of the genitofemoral nerve (L_1 and L_2) both of which are derived from the lumbar plexus.

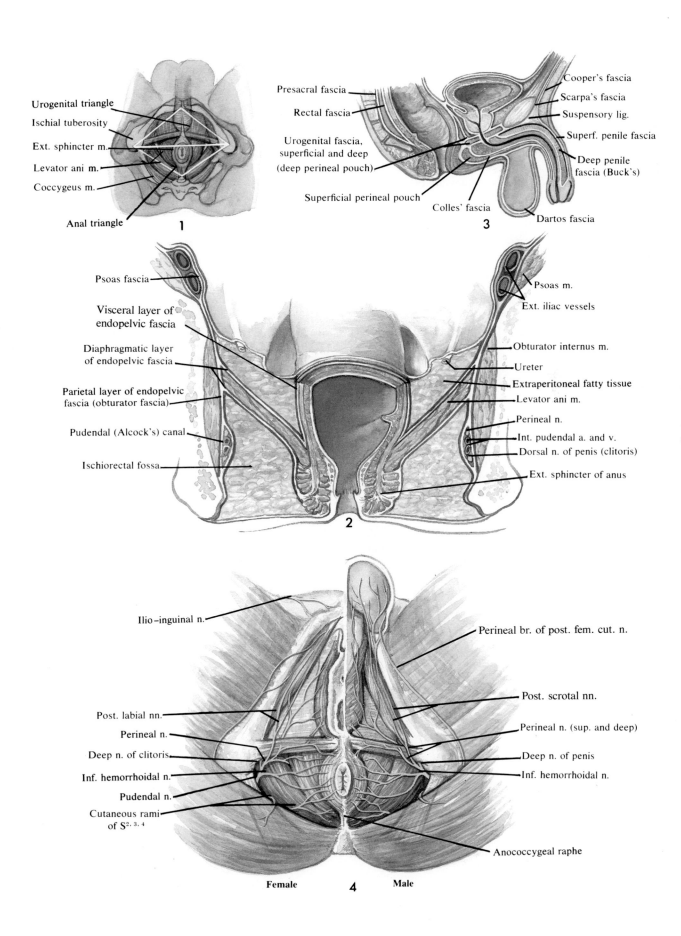

1

Urogenital triangle
Ischial tuberosity
Ext. sphincter m.
Levator ani m.
Coccygeus m.
Anal triangle

3

Presacral fascia
Rectal fascia
Urogenital fascia, superficial and deep (deep perineal pouch)
Superficial perineal pouch
Colles' fascia
Cooper's fascia
Scarpa's fascia
Suspensory lig.
Superf. penile fascia
Deep penile fascia (Buck's)
Dartos fascia

2

Psoas fascia
Visceral layer of endopelvic fascia
Diaphragmatic layer of endopelvic fascia
Parietal layer of endopelvic fascia (obturator fascia)
Pudendal (Alcock's) canal
Ischiorectal fossa

Psoas m.
Ext. iliac vessels
Obturator internus m.
Ureter
Extraperitoneal fatty tissue
Levator ani m.
Perineal n.
Int. pudendal a. and v.
Dorsal n. of penis (clitoris)
Ext. sphincter of anus

4

Ilio-inguinal n.
Post. labial nn.
Perineal n.
Deep n. of clitoris
Inf. hemorrhoidal n.
Pudendal n.
Cutaneous rami of S²⋅³⋅⁴

Perineal br. of post. fem. cut. n.
Post. scrotal nn.
Perineal n. (sup. and deep)
Deep n. of penis
Inf. hemorrhoidal n.
Anococcygeal raphe

Female   Male

6. **Urogenital Triangle** — the boundaries of the urogenital triangle consist of the symphysis pubis and the ischiopubic rami anteriorly, the ischial tuberosities laterally, and a line joining the two ischial tuberosities posteriorly (Fig. 1, page 255). The most superficial structures in this area, in both the male and female, are the external genitalia.

a. MALE EXTERNAL GENITALIA — are morphologically more simple in construction from an external view than the external genitalia of the female. They consist of the penis and scrotum (Fig. 5). The *scrotum* is a cutaneous pouch divided by a median septum into two compartments each containing the testis, epididymis, spermatic cord, and vas deferens (page 138). The *penis* consists of the root located in the superficial perineal pouch (see below) and the body which is pendulous and fully covered by skin. Immediately beneath the skin is the *superficial penile fascia*, continuous with the conjoined Camper's and Scarpa's fascia of the abdominal wall and the superficial perineal (Colles') fascia behind. This fascial layer is also continuous with the dartos fascia of the scrotum. A *deep penile (Buck's) fascia* surrounds the body of the penis and is the fascia propria of this structure. The remainder of the body is made up of three columnar parts which arise in the superficial perineal pouch and are surrounded by dense fibrous tissue (tunica albuginea). These three columns (corpora cavernosa) contain distendable venous cavities (hence the name) which account for the erectability of the organ. Two (the *corpora cavernosa penis*) are located side by side on the dorsal surface as extensions of the crura. The third (*corpus cavernosum urethra*) is smaller and located on the urethral surface of the penis (Figs. 2 and 3). At its distal end is an expansion, the *glans penis*, at the tip of which is located the *external urethral orifice*. The glans is covered by a double-layer of skin termed the *prepuce*, which is attached to the under surface of the orifice by a medial fold, the *frenulum* (Fig. 2).

b. FEMALE EXTERNAL GENITALIA (Fig. 1) — includes the labia majora, labia minora, clitoris, and vestibule. They are collectively called the *vulva* (L., a covering) or *pudendum* (L., to be ashamed).

The *labia majora* are bilateral folds of skin, homologous to the two compartments of the scrotum of the male. The lateral surface is related to the thigh, is pigmented and hairy, and is continuous anteriorly with the *mons veneris*, an eminence overlying the symphysis pubis. The medial surfaces are hair-free and join anteriorly beneath the symphysis to form the *anterior commissure*. The junction posteriorly, the *posterior commissure*, is much less distinct. Between the two labia majora is a cleft, termed the *rima pudendi*, which must be opened in order to view the other external genitalia. Deep to the skin of the labia is a poorly developed dartos fascia and adipose tissue. The round ligament of the uterus, whose male homologue is the gubernaculum testis, also inserts into this tissue after transversing the inguinal canal. Should the processus vaginalis (see page 136) persist, it is termed, in the female, the *canal of Nuck*.

The *labia minora (nymphae)* are two cutaneous folds which have smooth lateral surfaces which lie in contact with the labia majora and medial surfaces which bound the vestibule. Its homologue in the male is the urethral surface of the penis. The labia minora unite posteriorly to form the *frenulum of the labia* or *fourchette*. Anteriorly each labium splits around the clitoris and joins with each other. The fold anterior to the clitoris is the *prepuce* of the clitoris and the fold below the clitoris, the *frenulum of the clitoris*.

The *clitoris*, like its homologue, the penis, is an erectile organ located just beneath the symphysis pubis at the anterior part of the rima pudendi (Fig. 1). Like the penis, it possesses a body and root (Fig. 6). The *root* is located in the superficial perineal pouch, the *crura* of the clitoris. These two parts join, as the *corpora cavernosa clitoridis*, to form the *body* which turns upon itself in a downward and backward direction for a length of about 2.5 cm. It does not hang free as does the body of the penis but is embedded into the tissue of the vulva. Although the corpus cavernosum urethra of the penis is not represented in the clitoris, the body of the clitoris is capped by a small mass of erectile tissue, the *glans clitoris*, a homologue of the glans penis (Fig. 1).

The *vestibule* is an elongated area bounded on either side by the medial surfaces of the labia minora (Fig. 1). Anteriorly it is bounded by the frenulum of the clitoris and posteriorly by the fourchette. Its male homologue is the male urethra below the prostate utricle. In this area are the orifices of the urogenital systems and associated glands.

The most anterior opening is the *external urethral orifice* which is located approximately 3 cm. behind the clitoris and appears as a 4 to 5 mm. vertical slit. Posteriorly on either side of the urethral orifice are multiple, minute openings of the *paraurethral ducts of Skene* which represent the prostatic tubules of the male.

Just behind the urethral orifice is the *vaginal orifice* whose shape and size are extremely variable in appearance. In the virgin, it is partially closed posteriorly by a crescent-shaped *hymen* (Gr., membrane) which may be described as a tiny shred of human flesh about which love and pride have woven some of the weirdest imaginary schemes that the human brain ever conceived. After first coitus, the torn remnants remain as the nodular appearing posterior vaginal border, the *carunculae hymenales*. Posteriorly on either side of the vaginal orifice are the openings of pea-sized mucous secreting glands, the *greater vestibular glands of Bartholin* (whose male homologue is *Cowper's gland*). *Lesser vestibular gland orifices* are multiple and microscopic and are located in various parts of the floor of the vestibule. They are homologues of the urethral glands of Littré in the male.

That area of the vestibule between the vaginal

(Text continued on page 258.)

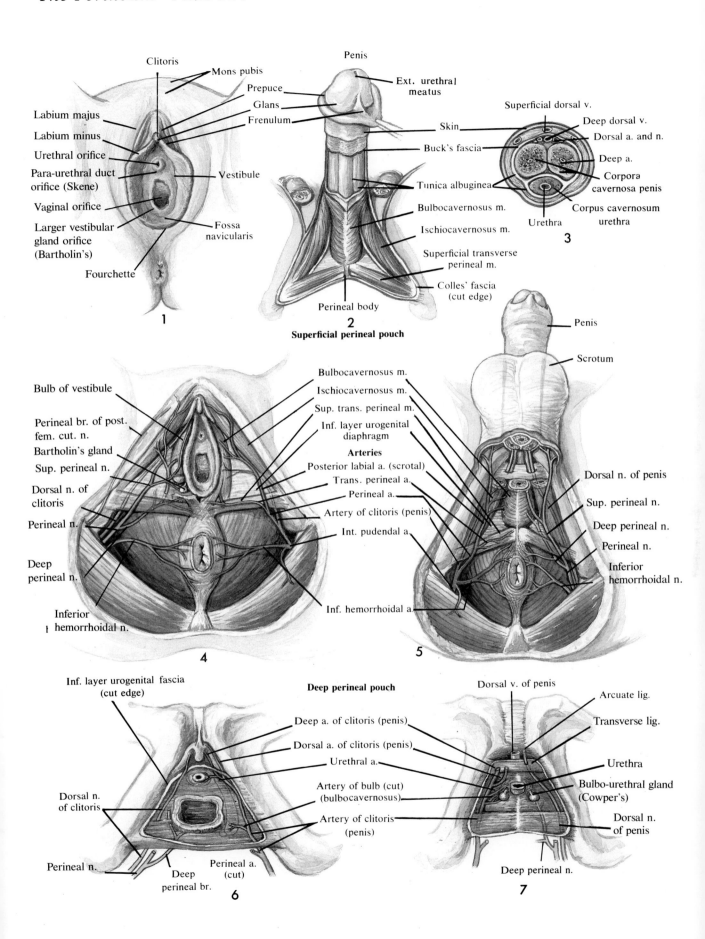

1

Clitoris
Mons pubis
Labium majus
Labium minus
Urethral orifice
Para-urethral duct orifice (Skene)
Vaginal orifice
Larger vestibular gland orifice (Bartholin's)
Fourchette
Prepuce
Glans
Frenulum
Vestibule
Fossa navicularis

2

Superficial perineal pouch

Penis
Ext. urethral meatus
Skin
Buck's fascia
Tunica albuginea
Bulbocavernosus m.
Ischiocavernosus m.
Superficial transverse perineal m.
Colles' fascia (cut edge)
Perineal body

3

Superficial dorsal v.
Deep dorsal v.
Dorsal a. and n.
Deep a.
Corpora cavernosa penis
Corpus cavernosum urethra
Urethra

4

Bulb of vestibule
Perineal br. of post. fem. cut. n.
Bartholin's gland
Sup. perineal n.
Dorsal n. of clitoris
Perineal n.
Deep perineal n.
Inferior hemorrhoidal n.

Bulbocavernosus m.
Ischiocavernosus m.
Sup. trans. perineal m.
Inf. layer urogenital diaphragm
Arteries
Posterior labial a. (scrotal)
Trans. perineal a.
Perineal a.
Artery of clitoris (penis)
Int. pudendal a.
Inf. hemorrhoidal a.

5

Penis
Scrotum
Dorsal n. of penis
Sup. perineal n.
Deep perineal n.
Perineal n.
Inferior hemorrhoidal n.

6

Inf. layer urogenital fascia (cut edge)
Dorsal n. of clitoris
Perineal n.
Deep perineal br.
Perineal a. (cut)

Deep perineal pouch

Deep a. of clitoris (penis)
Dorsal a. of clitoris (penis)
Urethral a.
Artery of bulb (cut) (bulbocavernosus)
Artery of clitoris (penis)

7

Dorsal v. of penis
Arcuate lig.
Transverse lig.
Urethra
Bulbo-urethral gland (Cowper's)
Dorsal n. of penis
Deep perineal n.

orifice anteriorly and the fourchette posteriorly is termed the *fossa navicularis*.

c. SUPERFICIAL PERINEAL POUCH — is a fascial compartment lying between Colles' fascia below and the inferior layer of the urogenital diaphragm (perineal membrane) above (Fig. 3, page 255).

In the female, three structures can be identified on either side of the pouch. The *crus of the clitoris* arises from the inferior ramus of the pubis and, under the symphysis pubis, joins its counterpart of the opposite side to form the body of the clitoris (Fig. 6). Adjacent to the vaginal orifice is the *bulb of the vestibule*. This is a mass of erectile tissue consisting of a venous plexus enclosed in a connective tissue covering. The bulb extends anteriorly as a slender prolongation along the sides of the urethra to the glans of the clitoris. The third structure on either side is *Bartholin's gland* or *major vestibular gland* (Fig. 4).

In the male, the *crus of the penis* can be identified (Fig. 5). This structure, although larger, is similar to the crus of the clitoris. It arises from the ischiopubic ramus and joins the crus of the opposite side beneath the symphysis pubis. The *bulb of the urethra* is also present in the superficial perineal pouch in the male. This midline structure is firmly attached to the perineal membrane and extends anteriorly into the penis as the corpus cavernosum penis and is transversed by the cavernous urethra. Its homologue in the female is the bulb of the vestibule.

The muscles of the superficial pouch are similar in name in both sexes. An *ischiocavernosus muscle* arises from the ischiopubic ramus and covers the crura. This muscle is of course much smaller in the female. A second muscle is the *bulbocavernosus muscle*. In the male, this muscle envelopes the bulb of the urethra, its right and left halves joining in a median raphe. In the female, the bulbocavernosus arises anteriorly and covers the outer side of the bulb of the vestibule and Bartholin's gland and inserts posteriorly in the perineal body. It is also referred to as the *sphincter of the vagina*. A third muscle in this compartment is the *superficial transverse perineal muscle*. This muscle arises from the ischial ramus and inserts into the perineal body.

The *perineal nerve*, a branch of the pudendal nerve, serves the superficial pouch. It divides in the region of the ischiorectal fossa into superficial and deep branches which enter the superficial pouch (Figs. 4 and 5). The *deep perineal nerve* carries the motor impulses to the muscles of this compartment and the sensory fibers from the mucous membrane of the urethra. The *superficial perineal nerve* enters the pouch and immediately divides into *medial* and *lateral posterior scrotal (labial) nerves* (Fig. 4, page 255).

The blood supply to the superficial perineal pouch is carried by the *perineal artery*, a terminal branch of the internal pudendal artery. Upon entering the pouch, the perineal artery gives rise to the *transverse perineal artery* which parallels the fibers of the superficial transverse perineal muscle. The terminal branches of the perineal artery are the *posterior scrotal (labial) arteries*. The arteries are accompanied by similarly named veins (Figs. 4 and 5).

d. DEEP PERINEAL POUCH — is that area between the inferior and superior layers of the deep perineal fascia (Fig. 3, page 255).

In the female, two structures traverse this space, the *urethra* and the terminal portion of the *vagina*. In the male, one finds the *membranous urethra* and the *bulbourethral (Cowper's) gland* (Figs. 6 and 7). The homologue of this gland in the female is Bartholin's gland which is found in the superficial perineal pouch. Cowper's glands are two small glands (4 to 8 mm. in diameter) located on each side of the membranous urethra. Their ducts pierce the inferior layer of the urogenital diaphragm, traverse the bulb, and empty into the cavernous portion of the urethra (Fig. 4, page 237).

Two muscles are located in the deep pouch, the *sphincter urethra* and the *deep transverse perineal muscle*. These muscles have been described on page 252 under Urogenital Diaphragm.

Like the muscles of the superficial pouch, these two muscles are also innervated by branches of the *deep perineal nerve*. Passing through the deep pouch is the *dorsal nerve of the penis (clitoris)*, a terminal branch of the pudendal nerve. Just below the pubic arch it pierces the superficial layer of the urogenital diaphragm and is distributed to the clitoris or to the dorsum of the penis, the glans, and the prepuce (Figs. 6 and 7).

The main artery of the deep pouch is the *artery of the penis (clitoris)*, a terminal branch of the internal pudendal artery. Within the deep pouch, the artery of the penis (clitoris) gives rise to the *artery of the bulb*. This branch passes medially, pierces the urogenital diaphragm, and supplies the bulb of the urethra in the male and the bulb of the vestibule in the female. This branch also supplies Cowper's and Bartholin's gland. A second branch, the *urethral artery*, also arises within the deep pouch. The artery of the penis (clitoris) terminates by dividing into the *deep artery of the penis (clitoris)* and the *dorsal artery of the penis (clitoris)*.

Most of the venous drainage of the area of the urogenital triangle is via tributaries of the *internal pudendal vein* which in turn empties into the internal iliac (hypogastric) vein. The venous drainage of the penis is by the large *dorsal vein of the penis*. It receives the deep tributaries from the organ, and beneath the pubic arch it passes between the *arcuate ligament* and *transverse perineal ligament* and enters the pelvis. Here it bifurcates and drains into the pudendal plexus of both sides.

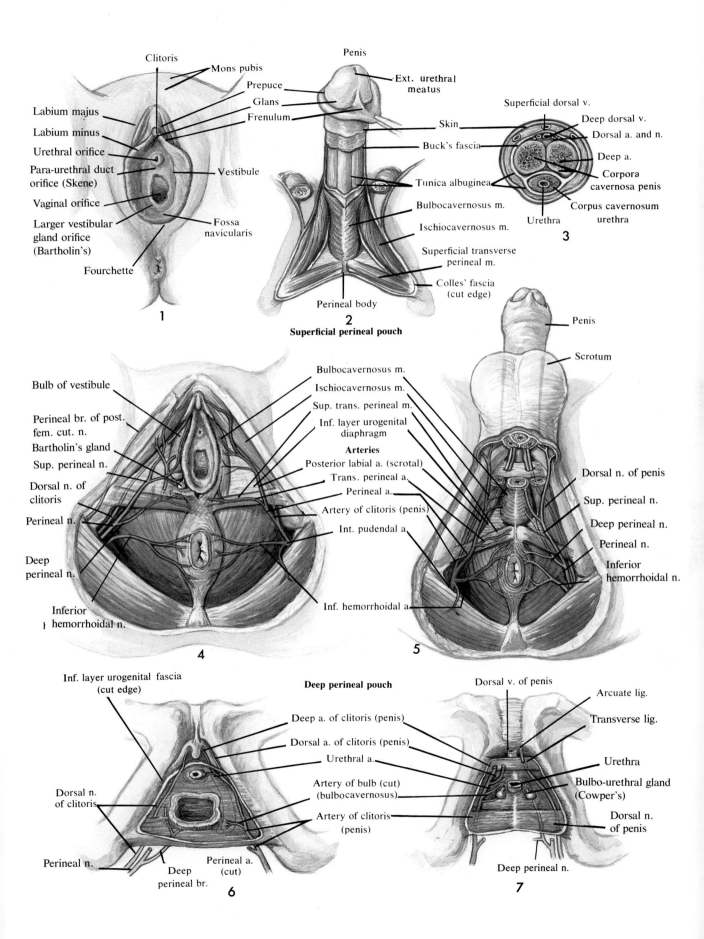

1

Clitoris
Mons pubis
Prepuce
Glans
Frenulum
Labium majus
Labium minus
Urethral orifice
Para-urethral duct orifice (Skene)
Vaginal orifice
Larger vestibular gland orifice (Bartholin's)
Fourchette
Vestibule
Fossa navicularis

2
Superficial perineal pouch

Penis
Ext. urethral meatus
Skin
Buck's fascia
Tunica albuginea
Bulbocavernosus m.
Ischiocavernosus m.
Superficial transverse perineal m.
Colles' fascia (cut edge)
Perineal body

3

Superficial dorsal v.
Deep dorsal v.
Dorsal a. and n.
Deep a.
Corpora cavernosa penis
Corpus cavernosum urethra
Urethra

4

Bulb of vestibule
Perineal br. of post. fem. cut. n.
Bartholin's gland
Sup. perineal n.
Dorsal n. of clitoris
Perineal n.
Deep perineal n.
Inferior hemorrhoidal n.
Bulbocavernosus m.
Ischiocavernosus m.
Sup. trans. perineal m.
Inf. layer urogenital diaphragm
Arteries
Posterior labial a. (scrotal)
Trans. perineal a.
Perineal a.
Artery of clitoris (penis)
Int. pudendal a.
Inf. hemorrhoidal a.

5

Penis
Scrotum
Dorsal n. of penis
Sup. perineal n.
Deep perineal n.
Perineal n.
Inferior hemorrhoidal n.

6
Deep perineal pouch

Inf. layer urogenital fascia (cut edge)
Dorsal n. of clitoris
Perineal n.
Deep perineal br.
Perineal a. (cut)
Deep a. of clitoris (penis)
Dorsal a. of clitoris (penis)
Urethral a.
Artery of bulb (cut) (bulbocavernosus)
Artery of clitoris (penis)

7

Dorsal v. of penis
Arcuate lig.
Transverse lig.
Urethra
Bulbo-urethral gland (Cowper's)
Dorsal n. of penis
Deep perineal n.

MALE PERINEUM:
CLINICAL CONSIDERATIONS:

The external genitalia occupy the area of the urogenital triangle of the perineum. There are many clinical considerations where knowledge of applied anatomy is most useful.

1. **Penis and Cavernous Urethra** — after piercing the urogenital diaphragm (membranous portion), the urethra enters the bulb of the penis and traverses the corpus cavernosum urethra (cavernous portion). The normal adult urethra is capable of allowing the passage of an instrument of approximately 8 mm. in diameter without undue stretching.

a. OBSTRUCTION OF THE URETHRA — is quite common and may be caused by congenital valves, hypertrophy of the verumontanum, or extrinsic pressure from an enlarged prostate. Congenital, traumatic, or postinflammatory strictures may obstruct any portion of this lower urinary tract.

Dilatation is the treatment of choice for urethral strictures. Metallic instruments called *sounds* are used to dilate the urethra. Sounds are graduated in the French scale. The numbers of the French scale are three times the diameter of the instrument in millimeters; therefore, a No. 24 French sound is 8 mm. in diameter. Should the external urethral meatus be too small to permit instrumentation, a *meatotomy* must be performed. In this procedure a small ventral midline incision is made in the external urethral orifice. Should the dilatation be unsuccessful in relieving the stricture, or if urgency is required, an *internal urethrotomy* should be performed. In certain instances an *external urethrotomy*, requiring a midline incision, may be necessary.

b. URETHRAL CATHETERIZATION — is a frequently used procedure to relieve a patient who is unable to void, to determine the amount of residual urine, to irrigate the bladder, to maintain continuous drainage, or to obtain an uncontaminated urine specimen. Catheterization is a relatively simple procedure in the female, but in the male the two major curvatures of the urethra must be dealt with. When maneuvering catheters, sounds, or cystoscopes the physician must take these curvatures into consideration.

c. RUPTURE OF THE CAVERNOUS URETHRA (Figs. 1 and 2) — particularly its bulbous portion, is rather common in straddle injuries. The bulbous portion of the urethra often tears when it is forcibly caught between a hard object, such as the horn of a saddle, the rail of a fence or a frame of a bicycle, and the equally hard unyielding pubic arch. Disruption can also result from inflammation or instrumentation of a stricture.

The urine, in an injury to the bulb, escapes into the superficial perineal pouch and passes into a fascial plane limited superficially by the attachments of Colles' fascia and contiguous counterparts, such as dartos, penile, and Scarpa's fasciae. The urine extravasates posteriorly under the urogenital diaphragm. Here it is limited at the posterior border of the diaphragm at the attachment of Colles' fascia. Laterally it is stopped at the attachment to the ischiopubic ramus. It may extend anteriorly and inferiorly into the scrotum between dartos fascia and the external spermatic fascia. It may extend into the penis between the penile fascia and Buck's fascia and onto the lower abdominal wall deep to Scarpa's fascia. Here there is no anatomic barrier, and the urine may reach the level of the thorax if correct surgical management is delayed. It cannot extend down over the thighs since Scarpa's fascia attaches to the fascia lata just below the inguinal ligament.

d. CONGENITAL DEFORMITIES OF THE URETHRA — include absence, duplication, or atresia — all of which are rare. Congenital valves are limited to the prostatic portion. The most frequent deformity is *hypospadias*, in which, the urethral opening is in a more proximal position on the urethral surface of the penis or perineum (Fig. 3). Depending upon the location of the urethral opening, a number of anatomic varieties are described: glandular, penile, penoscrotal, scrotal, and perineal. In all varieties the prepuce is deformed and the frenulum is absent.

A more rare congenital deformity is *epispadias*. Here the external urethral orifice is located on the dorsum of the penis. It is frequently associated with other severe deformities of the urinary system such as exstrophy of the bladder.

2. **Scrotum** — the scrotum has been described on page 138. The testicle, epididymis, and the vas deferens constitute the visceral contents of this sac. Each of these structures are easily palpable within the scrotum.

a. TESTICLE — in cases of malignant tumors, this organ must be sacrificed (*orchiectomy, castration*). Other indications for its removal are the elective management of prostatic carcinoma, severe injuries, or advanced chronic granulomatous infections. It should be kept in mind that the testicle develops in the lumbar area, and its nerves, lymphatics, and vascular supply originate there. Pain arising from disease of the testes may be referred to the renal area; and conversely, renal disease may give rise to scrotal pain. Lymphatic spread of testicular disease extends not into the inguinal nodes as many assume, but rather into the upper lumbar chain of lymph nodes (page 208).

(Text continued on page 262.)

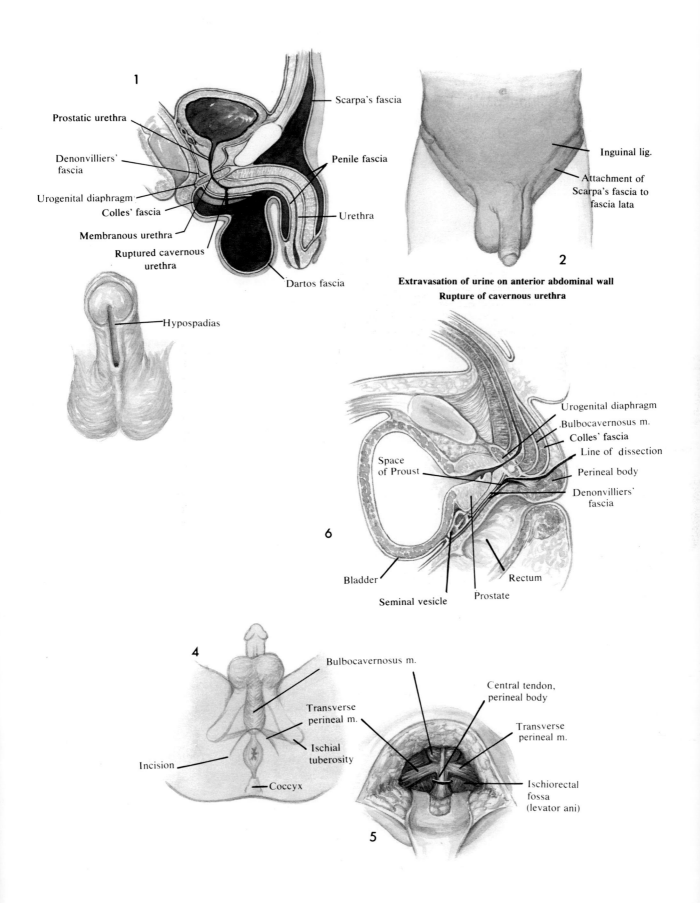

1

Prostatic urethra

Denonvilliers' fascia

Urogenital diaphragm

Colles' fascia

Membranous urethra

Ruptured cavernous urethra

Scarpa's fascia

Penile fascia

Urethra

Dartos fascia

Hypospadias

2

Inguinal lig.

Attachment of Scarpa's fascia to fascia lata

Extravasation of urine on anterior abdominal wall
Rupture of cavernous urethra

6

Urogenital diaphragm

Bulbocavernosus m.

Colles' fascia

Line of dissection

Perineal body

Denonvilliers' fascia

Space of Proust

Bladder

Seminal vesicle

Prostate

Rectum

4

Bulbocavernosus m.

Transverse perineal m.

Ischial tuberosity

Incision

Coccyx

5

Central tendon, perineal body

Transverse perineal m.

Ischiorectal fossa (levator ani)

A dilatation of the pampiniform plexus *(varicocele)* is usually idiopathic. Rarely, however, a rapidly developing varicocele may indicate a tumor of the left kidney, where invasion of the renal vein may obstruct the drainage of the left testicular vein.

b. EPIDIDYMIS — may be enlarged because of cyst formation, tuberculosis, or other acute or chronic infections, which may be indications for its removal *(epididymectomy)*. A cystic enlargement of the epididymis must be distinguished from a vaginal *hydrocele*. The latter is a fluid accumulation in the tunica vaginalis testis, either idiopathic or secondary to testicular disease. A hydrocele is related to the front and sides of the testis, whereas the epididymis lies above and behind the testis.

c. VAS DEFERENS — may be ligated bilaterally by an approach through the upper scrotal wall when sterilization of the male is indicated.

Hernias extending into the scrotal sac have already been discussed on pages 140 and 142.

3. **Perineal Prostatectomy** — has several advantages over other approaches (page 240). It permits complete removal of the gland under direct vision and provides for dependent drainage.

An inverted V incision is made with the apex about 3 cm. anterior to the anus, overlying the perineal body (Fig. 4). With the retraction of the skin and superficial fascia the bulbocavernous and superficial transverse perineal muscles are visible anteriorly. The perineal body is incised and the anterior rectal wall is exposed. By retraction, the external sphincter of the anus and the rectum are displaced posteriorly from the superficial transverse perineal muscles (Fig. 5).

In the fetus the peritoneum extends as a pouch to the pelvic floor in the region of the urogenital diaphragm. With the development of the pelvic visceral organs anterior and posterior to the pouch, the two layers of peritoneum are pressed together and loosely fuse leaving a potential space between them. The two layers are attached to the peritoneum above at the base of the rectovesical fossa and to the urogenital diaphragm and perineal body below. This double fascial layer is termed *Denonvillier's fascia (prostatoperitoneal fascia)*. The anterior layer is firmly attached to the prostate, and the posterior layer is only loosely attached to the rectum. The potential space between the two layers is the *retroprostatic space of Proust*. When the perineal body has been cut, the plane between the two fascial layers (space of Proust) must be identified. It is an essential step in protecting the rectum from injury and in minimizing bleeding, thereby improving exposure of the surgical field. It has been the lament of many that it is not always easy to find this passage between "wind and water" (Fig. 6).

When the anterior layer of Denonvillier's fascia is incised, the prostate gland and, in fact, the seminal vesicles are exposed.

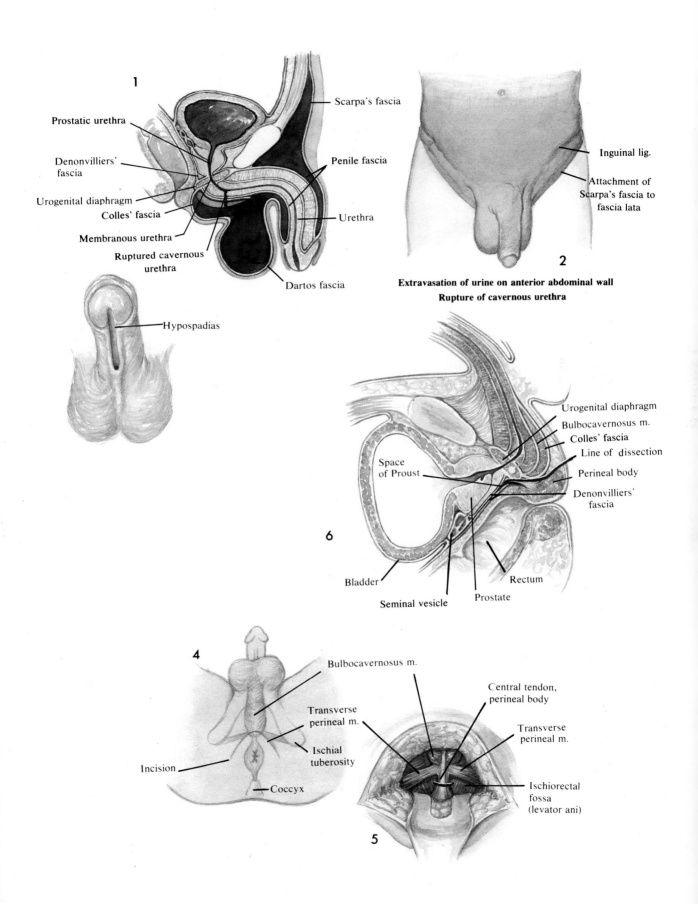

1

Prostatic urethra

Denonvilliers' fascia

Urogenital diaphragm

Colles' fascia

Membranous urethra

Ruptured cavernous urethra

Scarpa's fascia

Penile fascia

Urethra

Dartos fascia

Inguinal lig.

Attachment of Scarpa's fascia to fascia lata

2

Extravasation of urine on anterior abdominal wall
Rupture of cavernous urethra

Hypospadias

6

Space of Proust

Bladder

Seminal vesicle

Prostate

Rectum

Urogenital diaphragm

Bulbocavernosus m.

Colles' fascia

Line of dissection

Perineal body

Denonvilliers' fascia

4

Incision

Bulbocavernosus m.

Transverse perineal m.

Ischial tuberosity

Coccyx

Central tendon, perineal body

Transverse perineal m.

Ischiorectal fossa (levator ani)

5

FEMALE PERINEUM:
CLINICAL CONSIDERATIONS:

Operative procedures in the female perineum are primarily concerned with the vulvar structures.

1. **Urethra** — whereas *urethral stricture* is generally regarded as a disease of the male, it may also occur as a congenital deformity in the female. Acquired strictures may follow gonorrhea or lymphopathia venereum in the female. Management is simplified by the shortness of the passage and the ease with which instrumentation can be performed.

A *urethral caruncle*, a small red tumor-like growth usually located on the posterior wall of the urethra, may produce pain or bleeding.

2. **Bartholin's Gland** — is frequently the site of infection due to gonorrhea, resulting in a chronic cyst formation. The incision for removal of such a cyst is made over its most prominent part.

3. **Vagina** — certain procedures are performed in order to open or enlarge the vaginal orifice. An *imperforate hymen* prevents the outflow of the menses resulting in *hematocolpos*. A cruciate incision is made in the hymen and its four quadrants excised to the vaginal wall. In certain cases of *dyspareunia*, or painful intercourse, a plastic procedure must be performed to enlarge the vaginal orifice.

By far the most frequent surgery for enlargement of the vaginal orifice is an *episiotomy*. This has become almost a routine procedure in the delivery of all primiparae. The episiotomy is used to prevent unpredictable perineal tears during childbirth. It may be performed in a posterior midline or in a posterolateral direction.

In the *midline episiotomy* the incision is made through the posterior vaginal wall, the perineal skin, the perineal body, and the superficial fibers of the external sphincter muscle of the anus.

In a *posterolateral episiotomy* (Fig. 1) the incision divides the vaginal wall, the skin over the ischiorectal fossa and the bulbocavernosus and superficial transverse perineal muscles and extends into the anterior fibers of the levator ani (pubococcygeus) muscle. Repair of an episiotomy must be done carefully in order to reapproximate these anatomic structures. If this is not done properly a relaxed perineal floor may result.

Relaxation of the perineum may result from either laceration or stretching of the musculature as a result of childbirth. This relaxation produces an enlargement of the genital hiatus and therefore the vaginal orifice (Fig. 2). Descent of the anterior vaginal wall is always associated with some degree of descent of the floor of the bladder *(cystocele)*. Sagging of the posterior vaginal wall may allow the rectum to bulge forward into the vaginal vault, a defect termed a *rectocele*. When such defects are present and symptomatic, a plastic procedure is indicated in order to restore the pelvic floor to its normal supporting role. This procedure is termed a *perineorrhaphy* and is one of the most frequent operations in gynecology.

In an *anterior vaginoplasty* for the correction of a cystocele, connective tissue (the vesicovaginal ligament and perivesical tissue) and the smooth muscle fibers of the bladder floor are the only supportive tissues available. These structures must be plicated to correct the defect.

A *posterior vaginoplasty* used to correct a rectocele must always include plastic repair of the levator ani as well as restoration of the defective perineum. This nearly always narrows the genital hiatus. Precise reconstruction of the pelvic floor and perineum is an absolute necessity to correct this deformity. The muscles and fascia of the pelvic floor are exposed in the interval between the posterior vaginal wall and the anterior rectal wall. The approach is through an incision at the junction of the vaginal mucosa and the skin (Fig. 3). The ends of the external sphincter of the anus must be approximated if torn. The margins of the levator ani muscle (pubococcygeal fibers) are identified on either side and sutured together in the midline anterior to the anus. This procedure reduces the size of the genital hiatus in the pelvic floor and gives support to the anterior wall of the rectum (Fig. 4). The more superficial tissues which are made up of the scarred muscular and fascial structures of the urogenital diaphragm are then approximated by suture in the midline (Fig. 5). Redundant vaginal mucosa and skin are excised as the wound is closed.

In addition to these fundamental plastic procedures there are a great number of supplementary operations which utilize this vaginal perineal approach. Their selection depends upon the degree of descent, the size and position of the uterus, the age of the patient, and the desirability of future pregnancies.

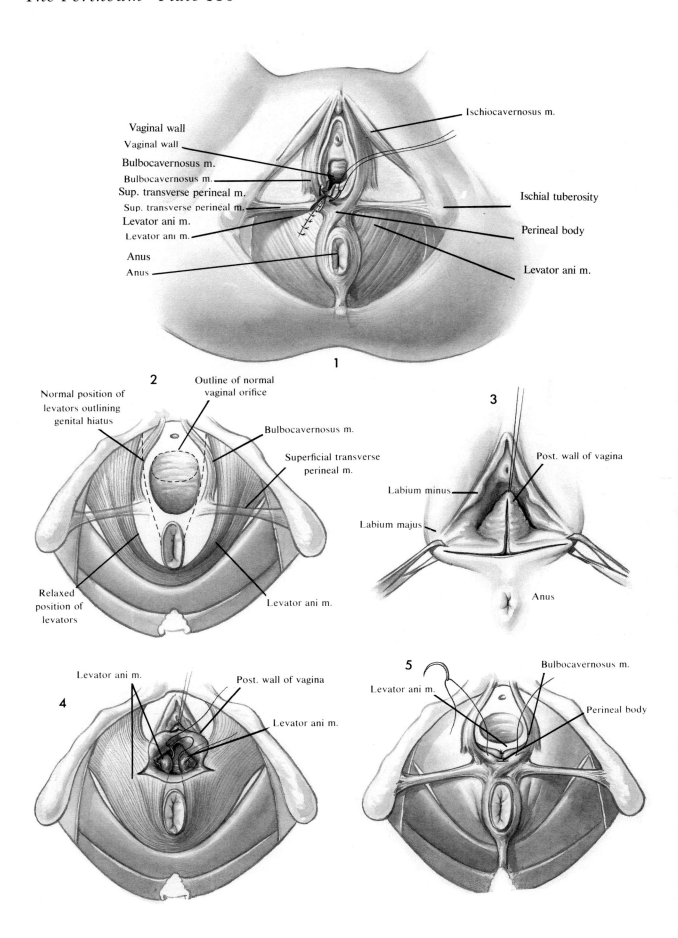

Vaginal wall

Vaginal wall

Bulbocavernosus m.

Bulbocavernosus m.

Sup. transverse perineal m.

Sup. transverse perineal m.

Levator ani m.

Levator ani m.

Anus

Anus

Ischiocavernosus m.

Ischial tuberosity

Perineal body

Levator ani m.

1

2

Normal position of levators outlining genital hiatus

Outline of normal vaginal orifice

Bulbocavernosus m.

Superficial transverse perineal m.

Relaxed position of levators

Levator ani m.

3

Labium minus

Labium majus

Post. wall of vagina

Anus

4

Levator ani m.

Post. wall of vagina

Levator ani m.

5

Levator ani m.

Bulbocavernosus m.

Perineal body

PERINEUM: CLINICAL CONSIDERATIONS OF THE ANAL TRIANGLE:

The anatomy of the anal triangle has been discussed on page 252. Consideration here is given to clinical conditions affecting the anus, anal canal, lower rectum, and the ischiorectal fossa.

1. **Perineal Anesthesia**—the skin and muscles of the perineum are innervated mainly by the *pudendal nerve*. Its course and distribution has been described on page 258.

Anesthesia of the perineum may be accomplished by several routes: subarachnoid (saddle block), epidural, paravertebral, presacral, and pudendal nerve block. We will limit discussion here to the pudendal nerve block, others will be considered on page 268.

a. PUDENDAL NERVE BLOCK—has its greatest value in operations upon the female external genitalia and in obstetrical practice when it may be used in the relief of pain during the second stage of labor caused by dilation of the birth canal, vulva, and perineum. The pudendal nerve may be blocked through either a perineal or transvaginal route.

In the *perineal route* the chief landmark is the ischial tuberosity. With the patient in the lithotomy position the ischial tuberosity is palpated and a skin wheal is raised just medial to the tuberosity. A needle is inserted perpendicularly for a distance of 2.5 cm. If the needle encroaches upon the tuberosity it is withdrawn slightly and redirected in a more medial direction (Fig. 1).

If the *transvaginal route* is used the chief landmarks are the ischial spine and the sacrospinal ligament. The ischial spine and sacrospinal ligament are palpated by a finger inserted into the vagina. The needle is introduced through the lateral vaginal wall to a point 1 cm. medial to the tip of the ischial spine and 1 cm. below the lower edge of the sacrospinal ligament.

In both perineal or transvaginal routes it is, of course, necessary to block both the right and left pudendal nerves.

If complete perineal anesthesia is required, it is necessary to supplement the pudendal block with an injection along the anterior margin of the vulva. This injection blocks the ilioinguinal nerve [anterior labial (scrotal) rami] and the filaments of the genitofemoral nerve (Fig. 1).

2. **Proctosigmoidoscopy**—examination by direct vision of the rectum and lower sigmoid by means of the sigmoidoscope is now considered an integral part of the rectal examination. By this examination alone some 70 per cent of all malignant tumors of the colon can be diagnosed. The technique is simple and the procedure safe if performed gently and correctly.

A *digital rectal examination must always precede* the introduction of the scope to exclude any obstruction which would prevent satisfactory passage of the instrument. The patient is placed in the knee-chest position (Fig. 2A) and the instrument introduced through the anus by steady pressure directed in line with the umbilicus (Fig. $2B_1$). Once beyond the sphincter, the obturator is removed and the remainder of the procedure is done under *direct vision*. After examination of the anal canal, the tip of the scope is redirected in an upward and backward direction (Fig. $2B_2$). Further examination of the sigmoid requires a more anterior direction of the scope to avoid the sacral promontory. *Great gentleness is required.* Severe pain indicates either inexperience of the operator or severe inflammation, both of which should indicate postponement of the examination.

3. **Anorectal Pathology**—a large variety of pathological processes may involve the anorectal area, only a few of which will be considered here. The congenital malformations have already been discussed on page 228.

a. RECTAL POLYPS (Fig. 3)—may be of two varieties: sessile or pedunculated. Sessile polyps have narrow stalks by which they are attached to the rectal mucosa. They may be palpated by digital examination or visualized by proctoscopic examination. All polyps should be considered as potentially malignant.

b. HYPERTROPHIED ANAL PAPILLA (Fig. 3)—is frequently misdiagnosed as a rectal "polyp." This entity is located at the pectinate line and can be equivocally diagnosed by proctoscopy.

c. HEMORRHOIDS (PILES)—also present as an anal-mass. Two types may be distinguished: internal and external hemorrhoids. An *internal hemorrhoid* arises as a varicosity of the internal hemorrhoidal plexus located above the pectinate line and covered by anal mucosa. An *external hemorrhoid* is a varicosity of the external hemorrhoidal plexus and is covered by skin (Fig. 3).

d. ANAL FISSURE (Fig. 4)—is a tear of the anal mucosa which in over 90 per cent of cases occurs posteriorly in the midline. An anatomic explanation for this location may be that the superficial portion of the external sphincter inserts posteriorly into the coccyx. At this point the mucosa is supported and may therefore be vulnerable to a tear should a hard fecal mass pass the site.

e. ANAL FISTULAE (Fig. 4)—usually arise secondary to infection of the anal crypts *(cryptitis)* located just above the pectinate line. The infected material invades the crypts and the vestigial anal glands associated with the crypts, then progresses either by lymphatic channels or by contiguous spread into the perianal areas to form a perianal abscess. With subsequent spontaneous rupture a secondary opening occurs in the perianal skin. Many varieties are described according to the course of the fistulous tracts. The subcutaneous and intrasphincteric types are shown in Figure 4.

In some cases a secondary opening may not occur, and the abscess persists. The abscess may be confined laterally to the ischiorectal fossa. It is imperative that such an *ischiorectal abscess* be incised and drained early in order to prevent its upward extension into the pelvis. An anal fistula may also extend upward and produce a *supralevator (pelvirectal) abscess.*

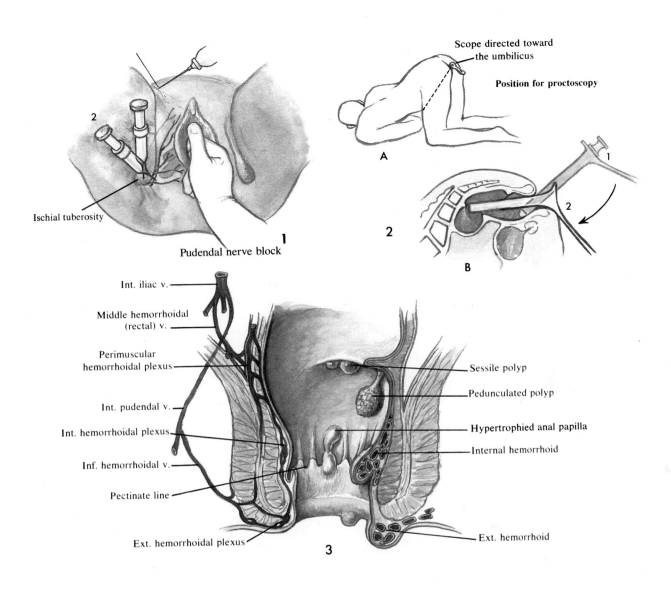

Scope directed toward
the umbilicus

Position for proctoscopy

A

B

2
1

2

1

2

Ischial tuberosity

Pudendal nerve block

Int. iliac v.

Middle hemorrhoidal
(rectal) v.

Perimuscular
hemorrhoidal plexus

Int. pudendal v.

Int. hemorrhoidal plexus

Inf. hemorrhoidal v.

Pectinate line

Ext. hemorrhoidal plexus

Sessile polyp

Pedunculated polyp

Hypertrophied anal papilla

Internal hemorrhoid

Ext. hemorrhoid

3

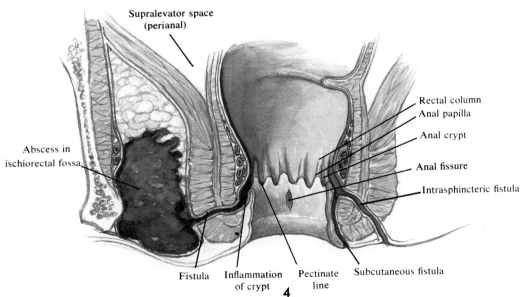

Supralevator space
(perianal)

Abscess in
ischiorectal fossa

Rectal column
Anal papilla

Anal crypt

Anal fissure

Intrasphincteric fistula

Subcutaneous fistula

Fistula   Inflammation   Pectinate
of crypt   line
4

The Lumbosacral and Gluteal Regions

THE LUMBOSACRAL REGION:

We will confine our discussion of the lumbosacral region to the relationship of the lumbosacral portion of the vertebral column and the spinal cord, its coverings and its related nerve trunks. The practical aspects of these relationships will be discussed as they apply to various techniques of regional anesthesia.

1. **Meninges** — three layers constitute the coverings of the spinal cord, which are collectively termed the meninges. They are the pia mater, the arachnoid mater, and the dura mater (Figs. 1, 2B, and 3).

a. Dura MATER — is a dense fibrous tissue layer which is the outer cover of the cord. The nerve roots which extend from the cord and pierce the dura receive a dural investment which is continuous with the epineurium or outer covering of the nerve sheath. The dura mater terminates as a cul-de-sac at the level of the second sacral vertebra.

b. Arachnoid MATER — is a delicate nonvascular membrane which, in the region of the spinal cord, is closely related to the overlying dura. Like the dura mater, it terminates at the level of the second sacral vertebra.

c. Pia MATER — is a thin vascular connective tissue layer which is intimately connected to the cord, extending into all its sulci and fissures. It is loosely connected to the overlying arachnoid by fine trabeculae. At the level of the disc between L_1 and L_2 the pia is spun out into a fine tubular structure, the *filum terminale*. This structure continues caudalward to the level of S_2 where it receives an investment of arachnoid and dura mater and finally attaches to the back of the first coccygeal segment of the vertebral column as the *coccygeal ligament*.

2. **Spinal Cord** — the cord lies within the vertebral canal covered by its investments described above. It begins above at the level of the foramen magnum. The level of termination of the cord is variable, occurring anywhere between T_{12} and L_3. In the majority of cases, it terminates at the level of the intervertebral disc between L_1 and L_2. Its tapered lower extremity is termed the *conus medullaris* (Fig. 1).

In the embryo, the 31 segmental nerves arising from the cord pass directly laterally to their respective intervertebral foramina. During later development there is a disproportionate growth between the vertebral column and the spinal cord resulting in an apparent ascent of the cord *(ascensus medullaris spinalis).* In the adult with the cord terminating at the level of L_1, the lumbar and sacral nerves have a long intradural course before reaching their intervertebral foramina. This group of descending nerve bundles, which resemble a horse's tail, is termed the *cauda equina.*

3. **Spinal Spaces** — several spaces related to the meningeal coverings of the cord are significant in regional anesthesia. They are the epidural, subdural, and subarachnoid spaces (Figs. 1, 2B, and 3).

a. Epidural (extradural) SPACE — in relation to the spinal cord, extends from the coccyx to the foramen magnum. It lies between the walls of the vertebral canal externally and the dura mater internally. The space varies in width, being widest in the lumbar region. It is occupied by the *internal vertebral venous plexus,* fat, and loose connective tissue.

b. Subdural SPACE — is located between the dura and the arachnoid. Because of the close adherence of these two layers in the region of the cord it is of little practical significance.

c. Subarachnoid SPACE — lying between arachnoid and pia mater contains the cerebrospinal fluid and is in direct continuity with the similar space in the cranial cavity. Below the termination of the cord (between L_1 and L_2) and the second sacral vertebral level this space is particularly large and contains the roots of the lumbar and sacral nerves, the cauda equina. Its practical significance is discussed below.

4. **Lumbar Puncture and Subarachnoid (Spinal) Anesthesia** — a needle may be inserted into the subarachnoid space in order to obtain a sample of cerebrospinal fluid for diagnostic purposes, to relieve increased intracranial pressure by withdrawing the fluid, or to inject certain therapeutic drugs into the subarachnoid space *(intrathecal injection).* Finally, anesthetic agents may be injected into the space to induce spinal anesthesia. Regardless of the purpose, the puncture technique is the same.

The patient is placed in a lateral decubitus position with the head flexed toward the knees and the knees flexed on the thighs (Fig. 2A). This is the position most frequently used and serves to widen the space between the adjacent lumbar spinous processes. In some in-

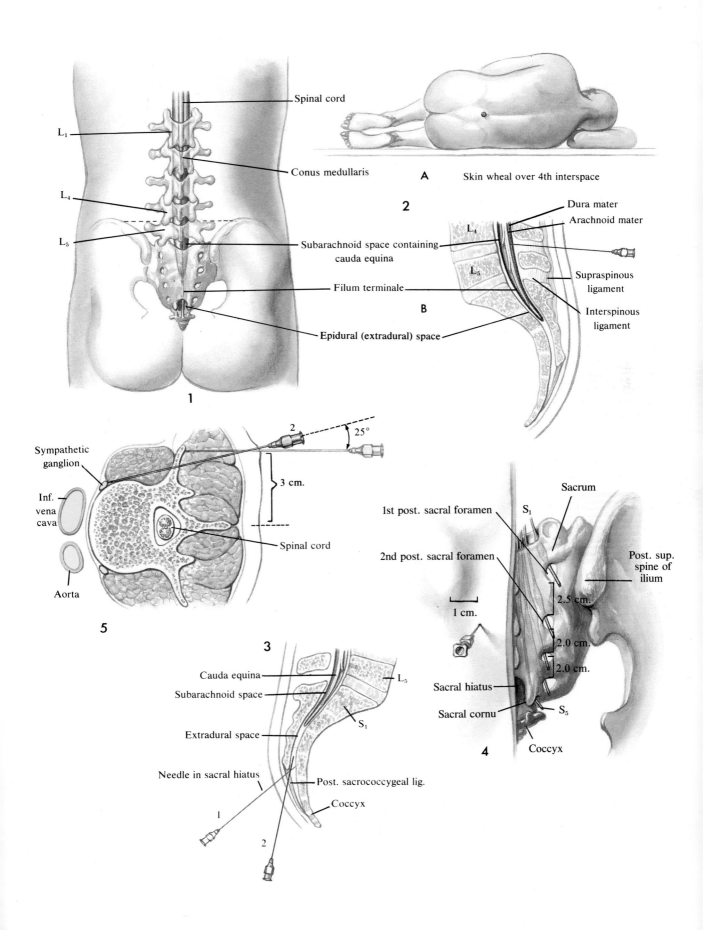

Spinal cord

L_1

Conus medullaris

L_4

L_5

Subarachnoid space containing cauda equina

Filum terminale

Epidural (extradural) space

1

A   Skin wheal over 4th interspace

2

Dura mater

Arachnoid mater

L_4

L_5

Supraspinous ligament

Interspinous ligament

B

Sympathetic ganglion

Inf. vena cava

Aorta

25°

3 cm.

Spinal cord

5

3

Cauda equina

Subarachnoid space

Extradural space

Needle in sacral hiatus

1

2

L_5

S_1

Post. sacrococcygeal lig.

Coccyx

Sacrum

1st post. sacral foramen

S_1

2nd post. sacral foramen

Post. sup. spine of ilium

2.5 cm.

1 cm.

2.0 cm.

2.0 cm.

Sacral hiatus

Sacral cornu

S_5

Coccyx

4

stances, a sitting position may be preferable, particularly if a low spinal or *saddle block* anesthesia is desired; that is, one in which the sacral nerves supplying the perineum are blocked.

A line drawn between the highest points of the iliac crest *(supracrestal line)* passes through the forth lumbar spine or the interspace between L_4 and L_5 (Fig. 1). A skin wheal is made in the midline over the desired interspace — the second, third, or fourth (Fig. 2*A*). A spinal needle is then inserted. In its course, the needle pierces the skin, superficial fascia, supraspinal ligament, interspinal ligament, epidural space, dura and arachnoid and then enters the subarachnoid space (Fig. 2*B*).

5. **Epidural (Extradural) Anesthesia** — in this method of regional anesthesia the spinal nerves are blocked in the space between the dura and the wall of the vertebral canal, the epi- or extradural space. The important landmarks are the tip of the coccyx and the sacral cornua. The needle is inserted into the sacral hiatus after piercing the posterior sacrococcygeal ligament (Fig. 3). The hiatus lies cephalad to the tip of the coccyx and between the cornua (Fig. 4).

6. **Paravertebral Block** — in this form of regional anesthesia an attempt is made to anesthetize the spinal nerves just as they emerge from the intervertebral foramen. This is usually done in the thoracic, lumbar, and sacral areas. In a *transsacral block* in the sacral area a posterior approach is used, and injection is made into the posterior sacral foramina. The posterior superior iliac spine is the important landmark in this technique. The second sacral foramen lies about 1 cm. medial to the spine and slightly below. Injection should begin at this site. The first foramen lies about 2.5 cm. above and the third about 2 cm. below the second foramen (Fig. 4).

7. **Lumbar Sympathetic Block** (Fig. 5) — in this block the needle is inserted into the skin about 3 cm. from the midline on the level of the desired vertebra. The needle is inserted perpendicular and advanced until it comes in contact with the transverse process; the distance is measured usually as 3.5 to 5 cm. The needle is withdrawn slightly and redirected in a medial and cephalad direction for a distance of 2.5 to 3 cm. beyond the previous measurement. This redirection overrides the transverse process and places the needle near the ganglion. Measurement of these distances is important, for too deep a penetration may injure the great vessels or other vital structures.

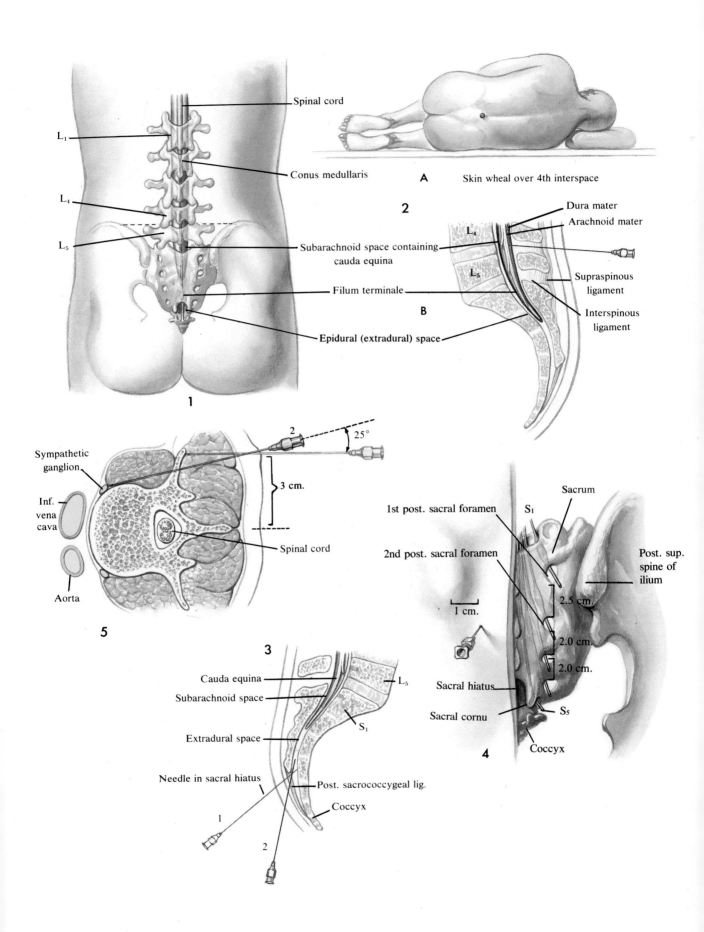

Spinal cord

L₁

Conus medullaris

L₄

L₅

Subarachnoid space containing cauda equina

Filum terminale

Epidural (extradural) space

1

A Skin wheal over 4th interspace

2

Dura mater

Arachnoid mater

L₄

L₅

Supraspinous ligament

Interspinous ligament

B

Sympathetic ganglion

Inf. vena cava

Aorta

5

Spinal cord

25°

3 cm.

3

Cauda equina

Subarachnoid space

Extradural space

Needle in sacral hiatus

1

2

L₅

S₁

Post. sacrococcygeal lig.

Coccyx

1st post. sacral foramen

2nd post. sacral foramen

Sacral hiatus

Sacral cornu

S₁

Sacrum

Post. sup. spine of ilium

2.5 cm.

2.0 cm.

2.0 cm.

1 cm.

S₅

Coccyx

4

THE GLUTEAL REGION:

The gluteal region actually is the uppermost portion of the posterior thigh. From its depth exit the muscular and neurovascular structures, from the pelvis to the lower extremity and perineum.

1. **Boundaries** — the gluteal region is bounded above by the crest of ileum and below by the gluteal fold of skin. Medially, it is bounded by the midline of the body and laterally by a line dropped perpendicularly through the tubercle of the ilium.

2. **Bony and Ligamentous Structures** (Fig. 1) — the ilium, ischium, sacrum, coccyx, and the upper end of the femur are located in this area. Two important ligamentous structures are also found here: the *sacrospinal* and *sacrotuberous* ligaments.

3. **Skin and Superficial Fascia** — the skin in this region of the body is thickened and highly sensitive because of the diffuse cutaneous nerve supply. The cluneal (Gr., gluteal) innervation is illustrated in Figure 2.

4. **First Layer of Muscle** — two muscles lie superficial in the gluteal region: the gluteus maximus and the tensor fascia lata.

a. Gluteus maximus (Fig. 2) — is a large rhomboid-shaped muscle arising from the posterior portion of the iliac crest, the lumbodorsal fascia, the sacrum and coccyx, and the sacrotuberous ligament. Its lower fibers insert into the gluteal tuberosity of the femur, and the upper fibers into a thickening of fascia lata termed the *iliotibial band*. It acts primarily as an extensor and a lateral rotator of the thigh. It also tenses the iliotibial band and thereby fixes the knee in extension. This muscle is innervated by the inferior gluteal nerve.

b. Tensor fascia lata — arises from the anterior portion of the iliac crest and inserts into the iliotibial band (Fig. 3, page 279). When the leg is free (lifted, as in walking), it flexes, abducts, and internally rotates the thigh. When the foot is in a fixed position (planted), it flexes, abducts, and laterally rotates the thigh. It, along with the gluteus maximus, helps keep the extended knee extended, but assists in flexion of the flexed knee. The superior gluteal nerve innervates this muscle.

5. **Second Layer of Muscle** — with the reflection of the gluteus maximus, a second muscular layer is revealed consisting of the gluteus medius and the piriformis (Fig. 3).

a. Gluteus medius — arises from the anterior portion of the iliac crest and from the outer surface of the wing of the ilium and is inserted into the greater trochanter of the femur. The muscle as a whole is a medial rotator of the hip and it steadies the pelvis while walking. It is innervated by the superior gluteal nerve.

b. Piriformis — takes origin from the ventral surface of the second to fourth sacral vertebrae and con-

stitutes one of the two muscles of the lateral pelvic wall (page 216). It exits from the pelvic cavity through the greater sciatic foramen and inserts on the greater trochanter of the femur. This muscle acts as a lateral rotator and abductor of the hips. Its innervation is via the sacral plexus branches S_1 and S_2.

As it exits through the greater sciatic foramen the piriformis divides the foramen into a suprapiriformis and an infrapiriformis recess.

(1) *Suprapiriformis Recess* (Fig. 3) — emits the superior gluteal artery, vein, and nerve. The *superior gluteal nerve* arises from the sacral plexus and innervates the gluteus medius and minimus and the tensor fascia lata. The *superior gluteal artery*, a branch of the posterior division of the internal iliac (hypogastric) artery, aids in the supply of the entire gluteal region. The *superior gluteal vein* is a tributary of the internal iliac (hypogastric) vein.

(2) *Infrapiriformis Recess* (Fig. 3) — is the point of exit for numerous pelvic vessels and nerves. From lateral to medial they are: the sciatic nerve, the posterior femoral cutaneous nerve, the inferior gluteal nerve, the inferior gluteal artery and vein, the internal pudendal artery and vein, and the pudendal nerve.

6. **Third Layer of Muscle** — is the deepest muscular layer of the gluteal region and consists of five muscles; four of which are lateral rotators of the hip joint (Fig. 4).

a. Gluteus minimus — arises from the anterior outer surface of the ilium and from the capsule of the hip joint and inserts on the greater trochanter of the femur. Its action is similar to the gluteus medius. The superior gluteal nerve innervates this muscle.

b. Obturator internus — like the piriformis, forms one of the muscles of the lateral pelvic wall (page 216). It has a wide origin from the pubic ramus, the obturator membrane, and the pelvic surface of the ischium between the ischial spine and obturator foramen. Its fibers converge in a fan-shaped manner and exit from the pelvis through the lesser sciatic foramen. It is the only pelvic structure that exits through this foramen. The muscle inserts into the trochanteric fossa of the femur, and, like the remainder of the muscles described at this level, it is a lateral rotator of the hip and is innervated by branches of the sacral plexus (page 274).

c. Gemellus superior — arises from the ischial spine and inserts into the trochanteric fossa in common with the obturator internus. The muscle belly lies just above the obturator internus tendon.

d. Gemellus inferior — arises from the ischial tuberosity and lies just below the tendon of the obturator internus and inserts on the femur as a common tendon with the aforementioned tendon.

e. Quadratus femoris — takes origin from the ischial tuberosity and inserts on the greater trochanter.

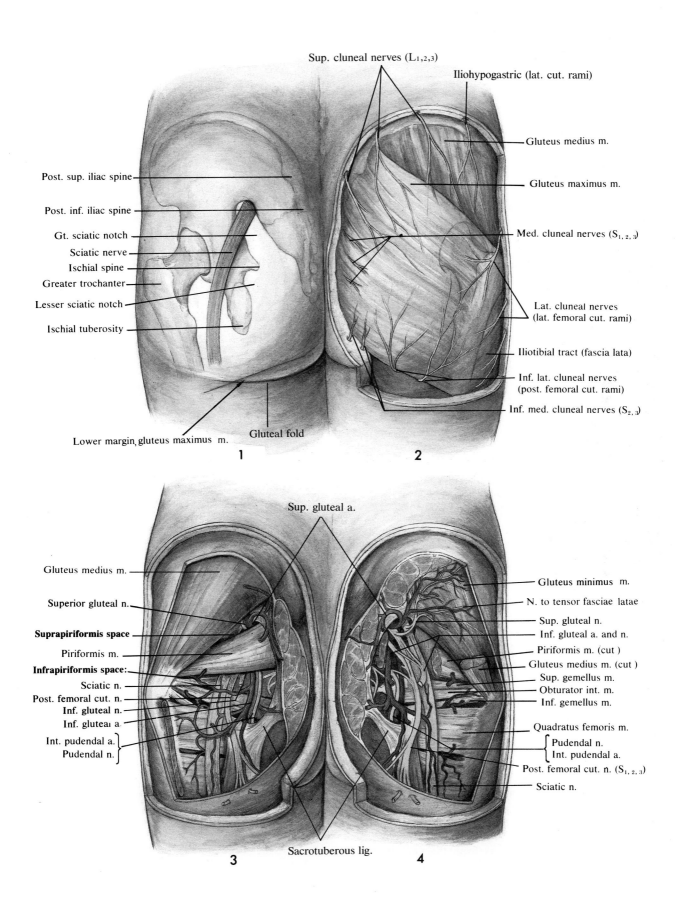

Sup. cluneal nerves (L₁,₂,₃)

Iliohypogastric (lat. cut. rami)

Gluteus medius m.

Gluteus maximus m.

Post. sup. iliac spine

Post. inf. iliac spine

Gt. sciatic notch

Sciatic nerve

Ischial spine

Greater trochanter

Lesser sciatic notch

Ischial tuberosity

Med. cluneal nerves (S₁,₂,₃)

Lat. cluneal nerves
(lat. femoral cut. rami)

Iliotibial tract (fascia lata)

Inf. lat. cluneal nerves
(post. femoral cut. rami)

Inf. med. cluneal nerves (S₂,₃)

Lower margin, gluteus maximus m.

Gluteal fold

1

2

Sup. gluteal a.

Gluteus medius m.

Superior gluteal n.

Suprapiriformis space

Piriformis m.

Infrapiriformis space:

Sciatic n.

Post. femoral cut. n.

Inf. gluteal n.

Inf. gluteal a.

Int. pudendal a.
Pudendal n.

Gluteus minimus m.

N. to tensor fasciae latae

Sup. gluteal n.

Inf. gluteal a. and n.

Piriformis m. (cut)

Gluteus medius m. (cut)

Sup. gemellus m.

Obturator int. m.

Inf. gemellus m.

Quadratus femoris m.

Pudendal n.
Int. pudendal a.

Post. femoral cut. n. (S₁,₂,₃)

Sciatic n.

Sacrotuberous lig.

3

4

7. Sacral Plexus (Figs. 1 and 2)—the sacral plexus of nerves is formed by the anterior primary divisions of L_4, L_5, S_1, S_2, and S_3. Although arising in the pelvis all the branches of the plexus exit through the greater sciatic foramen. With the exception of the superior gluteal nerve all these branches leave through the infrapiriformis recess (Fig. 3, page 273). The anterior primary divisions almost immediately divide into anterior and posterior secondary divisions. The branches of the plexus are depicted in the following table:

Anterior Primary Divisions		
ANTERIOR SECONDARY DIVISIONS	(SCIATIC NERVE)	POSTERIOR SECONDARY DIVISIONS
Tibial nerve	L_4, L_5, S_1, S_2, S_3	Peroneal nerve
Quadratus femoris nerve / Inferior gemellus nerve	L_4, L_5, S_1	Superior gluteal nerve
Internal obturator nerve / Superior gemellus nerve	L_5, S_1, S_2	Inferior gluteal nerve
Posterior femoral cutaneous nerve	S_1, S_2, S_3	Posterior femoral cutaneous nerve
	S_1, S_2	Piriformis nerve
	S_2, S_3	Inferior medial cluneal nerves

The *sciatic nerve* is the largest nerve in the body. It exits from the pelvis through the infrapiriformis recess and descends deep to the gluteus maximus to the posterior compartment of the thigh. It is actually two nerve bundles (the tibial and peroneal) enclosed in a common sheath.

The *posterior femoral cutaneous nerve* also leaves the pelvis through the infrapiriformis recess and supplies cutaneous innervation throughout the posterior thigh to the upper calf.

The *superior gluteal nerve* enters the gluteal region through the suprapiriformis recess and supplies the gluteus medius and minimus and the tensor fascia lata. The *inferior gluteal nerve* supplies the gluteus maximus after leaving the pelvis through the infrapiriformis recess.

8. Pudendal Plexus—arises from the anterior primary divisions of S_2, S_3, and S_4. Visceral, muscular, and terminal branches arise from this plexus.

a. VISCERAL BRANCHES—remain in the pelvis and are distributed to the pelvic viscera. They constitute the sacral outflow of the parasympathetic system and are collectively referred to as the *nervi erigentes* or *pelvic splanchnics*.

b. MUSCULAR BRANCHES—arise mainly from S_4 and innervate the muscles of the pelvic diaphragm (coccygeus and levator ani) and the external sphincter of the anus.

c. TERMINAL BRANCH—is the *pudendal nerve*, which is the most medial structure in the infrapiriformis recess. After passing over the ischial spine, this nerve passes through the lesser sciatic foramen and enters the pudendal (Alcock's) canal, a duplication of the parietal layer of endopelvic fascia.

9. Coccygeal Plexus—rami from S_4, S_5, and C_1 form the coccygeal plexus. These rami form cords lying on either side of the coccyx and coalesce to form the *anococcygeal nerve* (Figs. 1 and 2). The latter pierces the sacrotuberous ligament and innervates the skin surrounding the coccyx.

THE GLUTEAL REGION: CLINICAL CONSIDERATIONS:

The gluteal region is a frequent target for needle injections, superceded only by the antecubital fossa and deltoid region. Surgically, the gluteal region may be entered in order to afford a posterior approach to the hip joint.

1. Anatomy of Gluteal Injection—although the gluteal region is so frequently utilized for the intramuscular injection of various medications, little information can be obtained in standard textbooks regarding the proper injection procedure. Such an injection is not without risk of serious injury and may not infrequently lead to medicolegal problems. The most serious complication is injury to the sciatic nerve. Other complications include intravascular injection of drugs, embolism, abscess, periostitis, hematoma, and sloughing of the skin. The majority of these complications are directly related to the point of injection and the site where the medication is ultimately deposited.

a. TOPOGRAPHIC ANATOMY—of the gluteal region is illustrated in Figure 3. Frequently the gluteal area is incorrectly equated with the eminence of the gluteus maximus (the buttock or cheek). The proper topographic limits of the gluteal area consist of a superior line extending between the summits of the crest of the ilium. The inferior line coincides with the gluteal fold. A posterior vertical midline and a line dropped from the iliac tubercle forms a medial and lateral boundary. This area is then divided by a transverse and vertical line into four quadrants. Injections are made into the upper outer quadrant (Fig. 3).

A much simpler method is to draw an oblique line extending from the posterior-superior iliac spine to the upper border of the greater trochanter. Injection should be made into the gluteal area above this line which is well above the sciatic nerve.

2. Posterolateral Approach to the Hip Joint—the hip joint may be exposed by many approaches: anterior, lateral, or posterior. The posterolateral approach through the gluteal region may be utilized for open

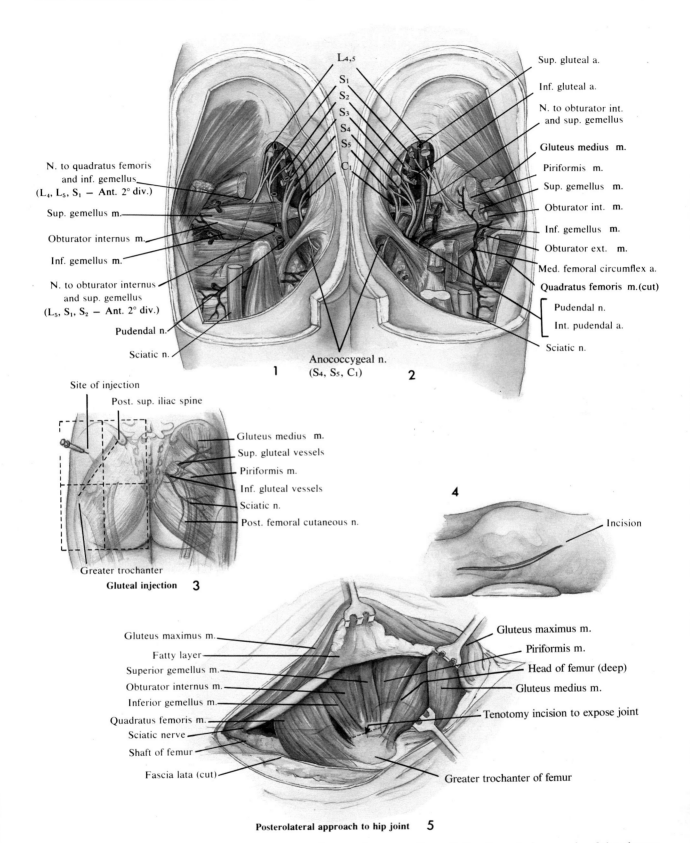

L₄,₅
S₁
S₂
S₃
S₄
S₅
C₁

Sup. gluteal a.

Inf. gluteal a.

N. to obturator int. and sup. gemellus

Gluteus medius m.

Piriformis m.

Sup. gemellus m.

Obturator int. m.

Inf. gemellus m.

Obturator ext. m.

Med. femoral circumflex a.

Quadratus femoris m.(cut)

Pudendal n.

Int. pudendal a.

Sciatic n.

N. to quadratus femoris and inf. gemellus (L₄, L₅, S₁ — Ant. 2° div.)

Sup. gemellus m.

Obturator internus m.

Inf. gemellus m.

N. to obturator internus and sup. gemellus (L₅, S₁, S₂ — Ant. 2° div.)

Pudendal n.

Sciatic n.

1

Anococcygeal n. (S₄, S₅, C₁)

2

Site of injection

Post. sup. iliac spine

Gluteus medius m.

Sup. gluteal vessels

Piriformis m.

Inf. gluteal vessels

Sciatic n.

Post. femoral cutaneous n.

Greater trochanter

Gluteal injection 3

4

Incision

Gluteus maximus m.

Fatty layer

Superior gemellus m.

Obturator internus m.

Inferior gemellus m.

Quadratus femoris m.

Sciatic nerve

Shaft of femur

Fascia lata (cut)

Gluteus maximus m.

Piriformis m.

Head of femur (deep)

Gluteus medius m.

Tenotomy incision to expose joint

Greater trochanter of femur

Posterolateral approach to hip joint 5

reduction of posterior dislocations, fracture dislocations of the hip, removal of benign or malignant lesions, the removal of loose bodies from the posterior region of the hip joint, or for hip replacement procedures.

An incision is made as shown in Figure 4, beginning about 5 inches below the greater trochanter and extend-

ing upward paralleling the anterior margin of the gluteus maximus. At the point at which the gluteus maximus inserts into the fascia lata an incision is made and the muscle reflected. The tendons of the piriformis, the gemelli, and the obturator internus muscles are transected and the capsule of the joint exposed (Fig. 5).

The Lower Extremity

THE THIGH

The *thigh* is limited above by the inguinal ligament anteriorly and the gluteal skin fold behind and extends below to the level of the knee. The shape of the thigh varies with the muscular development of the individual. The chief topographic landmarks are produced by the underlying muscular impressions upon the skin.

1. **Superficial Fascia** (Fig. 1) — in this layer on the anterior surface of the thigh one sees both vascular and neural structures. The arteries are branches of the common femoral artery. They are the *superficial circumflex iliac*, the *superficial inferior epigastric*, and the *superficial external pudendal arteries*.

a. GREAT SAPHENOUS VEIN — is the major superficial vessel in the anterior thigh. It arises from the dorsal venous rete on the dorsum of the foot and ascends over the medial malleolus of the tibia. In its ascent through the calf, it lies a finger's breadth medial to the medial border of the tibial shaft. At the knee, it lies approximately a hand's breadth medial to the patella and proceeds up the thigh and pierces the deep fascia in the region of the fossa ovalis to empty into the common femoral vein.

Its tributaries include three branches accompanying the aforementioned arteries; the *superficial circumflex iliac*, the *superficial inferior epigastric*, and the *superficial external pudendal veins*. In addition it receives the *lateral cutaneous* and *medial cutaneous (accessory saphenous) veins*.

b. SUPERFICIAL NERVES OF THE THIGH — are branches from the lumbar plexus. They consist of the *lateral femoral cutaneous nerve* which pierces the deep fascia of the thigh just below the anterior superior iliac spine. Pain and paresthesia over the distribution of this nerve is termed *meralgia paresthetica*, a common finding in patients with a shortened extremity. The femoral nerve gives rise to two major cutaneous branches from its superficial division; the *anterior* and *medial femoral cutaneous nerves*. The obturator nerve also gives rise to a cutaneous branch which is distributed to the medial aspect of the thigh. The *lumboinguinal branch of the genitofemoral nerve* innervates the skin of the midportion of the upper thigh. This branch serves as the afferent limb of the *cremasteric reflex*. Stroking the skin in its area of distribution results in contraction of the cremasteric muscle and elevation of the testicle through the efferent limb of the reflex via the external spermatic branch of the genitofemoral nerve.

2. **Subinguinal Area** — structures entering the anterior compartment of the thigh from the abdominal cavity must pass deep to the inguinal ligament. The fascial arrangement in this subinguinal area is such that two separate compartments are formed; a lateral muscular lacuna and a medial vascular lacuna (Fig. 2).

The abdominal wall is lined by endo-abdominal fascia, which (depending upon the muscle to which it is related) is given a specific name. In relation to the ventrolateral abdominal wall, it is the *transversalis fascia*; in relation to the posterior muscles of the false pelvis, the *iliopsoas fascia*. Where the bulk of the iliopsoas muscle passes laterally under the inguinal ligament in relation to the muscular lacuna these fascial layers fuse. At the medial border of the muscle the iliopsoas fascia is thickened extending from the inguinal ligament anteriorly to the iliopectineal eminence posteriorly located at the junction of ilium with the body of the pubis. This thickening of iliopsoas fascia is termed the *iliopectineal ligament*. It is this ligament which divides the subinguinal area into its two compartments.

a. MUSCULAR LACUNA (Figs. 2 and 3) — transmits the iliopsoas, the lateral femoral cutaneous and the femoral nerve. It is bounded by the inguinal ligament anteriorly, by the ilium posteriorly and laterally, and by the iliopectineal ligament medially.

The iliopsoas muscle forms the anterior group of iliofemoral muscles, the muscles of the gluteal region forming the posterior group. The muscles of the anterior group are innervated by branches of the lumbar plexus; the branches of the posterior group by the sacral plexus. The iliopsoas is formed by the iliacus and psoas major muscles. The *iliacus* arises from the iliac fossa, and the *psoas major* from the vertebral column, T_{12} through L_5. These muscles insert by a common tendon into the lesser trochanter of the femur. They act to flex the thigh at the hip and are innervated by the femoral nerve within the abdominal cavity.

b. VASCULAR LACUNA (Figs. 2 and 3) — allows passage of the femoral artery and vein. In this region, the iliopsoas fascia and transversalis fascia do not fuse beneath the ligament but are carried downward for a varying distance into the thigh forming the *femoral sheath*. The vascular lacuna is therefore bounded by the inguinal ligament in front, the pubis behind, the iliopectineal ligament laterally, and the lacunar ligament medially.

The extraperitoneal fatty tissue also extends downward with the femoral sheath and forms septa which divide the sheath into three compartments. The lateral compartment of the femoral sheath contains the common femoral artery and the middle compartment, the common femoral vein. The medial compartment unoccupied by vascular structures is referred to as the *femoral canal*. The canal is occupied by loose connective tissue, fat, and frequently, a deep femoral lymph node, the *node of Cloquet (Rosenmüller)*.

The abdominal opening of the canal is termed the *femoral ring*. It is in continuity with the extraperitoneal layer of fatty tissue of the abdominal cavity. Its boundaries are the inguinal ligament anteriorly, the femoral vein laterally, the pubic bone and pectineal (Cooper's) ligament posteriorly, and the lacunar ligament medially.

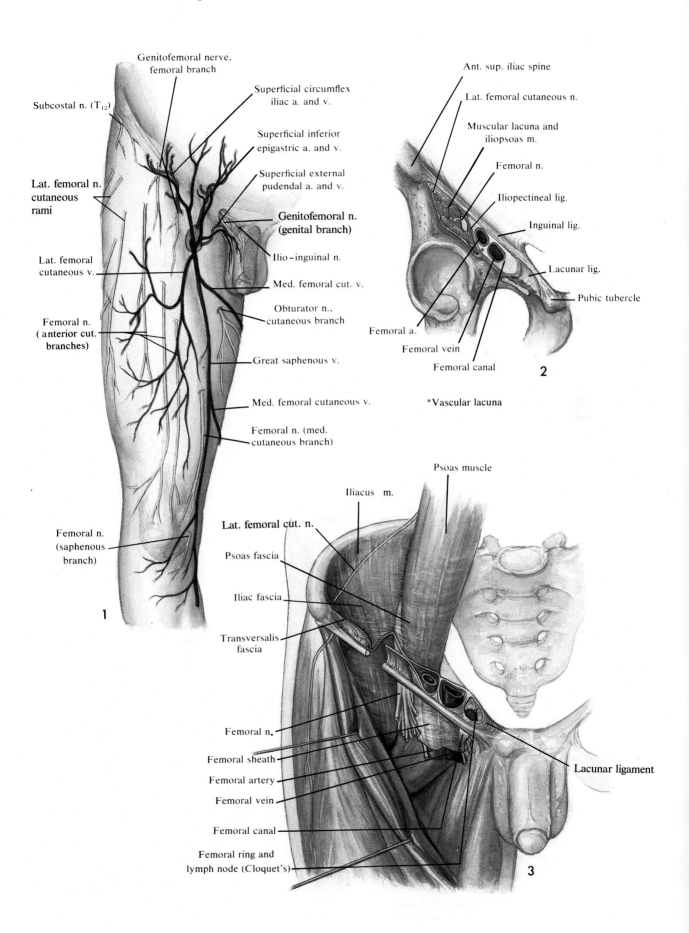

1

Genitofemoral nerve, femoral branch

Superficial circumflex iliac a. and v.

Superficial inferior epigastric a. and v.

Superficial external pudendal a. and v.

Subcostal n. (T₁₂)

Lat. femoral n. cutaneous rami

Genitofemoral n. (genital branch)

Ilio-inguinal n.

Lat. femoral cutaneous v.

Med. femoral cut. v.

Obturator n., cutaneous branch

Femoral n. (anterior cut. branches)

Great saphenous v.

Med. femoral cutaneous v.

Femoral n. (med. cutaneous branch)

Femoral n. (saphenous branch)

2

Ant. sup. iliac spine

Lat. femoral cutaneous n.

Muscular lacuna and iliopsoas m.

Femoral n.

Iliopectineal lig.

Inguinal lig.

Lacunar lig.

Pubic tubercle

Femoral a.

Femoral vein

Femoral canal

*Vascular lacuna

3

Iliacus m.

Psoas muscle

Lat. femoral cut. n.

Psoas fascia

Iliac fascia

Transversalis fascia

Femoral n.

Femoral sheath

Femoral artery

Femoral vein

Femoral canal

Femoral ring and lymph node (Cloquet's)

Lacunar ligament

3. **Compartments of the Thigh** — three muscle groups are described in the thigh. They are the anterior (extensor), the medial (adductor), and the posterior (flexor) group. In general, the anterior group of muscles is innervated by the femoral nerve, the medial group by the obturator nerve, and the posterior group by the sciatic nerve. Several muscles of the thigh receive dual innervation. Figure 1 is a diagrammatic representation of the musculature of the thigh on the basis of the innervation.

4. **Deep Fascia** — the deep fascia of the thigh is known as the *fascia lata*. It is a dense fibrous sheet which encases the musculature of the thigh. Laterally, it is greatly thickened to form a band extending from the iliac crest to the tibia, the *iliotibial band*. Superiorly, a muscle of the gluteal group, the tensor fascia lata, inserts into this band as does part of the gluteus maximus (page 272).

In the upper medial portion of the thigh there is an oval depression in the fascia lata just below the inguinal ligament, the *fossa ovalis*, which results from the parts of the fascia lata being at different depths (Fig. 2). A thin fascia, the *cribriform fascia*, covers this depression which is perforated by the entrance of the great saphenous vein, its tributaries with their accompanying arteries, and lymph channels. The fossa ovalis has a thick superior (*ligament of Hey*) and inferior (*ligament of Burns*) cornua which serve to protect the great saphenous vein from occlusion during flexion of the thigh.

5. **Anterior Group of Muscles** (Fig. 3) — are all innervated by the femoral nerve and consist of the sartorius and quadriceps muscles (rectus femoris and vastus lateralis, medialis, and intermedius). Although referred to as the extensor group, the sartorius is actually a flexor of the leg.

a. SARTORIUS — the longest muscle in the body, arises from the anterior-superior iliac spine and inserts into the ventromedial portion of the upper tibia. It serves to flex, abduct, and medially rotate the thigh and to flex and medially rotate the leg.

b. RECTUS FEMORIS — takes origin from the anterior-inferior iliac spine by its straight head and from the rim of the acetabulum by its reflected head. It inserts along with the other muscles of the quadriceps group into the patellar tendon which is discussed on page 312.

c. VASTUS LATERALIS — arises from the upper portion of the anterior surface of the shaft of the femur and from the lateral tip of the linea aspera (Figs. 1 and 2, page 289).

d. VASTUS MEDIALIS — takes origin from the intertrochanteric line and the medial lip of the linea aspera (Figs. 1 and 2, page 289).

e. VASTUS INTERMEDIUS — arises from the surface of the femur between the two aforementioned muscles and deep to the rectus.

Each of the muscles of the quadriceps femoris group inserts into the tibial tuberosity via the patellar ligament. They all act to extend the leg, but in addition the rectus flexes the thigh. These muscles are the chief stabilizers of the knee joint. They are prone to atrophy rapidly if immobilized, particularly the vastus medialis. For this reason a patient with an injury to the knee requiring

immobilization should be instructed in active quadriceps isometric exercises.

6. **Femoral Triangle** — this space in the upper thigh, also known as Scarpa's triangle, is bounded by the inguinal ligament above, by the sartorius laterally, and by the adductor longus medially. In the floor of the triangle on the medial side is the pectineus muscle and on the lateral side, the iliopsoas. It is covered by fascia lata and contains the femoral artery, nerve, and vein.

a. FEMORAL NERVE — is a branch of the lumbar plexus that crosses the false pelvis and innervates the iliacus and psoas major muscle (Fig. 3, page 277). After passing beneath the inguinal ligament it divides into a superficial and deep branch. The *superficial femoral nerve* gives rise to two cutaneous branches, the anterior and medial femoral cutaneous nerves; and two motor branches, one to the sartorius, the other to the pectineus muscle. The latter nerve passes deep to the femoral vessels to enter the muscle. The *deep femoral nerve* has one sensory branch and four motor branches. The motor nerves innervate the quadriceps muscle. The sensory branch is the *saphenous nerve*. It becomes superficial in the lower thigh and extends downward to the medial aspect of the foot (Fig. 1, page 299). It is the only branch of the lumbar plexus which extends below the knee.

b. FEMORAL ARTERY — a continuation of the external iliac, enters the thigh just beneath the midinguinal point. It gives rise to three superficial arteries previously described (page 276), the *superficial circumflex iliac*, the *superficial inferior epigastric*, and the *superficial external pudendal arteries*. It also gives rise to several small *inguinal branches* which supply the skin, subinguinal lymph nodes, and muscles in this region.

Its major branch is the *deep femoral (profunda femoris) artery*. It arises from the posterolateral surface of the femoral artery and extends distally in the thigh deep to the adductor longus muscle and sends perforating branches which supply the muscles of the posterior compartment of the thigh.

Arising from either the femoral directly or from the deep femoral is the *lateral femoral circumflex artery*. This branch passes laterally over the iliopsoas and deep to the rectus and divides into ascending, transverse, and descending branches. The ascending and transverse branches enter the cruciate anastomosis around the hip joint (Fig. 1, page 283), and the descending branch enters the popliteal anastomosis (Fig. 3, page 292).

Also arising from either the common femoral or the deep femoral is a *medial femoral circumflex artery* (Fig. 3) which passes deep between the iliopsoas and pectineus then over the adductor brevis and enters the gluteal region and forms part of the cruciate anastomosis (Fig. 1, page 283).

After giving rise to the deep femoral, the femoral artery continues through Scarpa's triangle as the *superficial femoral artery*. At the apex of the triangle this artery enters the adductor canal (page 280) and just before leaving the canal gives origin to the *supreme genicular artery* which also enters into the popliteal anastomosis (Fig. 3, page 292). The superficial femoral then enters the popliteal space as the *popliteal artery*.

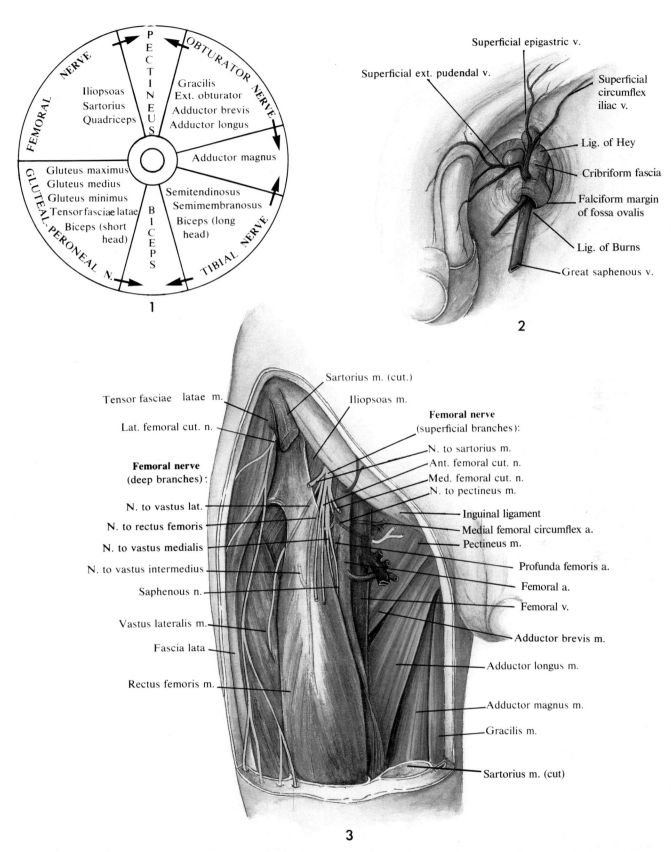

1

2

3

c. FEMORAL VEIN—is a continuation of the popliteal vein upward into the thigh. Its course is similar to that of the superficial and common femoral arteries. These relationships are considered on page 280. Its major tributaries during its ascent through the thigh are the deep femoral vein and the medial and lateral femoral circumflex veins. In the region of the fossa ovalis it also receives the great saphenous vein (Fig. 2).

7. **Medial Group of Muscles** (Figs. 1 and 2; Fig. 3, page 279) — all the muscles of this group arise from the bones of the pelvis and insert onto the posterior surface of the femur and tibia. They consist of the gracilis, pectineus, adductor longus, adductor brevis, adductor magnus, and obturator externus. They all act as adductors of the thigh; however, certain of these muscles may also act as flexors, extensors, or rotators of the thigh. All these muscles are innervated by the obturator nerve and L₄, but two of them (the pectineus and the adductor magnus) receive a dual innervation, the former from the femoral nerve and the latter from the sciatic nerve.

a. GRACILIS — is most superficial and most medial. It arises from the inferior ramus of the pubis and ischium and inserts just below the medial condyle of the tibia. It not only adducts but flexes and laterally rotates the thigh. It may also assist in flexion of the leg.

b. PECTINEUS — arises from the superior ramus of the pubis and inserts on the pectineal line of the femur (Fig. 2, page 289). This muscle both adducts and flexes the thigh.

c. ADDUCTOR LONGUS — also originates from the superior pubic ramus medial to the origin of pectineus. It inserts into the middle third of the linea aspera (Fig. 2, page 289) and acts as an adductor, flexor, and lateral rotator of the thigh.

d. ADDUCTOR BREVIS — takes origin from the inferior pubic ramus and inserts on the pectineal line and upper third of the linea aspera. It functions as an adductor, flexor, and lateral rotator of the thigh.

e. ADDUCTOR MAGNUS — has a rather extensive origin from the inferior ramus and tuberosity of the ischium and inserts along the entire length of the linea aspera and into the adductor tubercle of the femur. In addition to adducting the thigh, the upper fibers laterally rotate and flex. The lower fibers medially rotate and extend the thigh.

f. OBTURATOR EXTERNUS — arises from the outer surface of the ischial and pubic rami and the obturator membrane. It inserts into the trochanteric fossa and is a lateral rotator as well as an adductor.

8. **Obturator Nerve** — arises from the lumbar plexus, pierces the medial border of the psoas muscle, enters the pelvic cavity along its lateral wall in the extraperitoneal fatty tissue, and leaves the pelvis through the obturator foramen. Here it is accompanied in its exit by the obturator artery and vein (Fig. 2, page 217). In the proximal portion of the thigh at the upper border of the adductor brevis muscle it divides into an anterior and posterior branch (Fig. 1).

The *anterior branch of the obturator nerve*, after giving rise to an articular branch to the hip joint, gives off muscular rami to the pectineus, gracilis, adductor longus, and usually the adductor brevis.

The *posterior branch of the obturator nerve* innervates the obturator externus, the adductor magnus, and occasionally the adductor brevis. An important articular branch innervates the knee joint. Referred pain to the knee may be produced by pathologic changes in the hip joint since both joints are innervated by the obturator nerve.

9. **Obturator Artery** — is a branch of the anterior division of the internal iliac (hypogastric) artery (Fig. 1, page 219). It exits from the pelvis through the obturator foramen just below the nerve. Within the pelvis a constant *pubic branch* arises which ascends behind the lacunar ligament and anastomoses with the inferior epigastric or the external iliac. The artery at times may be of a large size. In approximately 40 per cent of individuals, the obturator will not arise from the hypogastric but rather as a direct branch of the inferior epigastric or external iliac, the so-called *aberrant obturator artery*.

Within the thigh, the obturator artery divides into an *anterior branch* and a *posterior branch*, which sends a branch to the hip joint and anastomoses with branches of the medial femoral circumflex artery (Fig. 1, page 283).

10. **Obturator Vein** — the tributaries of this vein correspond to the branches of the artery. After entering the pelvis through the obturator foramen it usually empties into the internal iliac vein. Like the artery, however, it may on occasions drain into the inferior epigastric or external iliac veins.

11. **Adductor Canal (Subsartorial or Hunter's Canal)** — is located in the middle third of the thigh and begins at the apex of the femoral triangle (Figs. 2 and 3).

a. BOUNDARIES — the canal is triangular in shape and is superficially covered by the sartorius muscle. The adductor longus and magnus muscles form the posterior wall, while the vastus medialis is related laterally and in front. Extending from the vastus medialis anteriorly and the adductor muscles posteriorly and forming the medial wall of the canal is a thickened aponeurotic fascial layer termed the *adductor membrane*. The canal extends into the upper portion of the popliteal space and exits by an opening in the adductor magnus muscle called the *adductor hiatus*. It is through this opening that the femoral vessels pass from the anterior compartment of the thigh to the popliteal space.

b. CONTENTS — through the entire length of the canal run the superficial femoral artery and vein. Two nerves enter the canal. They are branches of the deep femoral nerve; the nerve to the vastus medialis and the saphenous nerve. Neither of these nerves extend through the canal. The nerve to the vastus medialis pierces the lateral wall to enter the muscle at the midportion of the canal, while the saphenous nerve pierces the medial wall and descends into the superficial fascia of the lower thigh to the foot.

12. **Relationship of Femoral Artery and Vein** (Figs. 2 and 3) — there is a gradual change in the relationship between the femoral artery and vein as these vessels pass through the thigh.

a. IN THE FEMORAL TRIANGLE — at its base, the common femoral artery enters the thigh deep to the midinguinal point. Here it is very superficial and therefore easily palpable. At this point, the vein lies medial to the artery in the femoral sheath.

At the level of the apex of the triangle, the vein gains a position posterior to the artery. Directly posterior to the superficial femoral vein, with the adductor longus intervening, lie the deep femoral vein and artery in that order.

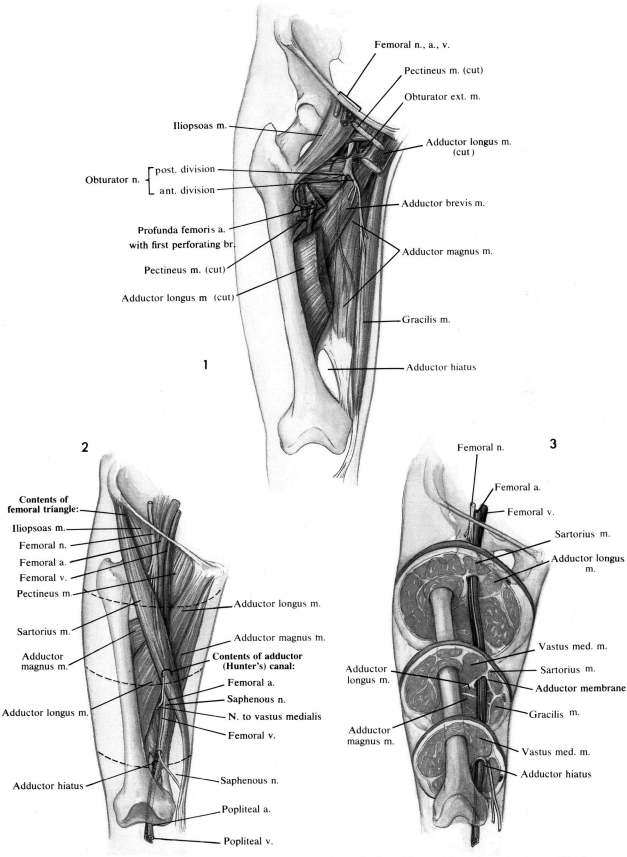

1

Femoral n., a., v.

Pectineus m. (cut)

Obturator ext. m.

Adductor longus m. (cut)

Adductor brevis m.

Adductor magnus m.

Gracilis m.

Adductor hiatus

Iliopsoas m.

Obturator n. { post. division / ant. division

Profunda femoris a. with first perforating br.

Pectineus m. (cut)

Adductor longus m (cut)

2

Contents of femoral triangle:

Iliopsoas m.

Femoral n.

Femoral a.

Femoral v.

Pectineus m.

Sartorius m.

Adductor magnus m.

Adductor longus m.

Adductor hiatus

Adductor longus m.

Adductor magnus m.

Contents of adductor (Hunter's) canal:

Femoral a.

Saphenous n.

N. to vastus medialis

Femoral v.

Saphenous n.

Popliteal a.

Popliteal v.

3

Femoral n.

Femoral a.

Femoral v.

Sartorius m.

Adductor longus m.

Vastus med. m.

Sartorius m.

Adductor membrane

Gracilis m.

Vastus med. m.

Adductor hiatus

Adductor longus m.

Adductor magnus m.

b. IN THE ADDUCTOR CANAL—proximally, the relationship of the superficial femoral artery and vein is similar to that in the apex of the femoral triangle; that is, the vein lies directly behind the artery. As they exit through the adductor hiatus to enter the popliteal space, the vein (although still posterior) runs toward the lateral side of the artery.

13. Cruciate Anastomoses (Fig. 1)—this arterial anastomotic network is formed by communication of branches of the internal iliac artery with those of the femoral artery. It serves as a collateral pathway after ligation of the external iliac or common femoral artery.

It is formed by medial and lateral transverse limbs, formed by the transverse rami of the medial and lateral femoral circumflex arteries (branches of the common or deep femoral arteries). These two arteries encircle the femur and anastomose behind the greater trochanter. A descending vertical limb is formed by a branch of the inferior gluteal artery, and an ascending vertical limb by the ascending ramus of the first perforating branch of the deep (profunda) femoral artery. The name of this anastomosis (cruciate) is derived from the arrangement of the contributing branches. Other arterial pathways supplement the cruciate anastomosis; they are the ascending ramus of the lateral femoral circumflex with the superior gluteal, the latter artery with the iliolumbar branch of the internal iliac, and the deep circumflex iliac branch of the external iliac with the iliolumbar (Fig. 1).

14. Superficial Fascia of the Posterior Thigh (Fig. 2)—in this area are located superficial veins and cutaneous nerve branches. The *medial femoral cutaneous vein (accessory saphenous)* drains the major portion of the posterior aspect of the thigh. The lateral aspect is drained by the *lateral femoral cutaneous vein*. Both vessels are tributaries of the great saphenous vein (Fig. 1, page 277).

The major cutaneous innervation of the posterior thigh is supplied by perforating branches of the posterior femoral cutaneous nerve. The main trunk of this nerve is derived from the sacral plexus (S_1, S_2, and S_3). After passing through the gluteal region it enters the posterior compartment at the lower border of the gluteus maximus and traverses the thigh deep to the fascia lata. In the lower part of the popliteal space it pierces the deep fascia and supplies the skin of the upper calf.

15. Posterior Group of Muscles (Figs. 3 and 4)—the muscles in the posterior compartment of the thigh consist of the biceps femoris, the semitendinosus and the semimembranosus. They are collectively termed the *"hamstring muscles."* By definition, a hamstring muscle is one which arises from the ischial tuberosity, inserts on one of the two bones of the leg, and is innervated by the tibial division of the sciatic nerve. The short head of the biceps fails to fulfill two of these requisites; it does not arise from the ischial tuberosity, and it is innervated by the peroneal division of the sciatic nerve. Strictly speaking, therefore, it is not a hamstring muscle.

a. BICEPS FEMORIS—its long head arises from the ischial tuberosity, whereas its short head takes origin from the lower half of the lateral lip of the linea aspera and from the proximal part of the supracondylar ridge of the femur. Their common tendon forms the lateral boundary of the popliteal space and inserts into the head of the fibula and the deep fascia of the leg.

The long head is innervated by the tibial and the short head by the peroneal division of the sciatic nerve. The long head acts on both the hip and knee joints, whereas the short head can act only on the knee. They

may extend, adduct, and laterally rotate the thigh as well as flex the leg.

b. SEMITENDINOSUS—arises from the ischial tuberosity in common with the long head of the biceps. Its tendon begins about midthigh and inserts into the medial condyle just behind the insertion of the gracilis and sartorius. These three tendons at the medial surface of the knee, each with a different innervation (tibial, obturator, and femoral nerves), are referred to as the *superficial goose foot (pes anserinus superficialis)*. The semitendinosus is innervated by tibial division of the sciatic nerve. It extends, adducts, and medially rotates the thigh and medially rotates and aids in flexion of the leg.

c. SEMIMEMBRANOSUS—takes origin from the tuberosity of the ischium and inserts into the medial condyle and the capsule of the knee joint (Fig. 4, page 313). Its innervation and action are identical to the semitendinosus.

16. Nerves—two nerves are located in the posterior compartment: the posterior femoral cutaneous and the sciatic nerve. The former nerve has been described above under Superficial Fascia.

a. SCIATIC NERVE (Figs. 3 and 4)—arises from the anterior primary divisions of L_4, L_5, S_1, S_2, and S_3. It enters the gluteal region deep to the gluteus maximus through the infrapiriformis recess, then descends into the posterior compartment of the thigh. In the thigh it is covered by the long head of the biceps and lies on the adductor magnus muscle.

The muscular branches to the hamstrings are given off from the medial side of the sciatic nerve in the upper thigh. They include a branch to the long head of the biceps, two branches to the semitendinosus, and a common trunk which innervates the semimembranosus and a portion of the adductor magnus. About midthigh a branch to the short head of the biceps arises from the lateral side of the sciatic nerve.

In the lower third of the thigh the sciatic divides into its two component parts: the tibial and common peroneal nerves. However, this division may occur at any point from its origin in the sacral region, in the gluteal region, or in the thigh.

17. Blood Supply (Figs. 1 and 4)—the *deep (profunda) femoral artery* supplies the posterior compartment of the thigh by four perforating branches. The deep femoral arises from the posterolateral surface of the common femoral about 4 cm. below the inguinal ligament. It descends between the adductor longis anteriorly and the adductor brevis posteriorly (Fig. 1, page 281). It gives rise to the four perforating arteries. The first three are related to the adductor brevis; the first at its upper border, the second which pierces the muscle, and the third at its lower border. The fourth perforating artery is the terminal branch of the deep femoral. Each of four arteries perforates the adductor magnus muscle and enters the posterior compartment to supply the muscles in that area. The *first perforating artery* by its ascending branch enters into the cruciate anastomosis. The *second* and *third perforating arteries* send off ascending and descending branches which anastomose with adjacent perforating arteries. The

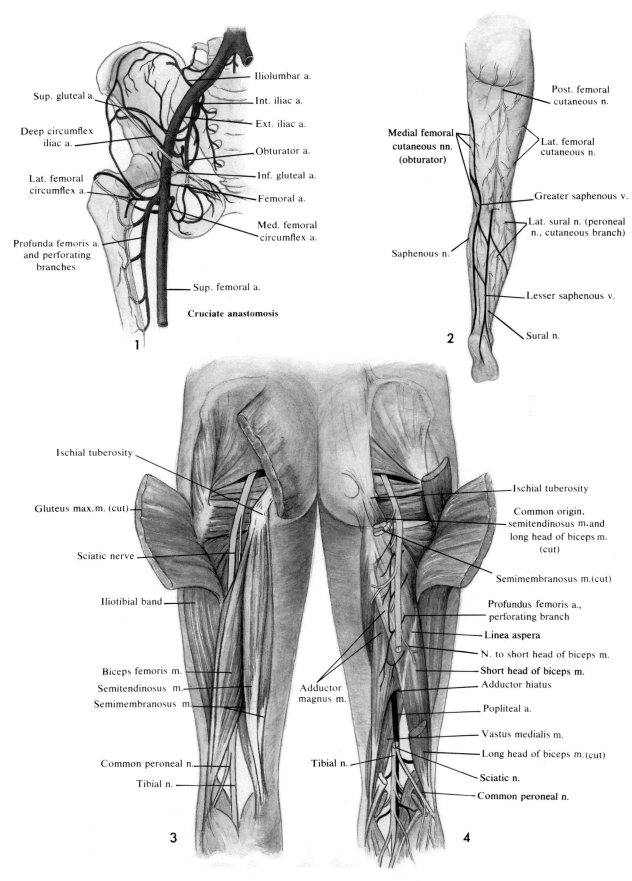

1

Iliolumbar a.

Sup. gluteal a.

Int. iliac a.

Deep circumflex iliac a.

Ext. iliac a.

Obturator a.

Lat. femoral circumflex a.

Inf. gluteal a.

Femoral a.

Med. femoral circumflex a.

Profunda femoris a. and perforating branches

Sup. femoral a.

Cruciate anastomosis

2

Post. femoral cutaneous n.

Medial femoral cutaneous nn. (obturator)

Lat. femoral cutaneous n.

Greater saphenous v.

Lat. sural n. (peroneal n., cutaneous branch)

Saphenous n.

Lesser saphenous v.

Sural n.

3

Ischial tuberosity

Gluteus max.m. (cut)

Sciatic nerve

Iliotibial band

Biceps femoris m.

Semitendinosus m.

Semimembranosus m.

Common peroneal n.

Tibial n.

Adductor magnus m.

4

Ischial tuberosity

Common origin, semitendinosus m.and long head of biceps m. (cut)

Semimembranosus m.(cut)

Profundus femoris a., perforating branch

Linea aspera

N. to short head of biceps m.

Short head of biceps m.

Adductor hiatus

Popliteal a.

Vastus medialis m.

Long head of biceps m.(cut)

Sciatic n.

Common peroneal n.

Tibial n.

descending branch of the *fourth perforating artery* communicates with muscular branches of the popliteal artery.

The deep veins of the posterior compartment accompany the perforating arteries as venae comitantes which drain into the deep femoral vein.

THE THIGH: CLINICAL CONSIDERATIONS

The new innovations in diagnostic and therapeutic procedures as well as the previously established procedures require that the physician possess an accurate knowledge of this area.

1. **Percutaneous Femoral Artery Puncture** — is utilized for the removal of an arterial blood sample and for the insertion of a catheter in order to perform a retrograde aortography, a selective arteriography of the aortic branches, or a femoral angiogram. The femoral artery is palpated at the base of Scarpa's triangle just below the midinguinal point where it lies superficial in position. The artery is immobilized between the index and middle fingers. The needle is inserted through skin and superficial fascia at which point it is essential to feel the pulse transmitted through the needle before entering the arterial wall.

2. **Femoral Artery Exposure** — is carried out by making a vertical incision beginning at the midinguinal point and descending into the thigh in alignment with the adductor tubercle, the hip being held slightly flexed and externally rotated. The common femoral artery occupies a separate compartment within the femoral sheath (Fig. 3, page 277). Such an exposure may be necessary in order to ligate the vessel following trauma or to insert a graft or venous by-pass to replace an arteriosclerotic segment. See Plate 125, page 287.

Aortofemoral anastomosis is indicated following resection of abdominal aortic aneurysm and in cases of aortoiliac occlusive disease (Fig. 1). The preclotted fabric prosthetic grafts may be woven, knitted, tubular, or bifurcation in type. The distal anastomosis may be end to end or end to side.

Extra-anatomic femorofemoral cross-over grafts are indicated in unilateral iliac occlusive disease (Fig. 2). Femoropopliteal by-pass is indicated in patients who have rest pain, incapacitating claudication, or gangrenous changes to the foot and toes, who would require amputation if a revascularization procedure were not performed. By-pass to the tibial or peroneal vessels is indicated in patients with necrosis and imminent limb loss.

Autogenous reversal saphenous vein grafts are the conduit of choice in by-passes to the popliteal, tibial, and peroneal arteries. Polytetrafluoroethylene (PTE) grafts can be used if veins are unavailable or if the patient is a poor risk and will not tolerate the extra time needed to harvest the saphenous vein. The PTE grafts and umbilical veins have been used as proximal segments of sequential by-passes to the popliteal and tibial arteries. Selective arteriograms are necessary to determine the site of occlusion and patency of the distal outflow tracts.

a. FEMOROPOPLITEAL BY-PASS ABOVE-THE-KNEE MEDIAL APPROACH (Fig. 3; see also Fig. 7, page 293) — an incision of approximately 15 cm. along the medial thigh parallel to the sartorius muscle behind the adductor mag-nus tendon is carried down to the medial condyle of the femur through the deep fascia. The sartorius muscle is retracted posteriorly and the vastus medialis muscle anteriorly, and the vessels are found posterior to the femur. For exposure of the popliteal artery below the knee, an incision is made from the medial epicondyle femur to the medial edge of the tibia; the fascia, the gracilis muscle, and the semitendinous and semimembranous tendons are divided from their tibial attachment and the medial head of the gastrocnemius is freed from the tibia. The popliteal vein will be found anterior and medial to the artery surrounded by adipose tissue. A tunnel through the popliteal space is created under the medial head of the gastrocnemius and carried under the sartorius muscle to the common femoral vessels (see Fig. 1, page 285).

The use of anterior tibial, posterior tibial, and peroneal artery by-pass procedures has improved salvage rates, as long as an outflow tract is patent.

b. FEMOROANTERIOR TIBIAL ARTERY RECONSTRUCTION — the anterior tibial approach through the anterior compartment of the leg (see Fig. 4, page 295, and Fig. 1, page 296). A mid-calf incision is made 3 cm. lateral to the tibia and carried down through the deep fascia. The anterior vessels are found on the interosseous membrane after retracting the tibialis anterior muscle medially and the extensor hallucis tendon posteriorly and laterally. After distal anastomosis, the graft is tunneled through the defect in the upper part of the interosseous membrane through the popliteal space.

c. FEMOROPERONEAL ARTERY RECONSTRUCTION (Fig. 4) — in the peroneal artery approach through the lateral compartment (see Figs. 1 to 4, page 295, and Figs. 3 and 6, page 297). An incision is made in the lateral compartment along the fibula. The peroneal muscles are retracted anteriorly, the soleus and gastrocnemius are retracted posteriorly, and 7 to 8 cm. of fibula is resected with a Gigli saw. The peroneal artery will be found medial to the fibula along the flexor hallucis muscle. The vessel is mobilized. The distal graft and anastomosis is completed and then tunneled through the popliteal space. An alternative approach through the posterior medial compartment of the right leg may be utilized.

In the posterior tibial artery approach through the posterior compartment (Fig. 5; see also Figs. 1 and 3, page 295, and Figs. 2, 3, and 5, page 297), a posterior compartment incision is made along the distal third of the leg. The gastrocnemius is retracted posteriorly. The soleus muscle is divided. The vessels are found along the tibialis posterior muscle and between the flexor digitorum longus muscle medially and the flexor hallucis longus muscle laterally. The distal graft anastomosis is completed and tunneled under the soleus along the posterior tibial artery to the popliteal space.

Other sites of ligation of the femoral artery are located at the apex of the femoral triangle and in the adductor canal (page 280).

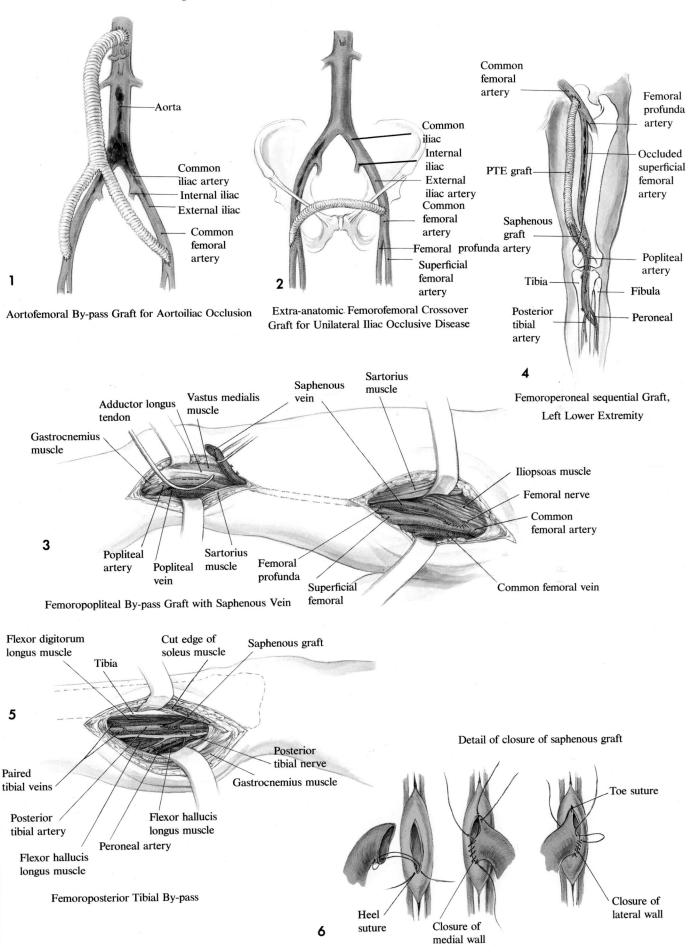

1 Aortofemoral By-pass Graft for Aortoiliac Occlusion

Labels for figure 1: Aorta; Common iliac artery; Internal iliac; External iliac; Common femoral artery

2 Extra-anatomic Femorofemoral Crossover Graft for Unilateral Iliac Occlusive Disease

Labels for figure 2: Common iliac; Internal iliac; External iliac artery; Common femoral artery; Femoral profunda artery; Superficial femoral artery

4 Femoroperoneal sequential Graft, Left Lower Extremity

Labels for figure 4: Common femoral artery; Femoral profunda artery; Occluded superficial femoral artery; PTE graft; Saphenous graft; Popliteal artery; Tibia; Fibula; Posterior tibial artery; Peroneal

3 Femoropopliteal By-pass Graft with Saphenous Vein

Labels for figure 3: Adductor longus tendon; Vastus medialis muscle; Saphenous vein; Sartorius muscle; Gastrocnemius muscle; Iliopsoas muscle; Femoral nerve; Common femoral artery; Popliteal artery; Popliteal vein; Sartorius muscle; Femoral profunda; Superficial femoral; Common femoral vein

5 Femoroposterior Tibial By-pass

Labels for figure 5: Flexor digitorum longus muscle; Tibia; Cut edge of soleus muscle; Saphenous graft; Posterior tibial nerve; Gastrocnemius muscle; Paired tibial veins; Posterior tibial artery; Flexor hallucis longus muscle; Peroneal artery; Flexor hallucis longus muscle

6 Detail of closure of saphenous graft

Labels for figure 6: Heel suture; Closure of medial wall; Toe suture; Closure of lateral wall

3. **Femoral Vein Exposure** (Fig. 1)—may be accomplished by making an incision similar to that which exposes the femoral artery. This vein lies in a compartment medial to the artery in the femoral sheath. After exposure of the common femoral vein at this site, the superficial and deep femoral veins and the greater saphenous tributary may be isolated. The superficial femoral vein is sometimes completely interrupted in the treatment of thrombosis of the vein.

For exposure of the greater saphenous tributary vein of the common femoral vein, an oblique incision is made about 2 cm. below and parallel to the inguinal ligament over the fossa ovalis. This vessel is ligated and divided for the treatment of varicosities of the saphenous vein or for harvesting the saphenous vein for by-pass procedures.

4. **Femoral Hernia** (Fig. 2)—results from the potential point of weakness in the medial aspect of the femoral sheath. Referring back to page 276 we note that the subinguinal region is subdivided into a muscular and a vascular lacuna. Within the vascular lacuna a prolongation of the transversalis and iliopsoas fascia extends into the thigh as the femoral sheath. This sheath contains three fascial compartments. The femoral artery occupies the lateral compartment, and the femoral vein the middle compartment. The medial compartment is normally occupied only by areolar tissue and lymph nodes. It is through this most medial compartment (femoral canal) that a femoral hernia may occur. Such a hernia is always acquired and is found most frequently in the female. Anatomically the latter may be due to the wider width of the female pelvis (therefore the larger the size of the femoral ring) and the more atonic abdominal musculature resulting from pregnancies.

The hernial sac descends through the femoral canal and consists of preperitoneal fat, parietal peritoneum, and omentum. Occasionally a loop of bowel (*Richter's hernia*) or a portion of bladder may herniate. The sac is restricted by the inguinal ligament anteriorly, the pectineal ligament posteriorly, and the lacunar ligament medially (Fig. 3). It may impinge upon the more resilient femoral vein laterally. Once achieving a position in the fossa ovalis, it may expand into the superficial fascia of the upper thigh. It can always be differentiated from an indirect inguinal hernia in that the neck of the femoral hernial sac is always below and lateral to the pubic tubercle.

The neck of the sac is always narrow, and this results in irreducibility and strangulation of the hernial contents. In order to reduce a femoral hernia, an operation is invariably required. This may be accomplished by either a subinguinal or inguinal approach. In either approach the anatomic boundaries of the femoral ring or entrance to the femoral canal must be recalled. The ring is bounded anteriorly by the inguinal ligament, medially by the lacunar ligament, posteriorly by the pubis and the peroneal ligament, and laterally by the femoral vein. If the subinguinal approach is used in a strangulated femoral hernia, the lacunar ligament may require division. But there is a high risk of dividing or damaging an *aberrant obturator artery*, which lies

deep to the lacunar ligament. From this approach there is no access to the vessel. This aberrant obturator artery, therefore, has been termed the *circle of death* (Fig. 4). There is normally an anastomotic branch between the pubic branch of the inferior epigastric and the pubic branch of the obturator. In some 40 per cent of cases, however, the obturator artery may arise directly from the inferior epigastric or external iliac rather than the hypogastric. For this and other surgical technical reasons the inguinal approach is preferred in the reduction of a femoral hernia.

5. **Amputation**—the thigh is a frequent site for amputation of the lower extremity. The indication for such operations may be congenital defects, infections, trauma, vascular disease, and cancer of the bone or soft tissue. All effort should be made to preserve as much of the length of the thigh as possible. The shortest possible length of stump which may be fitted properly into a prosthetic device is 7.5 cm. measured from the perineum. It is equally as important to amputate at a distance 7.5 cm. above the level of the center of the knee joint if a suction-socket type of prosthesis is to be used. The site of election of amputation above the knee (A-K amputation) is therefore at the junction of the middle and lower thirds of the femur.

A recent innovation in amputation is the *myodesis* technique in which the anterior, medial, and posterior muscle groups are sutured to the bone through holes drilled in the distal end of the bone. A rigid plastic dressing is applied at the operating table. This technique results in a much stronger, less edematous stump and permits ambulation of the patient within 48 hours.

A *supracondylar amputation* may be used. Figure 5, page 287, illustrates the structures severed at this level. At this same level a *Gritti-Stokes amputation* is performed (Fig. 6, page 287). In this procedure the patella is preserved, its articular surface removed, and the patella fitted over the amputated end of the femur in order to produce a bony union.

6. **Fractures of the Femur**—the femur, like other long bones of the body, is fractured as a result of direct or indirect violence or muscular action. Fractures involving the femur are divided into those involving the upper end, the shaft, and the lower end of the bone. Fractures of the upper end are discussed on page 308.

Fractures of the shaft usually involve the middle, occasionally the upper, and rarely the lower third of the bone. Fractures due to direct violence, usually crushing injuries, most frequently involve the lower third of the femur. Fractures due to indirect violence, such as falling upon the feet, most frequently occur in the upper third of the bone. Fractures due to muscular action which results from a sudden twist of the body with the foot in a fixed position usually disrupt the upper and occasionally the middle third of the femur.

The line of breakage resulting from direct violence is usually transverse. Fractures from indirect impact are usually oblique, while fractures due to muscular action are spiral in character. Oblique and spiral fractures are frequently compound fractures.

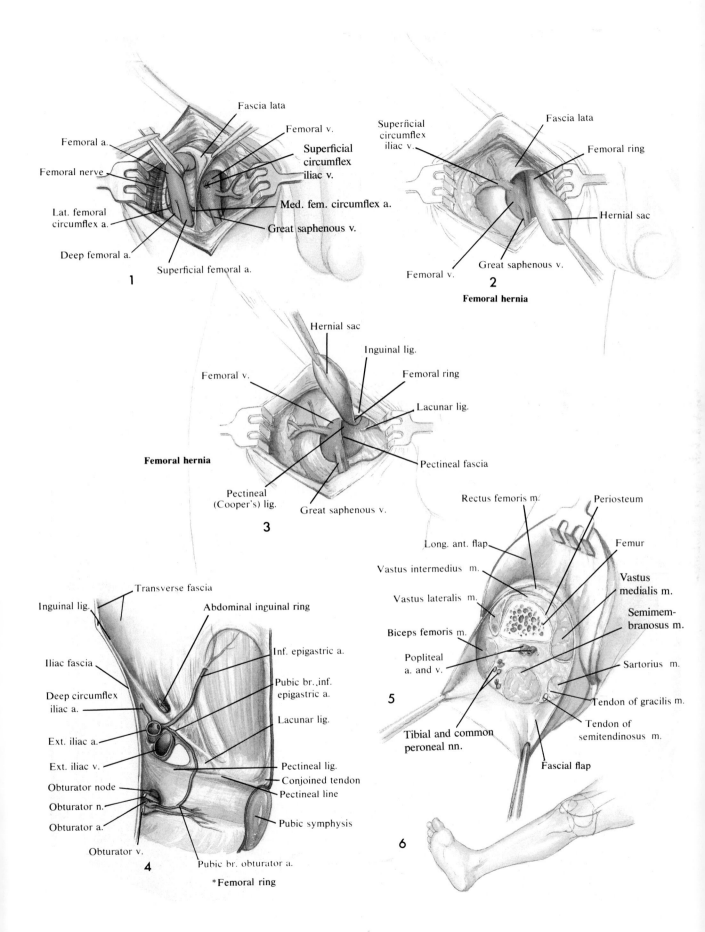

1

Femoral a.

Femoral nerve

Lat. femoral circumflex a.

Deep femoral a.

Superficial femoral a.

Fascia lata

Femoral v.

Superficial circumflex iliac v.

Med. fem. circumflex a.

Great saphenous v.

2
Femoral hernia

Superficial circumflex iliac v.

Fascia lata

Femoral ring

Hernial sac

Femoral v.

Great saphenous v.

3

Femoral hernia

Hernial sac

Inguinal lig.

Femoral ring

Lacunar lig.

Pectineal fascia

Femoral v.

Pectineal (Cooper's) lig.

Great saphenous v.

4

*Femoral ring

Transverse fascia

Inguinal lig.

Iliac fascia

Deep circumflex iliac a.

Ext. iliac a.

Ext. iliac v.

Obturator node

Obturator n.

Obturator a.

Obturator v.

Pubic br. obturator a.

Abdominal inguinal ring

Inf. epigastric a.

Pubic br.,inf. epigastric a.

Lacunar lig.

Pectineal lig.

Conjoined tendon

Pectineal line

Pubic symphysis

5

Rectus femoris m.

Long. ant. flap

Vastus intermedius m.

Vastus lateralis m.

Biceps femoris m.

Popliteal a. and v.

Tibial and common peroneal nn.

Periosteum

Femur

Vastus medialis m.

Semimembranosus m.

Sartorius m.

Tendon of gracilis m.

Tendon of semitendinosus m.

Fascial flap

6

Like fractures of the humerus, the displacements of the proximal and distal parts of the fractured femur are dependent upon the muscle attachments. Figures 1 and 2 depict the muscular attachments and insertions upon the femur.

The *iliofemoral muscle group* consists of an anterior and a posterior set. Anteriorly the iliacus and psoas major muscles insert into the lesser trochanter and act as hip flexors. Posteriorly, the gluteal muscles, piriformis, obturator internus, gemelli, and quadratus femoris, act to extend, externally rotate, and abduct the thigh. These muscles insert on the upper extremity of the femur.

The *adductors muscles*, the adductor brevis, longis, and magnus, all insert on the medial aspect of the shaft of the bone. One muscle of this group, the gracilis, attaches to the tibia.

Of the *quadriceps* muscle mass, three muscles have an extensive origin from the shaft of the femur. These muscles are the vastus medialis, lateralis, and intermedius. The rectus femoris arises from the pelvis. All insert via the patellar ligament.

The *hamstring muscles* also are involved in displacement of femoral shaft fractures. They consist of the semimembranosus, semitendinosus, and biceps femoris. All arise from the ischial tuberosity except the short head of the biceps, which arises from the posterior surface of the shaft. The hamstring muscles insert on one of the two bones of the leg.

Another important muscle in relation to femoral fractures is the *gastrocnemius*, which arises as lateral and medial heads from the condyles of the femur (Fig. 2, page 295).

7. **Fracture of the Upper Third of the Shaft** (Fig. 3) — results in a marked displacement of the proximal fragment due to the attachment of the iliofemoral muscle group. It is flexed by the pull of the iliopsoas muscle and abducted and externally rotated by the pull of the glutei, the gemelli, the obturator internus, and the quadriceps femoris. The distal fragment is displaced upward by the adductor and hamstring group of muscles.

8. **Fracture of the Middle Third of the Shaft** (Fig. 4) — results also in a flexion deformity of the proximal fragment due to the strong pull of the iliopsoas muscle upon the lesser trochanter. The abduction and external rotation of the proximal fragment seen in a fracture of the proximal third are less marked because of the counterbalance obtained by the attachment of some of the adductor muscles. The distal fragment is displaced upward and posterior owing to the pull of the adductors and hamstring muscles.

9. **Fracture of the Lower Third of the Shaft** (Fig. 1, page 291) — the displacement of the distal fragment is most significant in these *supracondylar fractures*. The nearer the fracture line is to the condyles, the greater will be the displacement. The distal fragment is angulated posteriorly by the gastrocnemius, and the popliteal artery is especially liable to injury because of its relation to the bone. The popliteal vein, medial popliteal (tibial) nerve, and lateral popliteal (common peroneal)

nerve are also vulnerable to injury. The hamstring and quadriceps muscles also displace this fragment upward. The pull of the iliopsoas and adductor muscles upon the proximal fragment results in a slight flexion and adduction deformity of this portion of the shaft.

10. **Fractures of the Condyles** — almost always extend into the knee joint resulting in a bloody effusion *(hemarthrosis)*. One condyle may be fractured and pulled upward by the attached thigh muscles. The distal fragment of some of the supracondylar fractures already described may split longitudinally converting them into either T- or Y-shaped *intercondylar fractures*. The condyles are separated from one another by the force of the gastrocnemius muscle. The quadriceps and hamstring muscles acting upon the leg pull these condylar fractures upward in a position in front of the proximal fragment of the fractured femur.

11. **Displacement of the Lower Femoral Epiphysis** — is most frequently seen in young males as a result of violent hyperextension injuries. The epiphyseal fragment is displaced anterior to the femoral shaft and pushes the shaft posterior in position. Vascular complications frequently result from compression or injury to the popliteal vessels by the proximal fragment of the femur. Reduction may be achieved by traction of the leg and flexion of the knee joint.

Treatment of femoral fractures requires anatomical realignment and immobilization. Realignment requires some form of traction to overcome the pull of the quadriceps, hamstrings, and adductor muscle groups. This may be achieved by simple skin traction or by skeletal traction techniques. Occasionally, the fractured fragments can only be anatomically reconstructed by operative means *(open reduction)*. Surgical intervention is especially necessary in the treatment of fractures of the upper and lower ends of the femur.

12. **Exposure of Femur** — the femur requires surgical exposure for a variety of reasons. The most frequent indication is the open reduction of recent fractures or the correction of delayed union or nonunion of femoral fractures. Other indications include ostectomy for the removal of benign tumors or osteomyelitis and osteotomy for the correction of congenital, traumatic, or arthritic deformities.

The surgical approach to the femoral head, neck, and trochanters is discussed on page 308. The femoral shaft may be approached by several routes.

The *lateral approach* to the femoral shaft is made in line with the lateral intermuscular septum. In the upper third of the thigh this interval is between the vastus lateralis anteriorly and the gluteus maximus posteriorly. Distally, the incision is made between the vastus lateralis anteriorly and the biceps femoris posteriorly. In each instance the periosteal incision is made anterior to the lateral intermuscular septum.

In an *anterior approach to the femoral shaft* one may enter the anterior muscular compartment either laterally or medially to the rectus femoris muscle. After the fascia lata is incised, the interval between the rectus femoris and vastus medialis is developed in the *anteriomedial approach*. Separation of these muscles

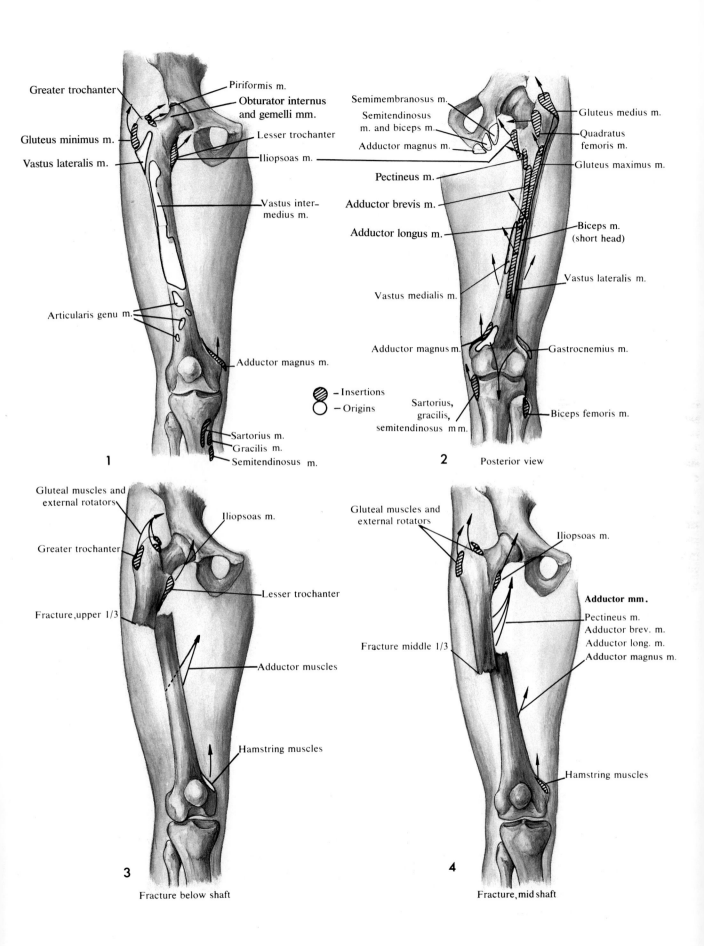

1

Greater trochanter

Gluteus minimus m.

Vastus lateralis m.

Piriformis m.

Obturator internus and gemelli mm.

Lesser trochanter

Iliopsoas m.

Vastus inter-medius m.

Articularis genu m.

Adductor magnus m.

— Insertions

— Origins

Sartorius m.

Gracilis m.

Semitendinosus m.

2   Posterior view

Semimembranosus m.

Semitendinosus m. and biceps m.

Adductor magnus m.

Gluteus medius m.

Quadratus femoris m.

Gluteus maximus m.

Pectineus m.

Adductor brevis m.

Adductor longus m.

Biceps m. (short head)

Vastus lateralis m.

Vastus medialis m.

Adductor magnus m.

Gastrocnemius m.

Sartorius, gracilis, semitendinosus mm.

Biceps femoris m.

3

Gluteal muscles and external rotators

Greater trochanter

Fracture, upper 1/3

Iliopsoas m.

Lesser trochanter

Adductor muscles

Hamstring muscles

Fracture below shaft

4

Gluteal muscles and external rotators

Fracture middle 1/3

Iliopsoas m.

Adductor mm.

Pectineus m.

Adductor brev. m.

Adductor long. m.

Adductor magnus m.

Hamstring muscles

Fracture, mid shaft

exposes the aponeurosis of the vastus intermedius. Incision through this aponeurosis and the periosteum exposes the femoral shaft.

In the *anterolateral approach* to the femoral shaft, the vastus lateralis is first separated from the rectus femoris. After this muscular separation, a neurovascular bundle is exposed in the upper portion of this muscular interval (Fig. 2). This bundle consisting of the nerve to the vastus lateralis and the lateral femoral circumflex vessels is carefully retracted. Incision is made through the aponeurosis of the vastus intermedius and periosteum. The femur may then be exposed by stripping the periosteum from the bone.

In an *anterior approach* to the femoral shaft care must be taken not to extend the lower portion of the incision through the vastus intermedius more than three fingers' breadth above the base of the patella. Such a precaution is necessary to prevent penetration into the suprapatellar extension of the synovial sheath of the knee (Fig. 7, page 313).

The femoral shaft may also be exposed by a *posterior approach*. After the fascia lata is incised an incision is placed lateral to the biceps femoris muscle along the posterior surface of the lateral intermuscular septum. The periosteal incision *must* be made close to the lateral intermuscular septum's bony insertion on the femur. It should be recalled that the blood supply of the posterior compartment comes from the perforating branches of the profunda femoris artery. These vessels enter the compartment by piercing the adductor magnus close to the medial border of the femur (Fig. 3). The sciatic nerve and its branches are protected by medial retraction of the biceps femoris muscle (Fig. 4, page 283).

13. **Veins of the Lower Extremity** — two systems of veins drain the lower extremity, a deep and a superficial system. The *deep veins* accompany the major arteries of the limb and lie beneath the deep fascia. They are named according to the artery they accompany. From the foot to the knee, two veins accompany each artery (venae comitantes). Above the knee, with the exception of the posterior thigh, a single vein accompanies the artery. They communicate with each other and with the superficial veins.

The superficial veins are referred to as the *saphenous venous system*. This is made up of the greater saphenous and lesser saphenous veins. The anatomic considerations of these vessels are discussed on pages 276, 292, and 294. Both vessels arise from the dorsal venous plexus of the foot. The *lesser saphenous vein*

passes behind the lateral malleolus, ascends through the calf, and terminates in the popliteal vein. The *greater saphenous vein* ascends in front of the medial malleolus of the tibia, proceeds through the subcutaneous tissue of the lower extremity, and drains into the common femoral vein. In the upper thigh, it receives the lateral and medial femoral cutaneous veins as well as the superficial epigastric, superficial external pudendal, and superficial circumflex iliac tributaries.

Several clinical features are important in regard to these vessels. The knowledge that the greater saphenous vein has a *constant* position anterior to the medial malleolus may be life-saving when emergency infusion or transfusion is indicated. Regardless of how young or how old or how thin or how obese an individual may be or how distended or how collapsed this vein may be, it can always be exposed by a cut-down at this site.

One of the most common afflictions of humans is the dilatation, elongation, and sacculation of the saphenous veins referred to as *varicose veins*. The essential cause of this entity is an increased back-pressure within these vessels. The contributing causes have been attributed to an hereditary defect of the valvular mechanism, an occupational hazard, proximal venous obstruction (as in pregnancy or pelvic tumors), or thrombosis of the deep veins of the lower extremity.

Because of these varicosities, stagnation of the blood flow in the skin of the lower limb results. This poor nutrition can lead to a breakdown of the skin of the leg even after minor trauma, thus producing a *varicose ulcer*. These ulcers are particularly prone to occur over the anteromedial surface of the tibia where even in the normal individual the blood supply is meager.

As is true with other common afflictions of the human body, the treatment of varicose veins is still quite variable and controversial. In determining necessary treatment, however, certain information about the functional anatomy of the saphenous system must be determined. The first principle is to rule out any possible proximal obstruction of the inferior caval system. A second principle is to determine which part of the venous system of the lower extremity is incompetent. Various compression tests are available to determine the latter. It is of particular importance to determine the competency of the communication between the superficial and deep veins, i.e., the *perforating veins*. If these valves are incompetent then little is achieved unless they are located, ligated, and divided regardless of what procedures are performed upon the greater saphenous vein.

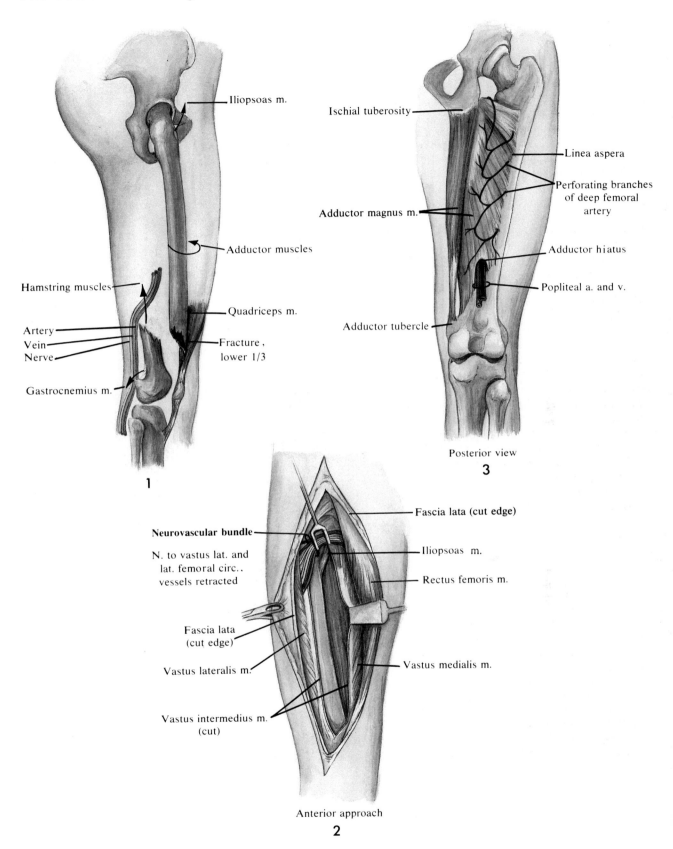

Iliopsoas m.

Adductor muscles

Hamstring muscles

Quadriceps m.

Artery
Vein
Nerve

Fracture,
lower 1/3

Gastrocnemius m.

1

Ischial tuberosity

Linea aspera

Perforating branches
of deep femoral
artery

Adductor magnus m.

Adductor hiatus

Popliteal a. and v.

Adductor tubercle

Posterior view
3

Fascia lata (cut edge)

Neurovascular bundle

Iliopsoas m.

N. to vastus lat. and
lat. femoral circ..
vessels retracted

Rectus femoris m.

Fascia lata
(cut edge)

Vastus lateralis m.

Vastus medialis m.

Vastus intermedius m.
(cut)

Anterior approach
2

THE POPLITEAL SPACE:

The *popliteal space (fossa)* is the transitional area between the thigh and leg located behind the knee joint. When the knee is flexed, the space presents as a hollow but when extended a bulge is produced by the fatty tissue contained in the fossa. With removal of the roof, the space appears as a rhomboid area possessing an upper femoral triangle and a lower tibial triangle.

1. **Boundaries** — the *roof* is composed of skin, superficial fascia, and deep (popliteal) fascia. The tendon of the biceps femoris muscle forms the *superiolateral wall*; and the tendons of the semimembranosus and semitendinosus constitute the *superiomedial wall*. The *inferiolateral* and *inferiomedial walls* are formed by the lateral and medial heads of the gastrocnemius muscle. From superior to inferior the *floor* is formed by the popliteal surface of the femur, the capsule of the knee joint, and the popliteus muscle. The *popliteus muscle* is triangular with its apex arising from the lateral epicondyle of the femur and its base inserting onto the popliteal line of the tibia. It is innervated by the tibial nerve and serves to flex and medially rotate the leg.

2. **Contents** — aside from the posterior femoral cutaneous nerve, the lesser saphenous vein, fatty tissue, and lymph nodes, the popliteal space contains the popliteal nerves and their rami, the popliteal vein and its tributaries, and the popliteal artery and its branches.

a. POSTERIOR FEMORAL CUTANEOUS NERVE — lies in the superficial fascia and has already been described on page 274.

b. LESSER (SMALL) SAPHENOUS VEIN — lies in the superficial fascia at the lower angle of the space. It begins from the lateral side of the venous arch on the dorsum of the foot. It ascends behind the lateral malleolus along the posterior aspect of the calf and, at the lower part of the popliteal space, pierces the deep fascia and empties into the popliteal vein (Fig. 1).

c. POPLITEAL NERVES (Fig. 1) — are the terminal divisions of the sciatic nerve. The *tibial (medial popliteal) nerve* within the space lies superficial in position and descends in the midline in a vertical direction. In the space it gives rise to several articular branches to the knee joint and a cutaneous branch, the *medial sural nerve*. The *common peroneal (lateral popliteal) nerve* extends along the medial border of the biceps tendon and at the lateral angle leaves the popliteal space crossing the plantaris muscle and the lateral head of the gastrocnemius. It gives off no muscular branches at this level but gives rise to articular branches to the knee and a cutaneous branch, the *lateral sural nerve*. The latter joins the medial sural branch of the tibial to form the *sural nerve*, which descends behind the lateral malleolus of the fibula and innervates the skin on the lateral aspect of the dorsum of the foot.

d. POPLITEAL VEIN (Figs. 1 and 2) — lies anterior and slightly medial to the tibial nerve within the space. It is formed at the lower border of the popliteus muscle by the confluence of the venae comitantes of the anterior and posterior tibial arteries. It ascends through the space and enters the adductor hiatus where it becomes the superficial femoral vein. The main tributary is the lesser saphenous, but it also receives from the lateral and medial surfaces *accessory popliteal veins*, which are common trunks of the sural and articular veins.

e. POPLITEAL ARTERY (Figs. 1, 2, and 3) — begins at the adductor hiatus as a continuation of the superficial femoral artery and terminates at the lower border of the popliteus muscle by dividing into an anterior and a posterior tibial artery. It is the deepest structure in the popliteal space. In addition to its two terminal branches, the popliteal artery gives rise to five important genicular arteries. These are the *superior medial, superior lateral, inferior medial, inferior lateral,* and *middle genicular arteries*. The branches enter into the formation of the patellar anastomosis.

f. PATELLAR ANASTOMOSIS (Fig. 3) — is formed by the communication of branches of the popliteal artery with those of the femoral artery. It forms the collateral pathway after ligation of the popliteal artery. The superior and inferior genicular arteries wind around the bones to the front of the knee and anastomose with each other. From above on the lateral side, the descending branch of the lateral femoral circumflex joins this anastomosis, while on the medial side the supreme genicular branch of the superficial femoral enters into it. From below, the anterior tibial recurrent artery contributes to it. Despite the apparent extensive collateral pathway, sudden ligation or occulsion results in gangrene in a high percentage of cases.

3. **Clinical Consideration** — in examining a swelling in the region of the popliteal space one should think anatomically in considering the differential diagnosis. It may be due to a tumor of the soft tissue, such as a lipoma or sarcoma. It could be a swelling related to the tendons or their bursa — a tendinitis or bursitis. The lump may be due to a localized varicosity of the lesser saphenous vein. An aneurysm of the popliteal artery may be the cause of a lump in this area. A joint effusion may present itself in this space, particularly in those cases of herniation of the synovial membrane through the joint capsule (Baker's cyst).

Because of the anterior-posterior relationship of the artery and vein, an arteriovenous fistula may result following a penetrating wound to this region.

The popliteal space may best be examined by placing the patient in a face-down position on the table with the knee in flexion. This maneuver relaxes the strong popliteal fascia and permits palpation of the contents of the popliteal space.

a. SURGICAL EXPOSURE OF THE POPLITEAL SPACE — may be necessary for the removal of malignant or benign tumors or in the treatment of an arteriovenous fistula, aneurysm, or injury to the popliteal vessels.

A *posterior approach* may be used as shown in Figures 4 and 5. A skin incision is made along the superior medial boundary of the space, extended laterally in line with the skin fold, and then inferiorly over the lateral head of the gastrocnemius. Retraction of the muscle boundaries expose the contents of the space. The retraction must be done with care so as not to injure the neural and vascular structures.

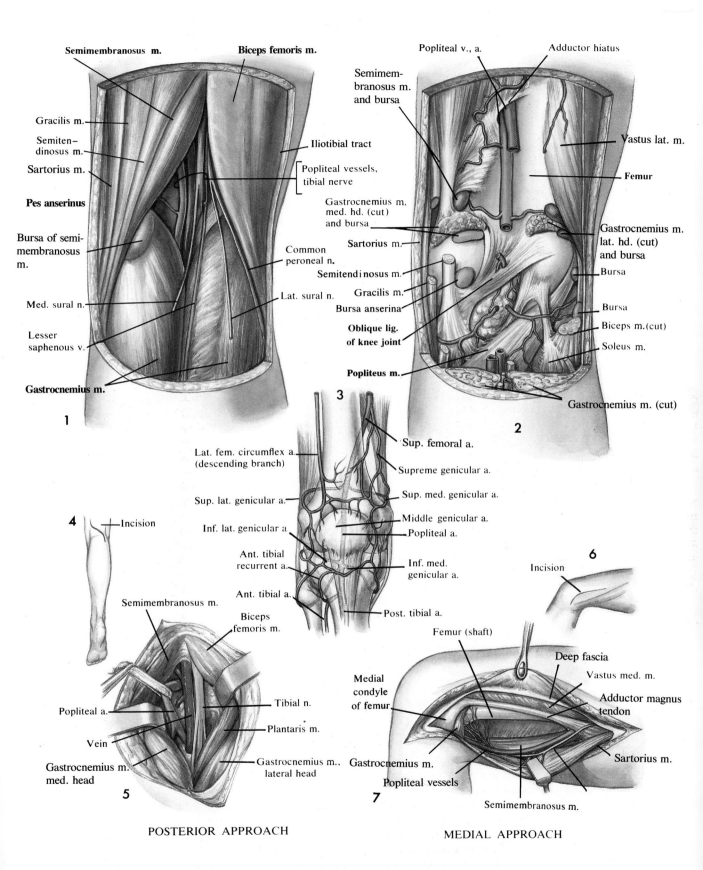

1

Semimembranosus m.

Biceps femoris m.

Gracilis m.

Semitendinosus m.

Sartorius m.

Pes anserinus

Bursa of semimembranosus m.

Med. sural n.

Lesser saphenous v.

Gastrocnemius m.

Iliotibial tract

Popliteal vessels, tibial nerve

Common peroneal n.

Lat. sural n.

2

Popliteal v., a.

Adductor hiatus

Semimembranosus m. and bursa

Gastrocnemius m. med. hd. (cut) and bursa

Sartorius m.

Semitendinosus m.

Gracilis m.

Bursa anserina

Oblique lig. of knee joint

Popliteus m.

Vastus lat. m.

Femur

Gastrocnemius m. lat. hd. (cut) and bursa

Bursa

Bursa

Biceps m.(cut)

Soleus m.

Gastrocnemius m. (cut)

3

Lat. fem. circumflex a. (descending branch)

Sup. femoral a.

Supreme genicular a.

Sup. lat. genicular a.

Sup. med. genicular a.

Inf. lat. genicular a

Middle genicular a.

Popliteal a.

Ant. tibial recurrent a.

Inf. med. genicular a.

Ant. tibial a.

Post. tibial a.

4

Incision

5

Semimembranosus m.

Biceps femoris m.

Popliteal a.

Tibial n.

Vein

Plantaris m.

Gastrocnemius m. med. head

Gastrocnemius m., lateral head

POSTERIOR APPROACH

6

Incision

7

Femur (shaft)

Deep fascia

Vastus med. m.

Adductor magnus tendon

Medial condyle of femur

Sartorius m.

Gastrocnemius m.

Popliteal vessels

Semimembranosus m.

MEDIAL APPROACH

The *medial approach* is popular for exposure of the popliteal artery (Figs. 6 and 7). The thigh is flexed, abducted, and laterally rotated and the knee placed in a flexed position. The incision is made just behind the adductor magnus tendon in a curved manner as illustrated.

THE LEG:

The leg extends between the knee and the ankle. Parts of both bones of the leg produce eminences and can be palpated in their subcutaneous position. The *head* of the fibula produces an eminence in the upper lateral part of the leg and the *lateral malleolus* in the lower lateral aspect of the ankle. The lower third of the fibular shaft is readily palpable beneath the skin. The entire anterior border of the tibia *(the shin)* presents a midline eminence at the upper portion of which the *tibial tuberosity* may be palpated. The entire antero-medial surface of the tibia is superficial in position and the lower portion of the surface produces an eminence at the medial aspect of the ankle, the *medial malleolus.* At its upper extremity the medial and lateral tibial condyles may be palpated.

The *patellar tendon* extending from the apex of the patella to the tibial tuberosity is prominent at the upper anterior surface of the leg. This tendon is the common insertion for the quadriceps muscles (page 312). At the inferior aspect of the posterior surface of the leg the *calcaneal (Achilles) tendon* is a distinct topo-graphical landmark. This tendon attaches to the cal-caneus and is a common tendon for the superficial muscles of the posterior compartment of the leg. The major portion of this same superficial muscle group produces posteriorly the major muscular eminence of the leg *(the calf).*

1. **Superficial Fascia** — in the subcutaneous tissue of the leg, branches of the saphenous system of veins and the major branches of the cutaneous nerves are found.

a. SAPHENOUS VEINS — arise from the venous rete over the dorsum of the foot. The *great saphenous vein* passes over the medial malleolus and ascends through the leg about one finger's breadth medial to the medial border of the tibia. Its course through the thigh and its termination in the common femoral vein is illustrated in Figure 1, page 277. The *lesser (small) saphenous vein* passes behind the lateral malleolus, ascends over the posterior surface of the leg, and pierces the deep fascia to empty into the popliteal vein. Numerous venous channels join these two major veins.

b. CUTANEOUS NERVES OF THE LEG — are branches of both the lumbar and sacral plexuses. The cutaneous supply of the anterior aspect of the leg is supplied mainly by the *saphenous nerve.* This is a branch of the deep femoral and is distributed over the anteromedial surface from the region of the knee to the ankle. The upper anterolateral surface is supplied by branches from the *lateral sural branch* of the common peroneal nerve. The lower anterolateral surface is innervated by the cutaneous portion of the *superficial peroneal nerve.* The posterior surface of the leg is supplied by the *sural nerve* with components from both the *tibial* and *common peroneal nerves.* Branches from the saphenous and posterior femoral cutaneous nerves also innervate this area.

2. **Deep Fascia and Muscular Compartments** — the musculature of the leg is encased in a strong fascial sheath termed the *crural fascia.* From this sheath two intermuscular septa arise dividing the leg into three muscular compartments: a posterior (flexor) compart-ment, an anterior (extensor) compartment, and a lateral (peroneal) compartment.

3. **Posterior (Flexor) Compartment** (Figs. 1, 2, and 3) — contains two groups of muscles: a superficial and a deep group, with three muscles to each group. The superficial group consists of the gastrocnemius, soleus, and plantaris, while the deep group consists of the flexor hallucis longus, flexor digitorum longus, and tibialis posterior. All these muscles are innervated by the posterior tibial nerve.

a. GASTROCNEMIUS — arises as a lateral and a medial head from the femur and the capsule of the knee. It inserts upon the posterior surface of the calcaneus.

b. SOLEUS — arises from the tibia and fibula and inserts in common with the gastrocnemius into the calcaneus by the calcaneal (Achilles) tendon.

c. PLANTARIS — takes origin from the posterior surface of the lateral epicondyle. Its muscle belly is very short and its tendon very long. The tendon in the lower leg becomes incorporated into the calcaneal tendon.

The muscles of the superficial group act chiefly to flex the knee and plantarflex the foot.

d. FLEXOR HALLUCIS LONGUS — arises from the distal two-thirds of the posterior surface of the fibula and inserts on the distal phalanx of the big toe.

e. FLEXOR DIGITORUM LONGUS — takes origin from the posterior surface of the tibia and inserts on the base of the distal phalanges of the lateral four toes.

f. TIBIALIS POSTERIOR — arises from the posterior surface of the interosseous membrane and the adjacent surfaces of the tibia and fibula. It has an extensive insertion on the plantar surface of the tarsal and meta-tarsal bones as shown in Figure 4, page 301.

All three of these muscles of the deep group plantarflex and invert the foot. In addition, the long flexors flex the distal phalanges.

The neurovascular structures of the posterior compartment consist of the posterior tibial nerve, artery, and vein. The *tibial nerve* arises in the popliteal space as a terminal branch of the sciatic nerve. At this level it gives off articular, cutaneous, and muscular branches. The muscular branches at this level innervate the popliteus and the superficial muscles of the posterior compartment (gastrocnemius, soleus, and plantaris). The tibial nerve passes deep to the soleus, descends through the posterior compartment where it is termed the posterior tibial nerve, and innervates the deep group of muscles. In the lower third of the leg it lies medial to the calcaneal tendon covered only by skin and fascia. Between the medial malleolus and cal-caneus the nerve terminates by dividing into the medial and lateral plantar nerves.

The *posterior tibial artery* is the larger of the two terminal branches of the popliteal artery. This division occurs at the lower border of the popliteus muscle. The posterior tibial artery then extends through the pos-terior compartment along with the posterior tibial nerve.

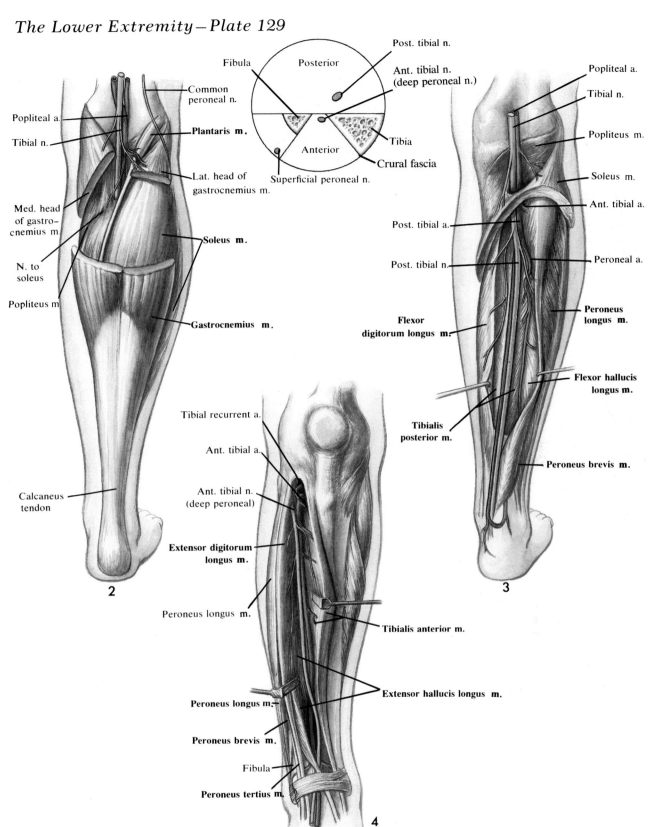

1. Post. tibial n.

Fibula
Posterior
Ant. tibial n.
(deep peroneal n.)

Common
peroneal n.

Popliteal a.

Tibial n.

Plantaris m.

Med. head
of gastro-
cnemius m

N. to
soleus

Popliteus m

Lat. head of
gastrocnemius m.

Tibia

Crural fascia

Superficial peroneal n.

Anterior

Soleus m.

Gastrocnemius m.

Calcaneus
tendon

2

Popliteal a.

Tibial n.

Popliteus m.

Soleus m.

Ant. tibial a.

Post. tibial a.

Post. tibial n.

Peroneal a.

**Peroneus
longus m.**

**Flexor
digitorum longus m.**

**Flexor hallucis
longus m.**

**Tibialis
posterior m.**

Peroneus brevis m.

3

Tibial recurrent a.

Ant. tibial a.

Ant. tibial n.
(deep peroneal)

**Extensor digitorum
longus m.**

Peroneus longus m.

Tibialis anterior m.

Extensor hallucis longus m.

Peroneus longus m.

Peroneus brevis m.

Fibula

Peroneus tertius m.

4

Like the nerve, it terminates by dividing into a medial and a lateral plantar branch. In addition to a muscular, a communicating, and a nutrient tibial branch, the posterior tibial gives off the *peroneal artery*. This artery descends along the medial margin of the fibula and sends branches to adjacent muscles including those of the lateral (peroneal) compartment. The arteries of the posterior compartments are accompanied by venae comitantes.

4. Lateral (Peroneal) Compartment (Figs. 1, 3, and 4)—contains two muscles both of which act to evert and plantarflex the foot. They are innervated by the superficial peroneal nerve.

a. PERONEUS LONGUS—arises from the upper half of the lateral surface of the fibula and adjacent intermuscular septa. Its tendon passes behind the lateral malleolus and inserts on the cuneiform and base of the first metatarsal on the sole of the foot.

b. PERONEUS BREVIS—takes origin from the middle third of the lateral surface of the fibula and inserts on the base of the fifth metatarsal.

The motor nerve to the musculature of this compartment is the *superficial peroneal nerve,* a branch of the common peroneal. The latter arises in the popliteal space where it gives rise to articular and cutaneous rami. It leaves the space by crossing the lateral head of the gastrocnemius, winds around the neck of the fibula, and enters the lateral compartment (Fig. 6). Here the common peroneal divides into a *recurrent articular branch* to the knee joint, a *deep peroneal (anterior tibial) nerve,* which immediately enters the anterior compartment, and the *superficial peroneal nerve.* This last nerve descends along the shaft of the fibula and at the junction of the middle and lower thirds of the leg pierces the deep fascia and is distributed to the skin of the lateral aspect of the leg and dorsum of the foot.

5. **Anterior (Extensor) Compartment** (Figs. 1 and 4, page 295)—there are three muscles contained in this compartment: the tibialis anterior, extensor digitorum longus, and extensor hallucis lungus. All these muscles dorsiflex the foot. The long extensors also extend the metatarsophalangeal and interphalangeal joints. The deep peroneal (anterior tibial) nerve is the motor nerve of the anterior compartment.

a. TIBIALIS ANTERIOR—arises from the proximal half of the lateral surface of the tibia and the interosseous membrane. Its tendon attaches to the medial surface of the first cuneiform and the base of the first metatarsal. It acts to dorsiflex and invert the foot.

b. EXTENSOR DIGITORUM LONGUS—lies superficial in the compartment along with the tibialis anterior. It arises from the upper three-fourths of the anterior surface of the fibula and adjacent interosseous membrane. Its tendons insert on the distal phalanges of the lateral four toes. A special portion of this muscle arising from the lower third of the fibula may be present and is termed the *peroneus tertius.* It inserts on the base of the fifth metatarsal. The muscle extends the metatarsophalangeal and interphalangeal joints and also aids in eversion of the foot.

c. EXTENSOR HALLUCIS LONGUS—lies deep in the compartment. Its origin is from the middle half of the fibula and its insertion is on the base of the distal phalanx of the big toe.

The neurovascular bundle of the anterior compartment contains the anterior tibial nerve and blood vessels (Fig. 4, page 295). The bundle begins in the upper leg in the muscular interval between the tibialis anterior medially and the extensor digitorum longus laterally. It lies on the interosseous membrane, and in the distal portion of the leg the bundle is crossed by the extensor hallucis longus.

The *anterior tibial (deep peroneal)* nerve arises as a branch of the common peroneal in the lateral compartment (Fig. 6). It pierces the extensor digitorum longus to enter the anterior compartment where it joins the anterior tibial artery and follows the course of the neurovascular bundle as previously described. During its course it gives rise to branches to the three muscles of the anterior compartment and to articular branches to the ankle joint. The anterior tibial nerve terminates on the dorsum of the foot by dividing into a *lateral*

terminal branch, which innervates the extensor digitorum brevis, and a *medial terminal branch,* which gives rise to the dorsal digital nerves on the adjacent sides of the first and second toes (Fig. 1, page 299). Anesthesia in this area is an early indication of anterior tibial nerve injury.

The *anterior tibial artery* arises as a terminal branch of the popliteal artery about 1.5 cm. below the popliteus muscle. At this point it passes above the interosseous membrane into the anterior compartment. An *anterior* and *posterior tibial recurrent* branch arise early and enters the patellar anastomosis (page 292). Muscular branches are given off during its descent through the leg, and *medial* and *lateral malleolar branches* in the lower leg. As the vessel passes anterior to the ankle joint, it becomes superficial and is referred to as the *dorsalis pedis artery.* Vena comitantes accompany the anterior tibial artery.

The origin of the muscles of the leg and insertions of some of the muscles of the thigh upon the tibia and fibula are illustrated in Figures 1 and 2.

6. **Clinical Considerations**—the superficial veins, bones, soft tissue of the leg, and neurovascular structures all are of clinical importance.

a. SAPHENOUS SYSTEM OF VEINS—has been discussed on pages 276, and 292, and their clinical significance on page 290.

b. COMPARTMENTAL EXPOSURE—may be required for a variety of pathological condition: for open reduction and nonunion of fractures, ostectomy for osteomyelitis of these bones, resection of benign tumors and, in the case of the tibia, for transplantation for bone grafts. Figure 3 illustrates the anatomical approach to the three compartments by anterior, medial, and posterolateral incisions. Acute compartment syndromes may be due to increased compartment contents from primary hemorrhage, edema, venous disease, soft tissue injuries, postischemic swelling from arterial thrombosis, embolism, and fractures. The decrease in compartment size may be due to constrictive casts, dressings, and tight closure of fascial defects. Diagnosis is established by the 6 Ps: Pain, Pressure, Pain with Stretch, Paresis, Paresthesia, and Pulses are present. The differential diagnosis should rule out arterial and nerve injuries. The treatment of choice is decompression by adequate fasciotomy.

c. COMMON PERONEAL (LATERAL POPLITEAL) NERVE—is most vulnerable to injury because of its superficial position as it winds around the neck of the fibula. It is particularly vulnerable in operative exposure of the proximal fibula (Fig. 6), but it may also be injured by tight bandages and casts and in severe adduction injuries of the knee joint.

d. FRACTURES OF THE TIBIA AND FIBULA—are most common. Should the fracture be due to indirect injury, the tibia usually fractures at the junction of the middle and lower thirds, and the fibula at the junction of the middle and upper thirds. In a direct injury they usually fracture at the same site. Because of the subcutaneous position of both bones, particularly the tibia, a compound fracture may result.

e. AMPUTATIONS—of the leg when electively indicated are performed approximately 15 cm. below the knee (Fig. 7). This insures the most ideal leverage for a good prosthetic fitting.

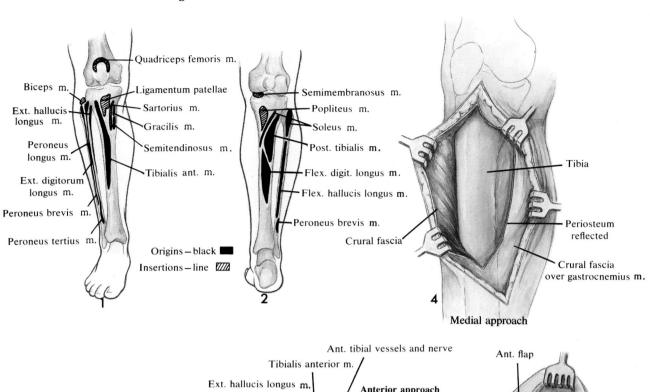

Quadriceps femoris m.

Biceps m.

Ligamentum patellae

Ext. hallucis longus m.

Sartorius m.

Gracilis m.

Peroneus longus m.

Semitendinosus m.

Ext. digitorum longus m.

Tibialis ant. m.

Peroneus brevis m.

Peroneus tertius m.

Semimembranosus m.

Popliteus m.

Soleus m.

Post. tibialis m.

Flex. digit. longus m.

Flex. hallucis longus m.

Peroneus brevis m.

Crural fascia

Origins — black ■
Insertions — line ▨

2

Tibia

Periosteum reflected

Crural fascia over gastrocnemius m.

4

Medial approach

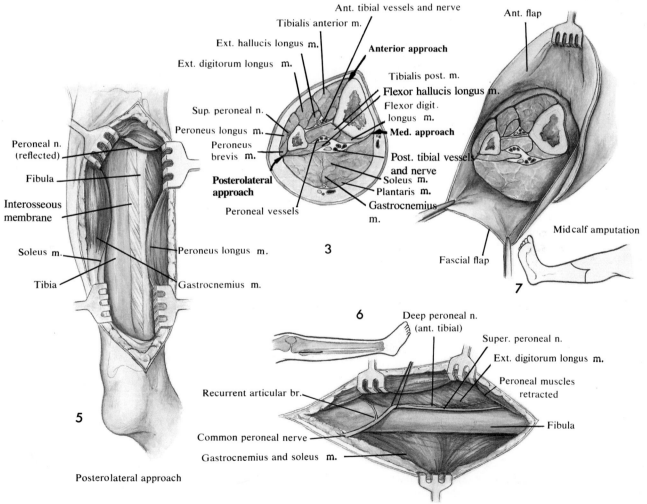

Ant. tibial vessels and nerve

Tibialis anterior m.

Ext. hallucis longus m.

Ext. digitorum longus m.

Anterior approach

Sup. peroneal n.

Peroneus longus m.

Peroneus brevis m.

Posterolateral approach

Peroneal vessels

Tibialis post. m.

Flexor hallucis longus m.

Flexor digit. longus m.

Med. approach

Post. tibial vessels and nerve

Soleus m.

Plantaris m.

Gastrocnemius m.

3

Ant. flap

Midcalf amputation

Fascial flap

7

Peroneal n. (reflected)

Fibula

Interosseous membrane

Soleus m.

Tibia

Peroneus longus m.

Gastrocnemius m.

5

Posterolateral approach

6

Deep peroneal n. (ant. tibial)

Super. peroneal n.

Ext. digitorum longus m.

Peroneal muscles retracted

Recurrent articular br.

Fibula

Common peroneal nerve

Gastrocnemius and soleus m.

Exposure of upper ⅓ of fibula

THE FOOT:

The foot may be considered as that part of the body topographically located below a line drawn through the tips of the malleoli of the tibia and fibula. A dorsal and a plantar surface may be described.

1. **Dorsum of the Foot** — the skin and superficial fascia over the dorsum of the foot are thin, and the deep fascia is not thickened. For this reason many of the superficial and deep structures are visible and palpable in this area, and dependent edema is prone to present itself early in this location.

a. SUPERFICIAL VEINS — of the dorsum of the foot begin as *dorsal digital veins* and form the *dorsal metatarsal veins*. These join to form the *dorsal venous arch*. Communicating veins between the two sides of the arch form the *dorsal venous rete*. From this rete arise the *greater* and *lesser saphenous veins* (Fig. 1).

b. SUPERFICIAL NERVE SUPPLY — to the dorsal surface of the foot is made up chiefly of the *superficial peroneal nerve*, a branch of the common peroneal (Fig. 6, page 297). As illustrated in Figure 1, this nerve supplies practically the entire dorsum of the foot except for a small area between the first and second toes, which is innervated by the *deep peroneal nerve*. On the lateral side of the foot the *sural nerve* contributes a *lateral dorsal cutaneous ramus*. Medially the *saphenous branch of the femoral nerve* contributes to the innervation of the skin of this area (Fig. 1).

c. DEEP FASCIA (Figs. 2 and 3) — in the region of the ankle the crural fascia is thickened to form several important ligaments which serve to retain in position certain of the tendons that pass from the leg to the foot. These are described as the extensor and peroneal retinacula, each of which is subdivided into a superior and an inferior portion. The *extensor retinaculum* consists of a superior *transverse crural ligament* extending between the tibia and fibula. From its deep surface a strong septum extends to the tibia dividing the underlying space into two osseofibrous canals: one medial for the passage of the tibialis anterior, the other lateral for passage of the long extensor tendons (Fig. 2). The inferior portion of the extensor retinaculum is termed the *cruciate ligament*. This ligament restrains the extensor tendons as shown in Figure 2.

The *superior peroneal retinaculum* extends from the lateral malleolus to the calcaneus, and the *inferior peroneal retinaculum* attaches to the lateral surface of the calcaneus (Fig. 3). These ligaments serve to hold the peroneus longus and brevis muscles in place.

A third ligamentous thickening of crural fascia is known as the *flexor retinaculum* or *laciniate ligament*. This is found on the medial side of the ankle extending from the medial malleolus to the calcaneus (Fig. 4).

d. EXTRINSIC MUSCLES OF THE DORSUM OF THE FOOT — extend from the leg to their insertion on the foot. In front of the ankle, deep to the extensor retinaculum, the tibialis anterior is most medial, passing to its insertion on the base of the first metatarsal and first cuneiform. Lateral to this tendon are the tendons of the extensor hallucis longus and extensor digitorum longus, which are readily visible in the dorsiflexed foot (Fig. 2). The peroneus longus and brevis pass behind the lateral malleolus. Behind the medial malleolus and deep to the flexor retinaculum, the deep flexor muscles of the posterior compartment of the leg with their accompanying neurovascular bundle enter the foot and extend into the plantar surface. From anterior to posterior these structures are the *t*ibialis anterior, flexor *d*igitorum longus, posterior tibial *v*ein, posterior tibial *a*rtery, posterior tibial *v*ein, posterior tibial *n*erve, and flexor *h*allucis longus (*T*im *d*oth *v*ex *a* *v*ery *n*ervous *h*orse — a convenient way of remembering these relationships) (Fig. 4).

e. INTRINSIC MUSCLES OF THE DORSUM OF THE FOOT — consist of but a single muscle, the *extensor digitorum brevis*. This muscle arises from the calcaneus and inserts by separate tendons onto the proximal phalanges of each of the toes. It is innervated by the deep peroneal (anterior tibial) nerve. It aids in the extension of the toes.

f. NEUROVASCULAR STRUCTURES — are the terminal branches of the anterior tibial artery and nerve. The *anterior tibial (deep peroneal) nerve* terminates by dividing in the foot into a medial branch that provides dorsal digital branches supplying adjacent sides of the first and second toes (Fig. 1). A lateral terminal branch supplies the extensor digitorum brevis.

The *anterior tibial artery* continues into the dorsum of the foot as the *dorsalis pedis artery*. It is palpable between the tendons of the extensor hallucis longus and extensor digitorum longus over the dorsum of the foot. Absence of the pulsation of this artery does not always imply vascular insufficiency. In about 15 per cent of normal individuals it may be absent. The dorsalis pedis artery gives rise to a medial and a lateral tarsal branch and descends over the dorsum to the level of the base of the first metatarsal where the *arcuate artery* arises. The latter runs laterally across the dorsum of the foot and gives rise to the second, third, and fourth *dorsal metatarsal arteries*. The dorsalis pedis artery terminates in the first interosseous space by dividing into the *first dorsal metatarsal artery* and the *deep plantar artery*, the latter entering the plantar arch.

2. **Plantar Surface of the Foot** — the anatomy of the plantar surface of the foot is very similar to the anatomy of the palm of the hand, for they are embryological counterparts. The major differences are: (1) an opponens muscle of the big toe is lacking; (2) there is an additional intrinsic muscle in the foot (quadratus plantae); (3) the lumbrical muscle innervation differs; and (4) the axis of action of the interosseous muscles is on the second toe, whereas in the palm the axis is the middle finger.

The skin overlying the heel, lateral surface, and ball of the toe is greatly thickened because these are weight-bearing areas. The remainder of the skin is highly sensitive and contains numerous sweat glands. The superficial fascia is also thickened over these weight-bearing surfaces.

a. DEEP FASCIA (Fig. 5) — of the plantar surface of the foot (*plantar fascia*) is similar to the palmar fascia of the hand (page 68). It is divided into three parts: a *medial plantar fascia* covering the intrinsic muscles of the big

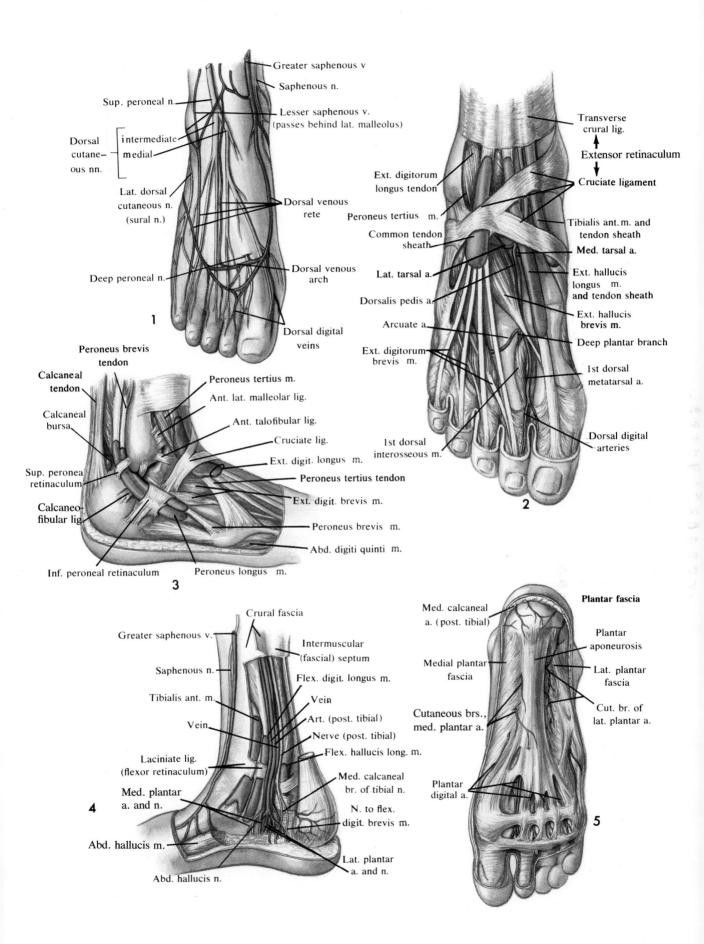

1

Greater saphenous v
Saphenous n.
Sup. peroneal n.
Lesser saphenous v.
(passes behind lat. malleolus)
Dorsal cutaneous nn. { intermediate / medial }
Lat. dorsal cutaneous n. (sural n.)
Dorsal venous rete
Deep peroneal n.
Dorsal venous arch
Dorsal digital veins

2

Transverse crural lig.
Extensor retinaculum
Cruciate ligament
Ext. digitorum longus tendon
Peroneus tertius m.
Common tendon sheath
Lat. tarsal a.
Dorsalis pedis a.
Arcuate a.
Ext. digitorum brevis m.
1st dorsal interosseous m.
Tibialis ant. m. and tendon sheath
Med. tarsal a.
Ext. hallucis longus m. and tendon sheath
Ext. hallucis brevis m.
Deep plantar branch
1st dorsal metatarsal a.
Dorsal digital arteries

3

Peroneus brevis tendon
Calcaneal tendon
Calcaneal bursa
Sup. peroneal retinaculum
Calcaneo-fibular lig.
Inf. peroneal retinaculum
Peroneus longus m.
Peroneus tertius m.
Ant. lat. malleolar lig.
Ant. talofibular lig.
Cruciate lig.
Ext. digit. longus m.
Peroneus tertius tendon
Ext. digit. brevis m.
Peroneus brevis m.
Abd. digiti quinti m.

4

Crural fascia
Greater saphenous v.
Saphenous n.
Tibialis ant. m.
Vein
Laciniate lig. (flexor retinaculum)
Med. plantar a. and n.
Abd. hallucis m.
Abd. hallucis n.
Intermuscular (fascial) septum
Flex. digit. longus m.
Vein
Art. (post. tibial)
Nerve (post. tibial)
Flex. hallucis long. m.
Med. calcaneal br. of tibial n.
N. to flex. digit. brevis m.
Lat. plantar a. and n.

5

Plantar fascia
Med. calcaneal a. (post. tibial)
Medial plantar fascia
Cutaneous brs., med. plantar a.
Plantar digital a.
Plantar aponeurosis
Lat. plantar fascia
Cut. br. of lat. plantar a.

toe (compare thenar fascia), a *lateral plantar fascia* over the muscles of the little toe (compare hypothenar fascia), and a thickened central portion, the *plantar aponeurosis* (compare palmar aponeurosis). The latter extends from the calcaneus and proceeds to each of the five toes. Each process inserts in part into the skin at the head of the metatarsal bones and into the fibrous tendinous sheaths of the digital tendons. From this aponeurosis vertical septa, the *lateral* and *medial intermuscular septa*, divide the sole of the foot into three compartments: medial, central, and lateral. The medial compartment contains the intrinsic muscles of the big toe and the lateral compartment contains the intrinsic muscles of the little toe. The central compartment is subdivided by transverse septa into four muscle layers.

b. PLANTAR MUSCLES—may be best described as being aligned in four layers. These intrinsic muscles of the sole primarily serve to support the longitudinal arches of the foot. Their action upon the digits is minimal except in aiding the long tendons in flexing the digits. Atrophy of these muscles due to aging or arthritic changes in the joints of the foot results in loss of support of the longitudinal arches, pronation of the foot, and postural strain from abnormal weight bearing.

The first layer of muscles (Fig. 1) consists of the *abductor hallucis* in the medial muscular compartment, the *abductor digiti quinti* in the lateral compartment, and the *flexor digitorum brevis* in the central compartment. They are important in maintaining support of the longitudinal arches. Their counterparts in the palm are the abductor pollicis brevis, the abductor digiti quinti, and the flexor digitorum sublimis.

The second layer of intrinsic muscles (Fig. 2) consists of the *quadratus plantae* (no counterpart in the hand) and the four *lumbrical muscles*. At this same level is the tendon of the *flexor digitorum longus* (flexor digitorum profundus), which sends a tendon to each of the lateral four toes, and the *flexor hallucis longus* (flexor pollicis longus), which inserts on the distal phalanx of the big toe. The lumbricals arise from the flexor digitorum longus tendon and insert on the medial side of the proximal phalanges. The quadratus plantae muscle arises from the calcaneus and inserts on the long digital flexor tendon. In addition to supporting the longitudinal arch it assists the long flexor muscle of the digit in aligning it on the digits parallel to the axis of the foot.

The third muscle layer (Fig. 3) is made up of the *flexor hallucis brevis*, the *flexor digiti quinti,* and the *adductor hallucis*. Each of these muscles has an equivalent in the palm. The flexor hallucis brevis arises from the tarsal bones. It has two bellies and two tendons that insert on either side of the base of the first phalanx. The tendon of the flexor hallucis longus passes between the tendons of the short flexor. The adductor hallucis (like its counterpart in the palm, the adductor pollicis) has an oblique and a transverse head. It inserts on the base of the proximal phalanx of the big toe. The flexor digiti

quinti inserts on the base of the proximal phalanx of the little toe.

The fourth layer of muscles of the plantar surface (Fig. 4) consists of the *interosseous muscles* of the foot. As in the hand, they consist of four *dorsal interossei* and three *plantar (volar) interossei muscles*. The axis of action of these muscles in the foot is the second toe, whereas in the hand these muscles act through the axis of the middle finger. The dorsal interossei abduct from and the plantar interossei adduct toward the axis of the second toe. At this same level, the insertion of the peroneus longus and tibialis posterior may be seen.

c. INNERVATION OF THE SOLE OF THE FOOT (Figs. 1, 2, 3, and 4)—is via the medial and lateral plantar nerves, the terminal branches of the tibial nerve. The medial plantar nerve has its equivalent in the medial nerve of the hand, and the lateral plantar nerve in the ulnar nerve.

The *lateral plantar nerve* arises at the lower border of the laciniate ligament and enters the sole deep to the abductor hallucis brevis. It supplies cutaneous branches to the little toe and the lateral half of the fourth toe (compare to ulnar cutaneous innervation of the palm). It supplies muscular branches to the abductor, flexor, and opponens digiti quinti, the quadratus plantae, the adductor hallucis, the lateral *three* lumbricals, and the interossei. It is the main muscular branch to the sole of the foot, as is its counterpart, the ulnar nerve, to the intrinsic muscles of the hand.

The *medial plantar nerve* supplies the cutaneous innervation to the medial three and one-half digits. Its motor fibers innervate the flexor digitorum brevis, the abductor hallucis brevis, the flexor hallucis brevis, and the first lumbrical muscle (compare with the median nerve innervation of the hand).

d. ARTERIAL SUPPLY OF THE SOLE OF THE FOOT (Figs. 1, 2, 3, and 4)—is carried by the terminal branches of the posterior tibial artery—the medial and lateral plantar arteries. These vessels along with their accompanying nerves emerge from the posterior tibial, into the sole deep to the abductor hallucis brevis muscle. The *medial plantar artery* is the smaller of these two terminal branches and, by way of a deep branch, supplies the muscle of the medial compartment. Its superficial branch sends small twigs that accompany the digital branches of the median plantar nerve. These twigs join the plantar metatarsal branches of the plantar arch. The *lateral plantar artery* accompanies the nerve of the same name to the lateral compartment of the foot. At the base of the first metatarsal bone, it sinks deep into the sole of the foot, bends medially, and anastomoses with the deep plantar branch of the dorsalis pedis to form the *plantar arch* (comparable to the deep volar arch of the palm). From this arch usually three *perforating branches* communicate with the dorsal metatarsal arteries. Four *plantar metatarsal arteries* also arise from the arch, each of which in turn gives rise to *plantar digital arteries*.

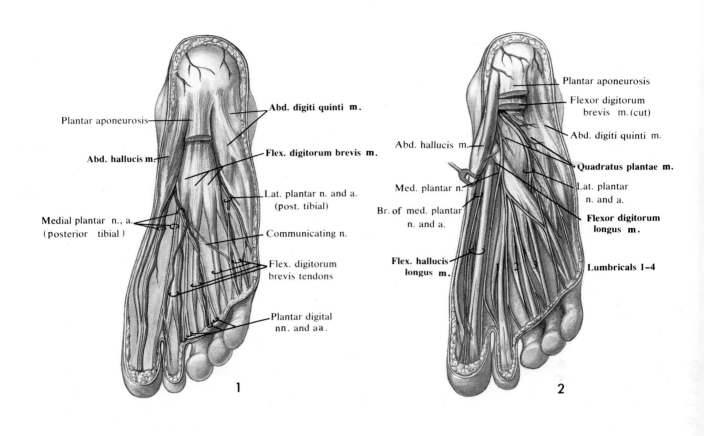

1

Plantar aponeurosis

Abd. hallucis m.

Medial plantar n., a.
(posterior tibial)

Abd. digiti quinti m.

Flex. digitorum brevis m.

Lat. plantar n. and a.
(post. tibial)

Communicating n.

Flex. digitorum
brevis tendons

Plantar digital
nn. and aa.

2

Plantar aponeurosis

Flexor digitorum
brevis m. (cut)

Abd. digiti quinti m.

Quadratus plantae m.

Lat. plantar
n. and a.

**Flexor digitorum
longus m.**

Lumbricals 1–4

Abd. hallucis m.

Med. plantar n.

Br. of med. plantar
n. and a.

**Flex. hallucis
longus m.**

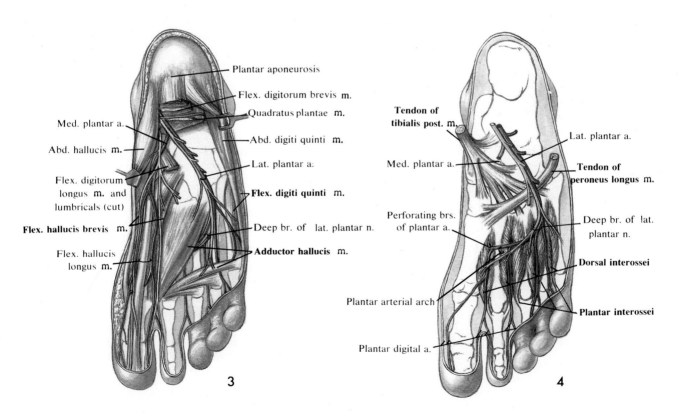

3

Med. plantar a.

Abd. hallucis m.

Flex. digitorum
longus m. and
lumbricals (cut)

Flex. hallucis brevis m.

Flex. hallucis
longus m.

Plantar aponeurosis

Flex. digitorum brevis m.

Quadratus plantae m.

Abd. digiti quinti m.

Lat. plantar a.

Flex. digiti quinti m.

Deep br. of lat. plantar n.

Adductor hallucis m.

4

**Tendon of
tibialis post. m.**

Med. plantar a.

Perforating brs.
of plantar a.

Plantar arterial arch

Plantar digital a.

Lat. plantar a.

**Tendon of
peroneus longus m.**

Deep br. of lat.
plantar n.

Dorsal interossei

Plantar interossei

CLINICAL CONSIDERATIONS OF THE FOOT:

The foot is probably the most overlooked structure of the human body in physical examination. Many common complaints arise from pathological changes in this anatomical area. These foot ailments are so common and so ignored by physicians that a nonmedical group, the podiatrists, is supported by this group of patients.

An obvious deformity is the congenital *club foot* or *talipes* (L., *talus*, an ankle, and *pes*, a foot) in which the patient walks on the outside of the foot. Infections *(osteomyelitis)* may affect the bones of the feet. Indolent painless ulcers *(mal perforant)* may affect the sole of the foot in the patient with syphilitic infection (tabes dorsalis). The heel is a frequent site of a *decubitus ulcer* resulting from mechanical pressure in bedridden patients. *Gangrene* of the toes is seen in the diabetic or arteriosclerotic patient. Aseptic necrosis *(osteochondritis)* of the navicular bone *(Kohler's disease)* or of the head of the second metatarsal *(Freiberg's disease)* is an obscure cause of foot pain and can be diagnosed by roentgen examination. A *plantar wart* is a common and extremely painful affliction affecting the sole of the foot.

Another common ailment of the foot is the *hammer toe*, a deformity of the second or third toe. It may be congenital or acquired as a result of wearing ill-fitting shoes. Another deformity that frequently results from the wearing of faulty footwear is *hallux valgus*. In this deformity the great toe is adducted toward the midline of the foot. When the bursa over the head of the first metatarsal becomes inflamed, a *bunion* will result. A *calcaneal spur* may produce a disabling pain in the heel. *Arthritis* of any variety may, of course, produce foot pain.

The most common cause of painful feet is faulty support of the arches. The longitudinal arch of the foot is flattened resulting in a *pronated (flat) foot*. The resultant postural strain may produce, in addition to the foot pain, night cramps in the leg and foot musculature and pain in the knee, hip, or lower back. Collapse of the transverse arch may result in *metatarsalgia (Morton's disease)*. The common digital branches of the medial plantar nerve become pinched between the heads of the metatarsal bones, resulting over a period of time in a neuroma. This usually involves the common digital nerve to the third and fourth toes.

1. **Arches of the Foot** — the entire weight of the body is supported by the foot. This weight is transmitted to the foot through the tibia to the talus, thence to the other bones of the foot. The bones are so constructed as to make up two arches — a longitudinal and a transverse arch.

a. LONGITUDINAL ARCH (Fig. 1) — is made up of two parts, a medial and a lateral section. The *medial longitudinal arch* consists of the talus, the navicular, the three cuneiform bones, the three medial metatarsals, and the corresponding phalanges. This arch because of its great convexity and elasticity sustains the violent impact of jumping and adds to the normal gait. The *lateral longitudinal arch* is made up of the calcaneus, the cuboid, the two lateral metatarsals, and the corresponding phalanges. This arch is less curved and more rigid and forms a firm support in the upright position. The main weight-bearing areas of this longitudinal arch are the calcaneus and the heads of the first and fifth metatarsal bones.

b. TRANSVERSE ARCH — is formed by the distal tarsal bones (the three cuneiform and cuboid bones) and the bases of the metatarsal bones. This arch is convex toward the dorsum of the foot.

c. SUPPORT OF THE ARCHES — is achieved by the bones of the foot, the plantar ligaments, the intrinsic muscles and fascia, and the extrinsic muscles. The *bones of the foot* are so shaped that they lend some strength to the arches. Several ligaments on the plantar surface aid in supporting the arches. The bones are held together by articular capsules and interosseous ligaments. In addition, four accessory ligaments are present (Fig. 2). The *long plantar ligament* extends from the calcaneus to the base of the lateral four metatarsal bones. The *short plantar (calcaneocuboid) ligament* binds the plantar surface of the calcaneus and cuboid. The *spring (plantar calcaneonavicular) ligament* is thick and elastic and is probably the most important supportive ligament of the foot. It extends from the sustentaculum tali to the plantar surface of the navicular. A *transverse capitular ligament* binds together the heads of the metatarsals and supports the transverse arch by preventing the spreading of these bones.

In addition to the bones and ligaments the arches are further supported by the plantar aponeurosis and the intrinsic muscles of the foot. The extrinsic muscles of the foot, particularly the peroneus longus, tibialis posterior, and tibialis anterior, contribute only by keeping the foot in proper balance between eversion and inversion.

2. **Amputations** (Fig. 1) — resection of a part of the foot may be necessary following trauma or in cases of cancer, arteriosclerosis, diabetes, or other peripheral vascular diseases affecting the phalanges or foot. Several levels are elective, two of which are illustrated in Figure 1. The *Lisfranc operation* transects the tarsal-metatarsal articulations. The *Chopart procedure* is a midtarsal amputation between the talus and navicular medially and the calcaneus and cuboid laterally.

3. **Surgical Approaches** (Figs. 3, 4, 5, and 6) — two approaches to the plantar surface of the foot are illustrated on the adjoining plate. In the *medial approach*, an incision is made through the skin and superficial fascia. The interval between the abductor hallucis and plantar aponeurosis and flexor digitorum brevis is then excised. In the *posterior approach* the calcaneus is

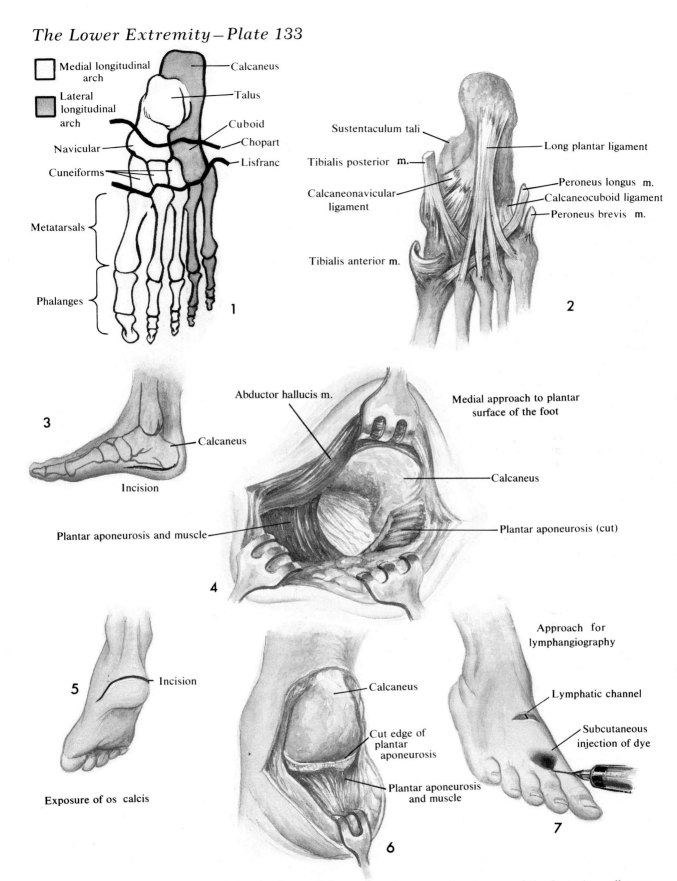

Medial longitudinal arch

Lateral longitudinal arch

Navicular

Cuneiforms

Metatarsals

Phalanges

Calcaneus

Talus

Cuboid

Chopart

Lisfranc

1

Sustentaculum tali

Tibialis posterior m.

Calcaneonavicular ligament

Tibialis anterior m.

Long plantar ligament

Peroneus longus m.

Calcaneocuboid ligament

Peroneus brevis m.

2

3

Calcaneus

Incision

Abductor hallucis m.

Medial approach to plantar surface of the foot

Calcaneus

Plantar aponeurosis (cut)

Plantar aponeurosis and muscle

4

5

Incision

Exposure of os calcis

Calcaneus

Cut edge of plantar aponeurosis

Plantar aponeurosis and muscle

6

Approach for lymphangiography

Lymphatic channel

Subcutaneous injection of dye

7

exposed and the plantar aponeurosis, the flexor digitorum brevis, and quadratus plantae muscles are stripped from the bone with an osteotome.

4. **Lymphangiography** (Fig. 7)—is now an accepted diagnostic procedure. A small amount of Evan's blue dye is injected subcutaneously between the first and second toes on the dorsum of the foot. A small transverse incision is made proximally over the medial venous arch. On careful dissection a lymphatic channel may be exposed and identified by the presence of the dye. This channel usually lies on the lateral side of the venous arch.

LYMPHATICS OF THE LOWER EXTREMITY:

As in other parts of the body, the lymphatics of the lower extremity begin as lymph capillaries in the tissue spaces. These capillaries empty into lymphatic vessels which drain the skin and subcutaneous tissue on one hand and the deep fascia, muscles, joints, and periosteum on the other. The lymphatic vessels drain into two sets of first echelon nodes in the lower extremity: the popliteal and inguinal lymph nodes.

1. **Popliteal Nodes** (Fig. 1) — are located in the fatty tissue of the popliteal space deep to the popliteal fascia. Three to six nodes constitute this group. They may be divided into anterior, middle, and posterior groups.

a. ANTERIOR GROUP — consists of a single node, the *juxta-articular node*, located anterior to the popliteal artery in relation to the middle genicular artery.

b. MIDDLE GROUP — includes three to four nodes located along the popliteal artery. A superior subgroup is located at the level of the superior genicular and an inferior subgroup at the level of the inferior genicular artery.

c. POSTERIOR GROUP — usually consists of an inconstant node, the *lateral saphenous node*, located lateral to the lesser saphenous vein at its entrance into the popliteal vein.

These nodes receive afferent lymph vessels from the deep and superficial lymphatic vessels of the leg and foot. Efferent channels from these nodes follow the femoral artery to the deep inguinal nodes (see below).

2. **Inguinal Nodes** (Fig. 2) — the principal nodes of the lower extremity are located in the upper region of the thigh in the area of the femoral triangle. They are divided into a superficial and a deep group. These nodes receive channels not only from the lower extremity, but from the lower abdominal wall, the gluteal region, and the perineum.

a. SUPERFICIAL INGUINAL NODES — vary in number; usually eight to 12 nodes are present lying in the superficial fascia. An arbitrary line drawn horizontally through the thigh at the level where the saphenous vein pierces the fascia lata divides this group into two subgroups. A superior nodal group, the *superficial inguinal nodes*, lies just beneath and parallel to the inguinal ligament. *Superficial subinguinal nodes* is the designation given those nodes of the inferior group.

A vertical line drawn upward in line with the saphenous vein to the inguinal ligament further divides the superior and inferior groups into medial and lateral subsidiary groups. As illustrated in Figure 2, the superficial lymphatics of the lower extremity drain into both the inferomedial and inferolateral group of superficial subinguinal nodes. Channels of the lower abdominal wall terminate in both the medial and lateral superficial inguinal nodes. Superficial lymphatics from the gluteal region terminate in the lateral group of nodes, and those from the perineal area drain into medial nodes of the superior and inferior groups of superficial inguinal and subinguinal nodes.

Efferent vessels from the superficial inguinal nodes pass to the lower external iliac nodes. From the superficial subinguinal nodes, vessels terminate in either the deep inguinal nodes or the lower external iliac nodes.

b. DEEP INGUINAL NODES — are located in the femoral canal medial to the femoral vein and average one to three in number (Fig. 3). The uppermost node is the most constant and is located at the femoral ring (*node of Cloquet* or *Rosenmüller*). These nodes receive the deep lymphatics of the lower extremities, vessels from the penis or clitoris, and vessels from the superficial subinguinal nodes. Their efferent channels extend to the external iliac nodes.

3. **Lymphatic Vessels of the Lower Extremity** (Fig. 4) — are divided, like the nodes, into superficial and deep groups.

a. SUPERFICIAL (CUTANEOUS) LYMPHATICS — drain the skin and superficial fascia of the lower extremity. Two major collecting systems are present. The medial is the larger of the two and follows the great saphenous vein in its ascent through the leg and thigh. From eight to 12 collecting channels constitute this medial group, which terminates in the inferomedial and inferolateral superficial subinguinal nodes.

The lateral collecting system consists of a number of channels that join the medial channels in either the leg or the thigh. Lateral collecting channels in the upper thigh empty directly into the superficial subinguinal nodes.

Two or three collecting channels follow the lesser saphenous vein. They originate from the posterolateral aspect of the heel and the posterior surface of the leg and terminate in the popliteal nodes. They communicate in part, however, with both the medial and lateral collecting vessels (Fig. 4) and therefore also drain into the subinguinal nodes.

The superficial lymphatics of the gluteal region terminate in the lateral nodes of the superficial inguinal and subinguinal group.

b. DEEP LYMPHATICS — drain the deep fascia, muscles, joints, and periosteum of the lower limb. These lymph vessels follow the course of the arteries of the lower extremity. The deep lymphatics of the foot and leg terminate in the popliteal nodes from which efferent channels ascend in association with the femoral artery and empty into the deep inguinal nodes. From the thigh, deep lymphatics follow branches of the femoral artery and end in the deep inguinal nodes while others by-pass these nodes and terminate in the external iliac nodes.

Some deep lymphatics of the thigh follow the obturator artery and those of the gluteal region follow the superior and inferior gluteal arteries to the hypogastric nodes.

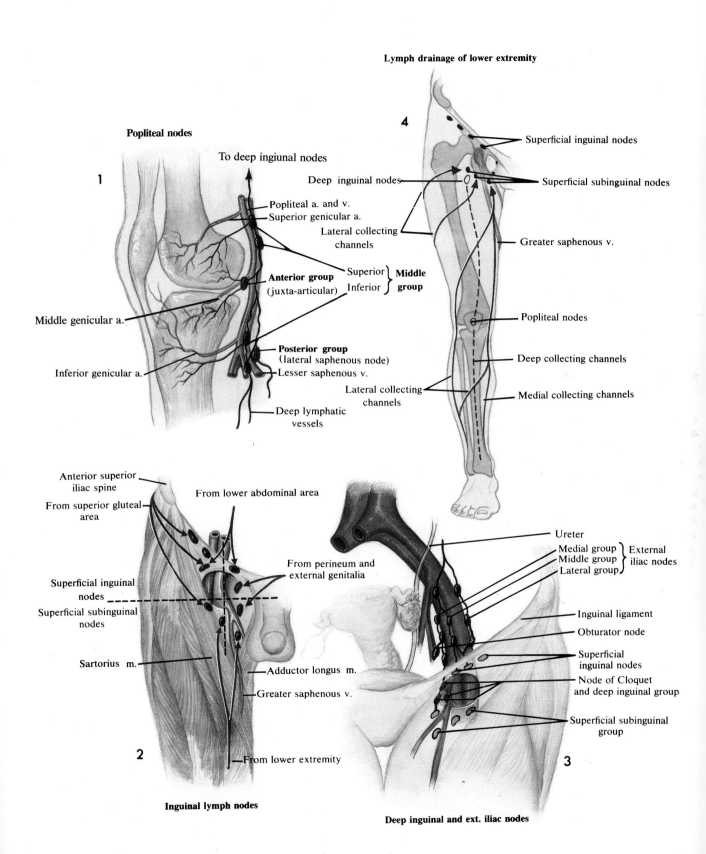

Lymph drainage of lower extremity

Popliteal nodes

1

To deep inguinal nodes

Popliteal a. and v.
Superior genicular a.
Lateral collecting channels

Anterior group
(juxta-articular)

Superior ⎱ **Middle**
Inferior ⎰ **group**

Middle genicular a.

Posterior group
(lateral saphenous node)
Lesser saphenous v.

Inferior genicular a.

Lateral collecting channels

Deep lymphatic vessels

4

Superficial inguinal nodes

Deep inguinal nodes

Superficial subinguinal nodes

Greater saphenous v.

Popliteal nodes

Deep collecting channels

Medial collecting channels

Anterior superior iliac spine

From superior gluteal area

From lower abdominal area

From perineum and external genitalia

Superficial inguinal nodes

Superficial subinguinal nodes

Sartorius m.

Adductor longus m.

Greater saphenous v.

2

From lower extremity

Inguinal lymph nodes

Ureter
Medial group ⎱ External
Middle group ⎰ iliac nodes
Lateral group

Inguinal ligament

Obturator node

Superficial inguinal nodes

Node of Cloquet and deep inguinal group

Superficial subinguinal group

3

Deep inguinal and ext. iliac nodes

THE HIP JOINT:

Like the shoulder joint (page 78), the hip joint is a diarthrodial joint of the enarthrodial (ball and socket) type. It possesses, therefore, two bony surfaces covered by articular hyaline cartilage, a capsule, and a synovial membrane. Flexion, extension, abduction, adduction, medial and lateral rotation, and circumduction of the thigh on the pelvis are permitted. It is the strongest joint in the body.

1. **Bony Parts** (Figs. 1 and 2)—of the articular surfaces consist of the spherical *head of the femur* and the deep *acetabular cavity of the innominate bone*. The ilium, ischium, and os pubis all contribute to the acetabulum. Unlike the shoulder joint where only a shallow receptive glenoid cavity exists for the head of the humerus, the acetabular cavity accommodates more than half of the femoral head. The acetabulum consists of a hemispheric articular (lunate) surface. Its sharp bony rim is deficient below, which produces the *acetabular notch*.

2. **Articular Capsule** (Figs. 1 and 2)—of the hip joint is one of the strongest ligaments of the body. Proximally, it is attached to the rim of the acetabulum. Distally, the capsule attaches anteriorly to the intertrochanteric line but posteriorly it crosses the middle of the neck of the femur. The entire anterior surface of the femoral neck, therefore, is intracapsular while only the medial half of the posterior surface lies within the capsule. In addition to its own strong intrinsic fibers, the capsule of the hip joint is reinforced by other ligaments.

a. Iliofemoral ligament—is a thickened portion of the anterior capsule (Fig. 3). It arises proximally from the anterior inferior iliac spine. Distally, it divides into two parts, which insert on the upper and lower portions of the intertrochanteric line. The medial limb prevents hyperextension in the erect position, whereas the lateral limb limits abduction and lateral rotation.

b. Pubocapsular ligament—strengthens the anterior and inferomedial part of the capsule (Fig. 3). Its proximal origin is from the obturator crest and superior pubic ramus. It inserts into the capsule where it blends with the medial fibers of the iliofemoral ligament. It serves to limit abduction of the joint.

c. Ischiocapsular ligament—reinforces the capsule posteriorly (Fig. 4). It is a triangular band arising from the body of the ischium and the ischial portion of the acetabulum and inserts into the capsule of the hip joint. It helps prevent too great a degree of medial rotation.

d. Ligamentum teres femoris (round ligament)—is a flat intra-articular ligament that extends from the acetabular rim and attaches to a depression on the head of the femur, the *fovea capitis*. It is intracapsular in position but extrasynovial, being completely surrounded by a tube of synovial membrane (Figs. 5 and 6).

e. Glenoid labrum—is a thick fibrocartilaginous ring attached to the circumference of the acetabulum. It serves to deepen the acetabular cavity.

f. Transverse ligament—may be considered as part of the glenoid labrum although no cartilage cells are present in its fibers (Fig. 5). It extends across the *acetabular notch* converting the three-quarter lunate articular surface into a complete hemispherical receptive area for the head of the femur. Deep to the transverse ligament, the acetabular notch becomes the *acetabular foramen* through which the nerves and nutrient vessels enter the joint (Fig. 6).

3. **Synovial Membrane** (Fig. 6)—lines the deep surface of the capsule. Proximally, it covers both surfaces of the glenoid labrum. In the region of the transverse ligament, the synovium forms a tube surrounding the ligamentum teres and also covers the acetabular fat pad (Haversian gland), which lies in the floor of the acetabulum. Distally, it is reflected upon the back of the femur.

4. **Musculotendinous Relations** (Figs. 1, 2, and 6)—muscle insertions add to the reinforcement of this intrinsically strong capsule of the joint.

Anteriorly, the psoas major muscle inserts on the lesser tuberosity of the femur fortifying this part of the joint capsule. It is separated from the joint by the *subpsoas bursa*. In some 10 per cent of individuals this bursa communicates with the synovial cavity through the interval between the iliofemoral and pubocapsular ligaments (Fig. 3). Posteriorly, the capsule is reinforced by the insertions of the piriformis, quadratus femoris, obturator internus, and the gemelli. Medially, the insertions of the obturator externus and pectineus add support to the capsule. Superiorly, the gluteus minimus and the reflected head of the rectus femoris reinforce the capsule.

It should be noted that there is no reinforcement of the joint capsule, either ligamentous or musculotendinous, to the inferior portion of the capsule. This area, therefore, is the most vulnerable site for the rare dislocation of the hip.

5. **Arterial Supply** (Fig. 6)—to the hip joint comes in part from the lateral and medial femoral circumflex arteries, branches of the femoral artery. They enter the joint near the greater and lesser trochanters. The obturator branch of the hypogastric artery enters the joint through the acetabular foramen and is the main supply to the femoral head. The inferior gluteal artery, also a branch of the hypogastric, enters the femoral neck posteriorly. From the first perforating branch of the profunda femoris artery, a nutrient branch supplying the diaphysis ascends to join these aforementioned vessels to form an anastomotic plexus in the region of the neck of the humerus after the epiphysis becomes united.

6. **Nerve Supply**—to the hip, as is true with other joints, follows *Hilton's law*; i.e., the nerves innervating the muscles acting on the joint also innervate the joint. The hip, therefore, receives branches from the obturator, femoral, and sciatic nerves. The same nerves innervate the knee joint. Primary disease in the hip frequently manifests itself by referred pain to the knee. Examination of the hip joint must never be overlooked in the patient complaining of pain in the knee.

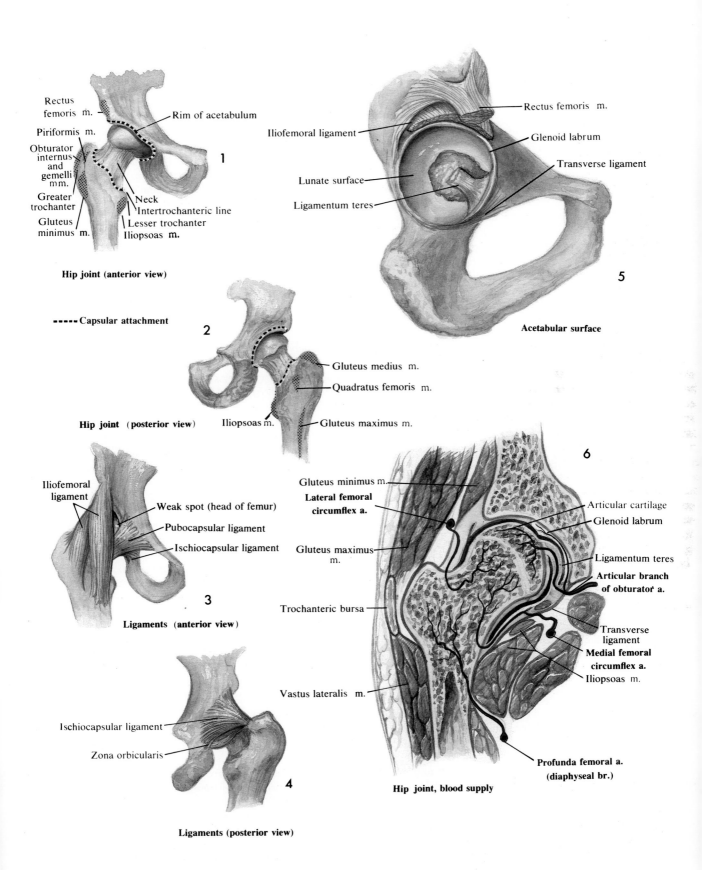

Rectus femoris m.

Rim of acetabulum

Piriformis m.

Obturator internus and gemelli mm.

Greater trochanter

Gluteus minimus m.

Neck

Intertrochanteric line

Lesser trochanter

Iliopsoas m.

1

Hip joint (anterior view)

- - - - - Capsular attachment

2

Gluteus medius m.

Quadratus femoris m.

Iliopsoas m.

Gluteus maximus m.

Hip joint (posterior view)

Iliofemoral ligament

Weak spot (head of femur)

Pubocapsular ligament

Ischiocapsular ligament

3

Ligaments (anterior view)

Ischiocapsular ligament

Zona orbicularis

4

Ligaments (posterior view)

Rectus femoris m.

Iliofemoral ligament

Glenoid labrum

Transverse ligament

Lunate surface

Ligamentum teres

5

Acetabular surface

6

Gluteus minimus m.

Lateral femoral circumflex a.

Gluteus maximus m.

Trochanteric bursa

Vastus lateralis m.

Articular cartilage

Glenoid labrum

Ligamentum teres

Articular branch of obturator a.

Transverse ligament

Medial femoral circumflex a.

Iliopsoas m.

Profunda femoral a. (diaphyseal br.)

Hip joint, blood supply

THE HIP — CLINICAL CONSIDERATIONS:

There are many pathological conditions affecting the hip joint—congenital, inflammatory, traumatic, and neoplastic. Several anatomical factors are important in the diagnosis and treatment of these disorders.

1. **Mensuration of the Lower Extremity**—pathological changes in the hip joint almost invariably reflect themselves in a change in length of the lower extremity. This length may be determined by a measurement of the affected extremity compared to its normal counterpart. Using a rigid tape measure, the proximal point is taken at the anterior-superior iliac spine. The tape is passed along the medial border of the patella and extended to the tip of the medial malleolus.

It is equally important to determine the angle with which the neck of the femur joins the shaft. Normally, this angle is 130 degrees. Pathological changes within the joint may affect a shortening *(coxa vara)* or a lengthening *(coxa valga)* of this normal angle of inclination (Fig. 7). Coxa valga is present in congenital hip dislocations or in poliomyelitis affecting infants. Adduction of the hip joint in these cases is very limited. Coxa vara is due to many causes, but in all such cases abduction is limited.

Two clinical guides are useful in determining alterations of this normal angle of inclination. One of these guides is *Nelaton's line* (Fig. 1). This is a line drawn from the anterosuperior iliac spine to the summit of the ischial tuberosity. In the normal extremity, the greater trochanter just touches this line. If the trochanter lies above this line it is an indication of a shortening of the limb due to pathology in the head or neck of the femur. Another useful guide is *Bryant's triangle* (Fig. 1). With the patient lying supine, a perpendicular line is drawn from the anterior-superior iliac spine to the table. A second line (equivalent to Nelaton's line) is drawn from the anterior-superior iliac spine to the summit of the greater trochanter. The base of the triangle extends horizontally from the tip of the greater trochanter to the perpendicular line. A shortening of the base of the triangle indicates derangement of the head or neck of the femur.

2. **Trendelenberg Test**—in the erect position the stability of the hip depends on the strength of the surrounding muscles and the integrity of the head and neck lever system within the joint. The patient is instructed to stand with total body weight bearing on one extremity. In the normal individual the hip abductors (gluteus medius and minimus and tensor fascia lata) act with such force that the pelvis rises on the opposite side. If, however, there is a defect in this musculature group (due to polio or disuse) or should there be an osseous deformity of the lever system of the head and neck of the femur (due to arthritis, a previous arthrosis, a dislocation, or a malunited fracture) the pelvis of the opposite side tilts downward. The latter result is referred to as a positive Trendelenberg test and indicates a defect in the osseomuscular stability of the hip joint.

3. **Dislocation of the Hip**—is rare because of the receptive compatibility of the head of the femur and acetabulum, the thickness of its capsule and intrinsic ligaments, and the strength of its related musculature. Auto accidents are the most frequent cause of dislocation of the hip. The thigh is flexed, adducted, and medially rotated, and direct violence results in a posterior dislocation. The capsule ruptures inferiorly and posteriorly. Should the thigh be abducted at the time of injury an anterior dislocation may result. In both varieties an associated fracture of the acetabular rim must be considered. Figure 2 depicts the characteristic deformity of the lower extremity in the more frequent posterior dislocation. The limb is flexed, internally rotated, and shortened. The foot is inverted.

4. **Fractures of the Proximal End of the Femur**—are frequent, particularly in the elderly patient. Almost invariably such fractures result in a deformity in which the thigh is flexed, externally rotated, and shortened. The foot is thrown into an everted position (Fig. 3).

Fractures at this site are anatomically divided into the intracapsular and the extracapsular varieties.

a. INTRACAPSULAR FRACTURES—include those involving the head and neck of the femur. Fractures of the head are extremely rare and are usually compression fractures. Fractures of the neck, on the other hand, are extremely common. Two types are usually distinguished, the subcapital and basal (Fig. 4). The anatomical considerations of the blood supply to this area are extremely important (Fig. 6, page 307). *Subcapital fractures* (Fig. 6) occur at the anatomical neck of the femur. The blood supply to the head is entirely dependent upon the obturator artery through the ligamentum teres. This supply is usually inadequate. *Basal fractures* occur in the neck of the femur below the anatomical neck. In this location, depending upon the portion of the capsule left intact, the blood supply to the proximal fragment of bone is still precarious. The closer the fracture is to the femoral head, the greater is the likelihood of avascular necrosis of the proximal segment.

b. EXTRACAPSULAR FRACTURES—of the proximal end of the femur occur in the region of the trochanters. In the *intertrochanteric fracture* the fracture line follows the anterior intertrochanteric line; the *pertrochanteric fracture* extends from the base of the greater trochanter to a point proximal to the lesser trochanter (Fig. 5). Although aseptic necrosis rarely occurs in these extracapsular fractures they do have a great tendency toward the development of a coxa vara.

All fractures of the head and neck of the femur after proper reduction are best treated by internal fixation. This fixation may be accomplished by means of nails, screws, plates, or, in fact, resection of the head and insertion of a prosthesis.

5. **Surgical Exposure of the Hip Joint**—is carried out for many reasons: for the correction of congenital and traumatic deformities, for arthroplastic procedures to correct arthritic deformities and dysfunctions, for amputation for malignant diseases, for ostectomy of benign tumors, but most frequently for the treatment of fractures of the head and neck of the femur. Anterior, lateral, or posterior surgical approaches may be utilized. Figures 8 and 9 depict the anterior iliofemoral approach.

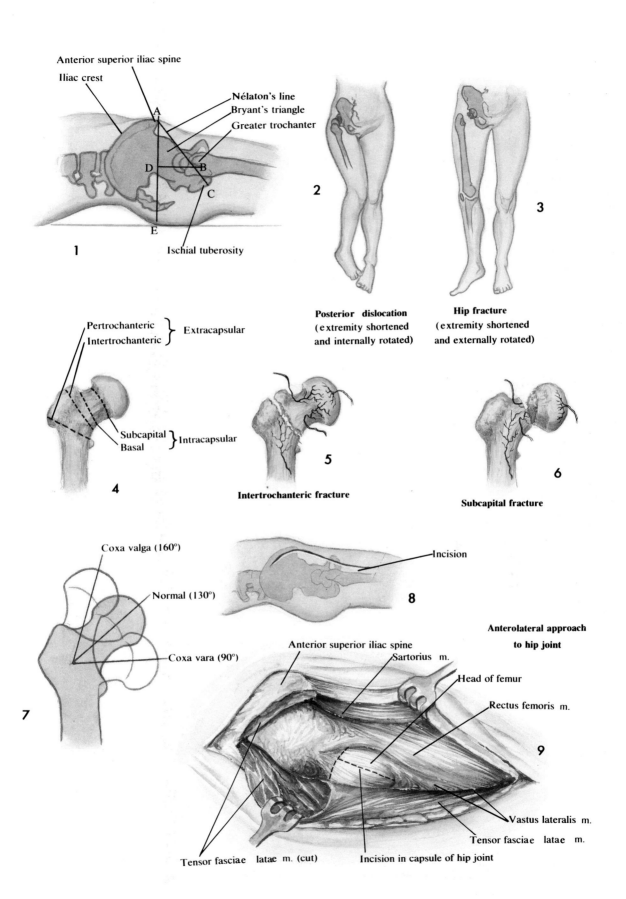

1

Anterior superior iliac spine
Iliac crest
Nélaton's line
Bryant's triangle
Greater trochanter
Ischial tuberosity

2 Posterior dislocation
(extremity shortened
and internally rotated)

3 Hip fracture
(extremity shortened
and externally rotated)

4
Pertrochanteric } Extracapsular
Intertrochanteric }
Subcapital } Intracapsular
Basal

5 Intertrochanteric fracture

6 Subcapital fracture

7
Coxa valga (160°)
Normal (130°)
Coxa vara (90°)

8 Incision

9 Anterolateral approach
to hip joint
Anterior superior iliac spine
Sartorius m.
Head of femur
Rectus femoris m.
Vastus lateralis m.
Tensor fasciae latae m.
Incision in capsule of hip joint
Tensor fasciae latae m. (cut)

With the improvement and development of synthetic biomaterials and better understanding of biocompatibility of alloys such as iron, cobalt, and titanium, total hip replacement has become a common and successful orthopedic procedure requiring frequent exposure of the hip joint. Total hip arthroplasty is most commonly indicated in patients with osteoarthritis, rheumatoid arthritis, malignancy, fractures and dislocations, or aseptic necrosis, and in those who have undergone previously unsuccessful hip operations requiring revision. Total hip arthroplasty involves resection of arthritic bone and cartilage from the femur and acetabulum. One of several alloys is implanted into the femoral component, which is fixed with acrylic cement and articulates with the acetabular component (polyethylene polymer). These components are fixed with methacrylate cement.

The surgical approach may be anterior, lateral, or posterior. Trochanteric osteotomy provides good exposure to the hip joint. An incision is made along the posterior (Fig. 2) aspect of the tensor fascia lata muscle and carried inferiorly along the posterior-superior aspect of the greater trochanter down the thigh for approximately 8 to 10 cm. After the superficial tissues and gluteus maximus muscles have been divided, the greater trochanter is exposed. Along the superior aspect are the gluteus medius and minimus fibers; inferiorly lie the vastus intermedius and lateralis muscles. After the tendon to the vastus lateralis is transected and trochanteric osteotomy is completed, muscles and capsular attachments to the trochanter are divided, the femoral head is dislocated, and the femoral neck transected. The acetabulum is exposed and the glenoid labrum excised. The acetabulum is reamed and curetted, anchor holes are drilled, methylmethacrylate cement is injected into the holes, and acetabuloplasty is completed.

To complete the femoral component of total hip arthroplasty, the femoral canal is opened, broached, reamed, and curetted and the prosthesis inserted (Fig. 3). After the femoral and acetabular components have been fixed with acrylic cement, the greater trochanter is transplanted over the femoral shaft and the trochanteric wires are secured; the vastus lateralis is reattached to the distal end of the greater trochanter.

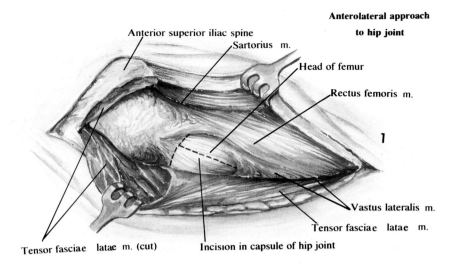

Anterolateral approach to hip joint

Anterior superior iliac spine

Sartorius m.

Head of femur

Rectus femoris m.

Vastus lateralis m.

Tensor fasciae latae m.

1

Tensor fasciae latae m. (cut)

Incision in capsule of hip joint

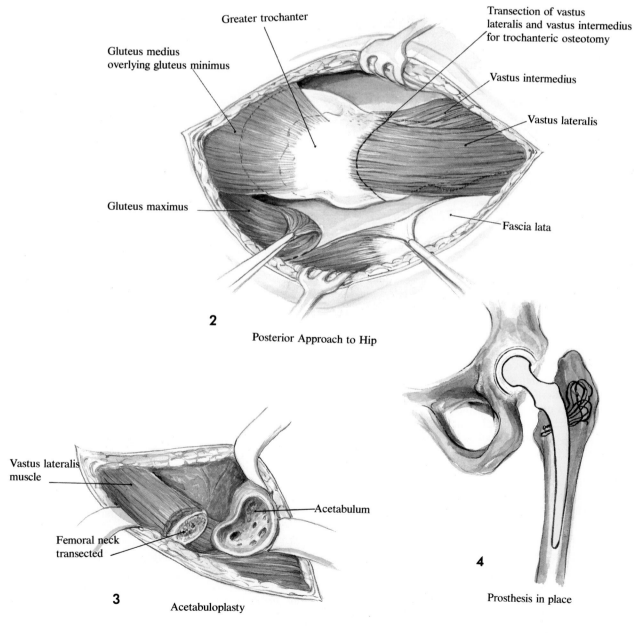

Greater trochanter

Gluteus medius overlying gluteus minimus

Transection of vastus lateralis and vastus intermedius for trochanteric osteotomy

Vastus intermedius

Vastus lateralis

Gluteus maximus

Fascia lata

2

Posterior Approach to Hip

Vastus lateralis muscle

Acetabulum

Femoral neck transected

3

Acetabuloplasty

4

Prosthesis in place

THE KNEE JOINT:

The knee joint, the largest and most complex joint of the body, is one of the most superficial and yet one of the weakest of our bony articulations. This latter fact is due primarily to the imperfect adaptation of the bony articular surfaces. This imperfection is corrected in part by the presence of strong intrinsic and extrinsic ligaments and the related musculature.

The knee is a diarthrodial hinge joint. Its movements are flexion and extension. Some rotation of the joint is possible if the knee is in a flexed position.

1. **Bony Parts** (Figs. 1 and 2) — consist of three bones that are involved in the articulation of the knee. They are the condyles of the femur and tibia and the patella. The *patella* is actually a sesamoid bone in the tendon of the quadriceps femoris muscle. It is triangular in shape, with the apex directed inferiorly. Its posterior surface articulates with the patellar surface of the femur, the *patellofemoral articulation*. The distal end of the femur is expanded into a *medial* and a *lateral femoral condyle*. The articular surfaces of the two condyles are continuous anteriorly to form the *patellar articular surface*. Distally, the articular surface of the femoral condyles coapt by means of internal ligaments with the articular surfaces of the *medial* and *lateral tibial condyles* to form the *femorotibial articulation.*

2. **Articular Capsule** (Figs. 1 and 2) — of the knee joint is loose and thin. It is attached below to the margins of the tibial condyles. Its femoral attachment lies above the articular surfaces of the bone and attaches to the medial and lateral margins of the patella. Strong external and internal ligaments reinforce this weak capsule.

3. **External Ligaments** (Figs. 3 and 4) — the quadriceps muscle tendons contribute significantly to the stability of the knee. Other fascial thickenings support the medial, lateral, and posterior portions of the capsule.

a. LATERAL PATELLAR RETINACULUM — is derived from the tendinous insertion of the vastus lateralis. These fibers insert mainly into the upper and lateral borders of the patella. Some of these fibers, however, extend inferiorly and attach to the oblique line of the tibia where they blend with the insertion of the iliotibial band of the fascia lata.

b. MEDIAL PATELLAR RETINACULUM — consists of those fibers from the vastus medialis that, in addition to their insertion to the oblique line, extend to the periosteum of the shaft of the tibia. These fibers blend with the medial collateral ligament.

c. PATELLAR LIGAMENT — is a strong, flat tendon extending from the inferior margins of the patella to the tibial tuberosity. Laterally, this ligament is continuous with the patellar retinacula.

d. MEDIAL (TIBIAL) COLLATERAL LIGAMENT — is a thick, flat, fibrous tissue structure extending from the medial epicondyle of the femur above to the shaft of the tibia below. It is attached to the internal ligaments of the knee on its under surface, a point of great clinical significance.

e. LATERAL (FIBULAR) COLLATERAL LIGAMENT — is a cord-like structure arising from the lateral femoral epicondyle and inserting on the head of the fibula. This structure is *not* attached to the capsule of the joint.

f. OBLIQUE POPLITEAL LIGAMENT — is located posterior in position and extends from the posterior aspect of the medial condyle of the tibia in a superior and lateral direction to insert on the lateral epicondyle of the femur.

g. ARCUATE POPLITEAL LIGAMENT — is also located on the posterior surface of the joint. It arises from the head of the fibula and inserts in common with the oblique ligament on the lateral epicondyle of the femur. It retains the popliteus muscle against the lateral epicondyle.

4. **Internal Ligaments** (Figs. 5 and 6) — consist of the cruciate ligaments, the semilunar cartilages, and the transverse ligament. The cruciate ligaments serve to prevent hyperextension and hyperflexion, whereas the semilunar cartilages tend to make the articular surfaces of the femur and tibia more receptive.

a. ANTERIOR CRUCIATE LIGAMENT — is so named because of its origin from the *anterior intercondylar fossa* of the tibia. It passes upward, posteriorly and laterally to the lateral condyle of the femur. This ligament prevents hyperextension of the knee.

b. POSTERIOR CRUCIATE LIGAMENT — arises from the *posterior intercondylar fossa* of the tibia — thus its name. It ascends in an anterior and medial direction to attach to the medial condyle of the femur. Hyperflexion of the knee is prevented by this ligament.

c. MEDIAL MENISCUS (MEDIAL SEMILUNAR CARTILAGE) — is the larger of the two menisci and is oval in shape. Its attachments on the tibia is in front of and behind the *intercondylar eminence* of the tibia. Medially this cartilage is firmly affixed to the medial collateral ligament. Injury to the medial collateral ligament frequently results in concomitant injury to the medial meniscus.

d. LATERAL MENISCUS (LATERAL SEMILUNAR CARTILAGE) — attaches likewise to the tibial plateau by anterior and posterior cornua related to the intercondylar eminence. It is smaller and more freely moveable than the medial meniscus. It is separated from the lateral collateral ligament by the popliteus tendon and bursa and is therefore less likely to be injured than the medial meniscus.

e. TRANSVERSE LIGAMENT — is a slender cord-like communication between the anterior fibers of the medial and lateral menisci.

5. **Synovial Membrane** — lines the inner aspect of the articular capsule. The synovial cavity of the knee is the largest in the body. It covers the femoral and tibial surfaces of the menisci and the anterior and lateral surfaces of the cruciate ligaments, rendering them intracapsular but extrasynovial. Superiorly, it is in communication with the *suprapatellar bursa*, which extends between the quadriceps femoris muscle mass and the femur. Posteriorly, it may communicate with the bursa of the popliteus, the bursa under the medial head of the gastrocnemius, and through it with the bursa of the semimembranosus.

The synovial membrane also covers the *infrapatellar fat pad*, which fills the space between the patellar

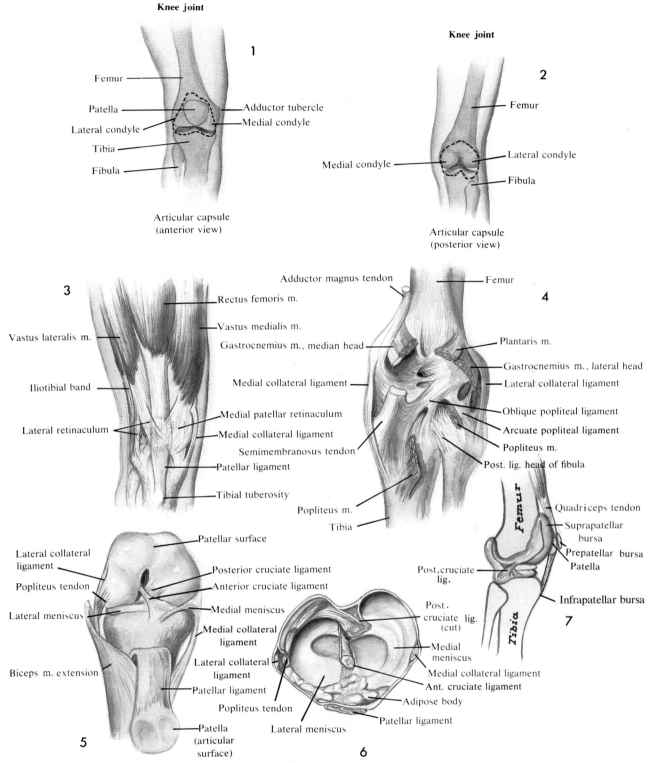

Knee joint

1

Femur

Patella

Lateral condyle

Tibia

Fibula

Adductor tubercle

Medial condyle

Articular capsule
(anterior view)

Knee joint

2

Femur

Medial condyle

Lateral condyle

Fibula

Articular capsule
(posterior view)

3

Vastus lateralis m.

Iliotibial band

Lateral retinaculum

Adductor magnus tendon

Rectus femoris m.

Vastus medialis m.

Gastrocnemius m., median head

Medial collateral ligament

Medial patellar retinaculum

Medial collateral ligament

Semimembranosus tendon

Patellar ligament

Tibial tuberosity

Femur

4

Plantaris m.

Gastrocnemius m., lateral head

Lateral collateral ligament

Oblique popliteal ligament

Arcuate popliteal ligament

Popliteus m.

Post. lig. head of fibula

Popliteus m.

Tibia

Patellar surface

Lateral collateral
ligament

Popliteus tendon

Lateral meniscus

Biceps m. extension

Posterior cruciate ligament

Anterior cruciate ligament

Medial meniscus

Medial collateral
ligament

Lateral collateral
ligament

Patellar ligament

Popliteus tendon

Patella
(articular
surface)

5

Lateral meniscus

Post. cruciate
lig.

Post.
cruciate lig.
(cut)

Medial
meniscus

Medial collateral ligament

Ant. cruciate ligament

Adipose body

Patellar ligament

6

Femur

Quadriceps tendon

Suprapatellar
bursa

Prepatellar bursa

Patella

Infrapatellar bursa

Tibia

7

ligament and the femoral intercondylar notch. The synovium covering the lateral free margins of this pad project into the joint as the *alar folds.*

Extracapsular bursae also are related to the joint. These are the *prepatellar bursa* and the *infrapatellar bursa.* The latter lies anterior to the tibial tuberosity. Both bursae lie subcutaneously in position and their involvement by inflammation (bursitis) is clinically referred to as *housemaid's knee.*

6. **Arterial Supply**—has been described on page 292.

7. **Nerve Supply**—again, following Hilton's law, a joint is supplied by the same nerves which innervate the muscles acting upon that joint. The knee joint, therefore, is supplied by branches of the sciatic, the femoral, and the obturator nerves. Emphasis has already been placed on the importance of referred pain to the knee in those cases in which the primary derangement is in the hip.

CLINICAL CONSIDERATIONS OF THE KNEE JOINT:

The knee, like the foot, is an anatomical area which is neglected in physical examination by the average physician. Its superficial location, on the other hand, makes it an ideal structure for clinical evaluation. An accurate knowledge of its anatomy is required, however, to make a definitive diagnosis of a derangement of function of this joint.

By simple inspection the common congenital deformities, such as *genu valgum (knock knee)* or *genu varum (bowlegs)*, are obvious. Inflammatory diseases produce excessive secretion of synovial fluid resulting in a *joint effusion*. Effusion may also result from postural strain due to poor body alignment and weight-bearing. Intracapsular bleeding from trauma results in *hemarthrosis* of the joint. Ballottement of the patella against the femur may give early evidence of joint effusion. Fractures, arthritis, and tumors affecting the articular surfaces of the bones of the knee or the synovial lining produce alterations of the normal anatomical configuration of the knee joint.

In every patient presenting the complaint of knee dysfunction, the quadriceps muscle should be carefully examined for both strength and girth. This muscle group is the chief stabilizer of the knee joint and wastes rapidly if normal knee function is impaired. It is most important that in the case of a patient in whom normal movement of the knee is limited, instructions be given in isometric contraction of this muscle mass. A most successful surgical repair of either the external or internal ligaments will result in failure unless this muscle group is restored to its normal strength.

The patellar ligament and retinacula, as well as the medial and lateral collateral ligaments, are readily accessible to the examining fingers. The stability of the collateral ligaments may be tested by fixing the thigh with one hand and, with the other hand, forcing the leg into adduction or abduction. Such movements are not possible if these ligaments are intact. Preternatural mobility toward abduction reflects derangement of the medial collateral ligament and toward adduction, derangement of the lateral collateral ligament.

In addition to the collateral ligaments, the cruciates and the cartilages must be tested. They constitute the three C's in the physical examination of the knee.

The stability of the cruciate ligaments is tested with the patient in a supine position, the knee flexed at a 90 degree angle, and the foot fixed upon the table. The leg is grasped by the examiner just below the knee and forced in a posterior direction. Increased backward mobility of the tibia suggests injury to the posterior cruciate ligament. To test the stability of the anterior cruciate ligament, the leg is forced in an anterior direction. Increased forward mobility implies derangement of the anterior cruciate ligament.

Physical examination of the menisci is more difficult than the other ligaments of the knee. These cartilages may be palpated on either side of the patellar ligament just above the tibial plateau with the knee in a flexed position. Localized tenderness and pain in this location and limitation of full extension indicate possible injury to the menisci. The medial meniscus, because of its intimate relation to the medial collateral ligaments, is the most frequently deranged internal ligament of the knee.

1. **Injection of the Knee Joint** (Figs. 1 and 2)—is done for both diagnostic, but mainly therapeutic, purposes. Aspiration of joint effusions is best performed with the patient sitting on the side of a table with the knee flexed and the leg hanging in a dependent position. The joint may best be approached laterally. Three points are palpated: the apex of the patella, the lateral-most tip of the lateral condyle of the tibia, and the anterior-most prominence of the lateral condyle of the femur. A needle is inserted into the midpoint of this triangular space and directed posteriorly and medially. In addition to the aspiration of serous and sanguinous fluids, steroids are also administered by this route in the treatment of knee pathology.

2. **Mechanism of Cartilage Tears**—athletic injuries, particularly football injuries, are the most frequent cause of trauma to the three C's: the cartilages, the collateral ligaments, and the cruciate ligaments of the knee. Figure 3 depicts the fundamental mechanism of injury to the medial meniscus. The foot of the victim is firmly fixed and the knee is semiflexed as in running. The offender throws an impact which forces the victim's body weight inward, causing the femur to be forcibly rotated medially (see arrow). Because of the fixation of the foot, the tibia is forced into abduction. Rupture of the medial collateral ligament ensues. Because the medial meniscus is firmly attached to the collateral ligament, it is torn as the end result.

3. **Surgical Approaches**—of the knee joint are carried out for a variety of reasons. These include the removal of menisci or loose bodies in the joint, the debridement of the articular cartilages in advanced arthritis, synovectomy, and the removal of benign tumors of the joint.

a. MEDIAL PARAPATELLAR APPROACH—is the most popular. The incision begins along the medial border of the rectus femoris about 1½ inches above the patella. It is gently curved downward around the medial border of the patella to the level of the tibial tuberosity (Fig. 4). The rectus femoris tendon is separated by sharp dissection from the vastus medialis and the capsule and synovium are incised to expose the joint cavity. The patella is retracted laterally (Fig. 5).

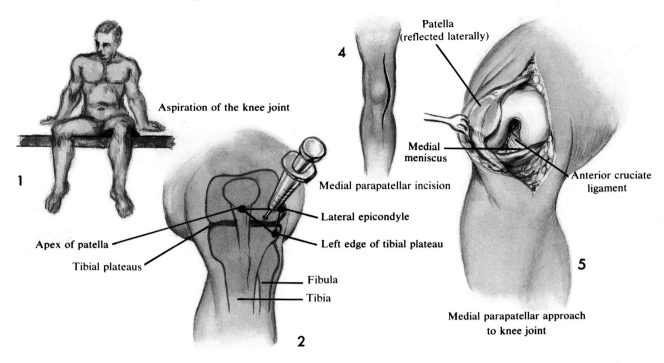

1 Aspiration of the knee joint

2 Apex of patella

Tibial plateaus

Lateral epicondyle

Left edge of tibial plateau

Fibula

Tibia

4 Medial parapatellar incision

Patella (reflected laterally)

Medial meniscus

Anterior cruciate ligament

5 Medial parapatellar approach to knee joint

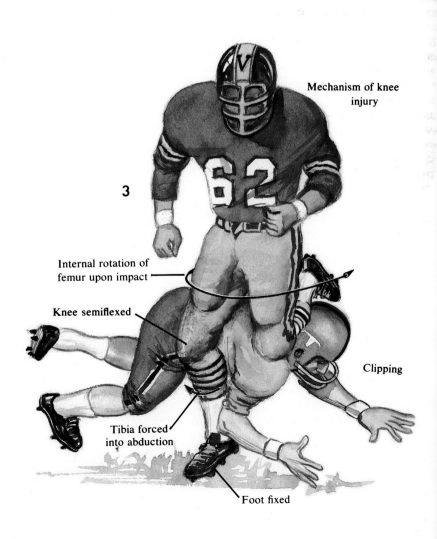

3 Mechanism of knee injury

Internal rotation of femur upon impact

Knee semiflexed

Tibia forced into abduction

Clipping

Foot fixed

Right Knee Arthroscopy —the arthroscope is a useful orthopedic diagnostic and surgical tool that can be used in various joints and allows wide visualization of the interior of the joint space. Right knee arthroscopy is a common procedure that can be done on an outpatient basis with minimal morbidity. It shortens the period of rehabilitation, which is especially important in industry and sports medicine. Various specially designed instruments (biopsy forceps, graspers, scissors, cutters, knives, and abrasers) permit tissue biopsy excision of meniscal or ligamentous lesions, retrieval of loose bodies, chondroplasty, and synovectomy to be successfully performed without formal arthrotomy.

Knee arthroplasty entails the use of a femoropatellar and tibial component and is indicated in patients with rheumatoid and osteoarthritis to relieve pain and improve function.

The femoral component (cobalt-chrome), the tibial component (high-density polyethylene prosthesis), and the patellar prosthesis are designed to fit the anatomic surfaces of these bones. Methylmethacrylate cement interface fixes the prosthesis to trabecular bone.

Through a long medial parapatellar incision, the vastus medialis with its tendinous attachment is reflected medially. The capsule is incised and the joint explored. Complete synovectomy is performed; the menisci, cruciate ligaments, and bone that are involved in the arthritic process are excised. Depending on the components involved, the tibial and femoral prosthesis are inserted and knee arthroplasty is completed.

b. LATERAL PARAPATELLAR APPROACH —begins at the base of the patella, parallels the lateral margin of the patella, and extends to the level of the tibial tuberosity (Fig. 6). The lateral retinaculum, joint capsule, and synovial membrane are incised to expose the joint.

c. POSTERIOR POPLITEAL APPROACH (Fig. 7) —has already been described

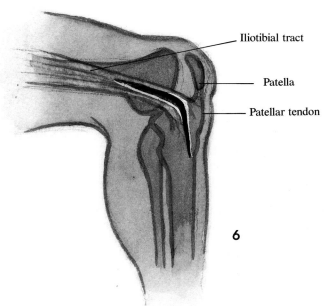

Iliotibial tract

Patella

Patellar tendon

6

Lateral approach to knee joint

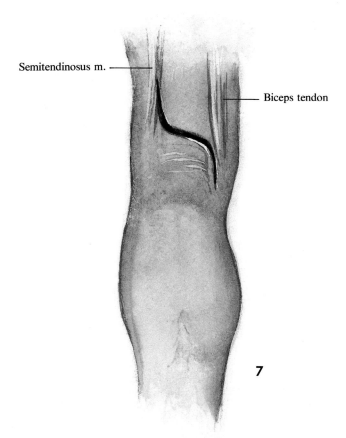

Semitendinosus m.

Biceps tendon

7

Posterior approach to knee joint

THE ANKLE JOINT:

The ankle (talocrural joint) is a diarthrodial joint of the ginglymus or hinge-joint type. Its movements are limited to dorsiflexion (extension) and plantarflexion (flexion) of the foot. Eversion or inversion of the foot is *not* a movement of the ankle but of the *intertarsal joints.* The latter consist of the *talocalcaneal,* the *talocalcaneonavicular,* and the *calcaneocuboid articulations.*

1. **Bony Parts**—of the ankle consist of the inferior and malleolar articular surfaces of the tibia and the malleolar articular surface of the fibula joining the superior and malleolar surfaces of the talus.

2. **Articular Capsule**—of the ankle joint attaches closely to the articular margins of the bones described above. As is true in any hinge joint the capsule is thin anteriorly and posteriorly in order to facilitate its functional movements, but reinforced medially and laterally by ligaments.

a. MEDIAL COLLATERAL LIGAMENT OF THE ANKLE (Fig. 3)—is also referred to as the *deltoid ligament* and is made up of four component parts. This ligament is triangular in shape with the apex arising from the medial malleolus and the base fanning out to attach to the tarsal bones. The anterior fibers form the *anterior talotibial ligament* and the posterior fibers, the *posterior talotibial ligament.* The intermediate fibers attach anteriorly to the navicular bone (*tibionavicular ligament*) and posteriorly to the calcaneous (*calcaneotibial ligament*).

b. LATERAL COLLATERAL LIGAMENT OF THE ANKLE (Fig. 4)—consists of three distinct fibrous bands and are the most frequently injured in traumatic injuries of the ankle joint. They are the *anterior talofibular ligament*, the *posterior talofibular ligament*, and the intermediate *calcaneofibular ligament.*

3. **Synovial Membrane**—lines the inner aspect of the joint capsule but may extend upward between the tibia and fibula to the lower border of the interosseous ligaments. Effusions within the joint readily expand anteriorly and posteriorly because of the laxity of the capsule in these areas.

4. **Musculotendinous Relations**—the related muscles and tendons add little to the support of the ankle joint. The tendons of the tibialis posterior, flexor digitorum longus, and flexor hallucis longus cross the posterior portion of the deltoid ligament. The peroneus longus and brevis muscle tendons cross the lateral collateral ligament.

The principal muscles acting on the ankle consist of the tibialis anterior, the extensor digitorum longus, and the extensor hallucis longus for dorsiflexion and the gastrocnemius, soleus, tibialis posterior, flexor hallucis longus, and flexor digitorum longus for plantarflexion.

5. **Nerve Supply**—to the ankle comes by way of the saphenous branch of the femoral nerve, the anterior tibial nerve, and the deep peroneal nerves.

6. **Blood Supply**—to the ankle joint is carried by the perforating branch of the peroneal artery and by malleolar branches of the anterior and posterior tibial arteries.

CLINICAL CONSIDERATIONS OF THE ANKLE JOINT:

The total weight of the body is supported by the ankle (talocrural) joint in the upright position. It is obvious, therefore, that this joint will be subjected to many postural and traumatic pathological changes.

1. **Postural Strain**—is probably the most frequent clinical entity affecting this joint. Such strain may result from pronated feet, neuromuscular disease affecting anatomical structures of the lower extremity or trunk, congenital skeletal disorders of the spine, arthritis, or a multitude of other disorders. Abnormal weight-bearing places great strain on the medial and lateral collateral ligaments of the ankle and upon the plantar aponeurosis. Tenderness on palpation of these areas without history of local trauma is usually indicative of postural strain upon the foot and ankle.

2. **Effusion**—of the ankle joint most frequently is a result of trauma, but may also stem from inflammatory disorders (arthritis) or postural strain. *Aspiration* of the joint to remove the excess synovial fluid or to inject anti-inflammatory medicines is frequently indicated. The technique of injection is simple because of the superficial position of the joint. The foot is placed in a slightly plantarflexed position. The tip of the medial malleolus is palpated and the anterior border of the malleolus followed upward for approximately 1 cm. The needle is injected just lateral to this point and directed posteriorly and slightly upward to a depth of about 3 to 4 cm. Care must be taken to avoid injury to the greater saphenous vein.

3. **Sprain**—of the ankle is a common occurrence. Such an injury may rupture only a part of or all the fibers of a ligament. The latter results in instability of the joint. Avulsion of the bony attachments of the ligaments produce a *sprain fracture* of the joint.

Sprains may be of two types, an inversion or an eversion sprain. Figure 5 shows the mechanism of production of an *inversion sprain,* which is by far the most common type. In this injury the foot is fixed against some object and thrown into an inverted position and the body weight violently transferred to the lateral collateral ligament. The calcaneofibular ligament tears, often along with the anterior talofibular ligament. An *eversion (abduction) sprain* involves the medial collateral ligament. In this type of sprain, the *anterior tibiofibular ligament* may also be ruptured.

4. **Fractures of the Ankle**—often accompany severe sprains of this joint. These fractures involve the medial and lateral malleoli of the tibia and fibula. Because of the strength of the deltoid ligament the medial malleolus is most frequently involved.

5. **Dislocation of the Ankle**—in an anterior or posterior position is rare despite the laxity of the joint capsule. Dislocations usually are associated with

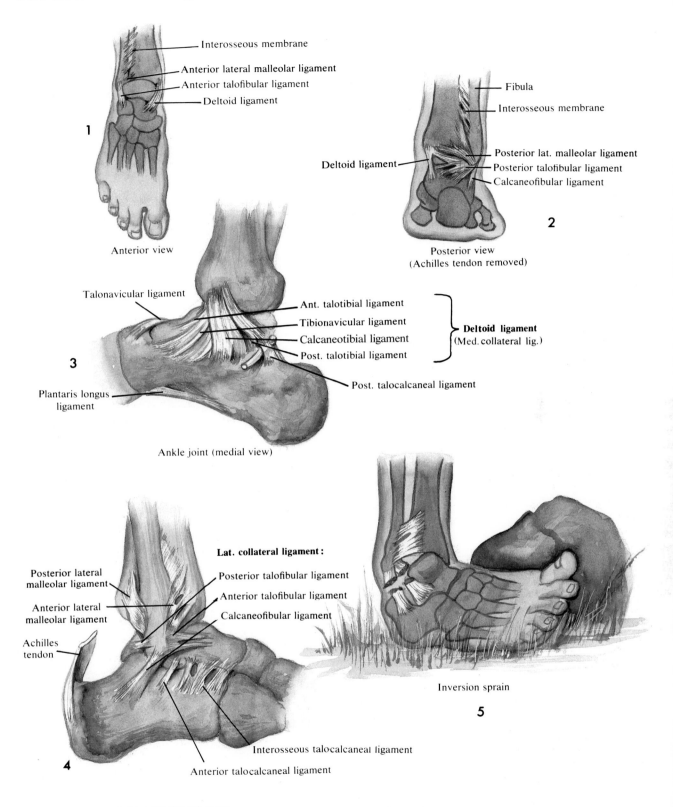

1

— Interosseous membrane
— Anterior lateral malleolar ligament
— Anterior talofibular ligament
— Deltoid ligament

Anterior view

2

Fibula
Interosseous membrane

Deltoid ligament —
Posterior lat. malleolar ligament
Posterior talofibular ligament
Calcaneofibular ligament

Posterior view
(Achilles tendon removed)

3

Talonavicular ligament

Ant. talotibial ligament
Tibionavicular ligament
Calcaneotibial ligament
Post. talotibial ligament

} **Deltoid ligament**
(Med. collateral lig.)

Post. talocalcaneal ligament

Plantaris longus
ligament

Ankle joint (medial view)

4

Posterior lateral
malleolar ligament

Anterior lateral
malleolar ligament

Achilles
tendon

Lat. collateral ligament:

Posterior talofibular ligament
Anterior talofibular ligament
Calcaneofibular ligament

Interosseous talocalcaneal ligament
Anterior talocalcaneal ligament

Ankle joint (lateral view)

5

Inversion sprain

malleolar fractures and are more frequently lateral rather than medial, again because of the strength of the medial collateral ligament.

6. **Amputation**—through the ankle is usually a procedure described as the *Syme's amputation*. The ankle is disarticulated and the articular surface of the tibia and the malleoli are removed. It is extremely difficult to fit a prosthesis to the stump.

Index

Note: Numbers in *italics* represent illustrations.

Index

Index

Index

Index